MEDICAL-SURGICAL
NURSING

$\mathcal{M}$EDICAL-SURGICAL NURSING

CHARLENE J. REEVES, M.S.N., R.N., C.N.S., F.N.P.

Assistant Professor
Hardin-Simmons University/North Abilene
Christian University/McMurray University
Abilene, Texas
Nurse Analyst and Nursing Supervisor
United Regional Health Care System
Wichita Falls, Texas

GAYLE ROUX, Ph.D., R.N., C.N.S.

Assistant Professor of Nursing
University of Southern Indiana
School of Nursing and Health Professions
Evansville, Indiana

ROBIN LOCKHART, M.S.N., R.N.

Doctoral Student, Texas Woman's University
Assistant Professor of Nursing
Midwestern State University
Wichita Falls, Texas

McGraw-Hill

Health Professions Division
McGRAW-HILL NURSING CORE SERIES

New York St. Louis San Francisco Auckland Bogotá Caracas Lisbon
London Madrid Mexico City Milan Montreal New Delhi San Juan
Singapore Sydney Tokyo Toronto

McGraw-Hill

A Division of The **McGraw·Hill** *Companies*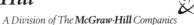

MEDICAL-SURGICAL NURSING

1 2 3 4 5 6 7 8 9 0 DOW DOW 9 9 8

ISBN 0-07-105480-4

This book was set in Sabon by V&M Graphics, Inc.
The editors were John Dolan and Peter J. Boyle;
and the production supervisor was Richard Ruzycka;
the text was designed by Patrice Sheridan;
the cover was designed by Joan O'Connor.
The index was prepared by Patricia Perrier.
R.R. Donnelley and Sons was printer and binder.

This book is printed on acid-free paper.

Cataloging-in-Publication Data is on file for this title at the Library of Congress.

CONTENTS

CONTRIBUTORS

Catherine Dingley, M.S.N., R.N., C.F.N.P.
Private Practice
Family Medicine
Denver, Colorado
Chapter 8

Pam Bragan Koob, Ph.D., R.N., C.F.N.P.
Jennie Stuart Medical Center
Drs. Peter Isele and Travis Calhoun
Primary Care/Internal Medicine
Hopkinsville, Kentucky
Chapter 9

Robin Lockhart, M.S.N., R.N.
Doctoral Student, Texas Woman's University
Assistant Professor of Nursing
Midwestern State University
Wichita Falls, Texas
Chapters 4, 7, 13, and 14

Charlene J. Reeves, M.S.N., R.N., C.N.S., F.N.P.
Assistant Professor
Hardin-Simmons University
Abilene, Texas
Nurse Analyst and Nursing Supervisor
United Regional Health Care System
Wichita Falls, Texas
Chapters 1, 2, 3, 5, 6, 10, 11, 12, 15, and 16

Gayle Roux, Ph.D., R.N., C.N.S.
Assistant Professor of Nursing
University of Southern Indiana
School of Nursing and Health Professions
Evansville, Indiana
Chapters 1, 2, 3, 5, 6, 10, 11, 12, 15, and 16

FEATURES

Medical-Surgical Nursing is part of the McGraw-Hill Nursing Core Series. It is the second book in the series to publish after *Community Health Nursing: An Alliance for Health* by Klainberg, Holzemer, Leonard, and Arnold. Future titles include Psychiatry, Pediatrics, and Maternity Nursing. The book is to be used in the classroom or clinical practice site in a medical-surgical context.

The book emphasizes professionalism in achieving the best client outcomes. By using a combination of case studies, margin notes, and practice questions, the authors have distilled complex information into a concise and approachable text.

In addition to the affordable text, an Instructor's Test Bank is available.

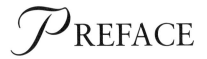

$\mathscr{P}$REFACE

To create is to raise a son, plant a tree, and write a book.
Old Mexican Proverb
To create is to raise a daughter, plant a tree, and write a book.
New Feminist Proverb

We have raised three daughters and a son, planted trees, but we had never written a book. Thus, we embarked on a creative mission to write this medical-surgical text. The idea of this book was conceptualized by nursing students, clinical nurses, publishers, and authors to serve a need for a concise, reader-friendly medical-surgical text. As authors, we joked that our goal was a text that weighed less than 40 lbs, was small enough to be hidden in a lab coat, and could be read in the bathtub without suffering muscle strain!

The style of the writing is direct and staccato. The content is written in a concise format, meant to appeal to nurses who are creative and intelligent practitioners or students. The language is that which is used to discuss clients with our peers or with students during clinical rotations. Thus, we use fewer formal references, all of which are cited and annotated for each chapter. The essentials of information given in the text are designed to give you the necessary details to think critically, make sound clinical judgments, and create therapeutic plans of care. The basics are here: go forth and create.

To get the most benefit from this book, of course, is to read it and use it! Keep this text handy in your clinical practice site; carry it in your car; read it at the pool; and write notes all over the margins meant for that purpose. This text was intended for practical use. One of the best "teachable moments" is at the time a question arises in clinical practice. Because we have condensed the information down to the basics, you *do* have time to "look things up" and read the concise explanations, but also take the time to master an entire chapter or body system in a more leisurely atmosphere.

Based on the premise that you will be using other resources to achieve excellence in practice, we have included annotated references and Internet sites where you can obtain additional information. Occasionally, organizations change Internet addresses, and we apologize if any sites listed are not current.

The case studies throughout the chapters and the questions at the end of the chapters were designed to stimulate and simulate your clinical decision making. The questions are taken directly from material in the text, so if you cannot answer the questions correctly, reread and rethink the material in the chapter. Discuss the questions and the specific practice issues with your peers.

So, did we achieve the stated purpose of this text? This is a question that we have asked ourselves over and over again. The most intriguing and heated question that arose among authors, editors, publishers, and nurses was, "What essential nursing care needs to be included in the text?" Indeed, the editor initially asked the question, "Is the nursing care detailed enough?" After intense reflection, further reading, and constructive debate, the authors answered this question as follows. The nurses or nursing students who will use this text are always in a hurry but never in such a hurry that they do not demonstrate professionalism and caring. The nurses who will use this text are concerned about working with other disciplines to achieve the best client outcomes in the shortest time and at the least cost. Therefore, more detail is given on nurses' responsibilities regarding various settings where the client could be treated, treatment costs, and strategies to promote collaborative and preventive health practices. We want to emphasize to the reader that taking the complex and making it concise was a very challenging mission.

But who are we (the authors)? Collectively, we have over 70 years of nursing experience: one of us entered practice as a licensed vocational nurse, and one of us began as a diploma graduate. Two of us have been single parents; all of us have worked hard to provide for our families. While we have all been very highly regarded in our respective nursing communities, our biggest distinction in authoring this book is that we share in the rewards and frustrations of clinical nursing, and we have all been life-long learners. Above all, the three of us have shared many personal and professional moments. In short, we are mothers, wives, nurses, scholars, nurse researchers, and friends who are always striving to improve.

In closing, we would like to request that our readers tell us something about themselves. We would also like to hear from you about this text via e-mail. Your messages can be clinical questions, things you found helpful about the book, or suggestions for areas that need improvement. Tell us about new trends or innovative clinical strategies that you have found to be successful. We will incorporate your ideas and suggestions into the next edition. We would enjoy hearing from you and feel that it is our nursing responsibility to create a learning partnership with you. Our e-mail addresses are: Gayle Roux: groux.ucs@smtp.usi.edu and Robin Lockhart: flckhrtr@nexus.mwsu.edu.

ACKNOWLEDGMENTS

It is with great appreciation that the authors thank Jane Edwards and Lisa Davis, the editors behind the authors. A special thanks to Mary Jo Distel, R.N., M.S., for her contribution to the gastrointestinal chapter and to Denise Blair, R.N., C.D.E., for the wound care protocol.

Charlene Reeves would like to thank: My son and daughter-in-law, Norman and Lenaya Reeves, for their love and support; my sister and brother-in-law, Betty and Ron Cettie, for their encouragement; and Dr. Jolene Walsh and Betty Henry for their special friendships.

Dr. Gayle Roux would like to thank: All of those people who encourage me to create, Mom, Mike R., Bill, Vicky, Jan, Blake, Angela, Janelle, Mike C., Marian, Nick, Jess, Dr. Patsy Keyser, and Dr. Helen Bush.

To my mom and dad, Leona and Charles Toussaint.
—CR
To my husband, Dimitri, and my daughters, Yvonne and La Roux.
—GR
To my family, Ron and Jessica.
—RL

In memory of Dr. Lillian Waring.

SENSORY SYSTEM: EYES AND EARS

CONDITIONS OF THE EYE

Overview

The eye has been referred to as "the most important square inch of the body surface" (Havener, 1979, p. 1). It is a sensory organ that enables human beings to view such wonders of the world as the Grand Canyon and the birth of a newborn. The eye is literally a window to the brain, as 90% of information reaches the brain through the eyes (Fig. 1-1). The eyes also give important physical clues to the general health of the body. For example, testing the cranial nerves provides important diagnostic information about the central nervous system (CNS). The eye examination evaluates cranial nerves (CN) II through VIII and assesses the optic disc for swelling (papilledema) when the intracranial pressure (ICP) is increased for any reason. Unilateral dilation of the pupil following a head injury or meningitis has diagnostic value because of the sensitivity of CN III to pressure. Complications from specific diseases like hypertension and diabetes mellitus (DM) result in recognizable structural retinal damage. DM causes common ocular complications such as diabetic retinopathy, cataracts, and refractive errors. As developing practitioners, nurses should learn how to assess and manage conditions of the eye.

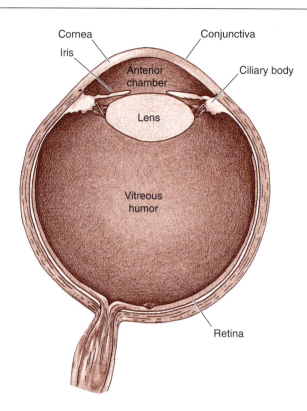

FIGURE 1-1 ◙

The normal eye.

The eyes, like all other organs, undergo changes as people age. However, unlike the rest of the aging process, changes in the eyes occur universally. It is essential that nurses be knowledgeable about these changes. Almost 100% of middle-aged people need eyeglasses. Decreased flexibility and elasticity of the lens are the first signs of aging. The decreased ability of the eye to focus (accommodate) for near and detailed work is termed *presbyopia*. As the lens turns yellow with advancing age, this causes difficulty in distinguishing colors at the blue end of the spectrum. In the elderly, a smaller pupil (*senile miosis*) adds to the distortion of color. This miosis also affects the amount of light reaching the retina and results in problems adapting to dim light and darkness.

As people age, changes occur in almost all structures of the eye. Aqueous humor production decreases in the sixth decade of life. The quantity and quality of tears decrease with age. As a result, the eyes of the elderly tend to feel dry and scratchy. The drainage of tears is less efficient, resulting in dripping of tears. Arcus senilis, a visible gray ring that circles the periphery of the cornea, is the result of accumulated calcium and fat deposits in the cornea. As the cornea flattens over time, images become blurred and distorted. This condition is known as astigmatism.

The nurse needs to be aware of the following interventions to promote eye health in the aging population: As people age, they need more light to see. Therefore, changes must be made to improve lighting in homes, offices, restaurants, and geriatric centers. Decreased lens transparency begins in the fifth decade of life and leads to cataracts. Glaucoma is present in approximately 2% of the population over 40 years of age, and often visual loss with undiagnosed glaucoma is permanent. Because of these and many other changes that occur with aging, an annual eye examination is recommended for all people over 40 years of age.

All people fear blindness. This fear is often magnified as clients age and lose their vision. Blindness is defined as a visual acuity of 20/200 in the better eye with optimal correction or a visual field below 20 degrees (a normal field is 180 degrees). A person who is totally blind can perceive absolutely no light. Optical aids such as magnifying glasses and special reading lights may be helpful for clients with minimal vision.

Like all specialized areas of health care, ophthalmology has some unique terminology. The nurse must be familiar with these terms to provide better care for clients with eye conditions. These definitions (given in alphabetical order) should be reviewed before reading the section on common eye conditions:

- **Blepharospasm.** A spasm of the eyelid in which the client is unable to open his or her eye.
- **Chalazion.** An infection or retention cyst of the meibomian glands caused by an untreated sty. The meibomian glands are the sebaceous glands located in the edges of the eyelids. The swelling is firm to the touch but not painful.
- **Conjunctivitis.** An infection of the conjunctiva; the most common eye disorder. Photophobia (sensitivity to light), tearing, and discharge (watery, purulent, or mucoid) occur. The etiology of conjunctivitis is bacterial, fungal, viral, allergenic, or from a chemical irritant.
- **Corneal infections and inflammations.** These can cause corneal scarring or ulceration. Early diagnosis and treatment are essential because corneal infections and inflammations are two major causes of blindness.
- **Corneal ulcer.** This results in local necrosis of the cornea. The ulcer occurs from wearing contact lenses, infection (herpes is the usual cause), or trauma. This is a medical emergency in which partial or total loss of vision may occur.
- **Ectropion.** A rolling outward of the lower eyelid that occurs when the muscles that allow the lids to close lose their strength.
- **Entropion.** An inversion of the lower lid as the result of a muscle spasm.
- **Hordeolum (sty).** An acute localized inflammation of a hair follicle or sebaceous gland. Sties result from a staphylococcal infection and can be quite painful.
- **Keratitis.** An inflammation of the cornea.
- **Keratoconjunctivitis.** In this condition, both the cornea and the conjunctiva are inflamed.
- **Ptosis.** Drooping of one eyelid. Ptosis may be caused by a stroke, a congenital defect, or a neuromuscular disorder.
- **Uveitis.** Inflammation of all or part of the vascular portion of the eye (choroid, ciliary body, iris). The etiology is either ankylosing spondylitis, autoimmune responses, tuberculosis, or syphilis. Uveitis causes severe eye pain and photophobia.
- **Xanthelasma.** In this disorder, yellow plaques accumulate on the lid margins. High lipid levels may cause the condition.

In the past, the only duty of the nurse was to check if the batteries were working in the ophthalmoscope and then hand the instrument to the physician, but those days are over! Now, nurses must develop excellent skills in taking health histories and in performing the basic eye examination. This should include a test for visual acuity, an external examination of the eye, testing of the cranial nerves and extraocular muscles, and an examination with an ophthalmoscope. When an eye disease is suspected or when examination by an ophthalmologist is required, the eye examination often includes the following diagnostic tests:

- **Pupillary dilation.** Mydriatic eye drops are instilled in the eye to dilate the pupil. This allows for improved visualization of the retina and internal eye structures.
- **Fluorescein stain with slit-lamp examination.** This allows visualization of any corneal ulcers or abrasions.
- **Culture and sensitivity.** This assesses any infection that may be present.
- **Glaucoma screening.** This procedure measures the intraocular pressure.

Conjunctivitis

Conjunctivitis without complications is a common eye infection that can be treated and diagnosed by a nurse practitioner or family physician. Clients who do not respond to treatment, clients with AIDS, and clients with a corneal infection should be referred to an ophthalmologist for immediate treatment.

Treatment of Conjunctivitis or Keratitis Treatment involves applying topical antibiotic drops or ophthalmic ointment. Erythromycin, gentamicin, penicillin, bacitracin, or amphotericin B is commonly used. Warm saline compresses are applied for 15 minutes three times a day for comfort. Frequent eye irrigations are performed with sterile saline. The client is urged to practice a scrupulous hand-washing technique to minimize reinfection or spreading infection to the unaffected eye. The eyes are covered with a patch to reduce eye movement if the infection is severe. The client is encouraged to use sunglasses. Severe infections require intravenous antibiotics. Finally, corticosteroids are given for keratitis when it is related to systemic infections.

Corneal Transplant

A corneal transplant, or keratoplasty, has a success rate of 90%. The cornea is harvested from donor clients younger than 65 years of age. Because the cornea is avascular, this transplant does not carry the usual risks and problems of other transplanted tissue. A corneal transplantation that restores the vision of a blind client is a marvelous example of the gift clients receive when people generously donate their tissues after death.

The nurse should report any signs of potential graft rejection such as inflammation, cloudiness of the graft, or increasing pain. The client should wear an eye shield at night and avoid straining, bending, coughing, sneezing, or heavy lifting.

Corneal Abrasion

A corneal abrasion is a common injury that causes a disruption of the superficial epithelium of the cornea. It is caused by dry eyes, contact lenses, dust, or dirt. The treatment includes sterile saline eye washes and removing the contact lenses until the cornea heals. Abrasion of the cornea is very painful, but the cornea usually heals without scarring within 24 hours once the causative agent is removed. Photophobia and tearing are common. An eye patch may be applied to allow the cornea to rest.

Chemical Burns to the Eyes

These burns require immediate emergency care. The eye should be flushed with copious amounts of fluid. Normal saline is preferred, but if it is not available, water may be used. Normal saline causes less edema of the cornea. The eyes are irrigated continuously until the client arrives at the emergency room. A topical ophthalmic antibiotic ointment is applied, and a topical anesthetic such as tetracaine or proparacaine (Alcaine) is given for pain relief. If applied immediately and for a long time, direct irrigations from the inner to the outer canthus should prevent permanent corneal scarring. Every second counts in preventing damage to the cornea from strong caustic agents such as acids, alkalis, and cleaning agents.

Penetrating Wounds to the Eye

These also require immediate first aid. No pressure dressings should ever be applied. The eye should be loosely covered with gauze, and the penetrating object should never be removed until the surgeon evaluates the injury. The object is immobilized with a shield or paper cup, and the client is given antiemetics to reduce vomiting, and this inhibits increasing intraocular pressure. A carbonic anhydrase inhibitor such as acetazolamide (Diamox) is given to decrease intraocular pressure. Cefazolin (Ancef) or gentamicin is given intravenously to prevent infection. The patient is kept in the semi-Fowler's position and transported to the nearest center for emergency ophthalmic surgery.

Indications for Cataract Surgery. Cataract surgery is an elective procedure. It is generally indicated when the cataract has reduced visual function so that it compromises the client's safety and activities of daily life. "The indication for surgery is founded on the patient's requirement for better vision and the patient's reasons for undergoing surgery" (Agency for Health Care Policy and Research [AHCPR], 1993, p. 70).

Cataracts

A cataract is a clouding of the lens. It is one of the most common eye conditions for which elderly clients seek treatment. Located just behind the iris, the lens is the focusing mechanism of the eye. The lens, conjunctiva, and cornea contain the refractive media of the eye that must remain translucent for the light to refract accurately and for the client to maintain visual acuity. Clients describe their cataract-impaired vision as being like looking through a glass smeared with butter.

The types, or stages, of cataracts include senile, immature, and mature. With senile cataracts, as the fibers and proteins of the lens change and degenerate, the client loses clarity of vision. In a client with immature cataracts, only a portion of the lens is affected. Mature cataracts are gray or white in color, and the entire lens is opaque.

Etiology Cataracts are either congenital or acquired. The most common cause of acquired cataracts is aging, although the exact mechanism is unknown. Corticosteroid and thorazine use, DM, and trauma to the eye are other causes of acquired cataracts. Congenital cataracts occur with conditions such as maternal rubella during pregnancy. Cataracts occur in both eyes, but one lens is usually worse than the other. The diagnosis of cataracts includes a decrease in visual acuity, absence of the red reflex, and visualization of opacities in the lens upon examination.

Treatment Surgical removal of the lens is the preferred treatment for cataracts. An intraocular implant is usually required. If an implant is not performed, prescription eyeglasses with very thick lenses are needed to replace the function of the lens. There have been dramatic improvements in the surgical procedure for lens removal. Clients now undergo this procedure as outpatient surgery and are discharged in 3–4 hours. There are two types of lens extraction. *Intracapsular extraction* is the removal of the entire lens, and *extracapsular extraction* is the removal of the lens material without the capsule.

Preoperative nursing care includes documenting the visual acuity of both the surgical and nonsurgical eyes. A general physical examination, including an electrocardiogram (ECG) and blood chemistries, is performed, as elderly clients often have preexisting medical conditions. The nurse also explains the surgical procedure to the client and orients him or her to the surroundings. The nurse should caution the client to avoid lifting anything over 5 lb and to avoid coughing, sneezing, or bending over at the waist after surgery. The nurse instructs the client to remove all makeup preoperatively. In addition, mydriatic drops to dilate the pupils and cyclopegic drops to paralyze the ciliary bodies are administered as ordered to decrease intraocular pressure.

Postoperative nursing care includes monitoring vital signs, assessing the level of consciousness, checking the eye dressing, maintaining the eye patch and shield, and monitoring eye complications. The client should be positioned on the affected side (semi-Fowler's position) to decrease intraocular pressure. Antiemetics and sedation are administered as needed. If sudden eye pain occurs after surgery, hemorrhage may be the cause. This should be reported to the physician immediately. Flashes of light, "floaters," or the sensation of a curtain being pulled over the eye may signal possible retinal detachment and also should be reported immediately. If the patient has a known or suspected detached retina after surgery, this is another reason to position the client on the affected side.

Snellen Visual Acuity Test. While not based on strict scientific evidence, the general clinical consensus and guidelines of the AHCPR suggest a visual acuity in the affected eye of 20/50 or worse as the objective criterion justifying cataract surgery (AHCPR, 1993).

Referral to a Home Health Nurse. As outpatient eye and ear surgery has increased, clients are referred more frequently to a home health nurse. The nurse must ensure that the client and family understand and comply with discharge instructions. Clients with sensory system problems frequently have physical limitations that make reading or following discharge instructions difficult.

The nurse should always approach clients from the unaffected side and provide explanations of what they can expect. The client should be instructed to wear sunglasses to prevent photophobia and should also be reassured that vision will improve over time. The word cataract often frightens elderly clients; however, it is actually one of the least serious disorders known to cause loss of vision and is reversible. Replacing the opaque lens with a lens implant is almost always a successful operation.

Glaucoma

Increased intraocular pressure causes glaucoma. It is one of the most common causes of blindness. The normal intraocular pressure is approximately 15 mm Hg, with a range of 12–20 mm Hg (Guyton, 1991). Glaucoma occurs when the intraocular pressure reaches a pathological level of 60–70 mm Hg. Pressure levels of 20–30 mm Hg can result in a loss of vision over time. With acute glaucoma, the extreme pressure can cause blindness within hours.

Intraocular fluid, which is formed in the ciliary body of the eye (Fig. 1-2), flows between the ligaments of the lens, through the pupil, and into the anterior chamber of the eye (the chamber between the cornea and iris). The fluid then flows in the angle between the cornea and iris through a meshwork of minute openings termed trabeculae. Finally, the fluid flows into the canal of Schlemm and empties into the extraocular veins (Fig. 1-3). In the normal eye, the intraocular pressure remains constant, typically varying within a range of 2 mm Hg. Intraocular pressure is balanced between the production of aqueous humor in the ciliary body and the outflow through the pupil to the trabecular meshwork and canal of Schlemm. An increase in pressure can cause ischemia or death of the neu-

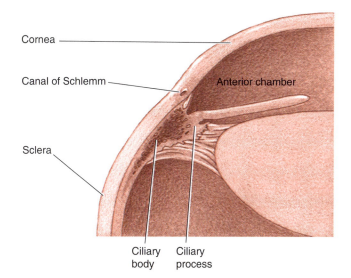

Cornea

Canal of Schlemm

Anterior chamber

Sclera

Ciliary body

Ciliary process

FIGURE 1-2

Structures of the ciliary body and anterior chamber.

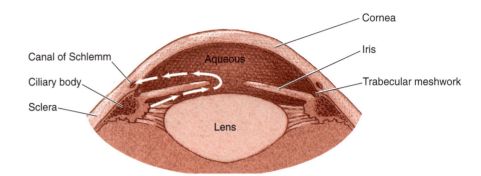

FIGURE 1-3

◙

Normal flow of aqueous humor.

rons of the eye, resulting in degeneration of the optic nerve and ultimately loss of vision.

All eye examinations should include a measurement of intraocular pressure. Because loss of vision can occur without symptoms, the early diagnosis and treatment of glaucoma are essential. All people over 40 years of age should have intraocular pressure measured annually. There are two common diagnostic measurements of intraocular pressure:

1. **Tonometry** is an indirect measurement of intraocular pressure. Once local anesthetic eye drops are administered, the footplate of the tonometer is placed on the cornea to measure the pressure.
2. **Gonioscopy** assesses the angle of the anterior chamber of the eye and measures the depth. Gonioscopy differentiates between open-angle and angle-closure glaucoma.

Types of Glaucoma

Primary Glaucoma Primary glaucoma usually occurs in patients over 60 years of age. It may be congenital in infants and children. There are two forms of primary glaucoma.

Open-angle glaucoma, the most common type, is chronic, simple glaucoma. In this condition, drainage through the canal of Schlemm is impaired, but as the name implies, the angle between the iris and cornea where the outflow of aqueous fluid occurs remains open. Open-angle glaucoma usually occurs in both eyes. Signs and symptoms include a loss of peripheral vision, mild headache, seeing halos around lights, and difficulty adapting to light. The disease progresses gradually. The client often remains asymptomatic even after visual loss has occurred.

Angle-closure glaucoma occurs when the outflow angle between the iris and cornea narrows or closes. The intraocular pressure increases rapidly, and permanent loss of vision occurs. This usually only occurs in one eye. As the anterior chamber angle narrows and the iris bulges into the anterior chamber, fluid outflow to the canal of Schlemm is restricted (Fig. 1-4).

Signs and symptoms of angle-closure glaucoma include eye pain, decreased visual acuity, nausea and vomiting, seeing colored halos around lights, red conjunctiva, and cloudy cornea. Angle-closure glaucoma is

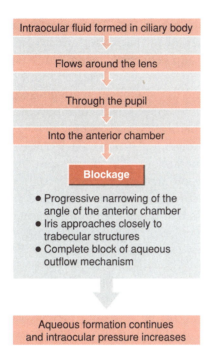

Intraocular fluid formed in ciliary body

Flows around the lens

Through the pupil

Into the anterior chamber

Blockage

- Progressive narrowing of the angle of the anterior chamber
- Iris approaches closely to trabecular structures
- Complete block of aqueous outflow mechanism

Aqueous formation continues and intraocular pressure increases

FIGURE 1-4

Blockage of fluid in angle-closure glaucoma.

treated both pharmacologically and surgically. Topical miotics or beta blockers are administered. Laser iridotomy is performed to reestablish the outflow of intraocular fluid.

Secondary Glaucoma Secondary glaucoma results from an infection, cataracts, tumor, or hemorrhage. Following a hemorrhage or intraocular infection, debris accumulates in the aqueous humor and is trapped in the trabecular meshwork leading to the canal of Schlemm. Accumulation of blood or infection increases pressure as a result of both occupying space and clogging the trabecular meshwork.

Surgical Management When drug therapy is not successful in managing intraocular pressure or when the glaucoma is acute, operative techniques are necessary to open the spaces of the trabeculae or to create outflow tracks for the fluid. Common surgical procedures for glaucoma include the following:

1. **Laser trabeculoplasty** is outpatient surgery that uses a laser to open the minute spaces of the trabecular network.
2. **Trabeculectomy** is a procedure performed under general anesthesia that forms a permanent fistula to drain aqueous humor from the anterior chamber.
3. **Photocoagulation (laser heat) and cyclocryotherapy (frozen tissue)** are used to decrease the production of aqueous humor by the ciliary body.
4. **Laser iridotomy** is a laser procedure that perforates the iris to allow for increased drainage.
5. **Iridectomy** is a procedure in which a small segment of the iris is removed to increase outflow.

Pharmacological Management Pharmacological and antiglaucoma agents are very important in the management of glaucoma. There is no physiological relationship between glaucoma and hypertension. Their only similarity is that clients with these diseases require life-long pharmacological management. Once the client is diagnosed with glaucoma, it is essential for the nurse to emphasize the importance of daily medication and annual eye examinations.

Clients who are taking antiglaucoma agents need to be particularly concerned about drug interactions. The nurse must instruct clients to avoid any over-the-counter cold and sleep remedies. Clients with narrow-angle or angle-closure glaucoma should avoid atropine and other anticholinergics such as mydriatics that dilate the pupils. Commonly used medications for glaucoma include miotics, mydriatics, beta-adrenergics, and carbonic anhydrase inhibitors.

Miotics After administering the miotic eye drops, the nurse should apply pressure to the lacrimal sac for 1–2 minutes to increase the local effect by preventing the drops from entering the systemic circulation. Cholinergics constrict the pupil to facilitate the aqueous humor outflow. The absorption of fluid into the canal of Schlemm decreases intraocular pressure. The decrease in intraocular pressure occurs when the iris is drawn away from the filtration angle, thus facilitating the outflow of aqueous humor (Wilson, Shannon, & Stang, 1998). Miotics such as acetylcholine, carbachol, and pilocarpine (Ocusert-Pilo) are used in open-angle and angle-closure glaucoma. Pilocarpine (Ocusert-Pilo) is an ocular system that is placed in the upper lid in the conjunctival sac and is changed weekly. It may blur the client's vision. The system is given at bedtime, and the drug peaks in two hours. Side effects include brow pain, headache, and increased tearing.

Mydriatics Mydriatics such as epinephrine are sympathomimetics that dilate the pupil and decrease production and increase absorption of aqueous humor. These actions decrease the intraocular pressure in open-angle glaucoma. The adrenergic drug should be discontinued if central nervous symptom (CNS) side effects, such as nerve and muscle tremors, occur. While taking mydriatics, the client should avoid over-the-counter cold and sinus medications.

Beta-Adrenergic Receptor Blockers Beta-adrenergic blockers such as betaxolol (Betaoptic), levobunolol (Betagan), and timolol (Timoptic) decrease intraocular pressure by slowing the production of aqueous humor. Doses are administered twice daily as the drugs have a long duration. The nurse must report any adverse effects such as decreased visual field, dyspnea, decreased exercise tolerance, diaphoresis, or flushing.

Carbonic Anhydrase Inhibitors Carbonic anhydrase inhibitors like dichlorphenamide (Daranide) and acetazolamide (Diamox) decrease the production of aqueous humor to lower intraocular pressure. They are given orally as adjunctive therapy. For a client with open-angle glaucoma, a carbonic anhydrase inhibitor is given intravenously prior to surgery to decrease intraocular pressure. The nurse should administer inhibitors in the morning because of their diuretic effect. They should be given with food to prevent nausea.

As with anyone taking a diuretic, nurses should urge clients to drink 2–3 L of fluid to avoid renal stones. The nurse should assess the client's daily weight and monitor fluid intake and output and vital signs for volume depletion. The nurse should monitor electrolytes as well as renal and liver function tests. The client may require a potassium-rich diet or potassium replacement. Adverse reactions include a rash, pruritus, purpura, pallor, and bleeding. The physician must be notified if the client develops a fever, sore throat, numbness, tingling, or flank pain (Wilson, Shannon, & Stang, 1998).

CASE STUDY: THE EYE

Mrs. B. has been experiencing headaches for the past two days over the frontal and temporal areas. She has also experienced pain in the right eye, decreased visual acuity, colored halos around lights, and nausea. The symptoms are becoming progressively worse, and she has contacted her ophthalmologist for an appointment.

The nurse at the ophthalmologist's office must recognize the symptoms as described by the client as being potentially very serious; he or she must then assist the client in obtaining an immediate appointment. The nurse should give brief, simple instructions to the client to assist her in understanding the need for immediate treatment to preserve vision. The client should be instructed to have someone drive her to the ophthalmology center immediately.

Upon examination, the ophthalmologist diagnoses angle-closure glaucoma. In preparation for an immediate laser iridotomy, the ophthalmologist perforates the iris to allow the aqueous humor to drain.

Postoperatively, the nurse gives instructions to the client to avoid bending, coughing, sneezing, or lifting anything over 5 lb. The client should be provided with an antiemetic, to be taken if she becomes nauseated at home, as vomiting tends to increase intraocular pressure. The nurse must instruct the client to call the physician immediately if eye pain occurs or if the same symptoms occur in the opposite eye. At the postoperative follow-up appointment, the nurse reinforces the information on any medication regimen and the need for follow-up eye examinations every 6–12 months.

The client will have the diagnosis confirmed and laser iridotomy performed by an ophthalmologist. The nurse is usually responsible for the pre- and postoperative education. Once the client has been discharged from the care of the ophthalmologist, she may be followed on a routine basis by her family practice physician or nurse practitioner. The client should have an eye examination in both eyes with measurement of the intraocular pressure every 6–12 months by the ophthalmologist. Consistent information and reinforcement from these members of the health team will help the client accept and manage her glaucoma.

Retinal Detachment

Retinal detachment is defined as a separation of the retina or sensory portion of the eye from the choroid (the pigmented vascular layer). Retinal detachment can occur spontaneously or be caused by trauma. The condition should be treated as an emergency and will result in permanent vision loss if not detected early and treated. Early detection and prompt surgery can prevent irreversible blindness and restore the client's normal vision. Signs and symptoms of retinal detachment include floaters (black spots), lines or flashes of light, the sudden sensation of a curtain being pulled over the eye, and blurred vision. Pain is absent. The visual field defect is located directly opposite the detached portion of the retina.

Treatment A client with suspected retinal detachment should be transported to the nearest facility with an ophthalmologist present for examination and diagnosis. Once diagnosed, the condition must be corrected surgically. The surgical procedures include the following:

1. **Cryotherapy** or **laser photocoagulation** welds the retina and choroid layers together.
2. **Scleral buckling** is a fold that is created in the sclera by encircling the globe with a scleral bond. This holds the contents of the eye together.
3. **Pneumatic retinopexy** is a procedure in which air is placed in the vitreous cavity.

Nursing care includes positioning the patient on the affected side (usually) to shift the intraocular pressure and assist in making the layers of the retina adhere. The client's fears should be allayed, and explanations of the surgical procedures are required. Hospitalization, which was often lengthy in the past, nowadays may last only a day or two. Restoration of normal physical activity may occur in 3–6 weeks. While a detached retina usually occurs in only one eye, the client may be genetically predisposed to a detachment in the other eye. Nurses should instruct clients to seek emergency care immediately if the symptoms listed above occur. In a client who has had a retinal detachment, a retinal examination every 6–12 months is suggested. Other clients who are at risk for retinal detachment, such as those with myopia or diabetic retinopathy, should also have routine eye examinations.

Macular Degeneration

The macula is the area of greatest visual acuity in the retina. Macular degeneration can occur as the retina ages. It is the leading cause of blindness in the elderly. The exact cause of this change is not known. Clinical manifestations include distorted straight lines that appear as wavy lines or dark spots. There is no primary prevention, and no treatment currently exists. In general, if the client seeks treatment at the first signs of changes in vision, some treatments, such as laser therapy, may preserve vision.

Retinitis Pigmentosa

Retinitis pigmentosa is a hereditary, degenerative disease that causes retinal atrophy and loss of retinal function. Clinical manifestations include poor night vision in childhood, a slow, progressive loss of visual fields, photophobia, disrupted color vision, and tunnel vision. No treatment is available.

Diabetic Retinopathy

Diabetic retinopathy is a vascular disorder affecting the capillaries of the retina. This is a major complication of DM and a leading cause of blindness. Manifestations include blurred vision, floaters, cobwebs, and flashing lights. Maintaining blood sugar levels within the normal limits (70–120 mg/dL) may help to prevent this condition. All diabetic clients should have annual eye examinations by an ophthalmologist to detect and treat retinopathy early.

Cytomegalovirus (CMV) Retinitis

This type of eye infection occurs in clients with immunosuppression from acquired immunodeficiency syndrome (AIDS). CMV causes blindness. The treatment includes drug therapy with antiviral agents such as ganciclovir (Cytovene) and foscarnet (Foscavir) along with other AIDS drug therapies such as zidovudine (AZT) or didanosine (DDI or Videx). Regular ophthalmological examinations are necessary for AIDS patients.

Enucleation

Enucleation is the surgical removal of the eye. While every attempt is made to prevent enucleation, conditions such as penetrating eye wounds that cause irreparable damage and cancer (retinoblastoma) make it unavoidable. Postoperative nursing care includes monitoring the pressure dressings that are applied for the first 24–48 hours. Hemorrhage and infection are possible complications, and any fever, drainage, or eye pain should be reported to the physician. Within a week, a temporary prosthesis (conformer) is fitted into the empty socket. A permanent prosthesis is placed within a month or two after surgery. Nursing care includes washing the prosthesis with soap and water or normal saline. The eye socket is washed with a bulb syringe and clean water. The prosthesis should be stored in a plastic container wrapped in gauze sponges.

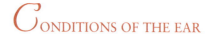
Conditions of the Ear

Overview

The ear receives sound waves, conducts sound from the tympanic membrane to the cochlea in the inner ear, and transmits auditory information to the CNS. The meaning of sound is deciphered in the brain (Fig. 1-5). The sense of hearing is intricately involved with the sensory system, enjoyment and quality of life, and the ability to communicate.

External and Middle Ear

Otitis Externa Clients with inflamed external ear canals have what is termed "swimmer's ear." *Pseudomonas* is the most common causative organism. Exostosis (bony growths) in a surfer's ears are attributable to the exposure to cold water and may also cause this condition. Clinical manifestations are ear pain and a feeling of fullness in the ears. When the client has otitis externa, pressing on the tragus or pulling on the pinna elicits discomfort or pain. The diagnosis of otitis externa is confirmed by an examination of the ear canal with an otoscope. On examination, the ear canal has a red, inflamed appearance, and clear or discolored drainage is often apparent.

Treatment Treatment includes topical or systemic antibiotics. A mixture of neomycin, polymyxin, and hydrocortisone (Cortisporin Otic) is often effective. When administering ear drops, the nurse should warm the solution by holding the bottle for five minutes prior to instillation. Medications should be at body temperature, as cold fluids in the ear can stimulate vertigo or nausea. The nurse should have the client lie on the unaffected side and remain there for five minutes after instillation. To keep the area sterile, a cotton ball may be placed in the canal for 15–20 minutes after instillation.

Impacted Cerumen and Foreign Bodies As a person ages, decreased cerumen with a firmer consistency is produced. As the cerumen hardens, it changes in color from yellow to brown or black. Conductive hearing loss occurs as the accumulated wax blocks the conduction of sound waves. This hearing loss may be accompanied by tinnitus (ringing in the ears). Cerumen may be softened and loosened by administering glycerine and hydrogen peroxide drops. The ear drops are used for a week or two. If the cerumen is impacted and needs to be removed, bacteriostatic saline should be used for irrigation of the ear canal if the tympanic membrane is intact. The ear should never be irrigated if the tympanic membrane is ruptured.

When a suspected or known foreign body is lodged in the ear canal, the ear should not be irrigated. The foreign body is capable of swelling upon contact with water, making removal more difficult. This occurs with

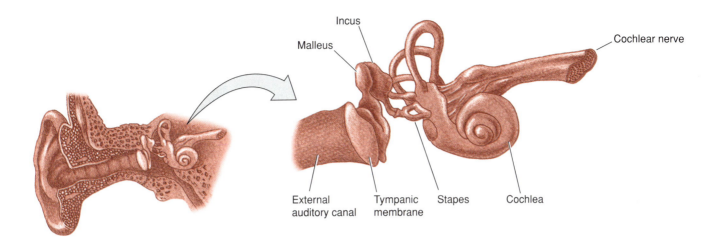

FIGURE 1-5 The normal ear.

objects such as peas, beans, and insects. A foreign body must be removed from the ear by a physician with the aid of a microscope. To remove an insect, the ear should be flushed with mineral oil, not water. The mineral oil kills the bug, which can then be removed by irrigation.

Otitis Media   Otitis media, a middle ear infection, is one of the most common infections in children younger than four years of age. The terms used to differentiate the types of otitis media are serous, acute, and chronic otitis media.

Serous Otitis Media   This occurs when the eustachian tube is obstructed and serous fluid accumulates in the middle ear. Signs and symptoms caused by the obstruction include snapping or popping sounds in the middle ear and bulging or retraction of the tympanic membrane. The etiology of serous otitis media is usually an upper respiratory infection or allergies.

Acute Otitis Media   This is caused by the sudden onset of a bacterial infection in the middle ear. Mucus and serous fluids accumulate in addition to various species of bacteria. The most common causative organisms are *Streptococcus pneumoniae*, *Streptococcus pyogenes*, and *Haemophilus influenzae*. The manifestations of acute otitis media include sudden ear pain, decreased hearing, fever, vertigo, nausea, and vomiting. Infants and toddlers are often irritable, waking up in the middle of the night crying and pulling at their ears. The diagnosis is confirmed by otoscope examination. On examination, the tympanic membrane is red and bulging and may have purulent drainage. The membrane has poor motility when air is infused by a pneumatic otoscope. Treatment includes decongestants or antihistamines to decrease the swelling of the mucosa in the middle ear and eustachian tube and prevent fluid accumulation in the middle ear. A course of antibiotics such as penicillin, erythromycin, amoxicillin, trimethoprim/sulfamethoxazole, and cefaclor is prescribed for 10–14 days. Analgesics such as acetaminophen (Tylenol) and ibuprofen (Advil) are used to promote comfort, allowing clients to sleep at night.

CASE STUDY: THE EAR

Jeff, a one-year-old, is brought to the pediatric clinic with an elevated temperature of 102°F of two days duration. The nurse practitioner takes a health history from the mother. The child's normal diet is four bottles of formula a day and three small meals with soft table foods. However, for the past two days the child has not been eating and is taking fluids sparingly. The nurse notes that the child is pulling at his ears, and the mother states that he has been waking up frequently during the night and crying. The child's immunizations are up to date, and he has had no previous illnesses. The child is not taking any routine medications. The mother has administered pediatric acetaminophen (Tylenol) for the temperature.

Upon examination, the nurse practitioner notes that both tympanic membranes are red and bulging. The tympanic membrane is intact, and no drainage is apparent. The oral mucous membranes and lips appear slightly dry. Lung sounds are clear upon auscultation. The diagnosis is acute otitis media.

The nurse realizes that the child will need a prescription for an antibiotic. The health history information that is essential to obtain from the mother includes the following:

1. Has the child taken any antibiotics before? If so, which ones?
2. Does the child have any known food or drug allergies?
3. What financial resources or prescription plan does the mother have to purchase an antibiotic?

The nurse learns that because the child has not had any previous illnesses, he has never taken antibiotics. The mother reports no known allergies. The mother is on a limited income, and she does not have health insurance or a prescription plan.

With no history of penicillin allergy, amoxicillin (Amoxil), a broad-spectrum antibiotic used for infections of the ear, nose, and throat, is often prescribed. The preparation is available in pediatric drops and is the most economical of all antibiotics.

The instructions to the mother should include the following:

1. Increase fluids, such as Pedialyte, immediately. Offer some liquids every hour. Pedialyte popsicles are also available at the grocery or pharmacy.

2. Administer antibiotics as directed. Provide an instruction sheet with side effect information. Provide a calibrated plastic dispenser or pediatric dropper to measure the antibiotic. A household spoon is not accurate enough to calculate dosage.

3. Call the clinic if the child does not improve within two days. Call immediately if a rash appears, as this could be an indication of a hypersensitivity reaction.

4. Continue to give acetaminophen (Tylenol) every four hours for comfort and fever, as needed.

5. Do not prop the feeding bottles; rather, hold the child and administer the bottle with the child in an upright position. Explain to the mother that placing the child in bed with a bottle may cause a backflow of fluid into the eustachian tube, predisposing the child to infection in the middle ear.

6. Complete the 10-day course of antibiotics. Return for a brief follow-up appointment for an examination of the middle ear to ensure that the infection has cleared.

Nurse practitioners frequently work with children and young families. Diagnosing and treating acute otitis media are within the scope of practice for a nurse practitioner. If the child does not improve, the nurse practitioner should consult with the physician. On follow-up, if the mother needed further financial or social services, the social worker would be a valuable resource for this family, and a referral would be made.

Chronic Otitis Media This condition results from repeated middle ear infections. When the infections recur, drainage and perforation can result. The child may have delayed language skills. Scarring of the tympanic membrane can also occur. In this condition, scars from previous perforations are seen as white, opaque areas on the tympanic membrane. Repeated ear infections that are frequently accompanied by perforation of the tympanic membrane may require a myringotomy. In this surgical procedure tubes are inserted in the tympanic membrane to allow fluid to drain, to keep the eustachian tube clear, and to decrease the incidence of repeated infections. It is performed on an outpatient basis, and the client is discharged on the same day with instructions to avoid getting water in the ears.

Acute Mastoiditis Acute mastoiditis is caused by the spread of infection from the middle ear. Infection and pus accumulate in the mastoid air cells. Currently, this seldom occurs because otitis media is diagnosed and treated at an early stage. However, with repeated middle ear infections, the infection can spread to the mastoids. Mastoiditis can occur 2–3 weeks after acute otitis media. Manifestations include ear pain, hearing loss, tenderness over the mastoid area behind the ear, tinnitus, and headache. The client may have profuse ear drainage that flows from the mastoid through the middle ear and exits through a perforation in the tympanic membrane.

The treatment includes intravenous administration of antibiotics such as penicillin, ceftriaxone (Rocephin), and metronidazole (Flagyl) for 14 days. If the client does not improve with antibiotics, a surgical mastoidectomy is performed. This procedure removes infected mastoid cells from the bone and drains pus. Some middle ear structures (incus and malleus) may also require resection. Tympanoplasty, the surgical reconstruction of the middle ear to preserve hearing, is also done. This is performed in an attempt to save the remaining ear structures and to preserve the client's auditory acuity. Following ear surgery, the client should lie on the unaffected side with the head of the bed elevated. Nose blowing, sneezing, and coughing are discouraged as these actions increase the pressure in the middle ear.

Cholesteatoma A cholesteatoma is a complication of chronic otitis media. Epithelial cell debris accumulates in the middle ear, forming a cyst that destroys the structures of the ear and diminishes hearing. As with mastoiditis, early detection and treatment of otitis media with antibiotic therapy have decreased the incidence of cholesteatoma. A cholesteatoma is benign and grows slowly, but if not removed, it can cause hearing loss. A mastoidectomy can remove a cholesteatoma; however, it remains controversial as to what is the best procedure to remove the cholesteatoma while still preserving as much hearing as possible.

Otosclerosis Otosclerosis is a hardening of the ear. In this condition, excess bone that forms over the stapes results in loss of movement of the stapes. The stapes becomes immobilized, causing a conductive hearing loss. It is a hereditary disorder that begins in adolescence. Signs and symptoms include an abnormal Rinne test, progressive loss of hearing, and a reddish-orange tympanic membrane. Treatment involves removal of the stapes followed by the insertion of a metallic prosthesis. This is termed a stapedectomy. A hearing aid may be needed postoperatively.

Presbycusis Presbycusis is the loss of ability to distinguish high-pitched sounds as the person ages. Most people suffer from some hearing deficit as they age. There is no treatment to prevent or cure presbycusis. If hearing loss is significant, a hearing aid may be needed.

Inner Ear

The inner ear generates nerve impulses in response to sound vibrations received from the middle ear. An inflamed inner ear is termed *labyrinthitis*. Causative organisms may be viral or bacterial from otitis media or an upper respiratory infection. Manifestations include vertigo, tinnitus, nystagmus (rapid involuntary eye movements), and temporary or permanent hearing loss. It is treated with antibiotics, antihistamines, and decongestants.

Meniere's Disease Meniere's disease is generally defined as a disorder of balance caused by a disturbance in the vestibular structures of the inner

Contraindications for Eye and Ear Surgery. The risks and benefits of surgery should always be considered, especially for elderly clients. Surgery should not be performed if the client does not want surgery, if aids such as glasses and hearing aids provide satisfactory function, or if the client has a preexisting condition that makes surgery or anesthesia high risk.

ear. Etiology may be genetic or viral. Classic signs and symptoms include vertigo with tinnitus, unilateral hearing loss, and nausea and vomiting. Fluid may be present in the inner ear. Clients complain of a feeling of fullness in the ears. This disorder cannot be cured but can usually be managed with drug therapy. The client should be cautioned to avoid sudden movements. The client must also avoid alcohol and caffeine. Clients are treated with various combinations of antihistamines, meclazine (Antivert), and vasodilators.

Vertigo Vertigo, strictly defined, is a symptom, not a diagnosis; however, because of the general nature of the client's symptoms and the difficulty in sharply defining it, vertigo is often used as a diagnosis. Vertigo is frequently accompanied by nausea, vomiting, and loss of balance. The sensation of being in motion in a fixed, unmoving environment is a subjective type of vertigo. This sensation occurs when clients feel like they are spinning in a still room. The sensation of being fixed and unmoving in a moving environment is an objective type of vertigo. This sensation occurs when the client feels like the room is spinning around him or her. Clients are treated with various drug combinations including diazepam (Valium), atropine, meclazine (Antivert), hydroxyzine (Vistaril), and prochlorperazine (Compazine).

When the client's chief complaint is dizziness, he or she is often unsteady, feels off-balance, and is at high risk for injuries as a result of falls. Clients are encouraged to lie in a supine position until the symptoms pass. In the hospital, the side-rails of the bed are raised for safety. Treatment also consists of decreasing the amount of sodium in the diet, furosemide (Lasix) or triamterene-hydrochlorothiazide (Dyazide) to decrease labyrinth pressure, and antiemetics for nausea and vomiting.

Labyrinthectomy, the removal of the labyrinth, is a treatment of last resort for clients with Meniere's disease or chronic vertigo who have not responded to medical therapy. After the labyrinthectomy, vertigo improves, but clients are still unsteady on their feet.

Acoustic Neuroma An acoustic neuroma is a benign tumor of CN VIII. Although the tumor is benign, growth from the internal ear toward the brain stem may cause life-threatening neurological problems. The tumor can grow into the internal auditory meatus and compress the auditory nerve. Manifestations include tinnitus, unilateral hearing loss, nystagmus, dizziness, and vertigo. The diagnosis is confirmed by computed tomography (CT) scans or magnetic resonance imaging (MRI). The tumor must be removed surgically. However, even with surgical removal, compression of the adjacent cranial nerves, especially the trigeminal and facial nerves, can occur. The gag reflex can then be affected and swallowing impaired following surgery. The client is given nothing by mouth until the physician determines that the client's ability to swallow has returned. Suction should be available during this time. Since complete removal of the tumor is usually not possible, the client should have follow-up CT scans or MRI annually to track the progress of tumor growth. Fortunately, these tumors grow slowly.

Developmentally Based Nursing Care. Nursing care is provided based on the developmental needs of the client, from the neonate to the elderly. The nurse must learn how clients function in their daily lives in order to care for them properly. Elderly clients, whose vision and hearing are impaired, often experience difficulties in walking and maintaining their balance. They often become isolated or depressed because of these limitations.

Summary

The function and health of the sensory system greatly impact an individual's quality of life, safety, mobility, and ability to communicate. The nurse must be skilled in taking the client's health history and performing the basic physical examinations of the eye and ear. When an abnormality of the eye is apparent, the nurse must be alert for other signs of disease. Complications from DM, hypertension, and neurological disorders may be diagnosed through examination of the eye and the early recognition of eye symptoms. To maintain eye health as well as overall health, clients older than 40 years of age should undergo an eye examination once a year by an ophthalmologist. Dramatic improvements in ocular surgical techniques have helped to preserve the vision and improve the well-being of clients. However, untreated glaucoma and diabetic retinopathy remain leading causes of irreversible blindness. Health education must continue to emphasize the importance of early diagnosis and treatment of eye disorders to reduce the incidence of blindness. The early detection of ear infections and treatment with antibiotics and decongestants have preserved hearing and decreased complications from conditions such as mastoiditis. Elderly clients frequently suffer from both vision and hearing loss; therefore, nurses must assist clients in adapting their homes to maintain a safe and functional environment.

Environment. Clients with sensory system problems are profoundly influenced by their environment. Potential hazards such as broken steps, throw rugs, cluttered pathways, and poor lighting must be identified and corrected in the home.

KEY WORDS

EYE

Accommodation	Enucleation
Angle-closure glaucoma	Hordeolum
Arcus senilis	Macular degeneration
Blepharospasm	Miotics
Cataract	Mydriatics
Chalazion	Open-angle glaucoma
Conformer	Presbyopia
Conjunctivitis	Ptosis
Cytomegalovirus retinitis	Retinitis pigmentosa
Diabetic retinopathy	Senile miosis
Ectropion	Uveitis
Entropion	

EAR

Acoustic neuroma	Meniere's disease
Acute mastoiditis	Otitis externa
Cerumen	Otitis media
Cholesteatoma	Serous otitis media
Chronic otitis media	Tympanoplasty
Labyrinthitis	Vertigo

QUESTIONS

1. Mr. S. has been diagnosed with a detached retina. Which one of the following symptoms should the nurse expect to occur during the acute phase?
   A. Curtain over the visual field
   B. Blepharospasm
   C. Distorted straight lines
   D. Total loss of vision

2. One clinical manifestation of open-angle glaucoma, the most common type of glaucoma, is
   A. rapid and permanent loss of vision.
   B. loss of peripheral vision.
   C. red conjunctiva.
   D. cloudy cornea.

3. Mrs. A. has undergone an enucleation of her right eye. The nurse should expect which of the following during the acute postoperative phase?
   A. Eye dressings on both eyes
   B. Excessive tearing from both eyes
   C. A pressure dressing on the right eye for 24–48 hours
   D. A permanent prosthesis in the right eye socket

4. Acute otitis media differs from serous otitis media in which of the following ways?
   A. The tympanic membrane is red and bulging.
   B. The tympanic membrane is always perforated.
   C. Pus cells are seen in the mastoid cells.
   D. Tympanoplasty must be performed.

5. Mr. G. has been diagnosed with Meniere's disease. The nurse should understand which of the following facts about this disease?
   A. Hearing loss is usually bilateral.
   B. Vertigo is not a usual complaint.
   C. Mr. G. should avoid sudden movements.
   D. A perforated tympanic membrane is the most common cause.

6. Mr. J. has a perforated tympanic membrane. An important precaution associated with this condition is
   A. not to allow water to enter the ear canal.
   B. to keep a cotton ball in the canal continuously.
   C. to instill normal saline into the ear canal twice a day to clear the canal of pathogens.
   D. to discourage coughing, sneezing, and nose blowing.

ANSWERS

1. *The answer is A.* As the two retinal layers separate and detachment becomes complete, blindness results because the macula detaches.

2. *The answer is B.* There is an increasing loss of vision as a result of increased intraocular pressure, and this begins in the periphery, followed by central loss.

3. *The answer is C.* Bleeding is a complication of this type of surgery. A double layer pressure dressing is commonly used to help prevent bleeding in the acute postoperative phase.

4. *The answer is A.* Serous otitis media occurs when fluid forms in the middle ear due to a blocked eustachian tube. Acute otitis media is an infection of the middle ear of sudden onset. Inflammation is apparent in the tympanic membrane.

5. *The answer is C.* This disease causes hearing changes, vertigo, and tinnitus. It is a disease of the inner ear involving the vestibular and semicircular canals. The client should be cautioned to avoid sudden movements, which may exacerbate symptoms.

6. *The answer is A.* Infection is always a concern when the tympanic membrane is perforated; thus, clients are warned not to allow water to enter the ear canal. Hearing loss is approximately one third of the normal range with a perforated tympanic membrane.

ANNOTATED REFERENCES

Agency for Healthcare Policy and Research (AHCPR). (1993). *Clinical practice guideline number 4. Cataracts in adults: Management of functional impairment.* Washington, D. C.: U. S. Department of Health and Human Services.

The AHCPR was established to enhance the quality, appropriateness, and effectiveness of health care services. This is an excellent guide written by a panel of experts. A copy may be obtained from the Director of the AHCPR, Executive Office Center, Suite 401, 2101 East Jefferson Street, Rockville, MD 20852.

Guyton, A. C. (1991). *Textbook of medical physiology.* Philadelphia: W. B. Saunders.

This is a classic reference text for human physiology. Understanding the underlying anatomy and physiology of a disease allows the nurse to understand the diagnosis and therapeutic plan for a client.

Havener, W. H. (1979). *Synopsis of ophthalmology*, 5th ed. St. Louis: C. V. Mosby.

This text reviews eye anatomy and the eye examination. It is also of historical interest because it provides an example that allows the reader to compare how ocular surgical techniques have advanced during the last 20 years.

Wilson, B. A., Shannon, M. T., & Stang, C. L. (1998). *Nurse's drug guide.* Stamford, CT: Appleton & Lange.

This drug guide for nurses contains pertinent drug information located by easily accessible headings.

INTERNET SITES FOR ADDITIONAL INFORMATION

Aging:
   http://www.portals.pdx.edu/~isidore/aging.html

AHCPR Clinical Practice Guidelines:
   http://text.nlm.nih.gov/ahcpr/guidesc.html

Blind Links:
   http://www.seidata.com/~marriage/rblind.html

Discharge Planning:
   http://www.med.ubc.ca/geriatrics/Geriatrics-andrew/homepage.html

Video Otoscopy Forum:
   http://www.li.net/~sullivan/ears.html

THE UPPER RESPIRATORY SYSTEM

INTRODUCTION

The respiratory system is divided into the upper and lower airways. The two systems function together as a unit but respiratory conditions, unique to each system, develop. The respiratory system facilitates gas exchanges, thereby maintaining cellular function. The system includes the respiratory tract, lungs, and adjacent structures. Its primary purpose is to obtain and move oxygen from the atmosphere to the alveoli, where gas exchange occurs and carbon dioxide is extracted from the blood. The upper airway structures include the nose, adenoids, pharynx, tonsils, epiglottis, larynx, and trachea (Fig. 2-1).

INFECTIONS OF THE UPPER AIRWAY

The entire respiratory system is lined with continuous mucosa and an infection or problem in one area can easily impact another part of the upper airway. Upper airway infections are also among the most common reasons why clients seek care in ambulatory or outpatient settings. It is important that nurses be prepared to provide care, education, and drug information to these clients. Despite every advance in medical technology, common clinical questions remain concerning effective strategies to prevent, diagnose, and treat upper airway infections. Some of these clinical questions are as follows:

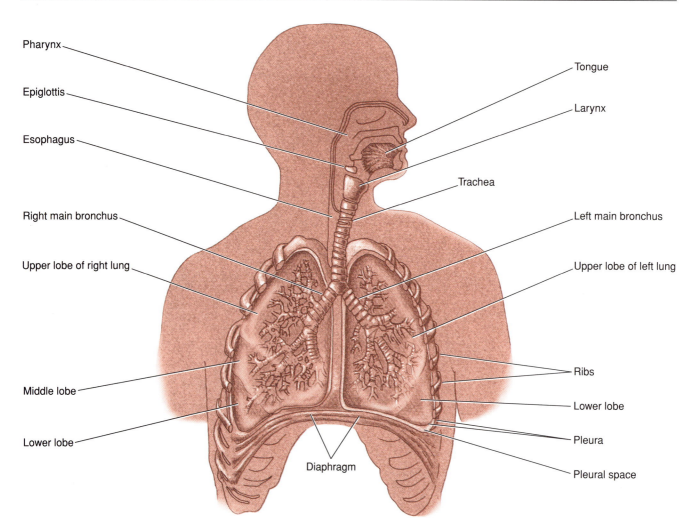

FIGURE 2-1 Anatomy of the lungs and upper and lower respiratory system

- What are the most effective ways to prevent upper airway infections?
- What are the best assessment criteria to distinguish bacterial from viral infections?
- What client education is needed regarding the danger of overprescribing antibiotics?
- Which antibiotic is the drug of choice for a bacterial infection of the upper airway?
- Which antibiotic is the most cost-effective?

There are no clear-cut answers to these questions.

Nursing management of infections of the upper respiratory tract, including sinusitis, rhinitis, pharyngitis, tonsillitis, and laryngitis, follows many typical patterns. Astute history, assessment, and examination techniques are vital to discriminate between a viral and bacterial infection. The nurse should assess and document the client's temperature and general energy level; the color, consistency, and odor of nasal and postnasal discharge; and the condition, color, and edema of mucous membranes lining the nose and pharynx. The nurse should perform palpation, percussion, and transillumination of the sinuses and look for evidence of swelling and exudate on the tonsils. The nurse should also assess the client's respiratory pattern. Most of these upper airway conditions are treated in an ambulatory setting or at home by the family physician or nurse practitioner. Nurses should help teach clients the care needed regarding increased fluid intake, hand washing, completion of antibiotics regimen, and the danger of taking antibiotics for viral infections. Clients who do not respond to treatment or who have chronic hoarseness or chronic infections such as chronic bacterial sinusitis need a referral to a specialist. The physician should be notified immediately if the client has respiratory distress or progressive difficulty breathing.

Sinusitis

Sinusitis may be either an acute or chronic condition. It is defined as inflammation of one or more of the paranasal sinuses. The sinuses are air-filled cavities lined with mucous membranes. Although the most common types of acute sinusitis are viral and allergic, an accurate diagnosis of bacterial or fungal sinusitis is essential for the well-being of the client and to prevent complications such as chronic sinusitis or spread of infection (e.g., meningitis).

Acute and Chronic Bacterial Sinusitis Acute bacterial sinusitis usually follows an upper respiratory infection. Common bacterial pathogens include *Haemophilus influenzae*, *Streptococcus pyogenes*, and *Streptococcus pneumoniae*. With chronic sinusitis scarring from repeat infections causes the membranes to thicken, and drainage becomes impaired. Bacteria, which are continually present, flourish in this type of environment.

The chief complaint of the client varies, but it is often related to pain and pressure over the sinuses accompanied by headache. Assessment includes palpation and percussion over the sinuses. Tenderness is usually elicited on palpation. With acute sinusitis, the client often experiences constant, severe pain. With chronic sinusitis, the pain is often dull and either constant or intermittent. Pressure and pain worsen 3–4 hours after waking as exudate accumulates in the sinuses. Other symptoms include fever, sore throat, postnasal drip, and nasal drainage. Diagnosis includes examination by transillumination. A flashlight is held over the maxillary sinuses and in the closed mouth to observe for the normal glow of the air-filled sinus. Dark areas indicate purulent secretions and blockage of the sinuses. Sinus x-rays or nasal endoscopy may be ordered, but this expense is usually deferred unless the client has repeated or chronic problems.

Treatment of acute bacterial sinusitis focuses on making the client comfortable and eradicating the bacteria. Based on the typical causative organisms and cost of the antibiotic, the drug of choice is penicillin or amoxicillin. For clients allergic to penicillin, erythromycin or azithromycin is used (Sanford, Gilbert, & Sande, 1998). Comfort is achieved by administering ibuprofen (Advil) or acetaminophen with or without codeine (Tylenol or Tylenol with codeine) to decrease pain. Decongestants such as pseudoephedrine or nasal spray are often effective for comfort. Antihistamines such as loratadine (Claritin–D) may help decrease drainage. Astemizole (Hismanal) and terfenadine (Seldane D) are no longer used due to the high incidence of drug interactions and side effects (Wilson, Shannon, & Stang, 1998).

When the client has a history and clinical picture of chronic bacterial sinusitis, the family physician or nurse practitioner may refer the client to an ear, nose, and throat (ENT) specialist. Treatment options include various surgical procedures to eradicate the infection and return the sinus structures to optimal function.

Rhinitis

Rhinitis is defined as an inflammation of the mucous membranes of the nasal cavity and nasopharynx. As with sinusitis, the condition may be acute or chronic, and the most common causes are viral and allergic. The chief complaint of the client is a runny nose (rhinorrhea). Rhinitis most often accompanies an acute viral upper respiratory infection known as the common cold. The virus is transmitted by droplets, usually from sneezing. Some experts believe that the best prevention of transmission of respiratory viruses is hand washing because droplets are transmitted to the respiratory tract via the hands. Allergies are another common cause of rhinitis. Allergic rhinitis, or hay fever, is caused by seasonal or random allergens. Other agents that irritate the nasal mucosa, such as smoke and temperature and humidity changes, cause nonallergic or environmental rhinitis.

The pathophysiology of rhinitis is an inflammation and swelling of the nasal mucosa that results in edema and discharge. Persistent rhinitis may result in fibrous scarring of connective tissues and atrophy of the glands that secrete mucus. Clinical manifestations include sneezing, thin and watery nasal discharge, cough, slight fever, sore throat, and malaise. On examination, the mucous membranes are red, swollen, and boggy. The client complains of itching and tearing of the eyes. Thick, mucoid, purulent, or greenish discharge may occur in chronic or bacterial infections. Secondary infections such as otitis media, bronchitis, or pneumonia must be ruled out.

Therapeutic management focuses on making the client comfortable. The client's symptoms are alleviated by rest and administering increased fluids to help mobilize secretions. Antipyretic and analgesic agents such as acetaminophen (Tylenol) or ibuprofen (Advil) are effective. (Aspirin is never given to children because of the correlation between aspirin and the incidence of Reye's syndrome.) Antibiotics are used only to treat secondary infections. Nurses must promote public health education concerning the differences between viruses and bacteria and the dangers of overprescribing antibiotics. A dramatic increase in antimicrobial resistance by common respiratory organisms is attributed to overprescribing and overuse of antibiotics.

Pharyngitis

Pharyngitis is an inflammation of the pharynx or throat. It is most often seen as a viral inflammation. However, it may be caused by bacteria such as hemolytic streptococci, staphylococci, or other bacteria. *Neisseria gonorrhoeae* may cause pharyngitis, and a culture must be performed to confirm this diagnosis. Gonococcal pharyngitis requires the same treatment as other sexually transmitted diseases. The client should be approached in a caring, nonjudgmental manner, and education should focus on the need to treat the sexual partner as well as the client and the practice of safer sexual practices. This condition must be reported to the health department.

Pharyngitis is also communicated by droplet transmission, and incubation may take a few hours to several days. On examination of the pharynx, the mucous membranes are inflamed and edematous with postnasal drainage, and the tonsils are frequently enlarged. Clinical manifestations common with streptococcal infection include a sore throat, severe pain and dysphagia, fever, dry cough, white plaques on the tonsils, and a red and edematous throat. Children may present with generalized symptoms of fever, poor eating and sleeping patterns, and vomiting.

The goals of therapeutic management again focus on keeping the client comfortable and eradicating bacteria if present. The nurse should instruct the client to rest and increase the intake of fluids. Analgesics, antipyretics such as acetaminophen (Tylenol), and throat lozenges are prescribed. An ice collar or warm saline gargle may relieve pain. Popsicles are soothing and help to increase fluid intake.

When bacterial pharyngitis is suspected, the practitioner will usually do a Quick or Rapid Strep Screen. This is a rapid diagnostic tool that confirms the presence of a streptococcal infection in ten minutes. If the Quick Strep is negative but a bacterial infection is still strongly suspected, a throat culture and drug sensitivity are performed. Penicillin is the least expensive antibiotic for pharyngitis-causing bacteria. As discussed previously, there are alternative antibiotics available for clients allergic to penicillin. If the client has valvular heart disease, such as mitral valve prolapse, prophylactic antibiotics are given to prevent subacute bacterial endocarditis.

CASE STUDY: UPPER RESPIRATORY INFECTION IN AN OLDER ADULT

Mrs. R. is a 75-year-old widow who presents with a nonproductive cough, headache, myalgia, low-grade fever, and a sore throat for two days. She does not smoke and has no other chronic conditions such as diabetes, heart, lung, or kidney disease.

On physical examination, lung sounds are clear. The pharynx demonstrates mild erythema. Slight enlargement of tonsillar lymph nodes is present, with no other lymph node enlargement evident. The chest x-ray is normal. The client is alert and oriented, but experiencing more fatigue than usual.

The diagnosis is viral pharyngitis and upper respiratory infection. This is generally a self-limiting condition of brief duration, but it can be a significant health risk in older adults, particularly if they have other chronic health conditions (Staab & Hodges, 1996). Treatment includes rest, increased fluids, acetaminophen (Tylenol) every 4–6 hours for myalgia, and saline and warm water gargles. Antibiotics are not prescribed, as most cases have a viral etiology. Taking special precautions due to the client's age, Mrs. R. is instructed to return for a follow-up appointment if the symptoms did not improve within 72 hours.

Tonsillitis

Tonsillitis is the acute inflammation of the tonsils and their beds. The most common causative organisms are *Streptococcus* or *Staphylococcus*. Infections in the nose or pharynx drain through the lymphatic system to the tonsils. Hypertrophy caused by repeated infections may cause the tonsils to become so enlarged that they occlude the airway. Clinical manifestations include enlarged tonsils; a red, edematous pharynx; sore throat; pain on swallowing; high fever; and gray-white exudate on the tonsils. An abscess may form on the tonsils. This complication is termed "Quinsy sore throat" or "peritonsillar abscess."

Therapeutic management includes performing a Quick or Rapid Strep Screen and a throat culture with a drug sensitivity panel. The same antibiotics are prescribed for both tonsillitis and pharyngitis. If a peritonsillar abscess is present, incision and drainage may be required. Over the years, the clinical practice of removing the tonsils and adenoids has changed. It is no longer thought to be an absolute necessity. The current criteria for performing a tonsillectomy are three to four documented episodes of tonsillitis or pharyngitis a year for two years. The tonsils may need to be removed 4–6 weeks after a peritonsillar abscess occurs.

Laryngitis

Laryngitis is an inflammation of the mucous membranes lining the larynx. The inflammation may be acute or chronic, and the etiology may be viral, bacterial, allergic, or environmental. Symptoms occur as a result of swollen vocal cords. The client may have a history of recent respiratory infection, smoking, loud vocal speaking, excessive alcohol intake, or recent endotracheal intubation. Common bacterial agents are *Streptococcus pneumoniae* and beta-hemolytic *Streptococcus*. Clinical manifestations include hoarseness or loss of voice (aphonia), fever, malaise, pain on swallowing, dry cough, and scratchy throat. In clients with severe laryngitis, stridor and dyspnea may occur. On examination, the true vocal cords should be white with rounded edges. In clients with laryngitis, the cords are red and swollen, and secretions are present. **Therapeutic management** focuses on relieving symptoms and eradicating any bacteria that are present. Antipyretics, analgesics, throat sprays, steam or cool mist inhalations, and rest are effective for client comfort. Antibiotics are prescribed when a bacterial infection is present.

Chronic Laryngitis The client with chronic laryngitis presents with progressive hoarseness that is worse in the morning and evening as a result of dried secretions. Clients clear their throat frequently and have a dry, harsh cough. Often the client has a history of smoking, alcohol abuse, excessive use of their voice (such as vocalists), or industrial exposure to fumes or chemicals. The American Cancer Society considers persistent hoarseness one of the seven classic warning signs of laryngeal cancer. When it is present, the physician or nurse practitioner should refer the client for laryngoscopy to rule out cancer of the larynx. Chronic polypoid laryngitis frequently develops in clients who smoke, but a biopsy must be taken to confirm whether the polyp is benign or malignant. Indirect laryngoscopy by mirror visualization is performed in the physician's office.

Acute Epiglottitis

Acute epiglottitis is an uncommon but life-threatening condition that occurs in children. Clients present with difficulty swallowing, and drooling is often evident. The child may be leaning forward with his or her mouth open to breathe. When epiglottitis is suspected, an examination of the throat must **not** be done, as stimulation from the examination may cause a spasm of the glottis resulting in occlusion of the airway and respiratory arrest. Clients with suspected epiglottitis must be transported by ambulance to the emergency room immediately. Tracheostomy or endotracheal intubation may be necessary.

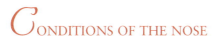

CONDITIONS OF THE NOSE

Deviated Septum

A deviated septum is a nasal obstruction caused by displacement of the nasal septum from the midline position. The etiology is typically nasal trauma or a congenital anomaly. This condition is not pathologic unless the nasal obstruction causes respiratory distress. Many people have some degree of septal deviation without any respiratory compromise. Clinical manifestations include nasal obstruction, snoring, noisy breathing, headache, epistaxis, postnasal drip, and sinusitis.

Surgery becomes necessary when the trauma or nasal obstruction causes respiratory compromise. The client is referred to a surgeon, plastic surgeon, or an ENT specialist. Common nasal surgeries for a deviated septum are:

1. **Submucosal resection.** An incision is made into the nasal mucous membrane, and the bone and cartilage causing the obstruction are removed.
2. **Nasal septoplasty.** This is a reconstruction of the nasal septum that may include rhinoplasty (reconstruction of the external nose). This is a common surgery used to treat a deviated septum.

Following nasal surgery, **nursing care** focuses on airway management, keeping clients comfortable, educating clients, and being observant for possible bleeding. The nurse must check the nasal packing frequently for bleeding. Clients often have a dressing, or nasal sling, under the nares. The nurse should frequently check for signs of airway obstruction, including frequent swallowing, changes in respiratory pattern, increased respirations, rapid pulse, and restlessness. The nasal and eye areas may have skin discoloration, edema, and localized pain. Surgeons frequently order the application of ice for the first 24 hours after surgery to decrease pain and bleeding. The nurse should elevate the head of the bed 30–45 degrees to decrease nasal edema and assist drainage and should warn clients not to blow their nose or sneeze vigorously and to avoid nasal drops and sprays. Clients are encouraged to increase fluid intake, and oral hygiene and mouth rinses should be performed frequently.

The nurse needs to document vital signs, respiratory pattern, lung sounds, any change on the nasal drip pad (which may be changed PRN), fluid and food intake, what clients have been taught and their understanding of the material, and the administration of analgesics. Any signs of hemorrhage or respiratory distress should be reported to the physician immediately and documented.

Nasal Polyps

Nasal polyps are smooth, round outgrowths of the nasal mucosa. The mucous membranes of the nose or sinuses change as a result of recurrent localized irritation and swelling often related to asthma, allergies, or chronic rhinitis. A polyp looks like a small pale tumor. Because clients' feelings of awkwardness, examination with a nasal speculum is a frequently omitted procedure during a physical examination. However, the condition of the nasal mucosa is important and should not be overlooked. Nasal polyps are diagnosed by viewing the inside of the nose with a lighted nasal speculum. If polyps are found, the client should be referred to a surgeon or ENT specialist for a nasal polypectomy. Following surgery, nasal polyps may grow back.

Epistaxis

Epistaxis, or nosebleed, occurs most frequently in the anterior portion of the nasal cavity. The anterior portion receives blood from the external carotid arteries. The usual causes include trauma, chronic infection, violent sneezing, and nose blowing or picking. Posterior epistaxis is more severe than anterior epistaxis and often occurs in elderly men. The posterior portion of the nasal septum receives blood from the ethmoid and maxillary arterial systems. Trauma is the most common cause of epistaxis. If there is no history of trauma or if other symptoms cannot be explained, systemic diseases that cause coagulation disorders, such as leukemia, thrombocytopenia, hemophilia, and purpura, must be excluded.

Management of Nosebleeds Most nosebleeds can be controlled with simple first-aid measures. However, when these measures are ineffective, care in the emergency room or medical management is necessary. In severe cases, blood loss can lead to death from volume depletion, hypoxemia, and shock.

First-aid care includes applying nasal pressure for 5–30 minutes to compress the soft tissue against the septum. Additionally, ice packs are applied to the nose and forehead. The client is positioned in an upright sitting position with the head tilted forward. The nurse must ensure that the client expectorates the blood and does not swallow it.

If bleeding does not cease within approximately 30 minutes or if bleeding increases, medical intervention is required. Cautery is effective when the site of bleeding is visible. For posterior epistaxis, nasal packing with sterile gauze may be necessary. Nasal packing may be left in place for 24–72 hours. **Nursing care** includes observation of the nasal drip pad for signs of bleeding and observing for signs of respiratory distress. In cases where the nasal packing slips out of position, the airway may become occluded, resulting in hypoxemia and death. A nurse should never remove nasal packing without a physician's order. Another treatment option is a balloon tamponade in which a catheter is threaded into the nasopharynx, inflated, and left in place for 2–4 days. Medication therapy includes administering vasoconstrictors to staunch the flow of blood to the nose. This is usually effective for anterior epistaxis. Cotton balls or a nasal pack with 1:1000 phenylephrine (Neo-synephrine) and pressure applied for five minutes may control bleeding. When measures such as vasoconstrictor medications and packs fail to control bleeding, surgical intervention to cauterize or ligate the involved vessels is necessary.

Nursing care focuses on maintaining the airway, observing for signs of shock, and decreasing the client's anxiety. The nurse should observe the client for changes in respiratory rate and pattern, tachycardia, decreased blood pressure, and confusion or restlessness. These signs may indicate decreased cardiac output or shock. As the client improves, the blood should change color from red to brown. Ear discomfort should be minimal. **Pulse oximetry** should be monitored continuously, and readings should be above 95%. If oxygen is required, the nasal cannula should be positioned in the mouth with an oxygen flow of less than 5 L/min., when ordered by the physician.

Nasal Fracture

Nasal fractures result from trauma such as occurs in fights, sports injuries, and motor vehicle accidents. Signs and symptoms include displacement of the nasal septum, edema, and bruising. Diagnosis is confirmed with x-rays.

Pulse Oximeter/Oximetry. This is a device used to measure oxyhemoglobin in the capillary blood. The oximetry measurement of oxygen saturation should generally be above 90%. This device is used widely as a diagnostic tool because it is noninvasive, inexpensive, and accessible in all types of settings, from the physician's office to the emergency room.

To reduce a unilateral nasal fracture, pressure is applied by the physician on the convex side of the nose. Most nasal fractures can be reduced in this manner if treated within the first 24 hours. An external metal splint may be used to immobilize the nose for ten days. After 24 hours or if the fracture is complicated, surgery for open reduction and internal fixation (ORIF) may be necessary. Surgery should be delayed until the edema decreases enough to allow the damage to be assessed. **Nursing management** includes maintaining a patent airway, checking for bleeding, and observing for the presence cerebrospinal fluid (CSF) leakage. The presence of glucose in the CSF drainage is detected by use of a Clinistix. CSF is a clear fluid. At this point, oral suction may be needed. The client is positioned with the head of the bed elevated, and ice packs are used.

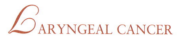

Laryngeal Cancer

Cancer of the larynx usually occurs in men between 55 and 70 years of age. Smoking and alcohol abuse are the highest risk factors for this disease; it is rare in people who do not smoke. Chronic laryngitis, voice abuse, and family history are also risk factors. The most common form of laryngeal cancer, squamous cell carcinoma, develops on the vocal cords. Carcinomas of the true vocal cords grow slowly because of the limited lymphatic supply. On the false vocal cords, tumors grow rapidly because lymphatic vessels are abundant. Clinical manifestations include hoarseness or a change in voice that lasts more than two weeks. Late symptoms include dysphagia, dyspnea, cough, hemoptysis, weight loss, pain in the thyroid area, and enlarged cervical lymph nodes. Diagnosis is made by computed tomography (CT) of the head and neck, direct laryngoscopy for visualization and biopsy, and other x-rays such as chest radiographs to determine the presence of metastases.

Therapeutic management begins by staging the tumor. The TNM system is a simple clinical way to stage any tumor: T indicates the tumor size and extent; N indicates the nodal size and location; and M indicates the presence of metastasis. Once the tumor is staged, treatment options are then discussed with the client and his or her family. Radiation therapy and surgical resection are the treatments of choice when the tumor is fixed and the vocal cord is moveable. Radiation therapy works by disrupting the deoxyribonucleic acid (DNA) structure of cells, causing cell death. When the tumor is diagnosed early and treated with surgical resection or radiation therapy, the rate of cure is approximately 80–96%. Side effects of radiation therapy include general malaise and changes in the tone and timbre of speech.

As for most types of cancer, various combinations of chemotherapy, radiation, and surgery are recommended, depending on the TNM results and the general health, age, and personal choices of the client. These treatment options need to be discussed in detail with the client, family, and health care team. Team members for a client with carcinoma of the larynx often include a medical oncologist, ENT surgeon, radiation oncologist, radiation technician, oncology clinical nurse specialist or nurse case manager, and social worker. When cancer of the larynx is more advanced, a total laryngectomy or radical neck dissection may be recommended. Since these procedures are complex, disfiguring, and involve the loss of voice and a tracheostomy, it is imperative that a thorough nursing plan of education and support be established with the client and his or her family or other people in the client's support system.

Surgical management includes performing a laryngectomy or hemilaryngectomy. In a hemilaryngectomy, only one vocal cord is involved and one-half of the larynx is excised through a vertical midneck incision. A temporary cuffed tracheostomy tube is inserted for five days, and a nasogastric tube is required for nutritional supplementation. A total laryngectomy is required for advanced laryngeal cancer of the true vocal cords. The client undergoes a permanent tracheostomy with loss of voice. The sense of smell is impaired by this procedure, and anorexia then becomes a concern. Total parenteral or enteral nutrition is necessary for 7–10 days after surgery to provide nutritional supplementation.

Radiation is often used to treat the primary tumor. A radical neck dissection with total laryngectomy may be performed for clients with metastases to the neck or when the risk of metastases is high. The cervical lymph nodes, internal jugular vein, sternocleidomastoid muscle, and spinal accessory nerve are removed to ensure the complete removal of the node and prevent nodal metastases. This radical surgical procedure (radical neck dissection) can also surgically remove cancers of the tongue, lip, tonsils, and thyroid. As a result of the radical nature of this procedure, the client experiences great physical and emotional distress; therefore, comprehensive intensive care from the entire health care team is required. There is a potential for respiratory distress and airway obstruction. Therefore, the nurse must monitor the client for increased respirations, decreased oxygen saturation, and rales on auscultation. The nurse must scrupulously maintain care of the tracheostomy and stoma, and a dietary consultation will aid the nurse in maintaining the caloric requirements of the client during the postoperative period. Prior to discharge, a metal or plastic laryngectomy tube (which is shorter and wider than a tracheostomy tube) is inserted. As the client recovers, the nurse should evaluate and document the need for home health care and the ability of the client to care for him- or herself. Clerical counseling and a support group for cancer clients should be offered.

Summary

The major categories of upper respiratory conditions are inflammation or infection, nosebleeds, nasal fractures, and laryngeal cancer. Nurses need to be skilled in assessment of upper airway conditions and remain up-to-date on trends in causative organisms and antimocrobial resistance for these organisms. Most upper airway infections are viral, but astute history-taking and assessment skills help to differentiate bacterial from viral infections. Special precautions need to be taken with respiratory infections in elderly clients who have preexisting medical conditions such as diabetes or heart disease. Most upper airway conditions are treated in an ambulatory setting and at home.

After diagnosing cancer of the larynx, the tumor is staged with the TNM system. This diagnostic information is shared with the client and family so they can make informed treatment decisions with the physicians. Treatment for a client with cancer of the larynx requires care from a multidisciplinary team of health care workers including the respiratory therapist, dietician, oncologist, and home health nurse. Antismoking campaigns and programs for smoking cessation remain the primary strategies to prevent cancer of the larynx.

KEY WORDS

Carbon dioxide
Epistaxis
Gas exchange
Laryngectomy
Oxygen

Quick or Rapid Strep Screen
Radical neck dissection
Squamous cell carcinoma
Upper respiratory infections

QUESTIONS

1. Mr. H. presents to the physician's office with a sore throat. He states that it has hurt to swallow for the last three days. The physician's diagnosis is posterior pharyngitis, the usual causative organism of which is viral. The nurse encourages the client to increase fluids, get plenty of rest, and do which of the following?
   A. Take antipyretics, gargle with saline and water, and eat a semisolid or liquid diet.
   B. Avoid blowing the nose, sneezing, or coughing.
   C. Refrain from talking and do not worry about transmission of the disease.
   D. Take antibiotics and antihistamines regularly.

2. Mrs. G. has been complaining of hoarseness for the past two days. Her physician's diagnosis is laryngitis. The nurse needs to encourage the client to do all of the following except
   A. use a cool mist humidifier.
   B. use analgesics.
   C. use a vaporizer.
   D. use antipyretics.

3. Nurse N. answers the phone in the emergency room, and Mrs. L. states that she has a nosebleed that has not stopped for the past two hours. The nurse tells Mrs. L. that she should come to the emergency room immediately but do which of the following first?

A. Put pressure on the bridge of the nose for 5–30 minutes, applying an ice pack, and sit with the head forward.
B. Apply heat to the bridge of the nose and do not eat.
C. Sit with the head back and use a towel to blot blood drainage.
D. When blood is felt in the nose, lightly blow the nose into a tissue.

ANSWERS

1. *The answer is A.* There is no reason for antibiotic therapy if the causative organism is viral. Antipyretics will decrease fever that is associated with viral infections; saline and water soothe the sore throat; and a liquid or semisolid diet will not irritate the throat.

2. *The answer is C.* A cool mist humidifier decreases swelling of the larynx and liquifies any secretions. Analgesics relieve pain, and antipyretics decrease fever and any associated inflammation. A vaporizer, which uses heat, would increase inflammation and edema.

3. *The answer is A.* The usual site of nose bleeding is the anterior portion of the nasal area. Applying pressure encourages coagulation of bleeding. Ice vasoconstricts vessels, thus decreasing bleeding, and putting the head forward facilitates any bleeding to drain out of the nose instead of draining into the stomach, causing nausea. Blowing the nose would dislodge any clot formation, which is not the desired outcome.

ANNOTATED REFERENCES

Sanford, J., Gilbert, D., & Sande, M. (1998). *Guide to antimicrobial therapy.* Dallas: Pfizer.

This pocket guide is a rapid reference for antimicrobials based on organism, diagnosis, or anatomic location of the infection.

Staab, A., & Hodges, L. C. (1996). *Essentials of gerontological nursing: Adaptation to the aging process.* Philadelphia: J. B. Lippincott.

This text emphasizes quality care for older adults in a variety of settings.

Wilson, B., Shannon, M., & Stang, C. (1998). *Nurses' drug guide.* Stamford, CT: Appleton & Lange.

This drug text includes nursing information needed for safe administration, patient teaching, and dosage. Information is also included on pregnancy category, contraindications, and side effects.

INTERNET SITES FOR ADDITIONAL INFORMATION

American Cancer Society:
  http://www.cancer.org/

Cancer Archives:
  http://cure.medinfo.org/lists/cancer/index.html

Cancer Guide:
  http://cancerguide.org/

ChronicIllnet:
  http://www.calypte.com/ci_home.html

THE LOWER RESPIRATORY SYSTEM

INTRODUCTION

The lower airway structures (Fig. 3-1), which work in conjunction with the upper airway structures, are contained primarily within the lung. The lower airway structures include the bronchi, bronchioles, alveolar ducts, and alveoli. These structures provide ventilation to maintain oxygenation of all cells, tissues, and organs (Fig. 3-2). Conditions that interfere with **ventilation** and pulmonary gas exchange lead to respiratory compromise of varying degrees. The client experiences a continuum of symptoms from feeling slightly short of breath to the critical point of respiratory failure.

The major categories of conditions that interfere with ventilation function and gas exchange are: chronic obstructive pulmonary disease (COPD), asthma, restrictive lung disease, respiratory failure, infectious diseases such as pneumonia and tuberculosis, lung cancer, and traumatic injuries. Unsuccessful treatment of these disorders can result in respiratory failure and death.

CHRONIC OBSTRUCTIVE PULMONARY DISEASE

In COPD, *expiratory* airflow is chronically obstructed, and the client experiences difficulty in exhaling. COPD is actually a major category of

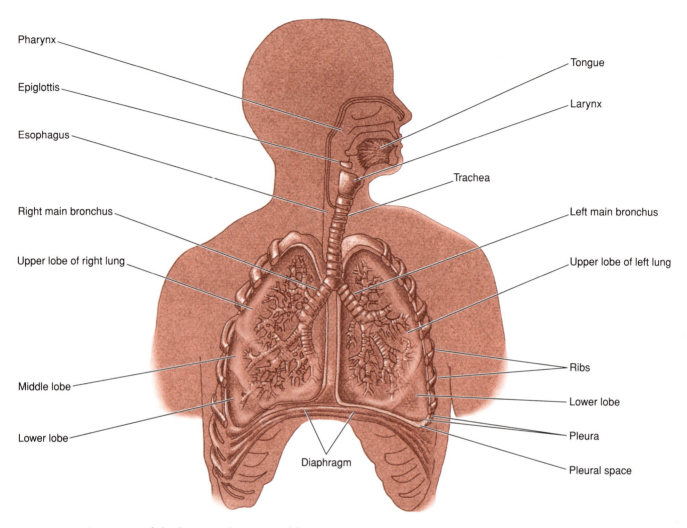

FIGURE 3-1 Anatomy of the lungs and upper and lower respiratory system.

Ventilation. This is the respiratory process by which gases are exchanged in the lungs.

lung disease and encompasses several different diseases. Emphysema and chronic bronchitis are two common examples of COPD in which altered breathing patterns occur.

Clinical Presentations

Emphysema Emphysema occurs when the air spaces distal to the terminal bronchioles enlarge (see Fig. 3-2). This causes destruction of the alveolar wall, which leads to malfunction of gas exchange. Clients with emphysema must learn to live with this irreversible condition; and they often benefit from rehabilitation programs. Typically, clients experience stable periods followed by exacerbations, which often occur as a result of respiratory infections. The nurse must observe and assess the client for signs and symptoms of deterioration, including increased sputum production, increased thickness of sputum with a color change to yellow or green, increased anxiety, decreased tolerance to activity, and increased rhonchi

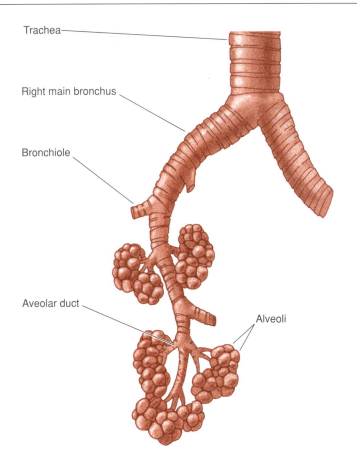

Trachea

Right main bronchus

Bronchiole

Aveolar duct

Alveoli

FIGURE 3-2

Anatomy of the alveolar unit.

and crackles on auscultation of the lungs. Obtaining a thorough history of the client is essential, keeping in mind that clients often do not report insidious changes because they are chronically ill.

Chronic Bronchitis Chronic bronchitis is defined by excessive tracheo-bronchial secretions that accumulate every day for at least three months a year for two consecutive years (Phipps, Cassmeyer, Sands, & Lehman, 1995). The client complains of a chronic cough with increased sputum production. Other causes of coughing such as laryngeal or lung cancer should be ruled out. Normally, secretions are produced at the rate of 10–150 mL/day. In chronic bronchitis, excessive secretions accumulate and are expectorated as thick, white sputum. Over time, enlargement of the bronchial mucous glands occurs, causing airway obstruction.

Etiology

COPD is caused by environmental and life-style factors that are largely preventable. Smoking accounts for 80–90% of cases of COPD. Other risk factors include a low socioeconomic and occupational status, environmental exposure from coal mining, second-hand smoke, or air pollution, and excessive alcohol intake. COPD is most frequently diagnosed in men between 30 and 40 years of age.

Pathophysiology

The pathophysiology of COPD is complicated and comprehensive, affecting all body systems as well as the client's life style. The disease process causes alveolar damage that alters respiratory physiology, thus affecting the oxygenation of the entire body. The pulmonary abnormalities of gas exchange are primarily related to three mechanisms:

Hypoxemia. This condition is characterized by a deficiency of oxygen (Pa_{O_2}) in the arterial blood. Oxygen levels in the arterial blood should be 95–100 mm Hg.

1. **Ventilation-Perfusion Mismatch.** This is the major cause of **hypoxemia,** or decreased oxygenation, in the blood. The normal equilibrium between alveolar ventilation and perfusion of pulmonary capillary blood flow is disturbed. The relationship of ventilation to perfusion is defined in terms of the ventilation-perfusion (V/Q) ratio. An increase in the V/Q ratio occurs when advancing disease causes the destruction of alveoli and the loss of capillary beds. In this situation, the perfusion decreases, but ventilation remains the same.

   A decreased (V/Q) ratio is seen in COPD clients whose airways are occluded by thick mucus or bronchospasms. Decreased ventilation occurs, but perfusion is the same or only slightly decreased. Many COPD clients have both emphysema and chronic bronchitis, and this may explain why they have regions of increased and decreased V/Q ratios.

2. **Shunting of Pulmonary Capillary Blood.** As unoxygenated blood is pumped from the right ventricle to the lung, some of the blood passes through the pulmonary capillary bed without picking up oxygen. This may be due to increased pulmonary secretions occluding alveoli.

3. **Impaired Gas Diffusion.** Impaired gas exchange usually occurs as a result of one or two conditions. There may be a decreased alveolar surface area available for gas exchange as a result of emphysema or increased secretions, making diffusion more difficult.

Signs and Symptoms

A progression of symptoms typifies COPD. Chronic malfunction of the respiratory system is initially manifested by cough and sputum production, especially upon arising in the morning. Mild shortness of breath with exertion progresses to extreme shortness of breath. Cough and sputum production (smoker's cough) deteriorate into a persistent cough with the production of large quantities of sputum. Frequent respiratory infections and weight loss occur, and eventually the client is unable to perform household tasks or occupational responsibilities. The client is easily fatigued and becomes physically disabled. Many COPD clients experience weight loss as a result of loss of appetite from excess sputum production, decreased strength, loss of socialization with meals (social isolation), and decreased digestion secondary to inadequate oxygenation of cells of the gastrointestinal (GI) tract (Dudek, 1997). The client with COPD burns many calories as a result of increased respiratory effort.

Complications

Three major respiratory complications (acute respiratory failure, pneumothorax and giant bullae) and one cardiac complication (cor pulmonale) commonly occur with COPD.

Acute Respiratory Failure (ARF)
ARF occurs when ventilation and oxygenation are inadequate to meet the resting needs of the body. **Arterial blood gas analysis** of COPD clients reveals an arterial oxygen partial pressure (Pa_{O_2}) of 55 mm Hg or less and an arterial carbon dioxide partial pressure (Pa_{CO_2}) of 50 mm Hg or greater. If the client or family desires life support measures, the client will require intubation and placement on a respirator for **mechanical ventilation**.

Cor pulmonale
Cor pulmonale, or right ventricular decompensation, is an enlargement of the right ventricle caused by the overloading that results from pulmonary disease. This cardiac complication occurs as a compensatory mechanism secondary to the lung pathology in COPD. Cor pulmonale is a good example of the body working as a whole. Once one organ system malfunctions, a cascade of malfunctions begins to occur in other organ systems. In COPD, chronic hypoxemia causes pulmonary vasoconstriction of the pulmonary capillary bed, which in turn increases pulmonary vascular resistance. The "domino effect" of these physiologic changes and the increase in pulmonary pressures cause the right ventricle to pump harder and hypertrophy (increase in size) (Fig. 3-3).

The treatment for cor pulmonale includes low-dose oxygen (limited to 2L/min), diuretics to decrease peripheral edema, and rest. Peripheral edema is another domino effect, as systemic or peripheral cardiac return is affected by the right ventricular hypertrophy and increase in right ventricular pressures. Digitalis is used only when the cor pulmonale is associated with left heart failure.

Pneumothorax
Pneumothorax is another serious complication of COPD. *Pneumo-* literally means air, and pneumothorax is defined as an accumulation of air in the pleural space. The pleural space is actually only a *potential* space, a thin layer of liquid between the visceral and parietal layers of the lung. The function of the pleural fluid is to promote a smooth, gliding movement of the lungs during ventilation. When air accumulates in the pleural space, the normal lung capacity for gas exchange is compromised, resulting in decreased vital capacity and hypoxemia.

Arterial Blood-Gas Analysis. This laboratory test is used to determine pH, oxygen, carbon dioxide, and bicarbonate levels. Arterial blood is usually drawn from an indwelling arterial blood-gas line, a central line such as a Swan-Ganz catheter, or from the radial artery.

Mechanical Ventilation. A respirator mechanically conducts the respiratory process of gas exchange. Patients are connected to the respirator for mechanical ventilation by an endotracheal or tracheostomy tube.

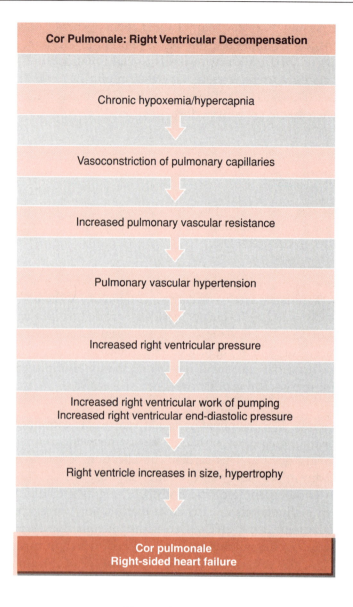

Signs and symptoms

- Hepatomegaly
- Peripheral edema
- Jugular vein distension
- Weight gain

FIGURE 3-3

⌧

The sequence of pathology with cor pulmonale.

Giant Bullae Pneumothorax is often associated with another complication of COPD: the formation of giant bullae. While air accumulates in the pleural space in a pneumothorax, bullae occur when air is trapped in the actual lung parenchyma. The alveoli become ineffective "air traps." Bullae alter respiratory function both by compressing lung tissue and by inhibiting gas exchange. Entrapment of air in the alveoli and the associated overstretching result in marked destruction of many of the alveolar walls.

Physical Assessment

Physical findings in clients with COPD include dyspnea; a pale or dusky color; rapid, shallow respirations through pursed lips; and use of accessory muscles to breathe. COPD causes an increase in the anterior-to-posterior diameter of the chest, which results in a barrel-shaped chest. Because of the difficulty in exhaling air, the client has a prolonged expiratory phase (greater than 4 seconds). Pulmonary function tests are used to diagnose COPD.

A typical client with COPD has decreased expiratory airflow and decreased forced expiratory volume (FEV). Chest x-rays are not used to diagnose early-stage COPD because radiographic studies are often normal in the early stages. As the disease advances, x-rays show flattening of the diaphragm and increased lucency.

Nursing Management

The plan of care of the patient with COPD focuses on maintaining the highest level of function and well-being possible for the client and his or her family. COPD is a progressive condition with no cure. Symptomatic relief centers on four main areas of intervention: drug therapy, life-style changes, respiratory therapy, and emotional support. A drug regimen commonly includes bronchodilators such as anticholinergics (ß-andrenergic agonists), and methylxanthines. In addition, corticosteriods, mucolytics, expectorants, and antibiotics are frequently necessary.

When the client is at home, continual oxygen therapy is used if the resting Pa_{O_2} decreases below 55–60 mm Hg or if the oxygen saturation decreases below 85% (Phipps, et al., 1995). The nurse should diligently assess the respiratory status of these clients whether they are in the hospital, in an ambulatory care center, or at home. Signs of deterioration include an increased rate and decreased depth of respiration, an increased production of greyish-green sputum, and a change in mental status.

The nurse must know the client's typical blood gas values and oxygen saturation in order to recognize a trend toward deterioration. A trend is more significant than a change in just one reading. The pulse oximeter is commonly used to monitor oxygen saturation. The pulse oximeter sensor probe, which monitors oxyhemoglobin saturation in the capillaries, is commonly placed on the ear lobe or finger. Desaturation, or a decrease in oxygen saturation, is defined as a decrease of more than 3% with activity or an oxygen saturation of less than 85%. A client with a constant oxygen saturation of less than 85% requires continuous 24 hr/day low-dose oxygen at 1–2 L/min. In addition, when the saturation is this low, it is accompanied by an increase in the heart rate, and alterations in the daily functioning of the client need to be addressed.

Meticulous respiratory therapy and respiratory hygiene are necessary to maintain the oxygenation and effectiveness of airway clearance. Chest percussion therapy every 2–4 hours is needed during exacerbations and is often a part of daily maintenance. In the hospital, the client can breathe more easily by leaning on a pillow placed on a table. This orthopneic position also aids in ventilation. Clients frequently sleep in a recliner at home.

The nursing staff is involved in a comprehensive program of support and education for the client and family. The COPD client often requires dietary supplements, emotional support, home health care assistance, and counseling regarding medical expenses. Oxygen therapy is administered at 1 to 2 L/min via a nasal cannula. High oxygen levels should not be administered routinely as these levels actually make the client retain more carbon dioxide. Clients require instruction on safety and administration techniques for continual oxygen therapy. Oxygen is given by three methods: compressed gas, liquid oxygen, and oxygen concentrators. Liquid oxygen is best for maximal portability; oxygen concentrators are best for home use; compressed gas is the least expensive. The client and family need a holistic palliative program of care and are often best managed by a nurse case manager or home health care team. Walking is the best exercise, and the client often benefits both physically and emotionally from a slowly progressive walking routine (Black & Matassari-Jacobs, 1997).

CO2 Narcosis. Clients with chronic respiratory diseases such as COPD often have physiologically accommodated themselves to increased levels of Pa_{CO_2} and decreased levels of Pa_{O_2}. These patients must not be given more than 2 L/min of oxygen or the impulse to breathe coming from the central nervous system will diminish or stop.

Asthma

Asthma, or reversible airway obstruction, occurs when the bronchi are affected by inflammation and hyperresponsiveness. This causes narrowing of the airways and difficulty breathing. Asthma is a reversible condition, distinct from the continuous irreversible airway obstruction of emphysema and chronic bronchitis.

Etiology

The etiology of asthma may be an allergic reaction that often occurs in clients under 30 years of age. However, the occurrence of asthma in adult clients over 30 years of age should always be taken seriously. Many irritants, such as airborne dusts, vapors, cleaning products, or fumes, may trigger this airway reaction. Additional triggers include cold air, upper or lower respiratory tract infections, and stress.

Pathophysiology

The pathophysiology of asthma begins with an inflammatory reaction of the airway that triggers the pathologic changes of hyperresponsiveness and bronchospasm. These changes interfere with gas exchange and ventilation. Most clients learn to manage their asthma successfully, but asthmatic clients always need to be taken seriously, as an asthmatic reaction can lead to respiratory failure and death.

Asthma is the cause of over 5000 deaths each year.

Signs and Symptoms

Signs and symptoms of asthma include dyspnea, wheezing, hyperventilation (one of the first symptoms), dizziness, tingling sensations, headache, nausea, increased shortness of breath, fatigue, diaphoresis, and anxiety. The severity of the asthma attack depends on the degree of airflow obstruction, the level of oxygen saturation, the nature of the breathing patterns, changes in mental status, and how the client perceives his or her respiratory status. An ominous sign of changing mental status is an increasing restlessness that is eventually followed by or alternates with drowsiness. Once the client gives up from exhaustion, this critical state often leads to acute respiratory failure. Some clients with an asthmatic reaction deteriorate slowly while others may deteriorate in minutes. Therefore, time is not a reliable parameter in deciding whether to call the physician or seek emergency help. All the indicators listed above need to be considered.

CASE STUDY: ASTHMA

Mr. N. is highly allergic to environmental pollens. He appears very anxious and is breathing in a rapid pattern. His vital signs are as follows: blood pressure (BP) 168/82 mm Hg; pulse, 132 beats/min; respirations, 46; and temperature, 100.8°F. Lung sounds exhibit expiratory wheezing. The physician's diagnosis is asthma.

The nurse should understand the following factors about this client: His systolic BP is too high, and he is tachycardic and tachypneic. His temperature is elevated. He is anxious and is experiencing shortness of breath. His muscles are working very hard to breathe, thereby increasing his metabolic rate, temperature, and stress. Mr. N. needs to have oxygen started due to the bronchospasm, and his condition necessitates an increased concentration of inspired oxygen. The nurse should encourage the client to sit up to maximize lung expansion. The nurse should also encourage hydration to thin secretions and facilitate expectoration. The physician will probably order an albuterol (Ventolin) inhaler to dilate the bronchioles since it is fast-acting. After the acute episode, it will be very important to determine environmental allergens to which Mr. N. is sensitive so they can be avoided.

Nursing Management

Therapeutic management centers on medication regimens, extensive education for the client and family on the management of asthma, life-style changes, and respiratory therapy. The mainstays of drug therapy for asthma include inhaled bronchodilators, β-adrenergic agonists, methylxanthines, and corticosteroids (Tables 3-1 and 3-2).

When the asthmatic client does not respond to the usual home drug therapy and management or if the severity of the reaction requires emergency treatment, the client is given three doses of inhaled or subcutaneous β-adrenergic agonists followed by systemic corticosteroids. Inhaled β-adrenergic agonists and theophylline are given for bronchodilation. Inhaled medications are also given via a nebulized breathing treatment. If the client does not improve after inhaling bronchodilators and receiving drugs, a condition termed status asthmaticus is present. The client is then intubated (i.e., an endotracheal tube is inserted) and placed on a respirator for mechanical ventilation.

Asthmatic clients receiving emergency or maintenance theophylline medications should have their serum theophylline levels (normal: 10–20

☒

TABLE 3-1

RESPIRATORY DRUG QUICK FACTS

Anticholinergics are bronchodilating agents that act by parasympathetic transmission.

- Atrovent inhaler: two inhalations four times a day, peaks in 1–2 hours, and lasts 4–6 hours; wait 15 seconds between puffs; not first choice agent because of slow action.

β-Adrenergic agonists cause relaxation of bronchial muscles resulting in dilation.

- Albuterol (Ventolin, Proventil) inhaler: acts in less than 15 minutes and lasts 3–4 hours.
- Metaproterenol sulfate (Alupent) inhaler: acts in less than 5 minutes and lasts 3–4 hours.
- Isoetharine HCL (Bronkosol) inhaler: acts in less than 5 minutes and lasts 1–3 hours.
- Isoproterenol HCL (Isuprel) inhaler.
- Epinephrine (Primatene): administered subcutaneously or by inhalation; acts immediately.

Methylxanthines or xanthines stimulate the central nervous system, decrease drowsiness, and stimulate the respiratory center in the medulla.

- Theophylline: helps ventricles to empty, acts as a bronchodilator, and clears mucociliary bodies.

Corticosteroids

- Beclomethazone (Vanceril) inhaler: two puffs 3–4 times a day.
- Dexamethasone (Decadron) inhaler: two puffs 3–4 times a day.
- Elunisolide (Aerobid) inhaler: two puffs twice a day.
- Triamcinolone acetonide (Azmacort) inhaler: two puffs 3–4 times a day.
- Hydrocortisone (Solu-Cortef): administered intravenously

mg/mL) tested periodically. This ensures that the client is receiving the maximum benefit from the bronchodilator and also guards against toxicity. Signs and symptoms of theophylline toxicity include GI upset with nausea and vomiting, restlessness, tachycardia, seizures, and tachyarrhythmias. Theophylline metabolism may be affected by fever, liver disease, congestive heart failure (CHF), and antibiotics such as erythromycin. Theophylline levels should be routinely tested every 6–12 months.

Routine assessment of the client with asthma and assessment during an asthmatic reaction include the rate of respiration, level of dyspnea, the client's perceptions of the asthmatic reaction, auscultation for air movement during inspiration and expiration, and the presence of audible or ausculatory wheezing. When available, diagnostic testing for oxygenation

---

TABLE 3-2
OXYGEN THERAPY QUICK FACTS

Room air is 21% oxygen and 78% nitrogen, which holds the alveoli open.

Simple mask. Never put the mask on with less than 5 L/min because if carbon dioxide is rebreathed, carbon dioxide narcosis may result, and the patient could die.

Nonbreather mask. This mask delivers up to 100% oxygen.

Venturi mask delivers a precise concentration of oxygen. It can be precisely regulated from 24–50% by dialing the concentration on the end piece.

Partial rebreather mask is used for hyperventilation, 40–70% oxygen, set at 5–15 L/min.

Nasal cannula:

Oxygen		Add 4% for each Liter		Oxygen in Atmospheric Air		Total Oxygen
1 L	=	4%	+	21%	=	25%
2 L	=	8%	+	21%	=	29%
3 L	=	12%	+	21%	=	33%
4 L	=	16%	+	21%	=	37%
5 L	=	20%	+	21%	=	41%

Liquid oxygen is economical to use. *Use only medical grade O2 USP* (green top on cylinder).

FIO2% is fractional-inspired oxygen.

Oxygen is a drug and should be given in the correct dose and by the correct method. Oxygen therapy is administered to clients when they experience shortness of breath. The nurse should assume that clients are hypoxic until proven otherwise. Restlessness and a change in mood are symptoms of respiratory distress. Oxygen releases endorphins from the brain that signal you to feel better.

should be performed using a pulse oximeter, peak flow meter, and arterial blood gas analysis.

In school, hospital, and community programs, nurses are valuable members of the comprehensive health care team involved in the care and education of asthmatics and their families. Nurses teach that life-style changes, such as avoiding known irritants, frequent changing of air conditioner filters, and avoiding smoking, are important. Nurses help clients develop skills and self-confidence by educating them about medication regimens, metered dose inhalers, peak flow meters and potential exercise routines. The goals of treatment include working toward decreased visits to the emergency room and hospitalizations, decreased number of days lost from work and school, and increased ability to participate in activities and hobbies. Other positive goals include reaching a Pa_{CO_2} below 40 mm Hg, oxygen saturation above 85%, a Pa_{O_2} above 60 mm Hg, and a normal respiratory rate and pattern.

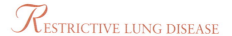

RESTRICTIVE LUNG DISEASE

Restrictive lung disease is a global term that describes many conditions in which lung volumes are decreased as a result of altered respiratory mechanics and gas exchange. In these conditions, reduced chest wall movement causes decreased ventilation. For example, if the diaphragm cannot fully descend in a pregnant woman at 36 weeks gestation because of the space occupied by the fetus, decreased ventilation and gas exchange result. Physiologic changes in elastic recoil, the work of breathing, and changes in pressure-volume relationships all play a part in conditions causing restrictive lung disease.

Etiology

The etiology at the site of restriction may be intrapulmonary, as in atelectasis, or extrapulmonary, as in nervous system diseases such as myasthenia gravis. Common intrapulmonary disorders include diseases of the lung tissue such as interstitial lung disease, atelectasis, and lung resection. Extrapulmonary disorders include abnormalities of the pleura, chest wall, and respiratory muscles. Spinal deformities, neuromuscular deformities, Guillain-Barré syndrome, muscular dystrophy, and spinal cord injury involve multiple body systems including the muscles of respiration. Interstitial lung disease causes idiopathic interstitial pulmonary fibrosis, a condition that is often related to occupational exposure to chemicals or fumes, immunologic diseases, or genetic disorders such as cystic fibrosis.

Pleural conditions that affect lung expansion include pleural effusion, pneumothorax, obesity, ascites, and pregnancy. An increased chest wall mass resulting from obesity, ascites, or pregnancy decreases the movement of the diaphragm and limits the volume of inspired air. Therefore, less oxygen is delivered to the alveoli and consequently to the tissues. Clients with these conditions experience dyspnea, increased fatigue, increased difficulty breathing, and possible carbon dioxide retention.

Pathophysiology

Pathophysiologic changes of restrictive lung disease occur as the total respiratory system becomes less compliant (stiffer). Normally, the lungs and chest wall exhibit good elastic recoil for respiration. With restrictive lung disease, the muscles need to work harder to inflate stiff lungs. The entire ventilation process is impeded; the effort expended to breathe increases; and more oxygen is used. **Hypoxemia** characterizes intrapulmonary disorders such as interstitial fibrosis and pneumonia. Hypoxemia is caused by a ventilation-perfusion (V/Q) mismatch. When **hypercapnia** occurs, the Pa_{CO_2} level rises above 45 mm Hg. The primary complication of chronic restrictive lung disease is cor pulmonale.

Hypoxemia. This condition is characterized by a deficiency of oxygen (Pa_{O_2}) in the arterial blood. Oxygen levels in the arterial blood should be 95–100 mm Hg.

Hypercapnia. This condition is characterized by excessive amounts of carbon dioxide (Pa_{CO_2}) in the blood. Normal Pa_{CO_2} levels in the arterial blood are 35–45 mm Hg.

Clinical Manifestations

Dyspnea is the primary sign and symptom of restrictive lung disease. Clinical manifestations arising from the original cause of the restrictive lung disease comprise the other signs. For example, respiratory distress may be severe when accompanied by a pneumothorax and atelectasis resulting from sudden changes in ventilation and perfusion. In other situations, such as chronic nervous system disorders, the loss of respiratory function and resulting hypoventilation may be insidious. An increased rate and decreased depth of respiration and decreased tidal volume are apparent whether the hypoventilation is sudden or chronic. Tidal volume is defined as the sum of alveolar ventilation, or the volume of air in milliliters inspired or exhaled during one respiratory cycle.

Nursing Management

Therapeutic management focuses both on treatment plans for the lung disease and the primary condition itself. Steroids are used to slow the progress of diffuse lung inflammation and injury. When hypoxemia is present, the nurse administers oxygen therapy. The overall treatment goal is to maintain an oxygen saturation of greater than 90% and a Pa_{O_2} of greater than 60 mm Hg. If clients desaturate or if the resting Pa_{O_2} on room air is below 55 mm Hg, the client will require oxygen supplementation.

The client with restrictive lung disease also must be taught ways to conserve energy to decrease oxygen demands. The primary conditions require various individualized treatments. If obesity is the cause, the client requires a comprehensive therapeutic plan that includes dietary education, counseling, and an exercise routine to lose weight. Obese clients are more prone to atelectasis and pneumonia as a result of decreased lung expansion. The Pickwickian syndrome is a condition of severe obesity that leads to an obesity-hypoventilation syndrome. Administering a respiratory stimulant (progesterone) improves oxygenation and ventilation. Oxygen is given at night when sleep apnea occurs. Nasal continuous positive airway pressure (CPAP) is a common treatment for Pickwickian syndrome. This treatment acts as a pneumatic splint by providing positive pressure to the upper airway to improve ventilation.

Mechanical ventilation is required when neuromuscular disorders such as myasthenia gravis result in paralysis of respiratory muscles. As respiratory muscles tire, the nurse should be alert for signs of paradoxic breathing, which occurs when there is outward movement of the chest and inward movement of the abdomen during inspiration and the opposite during expiration.

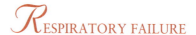

RESPIRATORY FAILURE

Respiratory failure is the inability of the respiratory system to maintain oxygen and carbon dioxide homeostasis. It causes significant morbidity and mortality. Respiratory failure can be acute or chronic, depending on the underlying cause and rapidity of disease progression. The diagnosis is established by blood-gas analysis, and changes in blood gases in addition to the clinical manifestations confirm it. In general, respiratory failure is defined by the blood-gas criteria of Pa_{O_2} of less than 60 mm Hg and Pa_{CO_2} greater than 50 mm Hg. Hypoxemia and changes in the pH are considered more significant markers of respiratory failure, as clients with chronic respiratory disease often live with preexisting hypercapnia. The pH determines whether the respiratory failure is acute or chronic. The criterion for acute respiratory failure is a pH below 7.30. In clients with COPD or other chronic respiratory conditions, the pH is often normal or close to normal as a result of compensatory mechanisms such as renal compensation. These clients are diagnosed as having chronic respiratory failure.

Respiratory failure is also categorized by cause. Ventilatory failure, oxygenation failure, or a combination of the two alter the ventilation and gas exchange functions, leading to respiratory failure. Common examples of oxygenation failure are pneumonia and pulmonary edema. These conditions do not allow enough blood to reach the alveoli for effective gas exchange to occur. Ventilatory failure occurs when the lungs fail as a pumping mechanism, as in central nervous system (CNS) disorders or malfunction of the respiratory muscles in clients suffering from drug overdose, poliomyelitis, or Guillain-Barré syndrome. Common conditions that put the client at risk for both oxygenation and ventilation failure include COPD and asthma. The current modalities of care for clients with pulmonary edema, acute respiratory distress syndrome, and pneumonia are discussed below.

Pulmonary Edema

Pulmonary edema is a serious cause of respiratory failure. It results primarily from physiologic changes in pressure in the lungs and heart. Occasionally this condition may arise as a medical emergency such as when blood or fluids are administered too rapidly, overloading a client's circulatory system. More often, pulmonary edema occurs as a result of cardiac disease. With left-sided CHF, the increase in pressure in the left ventricle causes a backflow increase in pulmonary venous pressure and, in turn, pulmonary capillary pressure. These pressure changes produce an increased pulmonary blood volume, and interstitial pulmonary edema results as serous fluid is forced into the alveoli. The increase in pressure and resultant edema produce diffuse pulmonary infiltrates, decrease lung compliance, and increase the work of breathing.

Clinical Manifestations Clinical manifestations include dyspnea, a productive cough with blood-tinged mucus, pulmonary crackles and wheezing, cyanosis, and tachycardia.

Nursing Management Clients with acute pulmonary edema are treated in the intensive care setting. Medical treatments are similar to those for CHF, as this pulmonary condition occurs in conjunction with left-sided heart failure. The client is given a regimen of digoxin and diuretic therapy with furosemide (Lasix). Immediate care focuses on the frequent assessment of respiratory status, administration of oxygen therapy, positioning the client in the orthopneic position, administering the prescribed medications, and reducing anxiety.

Acute Respiratory Distress Syndrome (ARDS)

ARDS is defined as oxygenation failure and severe hypoxemia that are caused by diffuse infiltrates. It is a diffuse noncardiac pulmonary edema characterized by increased permeability of the pulmonary capillaries. ARDS occurs as the result of a catastrophic event that triggers massive injury to the lungs. Possible causes include multiple blood transfusions, aspiration of gastric contents, sepsis, trauma, pneumonia, fat emboli, or a drug overdose. The injury to the lungs causes capillary membrane damage, leading to capillary leaking and pulmonary edema. Decreased surfactant (wetting agents of the pulmonary alveolar surfaces) and alveolar airway collapse cause poorly compliant lungs with right-to-left shunting and hypoxemia (Fig. 3-4). Clinically, the client exhibits signs and symptoms

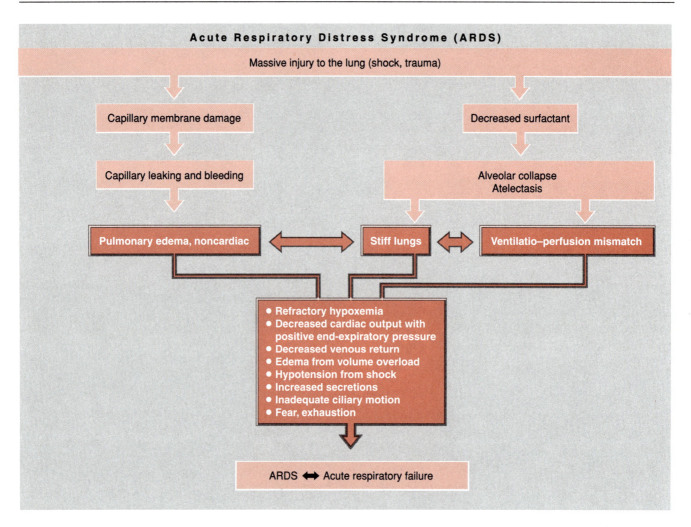

FIGURE 3-4 The sequence of pathology with acute respiratory distress syndrome.

of acute respiratory failure, including tachypnea, dyspnea, and hypoxemia. A chest radiography shows infiltrates, which appear as a "white-out."

Clinical Manifestations ARDS is a common and very challenging respiratory problem with a mortality rate of around 65%. A sudden onset of hypoxemia with no history of respiratory disease is the hallmark of ARDS. In many cases, the clients are young and otherwise healthy. They exhibit clinical manifestations of marked respiratory distress and hypoxemia. They are refractory to oxygen, meaning that they are hypoxemic even when given large amounts of oxygen therapy. Prolonged mechanical ventilation is almost always required (96% of clients). Despite advances in intensive care treatment and mechanical ventilation, clients who are over 30 years of age and have acquired immunodeficiency syndrome (AIDS), aspiration pneumonia, multiorgan failure, or disseminated intravascular coagulation have a poor prognosis.

Therapeutic Management The first goal of therapeutic management is to optimize gas exchange. Mechanical ventilation is initiated, and frequent blood-gas analyses are performed. Increased oxygen concentration is necessary initially (up to 100%). Later, positive end-expiratory pressure (PEEP) is used to lower the need for high concentrations of oxygen. If cardiac output is low or if blood pressure falls during PEEP, vasoactive drugs are administered.

Tissue perfusion is the second treatment goal in clients with ARDS. The client must be continuously monitored for both hypovolemia and hypervolemia. Fluid volume replacement and pulmonary and systemic pressures are monitored by the insertion of a central venous line such as a Swan-Ganz catheter. When the pressures and symptoms indicate hypervolemia, the client is treated with diuretics. When a decrease in pressure and urine output indicates hypovolemia, the client is treated with dopamine or dobutamine to increase cardiac output and thus oxygen transport. The client with low pressures may also be given plasma volume expanders.

Management of any underlying disease is the third goal of treatment. Sepsis or pneumonia is treated with parenteral antibiotics. Corticosteroids are not used because they cause fluid retention. Major **nursing responsibilities** include assessing the respiratory status of the client, maintaining oxygenation via mechanical ventilation, and monitoring tissue perfusion. Signs and symptoms of hypoxemia that the nurse must report to the physician include increased dyspnea, severe tachypnea, a change in mental status (the client is combative, confused, or restless), diaphoresis, and a change in the oxygen saturation or blood-gas analysis. The client is put on continuous cardiac monitoring, and vital signs are checked hourly. Cardiovascular warning signals that the nurse must report include dysrhythmias, tachycardia, raised arterial pressures, increased pulmonary artery pressures (PAP), and bradycardia, which may occur in clients with severe ARDS (Hudak & Gallo, 1994).

Monitoring tissue perfusion in vital organs such as the heart, kidneys, and brain is crucial. Nursing assessment of the neurologic system requires hourly documentation of the level of consciousness, pupillary reaction, movement and sensory responses of the client. Renal status is assessed by hourly urinary output, and serum creatinine and blood urea nitrogen (BUN) levels are followed closely. Myocardial function is monitored by heart rate and rhythm, skin color, peripheral pulses, blood pressure, and hemodynamic parameters such as PAP and pulmonary capillary wedge pressure (Hudak & Gallo, 1994).

Nursing Management Management of a client with any type of respiratory failure is challenging and requires collaboration among all members of the intensive care team, including the respiratory therapists, pulmonologists, radiologists, pharmacists, dietitians, and social workers. A client on mechanical ventilation, especially prolonged ventilation, requires drug therapy with bronchodilators such as intravenous aminophylline, corticosteroids, and with antibiotics. In addition, total parenteral nutrition (TPN) with lipids is provided to meet the caloric needs. A recent change in clinical practice involves the technique of positioning the client with ARDS in the prone position. This has been found to improve oxygenation by increasing ventilation. Further studies are required to document the effectiveness of this positioning practice. Nurses and social workers assist the client and family with emotional needs and life-support decisions that may arise. Spiritual care should always be offered, and the client and family may desire to see a minister, rabbi, or priest. Currently, emphasis is placed on preventive and palliative care to manage respiratory conditions before the client requires hospitalization or reaches the acute stage of respiratory failure. This benefits the client and reduces the cost and extent of hospital visits.

Weaning clients from mechanical ventilators is a gradual process. The ventilator settings are decreased incrementally and blood gases and respiratory status are assessed within 30 minutes to document the client's response to the change. The client is eventually weaned to a CPAP of 5 cm, and provided the respiratory response and blood-gas analysis are favorable, the client is extubated and given 40% oxygen by face mask.

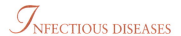

Infectious Diseases

Pneumonia

Pneumonia is defined as an infection of the lower respiratory tract that involves the lung parenchyma, including the alveoli and supportive structures. It is the fourth leading cause of death in clients over 65 years of age. Due to changes in pathogens causing pneumonia and the concern with antimicrobial resistance patterns, the nurse should be aware of the following classifications:

1. **Community-acquired pneumonia** begins as a common respiratory illness and progresses to pneumonia. Streptococcal pneumonia is the most common causative organism. This type of pneumonia usually occurs in the very young or the elderly.
2. **Hospital-acquired pneumonia** is also known as nosocomial pneumonia. Organisms such as Pseudomonas aeruginosa, Klebsiella, or Staphylococcus aureus are the most common bacterial causes of hospital-acquired pneumonia.
3. **Lobar and bronchopneumonia** are categorized on the basis of the anatomic location of the infection. Today, pneumonia is classified according to the organism rather than just the anatomic location.
4. **Viral, bacterial, or fungal pneumonias** are categorized on the basis of the causal agent. Sputum culture and sensitivity (C&S) are done to identify the offending organism.

Etiology Pneumonia is caused by virulent pathogens that are introduced into the body by aspiration, inhalation, or circulatory spread.

Aspiration pneumonia is caused primarily by bacteria. Inhalation pneumonia is communicated primarily by droplets from coughing and sneezing, and the causal agent is usually a virus. Pneumonia can result from hematogenous spread in clients with septicemia. The infection is usually caused by a bacterial or fungal agent. Older, chronically ill clients; clients on long-term steroid therapy; clients with AIDS, nutritional deficits, or drug and alcohol abuse problems; and immunosuppressed clients are more susceptible to pneumonia.

Bacterial Pneumonia Bacterial pneumonias comprise less than one-half of all pneumonias and usually occur in the elderly. However, 80% of clients who are hospitalized for pneumonia have a bacterial infection, often brought about by increasing severity of the illness and the age of the client (Phipps, et al., 1995). Gram-positive organisms that cause bacterial pneumonia are *Streptococcus pneumoniae, S. aureus,* and *Streptococcus pyogenes.* The incidence of pneumonia is highest in the winter or early spring and usually is a sequela of an upper respiratory tract infection. *Mycoplasma* pneumonia affects all age groups and spreads by droplet transmission. *Haemophilus influenzae* is the most common gram-negative organism. It is spread by droplet transmission and usually occurs in clients who have a preexisting respiratory disease such as COPD. *Klebsiella pneumoniae* and *P. aeruginosa* are usually acquired from the aspiration of airborne oral secretions or from respiratory equipment. Current trends toward decreased hospitalizations and reduced costs include programs such as promoting the early treatment of respiratory infections, administering antibiotic therapy at home, and admitting Medicare clients to subacute units. These strategies are used to treat clients with bacterial pneumonia who are not in respiratory distress.

Pneumonia was once known as a "friend of the elderly" because it brought a peaceful closure to an elderly client's life. It remains a prevalent disease today, and death rates for hospitalized clients with bacterial pneumonia are 15–20%. In clients older than 70 years of age, the mortality rate is 50–70%.

Viral Pneumonia Viral pneumonia, the most common type of pneumonia, is caused by an influenza virus spread via droplet transmission. Cytomegalovirus is the most common cause of viral pneumonia in immunosuppressed clients, where it has a high mortality rate. Clients with viral pneumonia should be treated symptomatically. The client may develop secondary bacterial pneumonia and thus should be monitored throughout the course of the respiratory infection.

Fungal Pneumonia Fungal infections such as histoplasmosis are spread by the inhalation of spores that are found in soil, bird droppings, and compost. Histoplasmosis infection is sometimes self-limiting and requires no treatment. When treatment is required, an antifungal agent (amphotericin B) is administered intravenously. Histoplasmosis must be prevented in pregnant women as the fungus may damage the developing fetus. Coccidiomycosis, commonly known as valley fever, is also spread by inhaling spores from contaminated soil and is endemic to well-defined geographical areas in the southwestern United States and parts of Argentina. Intravenous amphotericin B is the treatment of choice.

Pneumocystis carinii pneumonia (PCP), whose causative organism has been identified as both a protozoan and a fungus, occurs in immunosuppressed clients such as those with AIDS. Recent morphological studies of the organism indicate that it is more characteristic of a fungus. *P. carinii* pneumonia is an infection with worldwide distribution and is of utmost concern in the management of clients with AIDS. As with many opportunistic agents, infection in a normal host is usually asymptomatic. Prophylactic treatment of *P. carinii* pneumonia in clients with human immunodeficiency virus (HIV) has decreased the incidence of this fulminating pneumonia.

Pathophysiology   In pneumonia, the alveoli, bronchioles, and bronchi fill with suppurative exudate that prevents the ventilation of a portion of the lungs. This results in arteriovenous shunting and hypoxemia.

Clinical Manifestions   Typically, clients with pneumonia present with the abrupt onset of fever, shaking, chills, a productive cough, purulent sputum, and pleuritic chest pain. The primary manifestation of pneumonia is hypoxemia. Complications include metabolic acidosis, multilobar disease, dehydration, and respiratory failure. The most common causative organisms are *S. pneumoniae*, *H. influenzae*, and *K. pneumoniae*. The white blood cell (WBC) count is elevated, and chest x-rays show infiltrates. Atypical pneumonia often has a gradual, insidious onset and is less dramatic in clinical appearance. The client may complain of headache, sore throat, muscle soreness, and fatigue. A dry cough may be present; the client is afebrile; and the WBCs may not be elevated. The most common types include *M. pneumoniae*, viral pneumonia, and *Legionella pneumophila*. Occasionally clients who are long-term smokers or who have COPD may have atypical pneumonia, and it is more difficult to diagnose the changes in their health due to the chronic debility of their respiratory status.

Nursing Management   Therapeutic management of bacterial pneumonia is a full course of antibiotics prescribed in accordance with the suspected causal agent, cost, allergies, and any preexisting respiratory disease. Oxygen therapy is used to treat hypoxemia. Respiratory therapy treatments with chest percussion and postural drainage help to remove suppurative exudate. Every two hours the client should turn, cough, and breathe deeply. This is especially important for elderly clients who are immobile or have limited mobility. The head of the bed is elevated to assist in ventilation, and bronchodilators may be ordered. Nutritional supplements are necessary to maintain the caloric intake of elderly and immunosuppressed clients. Oxygen saturation is monitored with pulse oximetry. The level should be greater than 90%. Viral pneumonia is treated supportively. Nursing care focuses on relieving the client's signs and symptoms. Comfort measures for clients with pneumonia include increased fluid intake (warm tea), showers with steam, supporting the client with pillows during coughing spells, dental hygiene, and administering mucolytic agents.

Tuberculosis (TB)

TB is a systemic, highly contagious disease. It is caused by *Mycobacterium tuberculosis*, an acid-fast aerobic bacteria. TB is spread by airborne droplet transmission. The organism prefers tissues with a high oxygen concentration such as the lungs and kidneys. It can remain dormant until the immune system weakens. This process is known as *reactivation TB*. Most individuals remain asymptomatic and are noninfectious (a positive skin test and negative chest x-ray), but these clients are at risk for reactivation TB. Pulmonary TB left untreated results in liquefaction and destruction of the lung tissue.

Clinical Manifestations Presently TB concerns health officials as an opportunistic infection in the HIV-positive client and as a public health epidemic with drug-resistant strains. From 1985 to the present, the reported incidence of TB has increased, and some strains are now resistant to previously used antitubercular medications. Signs and symptoms include anorexia, weight loss, night sweats, fever, chills, persistent cough, hoarseness, and hemoptysis. Pleuritic pain is worse during inhalation or coughing.

When a client with known or suspected TB is hospitalized, isolation precautions must be taken. The client must be admitted to a private room with negative air pressure. Prefitted, particulate respirator masks are used by the staff and family. The doors are kept closed.

Nursing Management Diagnostic tests for TB include skin testing, chest x-rays, and a sputum smear and culture. For extrapulmonary TB, blood and stool cultures are done. The skin test may have a false-negative result, which is sometimes seen in clients over 50 years of age. If TB is still suspected, the test should be repeated in two weeks. This process demonstrates the *booster phenomenon*: the second test stimulates the immune response, indicating that the client actually is infected. A sputum specimen for acid-fast bacillus is ordered to confirm active TB and estimate the degree of infection. At least three specimens are ordered on three successive days, and the nurse should allow 2–12 weeks to read these cultures. The technique used to obtain the sputum specimen is important for an accurate diagnosis. The nurse should instruct the client to inhale and exhale deeply three times, and then inhale rapidly and cough forcefully into a sterile container. A positive sputum culture confirms the diagnosis of TB. Distinctive changes on the chest x-ray, notably enlarged hilar lymph nodes and the presence of a cavity or tubercle, are also evident in clients with pulmonary TB.

Clients both with and without clinically active disease are treated pharmacologically. The four primary drugs used are isoniazid (INH), rifampin, streptomycin, and ethambutol. The American Thoracic Society recommends that drug therapy continue for at least nine months or until at least six months have elapsed from the conversion of positive sputum to negative sputum. INH is given for 6–12 months to prevent TB in high-risk clients, such as those with a positive skin test and chest x-ray. A client is considered noninfectious after taking medications for two weeks. The emergence of drug-resistant TB has heightened the need to locate every client with TB and treat each with an entire course of the four-drug therapy. In an attempt to halt this epidemic, clients are now being monitored in their homes and at shelters and are even being placed in sanitariums to ensure their compliance with the drug therapy.

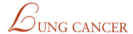 LUNG CANCER

Lung cancer remains a leading public health problem and cause of morbidity. Smoking causes 80% of all lung cancers. Occupational exposure to asbestos, chemical fumes, and second-hand smoke are also factors. Despite public health education programs, legislation requiring warning labels on cigarette packages, and restrictions on the sale of cigarettes to minors, the largest group of new smokers is teenage girls. In women, lung cancer has now surpassed breast cancer as the leading cause of death from cancer, making it the leading cause of death from cancer for both men and women (American Cancer Society, 1995). The peak incidence of lung cancer is in the fifth to sixth decade of life.

Etiology

Most cases of lung cancer are squamous cell carcinomas, which, because they grow slowly, have the best prognosis and account for 30–35% of all cases of lung cancer. Adenocarcinomas account for 25–30% of lung tumors. Large cell carcinomas account for 15% and grow rapidly. Small cell carcinomas represent 12–25% of lung tumors. They grow the most rapidly of all and metastasize the most frequently. Clients with small cell carcinomas have a survival rate of only 8–18 months (Phipps, et al., 1995).

Clinical Manifestations
Clinical manifestations of lung cancer include signs of local lung disease. Coughing is the most common presenting complaint. The cough is usually productive, and the client may complain of dyspnea or hemoptysis. Atelectasis and pleuritic pain may be present.

Lung cancer may be at an advanced stage or have metastasized before the client experiences symptoms or seeks medical attention. The most common sites of metastasis are to the thoracic cavity, CNS, and spinal cord. Fluid may accumulate in the pleural space, causing effusion and dyspnea. This fluid needs to be removed by a thoracentesis to maximize ventilation and make the client more comfortable.

Diagnostic tests for lung cancer include chest x-rays, sputum cytology, and **bronchoscopy**, or mediastinoscopy. Depending on the location and accessibility of the tumor, a biopsy specimen is obtained either by bronchoscopy, transthoracic needle biopsy, or exploratory thoracotomy. Imaging techniques such as magnetic resonance imaging (MRI) or computed tomography (CT) scans are performed to assist in staging the lung cancer and to detect areas of metastasis (Jaffe & McVan, 1997).

Therapeutic Management Therapeutic management depends on the type and stage of the cancer. In general, only 13% of all lung cancer clients, even those with an early diagnosis, survive five years after diagnosis.

Surgical Management The extent of surgical intervention is based on the location of the tumor, the stage of cancer, the presence of comorbid conditions, and the personal choice of the client. Surgical removal of the tumor, which is performed only if metastatic disease is not present, consists of removal of an entire lung (pneumonectomy) or a wedge resection. Lung surgery is typically performed through a thoracotomy, which is an incision in the intercostal spaces. A thoracotomy is commonly performed for a suspected or confirmed diagnosis of lung cancer. Pneumonectomy and lobectomy are the most common types of surgeries. A pneumonectomy is contraindicated in clients with COPD. Resection of a lung segment (segmental resection) may also be performed. In a wedge resection, a V-shaped wedge of tumor located near the surface of the lung is removed. Laser surgery by endoscopy allows a less invasive removal of peripheral lung tumors.

Complications following any type of lung surgery are serious, including atelectasis, empyema (an infection of the pleural fluid), bronchopleural fistula (the bronchial stump does not heal properly and communicates with the pleural space), and respiratory failure (particularly in clients with preexisting lung disease, such as COPD). **Nursing care** to prevent these complications or to detect them early and begin treatment requires close monitoring of the client's respiratory system. The nurse should have the client turn and cough frequently, and the incentive inspirometer is used as soon as the client is physically able. Respiratory treatments are given by the respiratory therapist every 2–4 hours. Following any thoracotomy surgery, chest tubes are inserted. The nurse should record the drainage hourly and note the color and amount. Drainage of more than 200 mL for more than 2–3 hours indicates postoperative bleeding, and the physician needs to be notified. The client is monitored for signs of dyspnea, fever, change in lung sounds, or a deterioration in chest x-rays, oxygen saturation, or blood gases. Postoperatively, the client should be placed on a cardiac monitor because dysrhythmias such as atrial fibrillation may occur. Atrial fibrillation is treated with digoxin (Lanoxin). After digitalization, the client is monitored for conversion to normal sinus rhythm.

Radiation Therapy Radiation therapy is frequently used to treat lung cancer. Radiation is used after surgery to improve tumor control, prevent metastasis to the brain, and to control signs and symptoms of pain. Toxic side effects of radiation include esophagitis, dysphagia, pneumonitis, and

Bronchoscopy. This procedure is a visual examination of the respiratory system by a physician. The vocal cords, trachea, and bronchial tree are viewed using a flexible fiberoptic bronchoscope. Biopsy specimens can be obtained during this procedure.

fibrosis. The nurse should instruct the client to report hoarseness, dyspnea, hemoptysis, pain on swallowing, or chest pain as these may be signs of complications either from the radiation or the cancer itself. Radiation therapy causes tracheobronchial secretions to thicken, which makes it difficult to expectorate. **Nursing measures** include raising the head of the bed, increasing fluid intake to thin the secretions, and teaching the client to use pursed-lip breathing.

Chemotherapy Chemotherapy, which also may be administered to provide systemic treatment of lung cancer, is most effective on small cell lung cancers. Pain management is crucial for any client living with cancer. Various combinations of radiation therapy, chemotherapy, and narcotic analgesia are components of adjuvant therapy for lung cancer clients. Nurses who work with these clients in a hospital, outpatient chemotherapy clinic, home, or hospice must frequently assess the levels of comfort, pain, and anxiety of their clients.

Prevention remains the only real hope of a cure for lung cancer. Individuals must stop smoking and wear protective equipment during any exposure to carcinogenic environmental or occupational substances.

CHEST TRAUMA

Penetrating or nonpenetrating chest trauma is another common cause of respiratory compromise. Nonpenetrating injuries can cause fractures of the rib cage and sternum, flail chest, pulmonary contusion, pneumothorax, and hemothorax. A penetrating injury also can cause a pneumothorax or hemothorax such as when a laceration of the lung parenchyma occurs in a motor vehicle accident, gunshot, or stab wound. Penetrating chest wounds due to gunshots or stabbings are common injuries seen in emergency rooms.

Penetrating and Nonpenetrating Injuries

Fractured Ribs Fractured ribs without accompanying lung contusion or trauma require no treatment as the bone heals in 3–6 weeks without intervention. The client may need mild analgesics or a rib splint for comfort.

Flail Chest Flail chest occurs when three or more adjacent ribs are fractured in two places. It is associated with severe chest trauma, and a pulmonary contusion is usually present. The affected portion of the chest wall is pulled in during inspiration and causes a mediastinal shift to the opposite side that interferes with venous return to the right side of the heart. A pulmonary contusion causes compression of the lung parenchyma. With severe trauma to the chest, atelectasis occurs as a result of blood shunting to the alveoli and interstitial spaces. Respiratory failure may occur as a complication of chest trauma. The nurse must monitor the client for dyspnea, cyanosis, decreased blood pressure, increased heart rate, decreased Pa_{O_2} and increased Pa_{CO_2}. Chest x-rays show areas of consolidation and large areas of infiltrates.

Pneumothorax A pneumothorax occurs when air collects in the pleural space between the visceral and parietal pleura. Pneumothorax is caused by trauma or is a sequela of COPD. The two types of pneumothorax are simple and tension. In a *simple pneumothorax,* air enters the pleural space and causes a partial or complete collapse of the lung. In a *tension pneumothorax,* air continually enters the pleural cavity and increases the intrapleural pressure above the alveolar pressure. A mediastinal shift occurs toward the unaffected side and compresses the other lung.

A specific sequence of pathophysiology occurs with a pneumothorax. The vital capacity decreases, ventilation decreases, venous return decreases, hypoxemia develops, and acute respiratory failure and death may occur if the pneumothorax is left untreated. The nurse must be alert to this condition and notify the physician immediately if he or she suspects a pneumothorax. Common signs of a pneumothorax are absent breath sounds over the affected lung, decreased blood pressure, and distant heart sounds. The client complains of dyspnea and chest pain; respirations are rapid and shallow; cyanosis is apparent; and the client may be quite restless (Fig. 3-5).

Hemothorax A hemothorax occurs when blood accumulates in the pleural space. It usually accompanies a pneumothorax or rib fracture and also can occur from bleeding in the pulmonary capillaries, thoracic aorta, or other vessels. Ventilation is decreased, and hypovolemic shock or hypoxemia may occur. Signs and symptoms include a decrease in blood pressure; tachycardia; rapid, shallow respirations; dyspnea; and chest pain. Arterial blood-gas analysis demonstrates a decreased Pa_{O_2} and an increased Pa_{CO_2}. Atelectasis or pneumonia may occur with a hemothorax. If fluid is not drained by a thoracentesis within 24–48 hours, bacteria that have grown in the fluid may cause empyema. Additionally, a bronchopleural fistula may form that drains purulent exudate from the pleural space to the airway. When this occurs the client expectorates purulent sputum.

Nursing Management Therapeutic management of clients with chest injuries varies. Many of these clients are stabilized in the emergency room and admitted to intensive care. Clients with flail chest may require mechanical ventilation to stabilize internally the floating segment of the rib cage. Pulmonary contusion often requires mechanical ventilation until the injury to the lung parenchyma has healed. First-aid treatment for an open "sucking" (segment pulls in and out with breathing) chest wound requires the placement of Vaseline-coated gauze over the wound to prevent a tension pneumothorax.

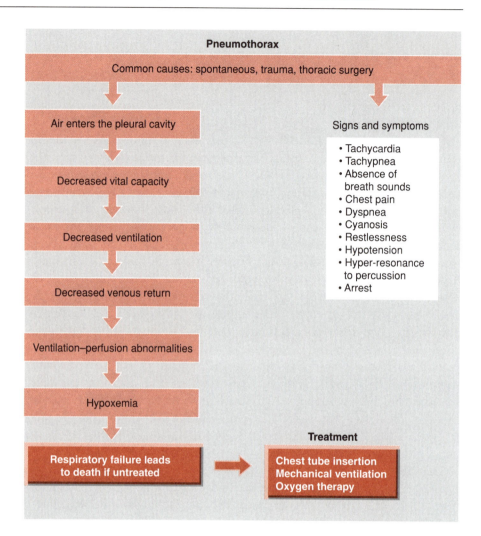

FIGURE 3-5

⬡

The sequence of pathology with a pneumothorax.

Chest Tubes. A chest tube has a large-bore drainage opening and is inserted through the thorax into the chest cavity to remove air, fluid, or blood from the pleural space. Chest tubes are necessary following chest or heart surgery or with the occurrence of a pneumothorax or hemothorax.

Chest tubes used for injuries to the chest have two primary purposes. First, the draining of air and fluid aids in the reexpansion of the lung, and second, they reestablish a negative air pressure in the pleural space. To treat a pneumothorax, chest tubes are inserted (chest tube thoracostomy) to drain the air and reestablish negative air pressure. To treat a hemothorax, the chest tube is inserted inferiorly to drain blood and secretions. In the treatment of a tension pneumothorax, a large-bore needle is inserted to decrease intrapleural pressure followed by the insertion of a chest tube.

For proper drainage, chest tubes are connected to a closed-chest drainage system. The most commonly used system in clinical practice is the Pleur-Evac, a plastic disposable unit. Nursing care for a client with a chest tube includes hourly documentation of the color and amount of drainage, monitoring for air leaks in the system, verifying that the system is continuously bubbling (in the suction chamber and not in the underwater seal chamber), and assessing the client for any signs or symptoms of respiratory distress. The client is monitored with pulse oximetry, blood-gas analysis, and daily chest x-rays.

SUMMARY

The major categories of lower respiratory conditions include infections, asthma, obstructive and restrictive lung disorders, respiratory failure, lung cancer, and chest trauma. Respiratory conditions cause compromised function in ventilation or gas exchange, varying from mild dyspnea to the critical point of respiratory failure; lung cancer; and chest trauma. **Nursing management** of clients with respiratory conditions requires the nurse to develop expertise in assessing the respiratory system, maintaining an unobstructed airway, and learning interventions that promote optimal airway function. Pharmacologic treatment is a major component of care. Therefore, the nurse must be able to educate clients on the major categories of respiratory drugs and be skilled in their administration. When the client is living with a condition such as asthma, COPD, or lung cancer, the nurse must focus on the needs of the client and family as they adapt to a chronic illness. The public needs additional antismoking programs for school-age children as well as smoking cessation programs for adults.

KEY WORDS

Arterial blood gases
Asthma-reactive airway disease
Bronchodilators
Chronic obstructive pulmonary disease
Dyspnea
Extubation
Hemothorax
Hypercapnia
Hypoxemia

Immunosuppression
Intubation
Lung cancer
Mechanical ventilation
Orthopnea
Pneumonia
Pneumothorax
Pulse oximetry
Wheezing

QUESTIONS

1. Mr. F. has been diagnosed with chronic obstructive pulmonary disease (COPD) for the last 10 years. He continues to smoke two packs of cigarettes a day. He requires oxygen to perform his daily activities. Which of the following therapeutic management modalities is necessary?

   A. Low flow oxygen is usually ordered.
   B. Oxygen flow is adjusted to a higher level if shortness of breath occurs.
   C. Petroleum jelly should be applied around the nares to prevent irritation.
   D. Oxygen flow rate is not a concern since he will feel better if the rate is high.

2. Mrs. R. has been diagnosed with acute asthma. She has been admitted to the hospital and all of the following instructions to the nurse are correct **except**

   A. the head of the bed should be in the high position to facilitate drainage and breathing.
   B. a cool and dry environment should be maintained.
   C. air conditioner filters should be changed often.
   D. oxygen should never be used as it could restrict airways more.

3. Nurse M. witnesses a motor vehicle accident. She stops to offer assistance and hears air rushing out of the driver's chest. She immediately suspects a pneumothorax and correctly does which of the following?

   A. Determines the entry wound area, covers it with clothing, and applies pressure until the ambulance arrives.
   B. Does not touch the driver since she could extend the pneumothorax.
   C. Attempts to insert a stick into the hole to stop the rush of air out of the chest.
   D. Encourages the driver to bend forward over the steering wheel to constrict the flow of air out of the chest.

ANSWERS

1. *The answer is A.* Oxygen therapy is required if the client is unable to maintain a $Pa_{O_2} > 55$ mm Hg or an oxygen saturation (O_2 Sat) $> 85\%$ at rest. Oxygen (1–2 L) is given to relieve pulmonary hypertension and decrease load on the right side of the heart. It should be used continuously. High flow oxygen elevates the Pa_{O_2} to a level that removes breathing stimulus.

2. *The answer is D.* Elevating the head of the bed facilitates drainage of secretions. A cool and dry environment decreases swelling of mucous membranes, expanding airway diameter to increase the amount of oxygen intake. Air conditioner filters are changed to remove pollens and environmental factors that may initiate an acute episode.

3. *The answer is A.* By covering the entry wound, the nurse is attempting to equalize intrathoracic pressure to facilitate lung inflation.

ANNOTATED REFERENCES

Black, J., & Matassarin-Jacobs, E. (1997). *Medical-surgical nursing,* 5th ed. Philadelphia: W. B. Saunders.

This text focuses on clinical management for continuity of care.

Dudek, S. (1997). *Nutrition handbook for nursing practice,* 3rd ed. Philadelphia: J. B. Lippincott.

This text uses the nursing process format and includes practical information on nutritional care in nursing. It is useful as a supplementary text.

Hudak, C. M., & Gallo, B. M. (1994). *Handbook of critical care nursing: A holistic approach.* Philadelphia: J. B. Lippincott.

This text is in outline format, which makes it easy to follow. The text includes step-by-step outlines for common critical care procedures and nursing care plans for critical care conditions.

Jaffe, M. S., & McVan, B. F. (1997). *Laboratory and diagnostic test handbook.* Philadelphia: F. A. Davis.

This is a reference guide to medical tests.

Phipps, W., Cassmeyer, V., Sande, J., & Lehman, M. K. (1995). *Medical-surgical nursing concepts and clinical practice.* St. Louis: C. V. Mosby.

This text gives detailed information on alterations in the systems of the body and nursing care for common problems in ill adults. It is useful for a more in-depth review.

INTERNET SITES FOR ADDITIONAL INFORMATION

Otolaryngology Resources:
http://www.bcm.tmc.edu/oto/others.html

Tuberculosis Resources:
http://www.cpmc.columbia.edu/tbcpp

American Lung Association:
http://www.lungusa.org

Asthma and Allergy Resource Page:
http://www.cco.caltech.edu/~wrean/resources.html

Asthma: Patient Teaching Guide:
http://www.meddean.luc.edu/lumen/Medicine/Allergy/
Asthma/asthmatoc.html

Cancer of the Lung (see also other cancer sites listed in Chapter 2):
Oncolink: http://cancer.med.upenn.edu
Oncology Nursing Society:
http://www.ons.org
Can Survive (Home Page):
http://www.avonlink.co.uk/amanda

CHAPTER 4

CARDIOVASCULAR DISORDERS

INTRODUCTION TO CARDIOVASCULAR DISEASE

Cardiovascular disease is one of the most prevalent health problems in the United States. Nurses must remember this, as most of the clients they see are either at risk for or have a cardiovascular disorder. The nurse should routinely assess for risk factors and clinical manifestations of cardiovascular disease when taking the client's history and performing a physical examination. Several factors contribute to the high incidence of heart disease in the United States, including a high-fat diet, sedentary life style, obesity, stress, smoking, pollutants, a family history of heart disease, and large populations of underserved minorities. When assessing clients for risk or presence of heart disease, nurses have three guidelines to aid them: the normal changes associated with aging, risk factors, and the cardinal symptoms of heart disease.

Normal Changes Associated with Aging

Age-related changes in the cardiovascular system typically have a slow, insidious onset. The muscles of the heart become less elastic and thus less effective in pumping blood (Stanley, 1995). Some stiffening of the valve tissues occurs (Stanley, 1995). **Structural changes** also occur in the heart's conduction system. As a result of these changes, the blood vessels dilate to allow for a greater volume of blood (Stanley, 1995). This compensatory

Cardiovascular changes that occur due to aging are related to **structural changes.** The tissues dilate and become less elastic, causing decreased pumping of the blood, decreased vessel pressure, and blood pooling.

effect exerts pressure on the venous valves, making them less effective or even unable to close.

The cardiovascular system also loses some function from the aging process. The ability to adapt to physiological demands for an increased volume of blood is reduced (Stanley, 1995). This affects the delivery of oxygen to the tissues and leads to the poor circulation associated with many vascular disorders. When the system attempts to compensate, systolic blood pressure increases progressively (Stanley, 1995).

Reactions to these age-related changes include poorly perfused tissues, muffled heart sounds, a shifting of the maximal impulse point from its usual position, and a systolic murmur. Elderly clients with heart disease may also develop pseudohypertension. To determine if pseudohypertension is present, the nurse should apply cuff pressure greater than the systolic blood pressure. The presence of pseudohypertension can result in an erroneous assessment of the client's blood pressure by as much as 10–15 mm Hg (Stanley, 1995). If the radial pulse remains palpable while the cuff is in place, significant atherosclerosis is most likely present (Stanley, 1995).

Risk Factors

Risk factors for cardiovascular disease are classified as **modifiable**, which includes smoking, obesity, a sedentary lifestyle, and stress, and **nonmodifiable**, which includes age, gender, race, and family history.

Risk factors are classified as **nonmodifiable** and **modifiable**.

Nonmodifiable Risk Factors Nonmodifiable risk factors include age, gender, race, family heredity, and diabetes. Diabetes is somewhat controversial, as it may be considered preventable in some people. After 55 years of age, the effects of age-related changes in the cardiovascular system become more pronounced. Men have a greater incidence of cardiovascular disease, but the incidence in women increases after menopause. Persons of African-American descent have a higher risk for developing cardiovascular disease than the general population. A family history of hyperlipidemia is another risk factor for developing cardiovascular disease. Uncontrolled diabetes damages blood vessels, increasing the risk of developing heart disease. Each of these areas should be explored to determine the client's nonmodifiable risk factors.

Modifiable Risk Factors Modifiable risk factors include increased levels of low-density lipoproteins (LDL), hypertension, smoking, obesity, a sedentary life style, and stress. When inquiring about a client's life style, the nurse should assess the actual levels of activity in which he or she participates during a typical day. Asking what a client's occupation is helps the nurse determine the activity level and the amount of job-related stress. The nurse should inquire if the client follows an exercise program, if he or she exercises consistently, and if any discomfort is experienced during or after the activity. A sedentary life style is conducive to obesity, which contributes to hypertension and hyperlipidemia. All of these problems lead to cardiovascular disease. It is generally thought that obesity is not a direct risk factor but a sign of a sedentary life style that may be related to a higher incidence of LDL in the blood. The body proportions of obese clients may be an important risk factor. To determine this, the nurse should assess the client's waist-to-hip ratio. This is done by measuring the circumference of the waist at the level of the umbilicus and then measuring the circumference of the hips at their fullest part. The waist measurement should be divided by the hip measurement. If the number obtained is greater than 0.8 for women or 1.0 for men, it may be a direct risk factor for developing cardiovascular disease.

The nurse can assess stress levels by inquiring about possible stressors such as the loss of a loved one, marital discord, job-related stress, fear, financial concerns, or other major events in the client's life. Major life events always add stress. If clients are experiencing prolonged levels of stress from an event or events in their lives, the stress may negatively affect cardiovascular health. The mechanism for this has not been determined.

The nurse must also assess whether the client smokes. Studies have shown that each year, one-third of the annual deaths from coronary artery disease are directly related to smoking (Hancock, 1991). It is not known how smoking affects the cardiovascular system. However, scientists have determined that nicotine stimulates the release of epinephrine and norepinephrine, which increases the heart rate and causes peripheral vasoconstriction (Haak, Richardson, Davey, & Parker-Cohen, 1994). This results in an increase in blood pressure that contributes to a greater cardiac workload and oxygen demand (Haak, et al., 1994). The increased level of catecholamines also releases fatty acids, which may contribute to higher levels of LDL in the blood (Haak, et al., 1995). Cigarette smoking is also associated with platelet aggregation that increases the risk of clot formation. It also has a long-term effect on tissue oxygenation. The risks of smoking decrease significantly when smoking is discontinued (Haak, et al., 1994).

Cardinal Symptoms of Heart Disease

The six cardinal symptoms of cardiovascular disease are dyspnea, chest pain or other discomfort, palpitations, edema, syncope, and excessive fatigue. The nurse should suspect a cardiac-related disorder if clients complain of insufficient energy to perform their typical daily activities. This can be difficult to assess, since changes that occur in the cardiovascular system often have a deceptively slow onset, and the client eventually learns to adapt to the changes. By inquiring about the client's daily activities at the time of and a few months prior to the current visit, the nurse can discern if the client is experiencing a change in his or her tolerance to activity. The need for increasing rest periods during the day may indicate an intolerance to activity or overwhelming fatigue. Dyspnea on exertion is associated with an intolerance to activity. The client experiencing dyspnea will complain of shortness of breath during daily activities. This can be a very limiting condition. For example, clients may be unable to walk to the bathroom without becoming short of breath. Some clients exhibit signs of air hunger. A barrel chest develops as the client continues to fight for air.

Some clients state they are most comfortable sitting in an upright position with their arms out at the elbows and their upper torso leaning forward over a table. This position gives additional room for lung expansion. It is important for the nurse to assess the client's respiratory rate and effort.

Some clients are able to discern when they are experiencing a dysrhythmia. These clients state they can feel their heart fluttering, racing, pounding, or skipping beats. The nurse may also be able to detect a dysrhythmia during the assessment of the client's heart sounds and pulse. An increased heart rate is termed tachycardia, and a decreased heart rate is termed bradycardia. Skipped and irregular beats are generally discernible during assessment.

Clients with certain cardiovascular diseases may experience pain associated with the disorder. Chest pain (angina) is felt as midsternal pain, jaw pain, left arm pain, or a general feeling of tightness or gripping in the chest. Chest pain may be indicative of an infarction. Peripheral vascular disease often presents as a deep, dull aching in the lower extremities. Pain that is elicited in the calf when the foot is flexed forward is suggestive of thrombus formation. This is termed a positive Homan's sign. Intermittent claudication is another painful response to a vascular problem. This pain occurs while ambulating and is relieved at rest. If there is pain in the extremities, the site of the pain should be assessed for signs of inflammation.

Edema is another symptom of cardiovascular disease. The client needs to be assessed for any recent weight gain. Clothes that fit tighter or leave indentations on the skin may be an indicator of edema. The nurse should assess for the presence of dependent edema by determining if the client has noticed edema in the legs and feet at the end of the day that improves by morning. Some clients complain that shoes or rings no longer fit. The nurse should also note if the client complains of edema in one area (e.g., one leg), in contrast to a more generalized edema (e.g., both feet). Edema can be caused by fluid retention associated with salt intake. The client's typical daily salt intake should be assessed.

If the client complains of periods of forgetfulness or time lapses, the nurse should be alert for the possibility of syncopal episodes. The presence of bruises may also indicate syncopal episodes. Orthostatic hypotension is a common problem for clients with cardiovascular diseases. Therefore, it is important for the nurse to determine if the client experiences light-headedness or syncope when rising from a prone to an upright position (Table 4-1).

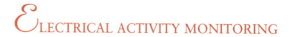

𝓔LECTRICAL ACTIVITY MONITORING

Electrocardiography (ECG)

Dysrhythmias are diagnosed with an ECG. This procedure consists of placing electrode leads on the client's skin that measure the electrical activity of the heart and display it in a waveform configuration. The number and placement of the leads depend on the number of views the health care provider wants to analyze. Generally this type of monitoring requires

TABLE 4-1
SIX CARDINAL SYMPTOMS OF CARDIOVASCULAR DISEASE

Symptom	Presentation
Dyspnea	The patient experiences shortness of breath and air hunger. It may increase gradually or have a sudden onset. It often occurs on exertion and may cause severe limitations to patient activity. Some patients will assume an air hunger position, sitting in a high Fowler's position with elbows out and leaning forward to breathe.
Chest pain or other discomfort	Chest pain may be felt as actual pain or a tightness in the chest wall. The pain may be gripping or dull. Patients also complain of left arm pain or jaw pain. Patients often cannot distinguish chest pain from indigestion.
Palpitations	A fluttering, pounding, or racing heart, or a feeling of skipped beats are words clients often use to describe their palpitations. The nurse may be able to palpate skipped beats and other dysrhythmias during the assessment of the patient's pulse.
Edema	Edema may be generalized or dependent. Assess if the edema is worse at night with improvement in the morning. The patient may complain of clothes, shoes, and jewelry being too tight. Salt intake may cause fluid retention. Restrictive clothes may leave indentations on the skin. Assess for recent weight gain.
Syncope	The patient may complain of lightheadedness, dizziness, or frequent falls. The presence of bruises may indicate syncopal episodes. The patient may flush and feel weak. Assess if the syncope occurs randomly or when standing up from a prone position.
Excessive fatigue	The patient may complain of being too tired to perform the activities of daily living. The onset is gradual, so the patient may adjust to it without realizing that it is a problem. Assess if the patient is taking frequent naps and inquire about changes in the patient's ability to function during a typical day.

either 3, 5, or 12 leads. Nurses most commonly use lead II. For a 3-lead system, lead II is used by placing the negative electrode at the right shoulder below the clavicle, the ground electrode at the left shoulder below the clavicle, and the positive electrode on the lower left torso, generally below the rib cage (Thelan, Davie, Urden, & Lough, 1994). The MCL1 is a widely used lead position because it identifies bundle branch blocks more accurately and distinguishes ventricular ectopy from aberrant ventricular conduction. For an MCL1 ECG tracing, the positive electrode should be placed at the fourth intercostal space to the right of the sternum, the negative electrode is placed at the left shoulder below the clavicle, and the ground electrode is placed at the right shoulder below the clavicle (Thelan et al., 1994 [Fig. 4-1].

Telemetry Monitoring

Telemetry monitoring is the continuous monitoring of the heart's electrical activity. A rhythm strip is produced that consists of waves, complexes, and intervals. The strip is printed on special paper containing small and large

Telemetry monitoring is the tracing of the electrical activity of the heart using a remote monitor.

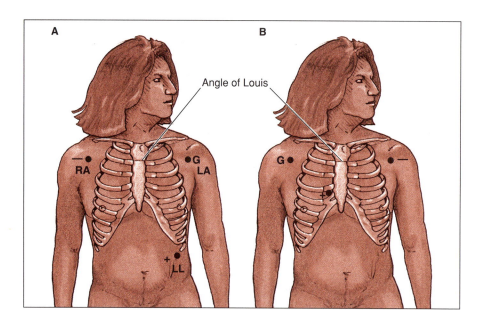

FIGURE 4-1

⌧

Electrode placement in a three-lead system for A lead II and B MCL1.

blocks that represent time. Each small block represents 0.04 seconds, and each large block represents 0.20 seconds. During atrial depolarization, the electrical activity of the heart is represented by a P-wave formation on the rhythm strip. P waves should be present for every QRS complex. They should not be higher or wider than three small blocks and should be upright. During ventricular depolarization, the electrical activity of the heart is represented by a QRS complex on the rhythm strip. These complexes should be upright, no more than 0.12 seconds in width, and should have a regular pattern. The regularity of the QRS complex is determined by assessing the consistency of the distances from R to R. During ventricular repolarization, the electrical activity of the heart is represented by a T wave on the rhythm strip. T waves should be upright and no more than 0.20 seconds in height.

The PR interval is from the beginning of the P wave to the beginning of the QRS complex. This represents the length of time from atrial depolarization to the beginning of ventricular depolarization. This interval should be present with each QRS and should be 0.12–0.20 seconds in length. A prolonged interval represents heart block. The ST interval, which should be at the baseline, represents ventricular systole. A depressed or elevated ST interval indicates the presence of tissue ischemia, most likely as a result of an acute myocardial infarction. Normal sinus rhythm is defined as a normal P wave followed by a normal QRS complex followed by a normal T wave, with regular intervals between the complexes. Sinus refers to the impulse initiation that occurs in the sinoatrial node (Fig. 4-2 and Table 4-2).

The presence of ectopic beats on the rhythm strip must also be assessed. These beats indicate that the impulse did not begin in the sinoatrial node. They can be atrial, junctional, or ventricular. Atrial ectopy presents as premature atrial contractions (PACs), paroxysmal atrial tachycardia (PAT), atrial fibrillation, and atrial flutter. PACs result from an ectopic focus in the atria and appear as early, abnormally shaped P waves. PAT is

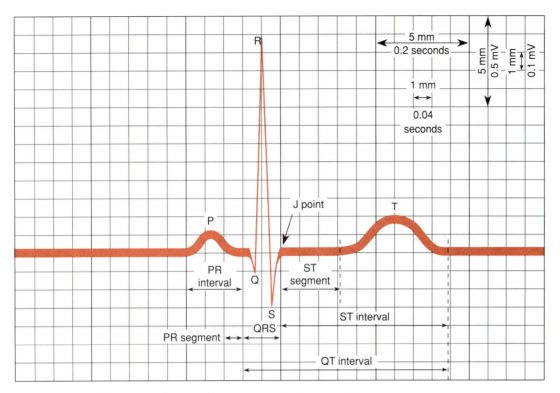

FIGURE 4-2 Deflection and intervals in a normal electrocardiogram.

a short-duration tachycardia with a sudden onset. Atrial fibrillation is an irregular rate in which the sites in the atria fire rapidly but ineffectively. On the rhythm strip, no P waves are seen, but in reality they are present and numerous. Atrial flutter is similar to atrial fibrillation in that the sites in the atria fire rapidly but ineffectively. The rhythm strip shows multiple P waves in a sawtooth pattern between QRS complexes.

In junctional ectopy the focus is either at the junction of the atrioventricular node and the atrium or at the junction of the atrioventricular node and the bundle of His. Depending on the site of impulse initiation, the rhythm strip shows a junctional rhythm as either an inverted P wave preceding a normal QRS complex or a P wave that is buried in the QRS or inverted following the QRS (Thelan et al., 1994). This dysrhythmia presents as premature junctional contractions (PJCs), junctional escape rhythms, or junctional tachycardia. Junctional escape rhythms occur when the heart is in bradycardia and the atrioventricular node fires to stabilize the rhythm.

Sinus, atrial, and junctional tachycardia are occasionally so rapid that it is difficult to distinguish a P wave. When this occurs the tachycardia is termed supraventricular tachycardia (SVT). This designation means that the tachycardia has originated from a site other than a ventricular pacemaker cell.

When impulse initiation occurs in a ventricular pacemaker cell, ventricular dysrhythmias result, and the QRS is altered. In PVCs, the QRS has a wide, bizarre pattern that is readily identifiable. Ventricular tachycardia

▨

TABLE 4-2

STEPS FOR INTERPRETING AN ECG RHYTHM STRIP

Step	Procedure	Interpretation
Rate	Estimate the heart rate by counting the number of QRS complexes in a 6-second strip and multiplying by 10.	Is the rate slow (bradycardia), fast (tachycardia), or normal?
Rhythm	Measure the R-to-R intervals in a 6-second strip by placing an index card across the top of the strip and making vertical marks at the point of two R waves. Then move the card across the strip and see if the R-to-R interval is the same as between each QRS interval.	Is the R-to-R interval regular or irregular?
P waves	Examine for the presence or absence of P waves. Measure the height and width of the P wave.	Are the P waves present or absent? Are they before each QRS, buried within the QRS, or after the QRS? Are they upright and no more than 0.12 seconds?
PR intervals	Count the number of small squares from the start of a P wave to the start of the QRS complex and multiply by 0.04 seconds.	Is the PR interval present? Is it normal (0.12–0.20 sec), shortened, or prolonged?
QRS complexes	Count the number of small squares between the Q and the S waves and multiply by 0.04 seconds.	Is the QRS upright? Is the QRS narrow or wide (> 0.12 sec)?
ST segments	Assess the appearance of the ST segment. Check if the ST segment is at the baseline of the strip.	Are the ST segments at the baseline, elevated, or depressed?
T waves	Assess if they are upright or inverted. Measure their height.	Are they upright or inverted? Are they normal in height (no more than 0.20 sec)?
Ectopic beats	Assess for indications that the impulse did not start from the sinoatrial node.	Are there atrial, junctional, or ventricular abnormalities?

presents as a continuous pattern of wide QRS complexes without discernible P or T waves. Ventricular fibrillation presents as a mild deflection or bumpy-looking baseline with no discernible complexes (Fig. 4-3).

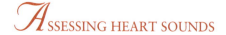ASSESSING HEART SOUNDS

Nurses often complain that it is difficult to assess heart sounds. The difficulty arises from uncertainty as to what one is actually hearing. In

(text continues on page 79)

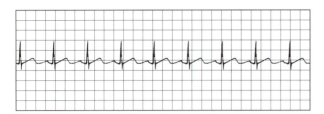

Normal sinus rhythm

Sinus node is the pacemaker, firing at a regular rate of 60–100 times per minute. Each beat is conducted normally through to the ventricles.

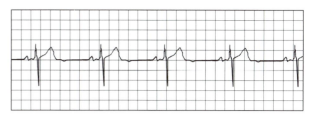

Sinus bradycardia

Sinus node is the pacemaker, firing regularly at a rate of less than 60 times per minute. Each impulse is conducted normally through to the ventricles.

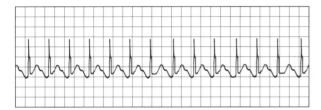

Sinus tachycardia

Sinus node is the pacemaker, firing regularly at a rate of greater than 100 times per minute. Each impulse is conducted normally through to the ventricles.

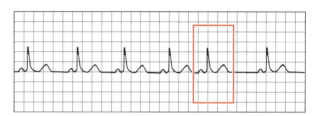

Premature atrial contraction

The pacemaker is an irritable focus within the atrium that fires prematurely and produces a single ectopic beat. Conduction through to the ventricles is normal.

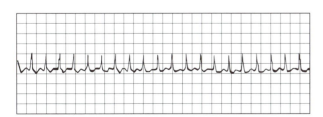

Atrial tachycardia

The pacemaker is a single irritable site within the atrium that fires repeatedly at a very rapid rate. Conduction through to the ventricles is normal.

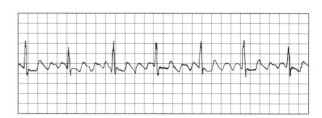

Atrial flutter

A single irritable focus within the atria issues an impulse that is conducted in a rapid, repetitive fashion. To protect the ventricles from receiving too many impulses, the atrioventricular node blocks some of the impulses from being conducted through to the ventricles.

FIGURE 4-3 Electrocardiogram (ECG) rhythm strip identification. (NOTE: From *Basic Arrhythmias* [3rd. ed.] by G Walraven, 1992, Englewood Cliffs, NJ: Prentice-Hall. Reprinted with permission.)

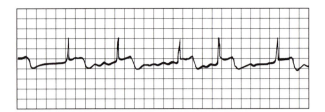

Atrial fibrillation

The atria are so irritable that a multitude of foci initiate impulses, causing the atria to depolarize repeatedly in a fibrillatory manner. The AV node blocks most of the impulses, allowing only a limited number through to the ventricles.

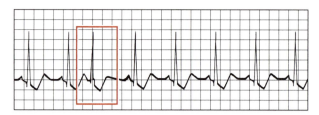

Premature junctional contraction

The pacemaker is an irritable focus within the atrioventricular junction that fires prematurely and produces a single ectopic beat. The atria are depolarized via retrograde conduction. Conduction through the ventricles is normal.

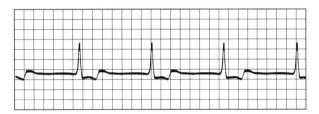

Junctional escape rhythm

When higher pacemaker sites fail, the atrioventricular junction is left with pacemaking responsibility. The atria are depolarized via retrograde conduction. Ventricular conduction is normal.

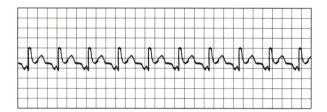

Junctional tachycardia

An irritable focus in the atrioventricular junction speeds up to override the sinoatrial nodes control of the heart. The atria are depolarized via retrograde conduction. Conduction through the ventricles is normal.

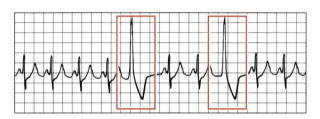

Premature ventricular contraction

A premature ventricular contraction is a single irritable focus within the ventricles that fires prematurely to initiate an ectopic complex.

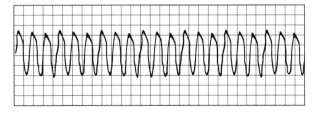

Ventricular tachycardia

An irritable focus in the ventricles fires regularly at a rate of 150–250 beats per minute to override higher sites for control of the heart.

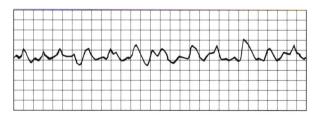

Ventricular fibrillation

Multiple foci in the ventricles become irritable and generate uncoordinated, chaotic impulses that cause the heart to fibrillate rather than contract.

FIGURE 4-3 Electrocardiogram (ECG) rhythm strip identification (*continued*).

assessing heart sounds, the nurse should use a systematic approach. Initially, the client should sit up and lean forward or lie in the left lateral recumbent position. The nurse should make sure the client is relaxed and warm. The nurse must take time to isolate each sound rather than attempt to hear all of the sounds of the cycle at once. The diaphragm of the stethoscope can be used to assess each area first, followed by the bell.

Mnemonic Device

As a simple approach, the nurse should memorize the mnemonic device, "**APE To Man**." Starting at the (A) aortic valve area found at the second right intercostal space to the right of the sternal border, listen for the S2 sound. S2 is of lower pitch and shorter duration than S1 and is louder than S1 in the aortic and pulmonic valve area. At the aortic valve area, the nurse should hear "**lub DUB**"; the "DUB" is the **S2** sound. The nurse should listen carefully while the client inhales and exhales to determine if the S2 is one or two sounds. A split S2 sound occasionally can be heard. This process should be repeated in the (P) pulmonic valve area, which is located at the second left intercostal space to the left of the sternal border.

The next area to be assessed is (E) Erb's point, the second pulmonic valve area. This area is located at the third intercostal space at the left sternal border. While assessing this area, the nurse must instruct the client to take a deep breath and hold it for a second. Listen for a possible split S2 sound during inspiration. This is normal.

The next area to be assessed is the (T) tricuspid valve area. This area is located at the fourth intercostal space along the lower left sternal border. The nurse should hear "**LUB dub**." The "LUB" is the S1 sound. S1 is loudest at the tricuspid and mitral valve areas. There should be no split sound in S1 such as that heard in S2. The next area to be assessed is the (M) mitral valve area. This area is located at the fifth intercostal space at the midclavicular line, which should be the apex of the heart. The S1 sound should be assessed in this area as well.

The mnemonic "**APE To Man**" can be used to remember the landmarks of heart sound assessment: "A," aortic; "P," pulmonic; "E," Erb's point; "T," tricuspid; and "M," mitral.

The heart sound **S1** is "**LUB dub**." **S2** is "**lub DUB**." **S3** is "**LUB dub dub**." **S4** is "**lub LUB dub**."

Extra Heart Sounds

Extra heart sounds that may occur, other than the normal S1 and S2 sounds, include S3, S4, snaps, clicks, murmurs, and rubs. S3 is an early diastolic heart sound immediately following S2. It is a ventricular gallop that is best heard by placing the bell of the stethoscope at the apex of the heart. **S3** has a "**LUB dub dub**" sound. It is caused by rapid ventricular filling that produces vibrations of the ventricular wall. S4 is an atrial gallop that is best heard by placing the bell of the stethoscope at the apex of the heart. It is caused by forceful atrial ejection into a distended ventricle. When present, the S4 sound is more readily discernible than the S3 sound. S4 is a late diastolic sound heard just before S1. **S4** has a "**lub LUB dub**" sound.

Snaps and clicks sound just like what their names suggest. A snap is heard when a stenotic mitral or tricuspid valve recoils abruptly. It is often confused with the S3 sound. Clicks occur as a result of the opening of deformed semilunar valves or because of mitral valve prolapse. Murmurs occur when blood is disrupted from its usual flow, producing a sound like a "gurgling brook." Murmurs may be so pronounced that a thrill in the chest wall is felt as well. Rubs sound like two tissues being rubbed together and are often heard in inflammatory processes such as pericarditis.

DIAGNOSTIC PROCEDURES

Recent advances in technology have improved the diagnosis and treatment of clients with cardiovascular disease. A number of laboratory tests, as well as ultrasonic, dynamic, and radiological studies can now be used to assist the health care provider in diagnosing cardiovascular disease. The nurse needs to be familiar with these procedures, as many of them require nursing expertise.

Laboratory Tests

Laboratory tests that measure CBC, ESR, PT, APTT, BUN, LDL and HDL, triglycerides, cholesterol, and the cardiac enzymes are frequently performed to assess the cardiovascular system.

Numerous laboratory tests are used to diagnose and as aids in the treatment of cardiovascular disease. A complete blood count (CBC) is often done. The red blood cell (RBC) count is decreased in subacute endocarditis and is increased with inadequate tissue oxygenation. The white blood cell (WBC) count is increased in acute and chronic heart inflammations and in acute myocardial infarctions.

The erythrocyte sedimentation rate (ESR) is increased in acute myocardial infarctions and in infectious heart disease. The prothrombin time (PT) is used to monitor warfarin (Coumadin) therapy. This test is reported as an international normal ratio (INR), which is used to measure the level of anticoagulation. The desired INR depends on the client's disease process. As a general rule, the INR should be 1.5–2.5 if the client is receiving warfarin. For a systemic embolism, the INR should be 2.0–3.0 (Fischbach, 1996). After cardiac stents are placed and to prevent thrombus formation in clients with mechanical valves, the INR should be 3.0–4.5 (Fischbach, 1996). The activated partial thromboplastin time (APTT) is used to monitor heparin therapy. Each laboratory determines its own normal and therapeutic values of this test, since multiple techniques can be used to obtain an APTT value. Currently, the dosage of heparin is adjusted frequently, using a sliding scale based on the level of anticoagulation determined by APTT.

The blood urea nitrogen (BUN) concentration increases with decreased cardiac output. A decreased cardiac output that results in renal compromise also increases the serum creatinine level. The serum protein levels decrease with edema.

Blood lipids are assessed as a risk factor for cardiovascular disease and to diagnose hyperlipidemia. The LDL concentration should be less than 160 mg/dL. A higher concentration means that the client is at high risk for coronary artery disease. The high-density lipoprotein (HDL) concentration should be greater than 35 mg/dL. If the levels are lower than 35 mg/dL, the client is at risk for coronary artery disease. LDLs are considered the bad lipoproteins, and HDLs are considered the good lipoproteins, as it is better to have less LDL and more HDL. Total cholesterol levels should be in the range of 150–240 mg/dL, and triglycerides should be in the range of 10–190 mg/dL. Higher concentrations increase the risk for developing coronary artery disease.

Cardiac enzymes from clients with coronary artery disease are also analyzed. These are assessed to determine if a client has experienced a myocardial infarction. The **cardiac enzymes** consist of serum aspartate aminotransferase (AST), creatine kinase (CK), creatine kinase MB (CKMB), CKMB mass, troponin I, and lactate dehydrogenase (LDH). The AST concentration increases following either an acute myocardial infarction or liver damage. Following an acute myocardial infarction, the level rises in 6–10 hours and peaks in 24–48 hours. If no additional infarction occurs, the level returns to normal in 4–6 days.

The **cardiac enzymes** are AST, CK, CKMB, CKMB mass, troponin I, and LDH.

Creatine kinase increases in response to damage to the heart and skeletal muscle. It increases within 4–6 hours post–myocardial infarction, peaks in 12–24 hours, and returns to normal within 3–4 days if no further damage occurs. The creatine kinase concentration elevates in response to muscle damage. To prevent a false-positive result, the client should not receive an intramuscular injection prior to providing a specimen for this test. Creatine kinase is divided into three separate isoenzymes. One of the three isoenzymes, CKMB, is specific to the heart. A CKMB level greater than 6% of the creatine kinase level strongly indicates a myocardial infarction. A CKMB mass can be assessed to measure the CKMB level without interferences from other isoenzymes associated with the CK.

LDH is an enzyme found in the heart, skeletal muscle, RBCs, liver, kidney, lungs, and brain. LDH levels increase 12–24 hours post–myocardial infarction, peak in 2–5 days, and remain elevated for 6–12 days. Since LDH levels remain elevated for a long period after a myocardial infarction, they are useful in diagnosing a subacute myocardial infarction. The LDH1:LDH2 ratio is the most sensitive indicator of myocardial damage. Normally, the LDH1 isoenzyme level is 14–26% of the LDH, and the LDH2 is 27–37% of the LDH. An opposite ratio in which the LDH1 level is higher than the LDH2 indicates that a myocardial infarction has occurred.

Troponin I is a contractile protein found exclusively in cardiac muscle. Elevations occur as early as 3–6 hours after onset of chest pain. The elevation may remain for up to 9 days.

Ultrasound Studies

Ultrasound studies allow the physician to visualize the structures of the heart and blood flow through the heart and peripheral vessels.

Ultrasound studies examine cardiovascular structure and blood flow.

Doppler Scans Doppler scans, which depend on sensitive measurements of the change in sound generated as blood moves past a point in a blood vessel, are also ultrasound studies. For example, a nurse assesses peripheral pulses with a Doppler probe. If a peripheral blood flow obstruction is suspected, the radiologist passes an ultrasound transducer over the peripheral blood vessels and then examines the image on a monitor for blood flow abnormalities.

Echocardiogram The echocardiogram is one of the most commonly performed studies designed to assess heart structure. This noninvasive procedure detects abnormalities of the heart, particularly structural abnormalities. It can detect abnormal pericardial fluid, valvular disorders, ventricular aneurysms, tumors, size of the cardiac chambers, stroke volume, cardiac output, and some myocardial abnormalities. During an echocardiogram, an ultrasound transducer is placed over the client's heart, and the image is viewed on a monitor.

Transesophageal Echocardiogram If the client has chronic obstructive pulmonary disease (COPD) or is obese, a transesophageal echocardiogram may be performed. A transducer connected to a flexible endoscope is inserted into the esophagus of the client. As COPD and obesity can interfere with the transmission of the image obtained by transthoracic echocardiography, this method allows for better visualization of the image. Some clinical indications for transesophageal echocardiography include aortic dissection, mitral valve prosthetic dysfunction, mitral valve regurgitation, infective endocarditis, congenital heart disease, intracardiac thrombi, and cardiac tumor. It is also used intraoperatively to assess left ventricular function and to determine whether a valve requires repair or replacement. Possible complications include esophageal perforation, pharyngeal bleeding, hypoxia, and cardiac dysrhythmias.

To prepare for a transesophageal echocardiograph examination, nurses must take a thorough client history to determine the presence of any esophageal abnormalities or past surgeries. The nurse should also assess for a history of allergic or adverse reactions to local anesthetics or sedatives. Most clients receive both a mild sedative and a local anesthetic before the device is inserted into their esophagus. The client should be given nothing by mouth for 4–6 hours prior to the procedure. The client's dentures and partial plates must be removed. An intravenous line (either a heparin lock or a keep vein open [KVO] infusion of normal saline) is generally started before the examination. Suction and resuscitation equipment should also be kept readily available.

Dynamic Studies

Clients wearing a **Holter monitor** must keep an activity log.

Holter Monitoring In this test the client's cardiac rhythm is assessed for 24 hours using a recording device. The client wears the monitor, which records the ECG rhythm strip continuously and automatically or when the client presses a button. Holter monitoring is used to detect intermittent dysrhythmias. The client needs to be taught how to operate the device and to wear it at all times. He or she should keep an activity log throughout the test. Some models have a button that clients can press to indicate when they have felt a dysrhythmia.

Stress Testing Stress testing is the process of applying stress to the heart and recording its reaction to it. The applied stress is either exercise induced or chemically induced (nonexercise).

Exercise Stress Test In an exercise stress test, the client exercises, usually on a treadmill, while being monitored. The client's blood pressure and heart rate are constantly monitored by an ECG. Occasionally, an echocardiogram is performed during the examination. Informed consent is required prior to exercise stress testing. The client should avoid caffeine the day of the examination. The client should also avoid smoking and taking nitroglycerin for two hours prior to the test. Digoxin (Lanoxin), propranolol (Inderal), and vasodilators should not be taken, as these may alter the test. The client may eat a light meal prior to the examination. The nurse should instruct the client to wear comfortable clothes and appropriate walking shoes. The client should also be instructed not to take a hot shower following the examination.

Clients scheduled for stress tests should not smoke or have caffeine the day of the exam. Nitroglycerin should be withheld for at least two hours prior to the exam.

Nonexercise Stress Test A nonexercise stress test is performed in the same manner as an exercise stress test except without exercise. The effects of exercise on the heart are chemically induced by adenosine, dipyridamole (Persantine), or dobutamine (Dobutrex). Dobutamine (Dobutrex) is a recent addition to the arsenal of medications that are given to induce the effects of exercise chemically. It more closely parallels the gradual myocardial effects of exercise (Thompson, Detwiler, & Nelson, 1996). The client must be treated the same way as for an exercise stress test. The nonexercise stress test replaces the exercise stress test if the client is either unable to exercise or the physician believes the exercise effects will be easier to control if chemically induced.

Imaging Studies

Thallium Scan Exercise stress tests are often combined with thallium imaging, a nuclear medicine study. Thallium is a nuclear agent that enhances visualization of the heart during a stress test. The client is given nothing by mouth until after the thallium is injected. The thallium is injected when the client reaches maximum heart stress on the treadmill. The distribution of the thallium is then visualized. It is diminished in areas of ischemia. This is generally a two-part test; a second scan is done after the heart has had time to rest.

Multiple Gated Acquisition (MUGA) and Positron Emission Tomography (PET) MUGA and PET scans are other types of imaging scans that are used to examine blood flow and myocardial metabolism. Unlike in thallium scans, in these studies the radioactive isotope stays in the bloodstream and is not picked up by the cardiac tissues. MUGA and PET are used to detect left ventricle ejection fraction, right ventricular infarction, aneurysms, and the effects of nitroglycerin and vasodilators on ventricular function.

The client history must assess the presence of implanted metal. Jewelry and implanted metal objects are contraindicated during a MRI scan.

Magnetic Resonance Imaging (MRI) MRI is used to detect aneurysms, cardiac output, and valve function. Prior to undergoing the study, the client should be warned that MRI machines emit a very loud knocking sound when in use. The client must also be told that he or she must lie within a small, cylindrical area and remain absolutely still for a long period of time. Many clients feel claustrophobic during this procedure, and it is not uncommon for it to be discontinued as a result of the client's anxiety. Since the MRI machine emits a magnetic field, the nurse should remove the client's jewelry and any other metal objects from the body. While taking the client's history, the nurse should determine if any past surgeries have left metal implanted in the client's body. MRI is not performed if the client has a pacemaker. It may not be performed if certain types of metal have been implanted during surgery or from some type of injury.

Angiogram An angiogram examines peripheral blood flow. It is used to determine the presence of a lower extremity obstruction. This examination is indicated when the client experiences the manifestations of decreased circulation such as edema, pain, coolness of the extremity, decreased pulses, and delayed capillary refill. The angiogram catheter is generally inserted into the right or left femoral artery. Contrast material is injected through the catheter, and a radiographic image is produced. Nonvisualization of part or all of a blood vessel indicates blockage.

Cardiac Catheterization Cardiac catheterization is similar to angiography. The catheter is inserted into the femoral artery, as in angiography. The dye, however, is injected into the coronary arteries. This allows visualization of blood flow through the arteries. The following case study illustrates this point.

CASE STUDY: CARDIAC CATHETERIZATION

A 59-year-old man is admitted to the hospital for possible coronary artery disease. He has been experiencing intermittent chest pains for the past two years. In the past, these episodes have been relieved with sublingual nitroglycerin. For the last month, however, his pain has occurred more frequently, and the nitroglycerin has been less effective in controlling the pain. He smokes one pack of cigarettes per day. The client underwent an exercise stress test in the physician's office two days previously and experienced chest pain during the examination. He is now scheduled for cardiac catheterization.

Nursing care Nursing requirements for both angiograms and cardiac catheterizations include the following points: The client must give informed consent prior to the examination. The groin area must be shaved and prepped. A client history should be obtained to determine if the client is allergic to the contrast dyes used in radiological studies. The client is usually given nothing by mouth until after the examination is completed.

An intravenous line (heparin lock access or infusion of normal saline) is often required during angiography or cardiac catheterization. A mild sedative is usually administered prior to the examination. Following the examination, the nurse must instruct the client that the extremity that was injected must be kept straight for 4–6 hours. The nurse should examine the insertion site frequently for signs of bleeding or hematoma formation. The nurse should frequently assess the client's vital signs, the pulses below the injection site, and capillary refill time. The extremities also should be assessed in terms of color, movement, temperature, and sensation (CMTS). When clients return to their rooms, they will have a small bandage over the insertion site and a sandbag may be placed over the site to provide pressure. Clients need to be informed that the head of the bed should not be elevated higher than 30 degrees.

A **peripheral circulation assessment** includes color, motion, temperature, sensation, pulses, and capillary refill of the extremity.

The client in the case study is likely to be concerned about both the cardiac catheterization and the final diagnosis. Cardiac catheterization has a number of risks, including perforation of a vessel, infarction, bleeding, hematoma formation, dysrhythmias, and cardiac arrest. The nurse should allow the client to explore his or her feelings of fear and anxiety openly. During the preparation for this examination, the nurse can assess the client's understanding of the procedure. It is also important that the nurse inform the client of the procedures he or she will undergo following the catheterization.

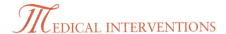MEDICAL INTERVENTIONS

Several medical therapies can be used when caring for a client with a cardiovascular disorder. Risk factor modification, pharmacotherapies, implantable and external regulatory devices, and invasive and noninvasive procedures are all used to manage cardiovascular diseases. Deciding which therapy to use depends on the client's overall condition, the availability of the therapy, and the client's response to the various therapies.

Risk Factor Modification

Risk factor modification is used as an adjunct to other therapies and for clients who are at risk but not exhibiting the symptoms of cardiac disease. Clients who use risk factor modification must understand what the risk factors are for developing cardiovascular disease. Many clients who are experiencing cardiovascular disease think, incorrectly, that since the disease is already present, there is no point in changing life-style patterns. For example, the client in the above scenario is a smoker. By quitting smoking, his condition may improve within the first year. Client education is an important part of the **nursing responsibilities** that this therapy entails.

Risk factor modification is physically, psychosocially, and culturally difficult.

Dietary Changes Clients who practice risk factor modification require assistance to make the necessary changes in their diet. A dietician may be consulted to develop a plan for dietary management. As a general rule, clients are encouraged to limit their fat and cholesterol intake. Polyunsaturated and saturated fats should comprise less than 10% of total caloric intake. Monounsaturated fats should comprise 10–15% of total calories, and cholesterol intake should be less than 300 mg per day. This type of life-style change is never easy. Since different cultures are partly identified by the foods they consume, nurses have little success in changing clients' food choices. It is important for the nurse to recognize that restructuring a client's dietary habits is a slow, painstaking process.

Weight Control Other important behavior modifications to reduce risk factors include assisting the client in weight control; increasing levels of activity, especially aerobic activity; and reducing stress. Clients should perform aerobic exercise for at least 30 minutes, three times per week to attain and maintain cardiovascular health. Some clients find this impossible as a result of their physical condition, while other clients refuse to comply with an exercise regimen. Isometric exercise is generally discouraged for clients with existing cardiovascular disease. Nurses can assist clients by helping them find activities they enjoy and are likely to perform consistently. The nurse should encourage the client to celebrate successful life-style changes rather than focusing on periods of noncompliance. If the client complies with the dietary guidelines and exercise regimen, weight control is not likely to be a problem. Unfortunately, these elements are connected, and relapses in one area affect all three.

Stress Reduction Reducing stress is a difficult task. The client may have conflicts between family, work, and community responsibilities. Occasionally, the client needs intervention to deal with stress rather than control it. Therapies such as massage and guided imagery may help to reduce stress. Setting priorities and goals can also help. Nurses' priorities are to work with the client to set goals and to assist the client in finding resources to deal with stress. Forcing the client either to not work or to limit responsibilities often increases rather than reduces the client's stress. To modify the client's behavior, the nurse needs to work with and support the client, rather than be directive and forceful. The nurse only sees the client for a short period, and permanently altering a client's life style takes time.

Pharmacological Management

Several medications treat cardiovascular disorders. Hypertension, decreased circulation, congestive heart failure (CHF), hyperlipidemia, angina, and various dysrhythmias are generally managed with a variety of pharmacological therapies. Adjuncts such as diuretics and electrolyte replacements are often used in addition to the cardiovascular agent. It is important that the nurse be aware of the effects of the cardiovascular medications. Nurses often know the adverse effects but may not be aware of the therapeutic effects, which should be committed to memory as well (Table 4-3).

(text continues on page 92)

TABLE 4-3

CARDIOVASCULAR PHARMACOLOGY

Classification	Action	Examples of Agents	Adverse Effects	Nursing Considerations
Anticoagulants	Prevent enlargement of existing thrombus or formation of new thrombus. Allow the thrombus to be absorbed or to adhere to the vessel wall.	Heparin, warfarin (Coumadin)	Bleeding, thrombosis, thrombocytopenia, gastrointestinal distress, osteoporosis, skin necrosis, hyperaldosteronism	Tissue trauma precautions. Monitor APTT for heparin and PT for warfarin. Expect PTT and PT to be 1.5 times above normal for therapeutic effect. Heparin is incompatible with most other intravenous agents. Antidotes include protamine sulfate for heparin and vitamin K for warfarin.
Antiplatelets	Inhibit platelet adhesion to vessel walls.	Aspirin, dipyridamole (Persantine), pentoxifylline (Trental), ticlopidine (Ticlid)	Gastrointestinal distress, gastrointestinal bleeding, headache, hepatitis, anemia, thrombocytopenia, prolonged prothrombin time, tinnitus, hearing loss, rapid pulse, wheezing, hyponatremia, hypokalemia, hypoglycemia	Dipyridamole is given 1 hour before meals, aspirin is given 30 minutes before or 2 hours after meals. Medications must be taken long term. The client must avoid alcohol and smoking; antacids decrease absorption.
Inotropics	Improve myocardial contractility to increase cardiac output.	Digoxin (Lanoxin) amrinone lactate injection (Inocor), dobutamine (Dobutrex), dopamine (Inotropin), epinephrine, isoproterenol (Isuprel), norepinephrine (Levophed)	Digoxin toxicity results in tachycardia, angina, fatigue, anorexia, headache, arrhythmias, visual disturbances, nausea, and vomiting. Other agents result in arrhythmias, hypotension, thrombocytopenia, and flushing.	Monitor vital signs frequently, correct hypokalemia before administration. For digoxin, take an apical pulse; if < 60 beats/min, consult a physician before administration. Monitor digoxin level. Correct any underlying fluid deficits before administration. Intravenous routes are potentially life threatening, especially if the wrong dose is given. Know how to calculate intravenous rates (mg/min, μg/kg/min). Antidotes include digoxin-specific antibody (Digibind) for digoxin, atropine for norepinephrine, and phentolamine (Regitine) for dopamine infiltration. Intravenous digoxin must be diluted in at least 5 mL and given over 5 minutes with continuous ECG monitoring.

TABLE 4-3 (*continued*)

CARDIOVASCULAR PHARMACOLOGY

Classification	Action	Examples of Agents	Adverse Effects	Nursing Considerations
Nitrates	Reduce myocardial workload and the need for oxygen. Nitroglycerin is given for angina pain.	Nitroglycerin, isosorbide	Headache, orthostatic hypotension, nausea, vomiting, flushing, fast pulse, dermatitis, skin irritation	Monitor vital signs and ECG. Administer nitroglycerin in glass bottles with lipid-compatible tubing. Wear gloves when applying nitroglycerin patches. Nitroglycerin has a short expiration date.
β-blocker anti-hypertensives	Reduce peripheral vascular resistance.	Atenolol (Tenormin), metoprolol (Lopressor), nadolol (Corgard), propranolol (Inderal)	Fatigue, lethargy, depression, exercise intolerance, diminished mental acuity, hypotension, second- and third-degree heart block, dyspnea, impotence	Hypotension can occur when bathed in hot water. Client must avoid alcohol. β-blockers are contraindicated for clients with CHF or second- or third-degree heart block. Client intolerance is common.
ACE inhibitors anti-hypertensives	Decrease systemic vascular resistance by preventing breakdown of bradykinin. This results in dilation of arterial and venous vessels. It lowers blood pressure and decreases preload and afterload in clients with CHF.	Captopril (Capoten), enalapril (Vasotec), lisinopril (Prinivil)	Dry nonproductive cough, dizziness, mood changes, hyperkalemia, blood dyscrasias, headache, impotence, acute renal failure	ACE inhibitors interact with antacids, diuretics, NSAIDs, and lithium- and potassium-sparing diuretics. Monitor potassium levels.

Category	Examples	Action	Side effects	Nursing considerations
Calcium channel blocker antihypertensives	Diltiazem (Cardizem), nifedipine (Procardia), verapamil (Calan)	Inhibit calcium ion influx during cardiac depolarization, resulting in smooth muscle relaxation by preventing contraction. Coronary artery dilation lowers blood pressure, and an antianginal effect results from increased oxygen delivery in patients with vasopressic hypertension.	Hypotension, palpitations, tachycardia, rash, flushing, peripheral edema, wheezing, sexual difficulties	Interacts with digoxin, β-blockers, and H_2 blockers.
Adrenergic antihypertensives	Clonidine (Catapres)	Inhibit vasoconstriction, thereby reducing blood pressure.	Orthostatic hypotension, fatigue, dizziness, impotence	Medication comes in patch and oral form. Monitor for retinal degeneration. A rebound effect can occur if discontinued suddenly.
Thiazide diuretics	Hydrochlorothiazide (Hydrodiuril), chlorthalidone (Hygroton), zaroxolyn	Inhibit resorption of sodium in the ascending loop and distal tubule.	Hypokalemia, orthostatic hypotension, hyperglycemia, hyperuricemia	Thiazide diuretics are contraindicated if creatinine clearance < 30–50 mL/min. Weigh the client daily. Zaroxolyn is often given 30 minutes before furosemide to increase the diuretic effect.
Loop diuretics	Furosemide (Lasix), ethacrynic acid (Edecrin), bumetanide (Bumex)	Block absorption of sodium and chloride in the ascending loop.	Volume depletion, hypokalemia, reversible hearing loss, gastrointestinal upset	Weigh the client daily, administer with food or milk and monitor electrolytes. Nurses may want to give intravenous form well before bedtime to prevent excessive nocturia. The intravenous form can be administered at a rate of 20 mg/min.

TABLE 4-3 (*continued*)

CARDIOVASCULAR PHARMACOLOGY

Classification	Action	Examples of Agents	Adverse Effects	Nursing Considerations
Potassium-sparing diuretics	Block effect of aldosterone on the tubules.	Spironolactone (Aldactone), triamterene (Dyrenium)	Renal insufficiency, hyperkalemia, sexual dysfunction	Monitor fluid volume status, body weight, and electrolytes.
Magnesium replacement	Increases serum levels of magnesium and prolongs conduction time in the myocardium by decreasing sinoatrial node impulse.	Slo-Mag	Sweating, decreased deep tendon reflexes, flushing, hypotension	Monitor magnesium levels.
Antilipid agents	Restrict lipoprotein production.	Niacin, clofibrate (Atromid S), gemfibrozil (Lopid)	Gastrointestinal upset, increased liver enzymes, cholelithiasis, rash, fatigue, leukopenia, sexual dysfunction, bleeding, pulmonary emboli, angina, renal toxicity	Antilipid agents are contraindicated with present liver dysfunction. They interact with insulin, oral antidiabetic agents, and anticoagulants. Mix antilipid powders with noncarbonated drinks. Long-term use requires fat-soluble vitamin supplements.
Antilipid agents	Increase lipoprotein removal.	Cholestyramine (Questran), colestipol (Colestid)	Same effects as above	Same considerations as above
Antilipid agents	Control cholesterol production.	Lovastatin (Mevacor)	Same effects as above	Same considerations as above
Class I anti-dysrhythmics	Treat symptomatic ventricular and life-threatening dysrhythmias.	Moricizine	Nausea, vomiting, diarrhea, headache, blurred vision, can be pro-arrhythmia.	Monitor vital signs closely. Administer intravenous forms by intravenous pump. Monitor ECG and drug levels.

Drug class	Action	Examples		
Class IA anti-dysrhythmics	Treat atrial fibrillation, PAC, PVC, and ventricular tachycardia.	Procainamide (Pronestyl), disopyramide (Norpace), quinidine (Cin-Quin)	Same as above	Same as above
Class IB anti-dysrhythmics	Treat ventricular dysrhythmias.	Lidocaine (Xylocaine), mexiletine (Mexitil)	Same as above	Same as above
Class IC anti-dysrhythmics	Treat severe ventricular dysrhythmias.	Encainide (Enkaid), flecainide (Tambocor)	Same as above	Same as above
Class II anti-dysrhythmics	Treat SVT and ventricular dysrhythmias.	Atenolol (Tenormin), metoprolol (Lopressor), propranolol (Inderal)	Same as above	Same as above
Class III anti-dysrhythmics	Treat life-threatening ventricular dysrhythmias	Bretylium (Bretylol), amiodarone (Cordarone)	Same as above	Same as above. Take client's apical pulse for 1 full minute with sotalol hydrochloride (Betapace)
Class IV anti-dysrhythmics	Treat PAT and rate control for atrial fibrillation and atrial flutter.	Diltiazem (Cardizem), verapamil (Calan)	Same as above	Same as above

NOTE: ECG = electrocardiogram; APTT = activated partial thromboplastin time; CHF = congestive heart failure; NSAID = nonsteroidal anti-inflammatory drugs; ACEI = angiotensin-converting enzyme inhibitors; PAC = premature atrial contractions; PVC = premature ventricular contractions; SVT = supraventricular tachycardia; PAT = paroxysmal atrial tachycardia; PT = prothrombin time; PTT = partial thromboplastin time.

Nitroglycerin The client in the previously mentioned case study has been receiving nitroglycerin for angina. Nitroglycerin is a nitrate that is used to reduce myocardial consumption of oxygen. In angina, the associated pain may be the result of myocardial ischemia. The client should be taught to take one nitroglycerin tablet sublingually at the onset of chest pain. If the tablet is not effective (i.e., the chest pain is not relieved), the client should be instructed to take another tablet in 5 minutes. The client can take up to three tablets, 5 minutes apart, until the chest pain is relieved. If the chest pain is not relieved after three tablets, the client should contact his or her physician. Common adverse effects of sublingual nitroglycerin include headache and decreased blood pressure. Headache associated with nitroglycerin indicates that the client is receiving an excessive amount. Nitroglycerin remains stable for a very short period of time and is light sensitive. Therefore, clients should be instructed to check expiration dates carefully and keep the sublingual tablets in their original package. Clients are often given transdermal (patch) nitroglycerin that delivers a continuous dose. The patches are usually replaced every day and should be applied to the upper chest, upper back, or upper arms. They should not be applied to the lower extremities. The client in the case study most likely will receive a nitroglycerin patch, since the episodes of angina are occurring more frequently.

Antilipid Agents Antilipid agents are ordered frequently for clients with high lipoprotein levels that cannot be controlled by diet. These agents result in a high incidence of gastrointestinal (GI) distress, fatigue, and altered sexual function. Clients must be taught to notify the physician if shortness of breath occurs, as these agents carry a risk of pulmonary emboli. They are contraindicated in clients who have liver disease. The BUN, creatinine level, and liver enzyme concentrations should be monitored periodically while the client is taking these agents. They interact with insulin, oral antidiabetic agents, and oral anticoagulants. Fat-soluble vitamin supplements should also be administered to clients who must take these on a long-term basis.

Anticoagulation Agents The anticoagulation agents prevent existing thrombi from enlarging and prevent the formation of new thrombi. They do not dissolve existing thrombi. Clients who take anticoagulation agents are at greatest risk for abnormal bleeding. The coagulation studies are monitored regularly while the client receives an anticoagulant. Nurses must educate clients thoroughly concerning anticoagulants. For example, clients should be taught to take the dose as prescribed and to avoid alcohol and over-the-counter drugs. They need to be aware of the dangers of abnormal bleeding and to avoid situations that are likely to cause trauma to the body. Clients even need to be cautious when shaving or brushing their teeth. They should avoid foods high in vitamin K if on warfarin, because vitamin K is the antidote for warfarin. Foods high in vitamin K include tomatoes, dark green leafy vegetables, bananas, and fish. The client must wear a Medic Alert identification bracelet. Coagulation studies should be performed on a regular basis.

Antiplatelet Agents Antiplatelet agents inhibit platelet adhesion to the blood vessels and to each other. Some examples of antiplatelet agents include aspirin, dipyridamole (Persantine), pentoxifylline (Trental), and ticlopidine (Ticlid). These agents improve peripheral tissue perfusion, decrease the pain associated with ischemia, decrease the incidence of dizziness, and improve other neurological symptoms associated with the client's disease state. These agents are generally prescribed for clients with coronary artery disease and peripheral vascular disease. Adverse effects include GI distress and bleeding, headache, hepatitis, thrombocytopenia, tinnitus, hearing loss, wheezing, hypoglycemia, hyponatremia, and hypokalemia. The nurse must teach clients who are receiving antiplatelet agents to report any side effects, such as ringing in the ears, swelling in the lower extremities, dark urine, clay-colored stools, rashes, abdominal pain, blurred vision, or the perception of halos around objects. Clients undergoing antiplatelet therapy should avoid alcohol and smoking. The agents must be taken for a long time to have therapeutic effects. Aspirin should be given 30 minutes before meals or two hours after meals for maximum effectiveness. Dipyridamole (Persantine) should be administered one hour before meals. Administering pentoxifylline (Trental) with digoxin decreases the metabolism of digoxin; therefore, the digoxin levels should be monitored carefully.

Thrombolytic Agents The thrombolytic agents are used to dissolve blood clots. Some examples of these agents include streptokinase, alteplase (Activase, tissue plasminogen activator [TPA]), and urokinase. Urokinase is often used to dissolve a clot obstructing a central venous line. As the client receives streptokinase or alteplase, the nurse needs to monitor the client constantly for the therapeutic effects, which include improved tissue perfusion, decreased chest pain, decreased leg pain, improved shunt performance, and prevention of further myocardial damage. Thrombolytic agents improve perfusion to the myocardium.

A specific client selection process determines who will receive thrombolytics to improve perfusion during a myocardial infarction. As a general rule, alteplase is administered rather than streptokinase. The following criteria must be met before alteplase can be administered:

- The client should be symptomatic for less than six hours.
- The client should have angina for at least 20 minutes that is not relieved by nitroglycerin.
- The ECG should reveal 3 mm or greater ST elevation.

It is contraindicated in clients with active internal bleeding or severe uncontrolled hypertension. The nurse must monitor constantly for reperfusion dysrhythmias following the administration of these agents.

Inotropic Agents Inotropic agents increase myocardial contractility. They are used primarily either to treat or prevent CHF. Examples of inotropic agents include digoxin, amirinone (Inocor), milrinone (Primacor), dobutamine (Dobutrex), dopamine (Inotropin), epinephrine, isoproterenol (Isuprel), and norepinephrine (Levophed). Inotropic agents act to prevent

Early clinical manifestations of **digoxin toxicity** are anorexia, nausea, and lethargy.

or decrease the clinical manifestations of CHF. Clients taking these medications report less shortness of breath at rest and on exertion. The client has clear breath sounds and a decreased incidence of dependent edema. Several adverse effects are associated with these agents, and they have a high incidence of toxicity. As a result of this and the large number of people taking digoxin, nurses must be aware of the clinical manifestations of **digoxin toxicity**. The earliest symptoms of digoxin toxicity include lethargy, nausea, vomiting, and anorexia. Other symptoms are arrhythmia (bradycardia or tachycardia), headache, angina, blurred vision, and seeing greenish-yellow halos around objects. Before administering digoxin, the nurse should auscultate the client's apical pulse for 1 full minute; if it is less than 60 beats/min, he or she should notify the physician. The nurse should monitor the client's digoxin level, as toxicity occurs at a level of more than 2.0 mg/mL.

Underlying **hypokalemia** or **hypovolemia** should be resolved before using inotropic medications.

Any underlying **hypokalemia** or **hypovolemia** should be resolved before administering inotropic agents. The client's vital signs must be monitored frequently, as many of these agents are given intravenously during acute episodes of CHF. Telemetry should be used to monitor clients who receive these medications intravenously. The nurse also should monitor the client's response to these agents. Antidotes exist for both digoxin and norepinephrine (Levophed) toxicity. Digoxin-specific antibody (Digibind) is the antidote for digoxin, and atropine is the antidote for norepinephrine (Levophed).

Antihypertensive Agents Antihypertensive agents are divided into several functional classes. Since there are a large number of agents and more are constantly being developed, it is preferable to learn the therapeutic and adverse effects of the antihypertensive agents by functional class rather than individually (Fig. 4-4). The diuretics and beta-blockers are the most commonly prescribed antihypertensive agents. The preferred diuretics are the thiazides and the potassium-sparing agents. They are used either alone or in combination with each other. The loop diuretics are used for clients with CHF but are not generally used as antihypertensives. Thiazides inhibit the resorption of sodium in the ascending loop and distal tubule. Some examples of antihypertensive agents are hydrochlorothiazide (Hydrodiuril), chlorothiazide (Diuril), chlorthalidone (Hygroton), and zaroxolyn. These medications are contraindicated if the creatinine clearance is less than 30–50 mL/min. They can cause hypokalemia, orthostatic hypotension, hyperglycemia, and hyperuricemia. The client receiving these agents should be monitored for sudden weight loss or weight gain. The client's potassium level needs to be monitored periodically, and potassium supplements may be indicated. Potassium-sparing agents block the effect of aldosterone on the tubules. Spironolactone (Aldactone) and triamterene (Dyrenium) are two examples of these agents. The adverse effects of these agents include renal insufficiency, hyperkalemia, and sexual disturbances. The client is often given a combination agent containing a potassium-sparing diuretic and a thiazide diuretic. When combined, these agents potentiate the antihypertensive effect and may help counteract the adverse effect on the client's potassium level. Triamterene-hydrochlorothiazide

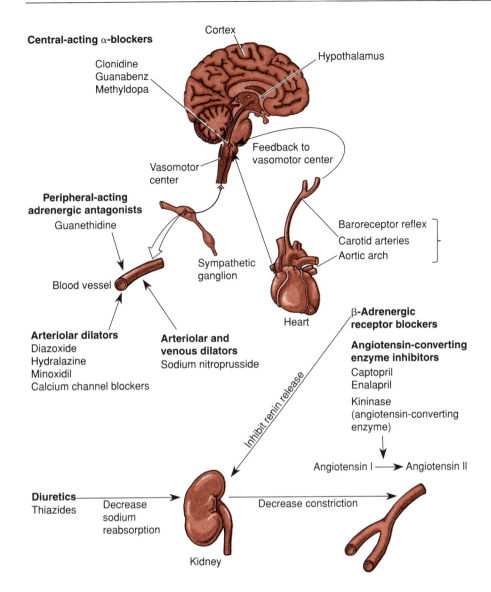

Central-acting α-blockers

Clonidine
Guanabenz
Methyldopa

Cortex

Hypothalamus

Feedback to
vasomotor center

Vasomotor
center

**Peripheral-acting
adrenergic antagonists**

Guanethidine

Baroreceptor reflex
Carotid arteries
Aortic arch

Blood vessel

Sympathetic
ganglion

Arteriolar dilators
Diazoxide
Hydralazine
Minoxidil
Calcium channel blockers

**Arteriolar and
venous dilators**
Sodium nitroprusside

Heart

**β-Adrenergic
receptor blockers**

**Angiotensin-converting
enzyme inhibitors**

Captopril
Enalapril

Kininase
(angiotensin-converting
enzyme)

Inhibit renin release

Angiotensin I ⟶ Angiotensin II

Diuretics
Thiazides

Decrease
sodium
reabsorption

Decrease constriction

Kidney

FIGURE 4-4 Effects of antihypertensive medications by organ site and method of action. (NOTE: From *Medical-Surgical Nursing: Assessment and Management of Clinical Problems* [4th ed., p. 876], by S. L. Lewis, I. C. Collier, & M. M. Heitkemper, 1996, St. Louis: C. V. Mosby. Reprinted with permission.)

(Maxzide) is an example of an agent that is comprised of a potassium-sparing diuretic and thiazide diuretic. The diuretics are among the few antihypertensive agents that do not inhibit sexual function. The beta-blockers, calcium channel blockers, and angiotensin-converting enzyme inhibitors (ACEIs) can cause sexual dysfunction.

Beta-Blockers ß-Adrenergic blocking agents (beta-blockers) are very effective in lowering peripheral vascular resistance. However, clients have shown a high incidence of intolerance to them. Specifically, beta-blockers often cause fatigue, lethargy, exercise intolerance, and impotence. The agents are often discontinued if the client develops any of these adverse effects. Other adverse effects of beta-blockers include depression, diminished mental acuity, severe hypotension, second- and third-degree heart block, dyspnea, wheezing, and bradycardia. Some examples of these agents are atenolol (Tenormin), metoprolol (Lopressor), and propranolol. Beta-blockers prevent the normal increase in heart rate that occurs during exercise. For this reason, clients should be told to not use heart rate to monitor signs of exercise intolerance. Another result of this physiological effect is that the client should avoid alcohol and hot baths, because the resulting hypotension may cause him or her to faint.

ACE Inhibitors ACE inhibitors decrease vascular systemic resistance by preventing the breakdown of bradykinin. This inhibits the release of angiotensin, a powerful vasoconstricting substance. Sodium and water resorption are prevented, but potassium is reabsorbed. ACE inhibitors are used to treat hypertension and CHF. Examples of these agents include captopril (Capoten), lisinopril (Zestril), and enalapril (Vasotec). They are often combined with hydrochlorothiazide (Hydrodiuril) to boost effectiveness. Several agents combine both an ACE inhibitor and hydrochlorothiazide (Hydrodiuril), including Lotensin HCT, Zestoretic, and Vasoretic. The adverse effects associated with these agents include a dry, nonproductive cough; hypotension; dizziness; mood changes; impotence; hyperkalemia; blood dyscrasias; and headache. These agents interact with antacids, diuretics, nonsteroidal anti-inflammatory drugs (NSAIDs), lithium, and potassium-sparing diuretics. Clients taking ACE inhibitors should have their electrolytes, especially potassium levels, monitored closely.

Calcium Channel Blockers Calcium channel blockers relax the smooth muscle by preventing contraction. Some examples of calcium channel blockers are diltiazem (Cardizem), nifedipine (Procardia), and verapamil (Calan). These agents have adverse effects, including hypotension, palpitations, tachycardia, constipation, nausea, rashes, flushing, peripheral edema, sexual difficulties, and wheezing. The adverse effects these agents cause are usually an overreaction to the therapeutic effects. The agents interact with digoxin, beta-blockers, and H_2 blockers. Research has shown that the rapidly released forms of these agents contribute to sudden death (Grossman, Messerli, Grodzicki, & Kowey, 1996). Therefore, they are usually given in a slowly released form.

Adrenergic Agent of Clonidine The adrenergic agent of clonidine (Catapres) inhibits vasoconstriction. It is administered either orally or by transdermal patch. The oral form of this medication rapidly lowers elevated blood pressure. Adverse effects include orthostatic hypotension, fatigue, dizziness, and sexual dysfunction. Clients who receive this medication should be informed that it must not be discontinued suddenly, because rebound hypertension may occur.

Medical Procedures

Cardiovascular disease is treated with surgery as well as other invasive procedures. The procedures are very technical, and the client is likely to be frightened. Nurses play an important role in managing the care for clients who must undergo these procedures. Specific nursing skills are required to prepare and educate the client properly. The nurse is usually responsible for assessing and monitoring the client's response to treatment.

Percutaneous Transluminal Coronary Angioplasty (PTCA) A client may undergo PTCA during a cardiac catheterization. Alternatively, the results of the cardiac catheterization may indicate that PTCA should be performed. PTCA is the process of dilating an occluded vessel to remove plaque blockage within the vessel (Fig. 4-5). The procedure is similar to cardiac catheterization, except that the physician dilates the vessel with a balloon. Occasionally, the physician will use a cutting device or laser to remove plaque from the artery. Stents are mesh-like devices that are inserted into the vessel at the site of plaque build-up and then expanded with a balloon to keep the vessel open (Figs. 4-6 and 4-7). There are a number of possible complications of PTCA; among the most serious are coronary artery occlusion, arterial dissection or rupture, and myocardial infarction, all of which can lead to emergency cardiac surgery. Pre- and postprocedure care are the same as for cardiac catheterization. The nurse must monitor for hematoma at the insertion site, the development of circulatory problems, and the development of emergent cardiac problems. The client in the case study underwent PTCA following cardiac catheterization. Two coronary arteries were dilated, and a stent was placed in one vessel. This procedure improved perfusion to the cardiac tissues to prevent irreversible ischemic damage. The frequency of chest pain episodes should decrease as well, since more oxygen is being delivered to the tissues. The client continues to experience angina, but the frequency of events has decreased.

Intra-aortic Balloon Pumps (IABP) An IABP is a temporary procedure that increases myocardial oxygen supply and decreases cardiac afterload. A balloon pump is a balloon attached to a catheter that is placed in the femoral artery and then threaded into the thoracic aorta. The catheter is connected to a pump that inflates and deflates the balloon. The pump exerts cyclic pressure to augment the diastolic blood pressure. Boosting the diastolic blood pressure enhances the cardiac output. This device is used on clients who have experienced a severe decrease in cardiac output as a result of CHF. If the balloon pump is effective, the client should experience improved sensorium; stable vital signs; and warm, dry skin (Fig. 4-8).

Pacemakers Pacemakers are applied to the heart or inserted within it to augment cardiac rate and rhythm (Fig. 4-9). They are generally used to correct sick sinus rhythm, bradycardia, tachycardia, or heart block. A pacemaker is composed of a pulse generator and pacing wires. The pulse generator electrically stimulates the sinoatrial node at a preset rate, and

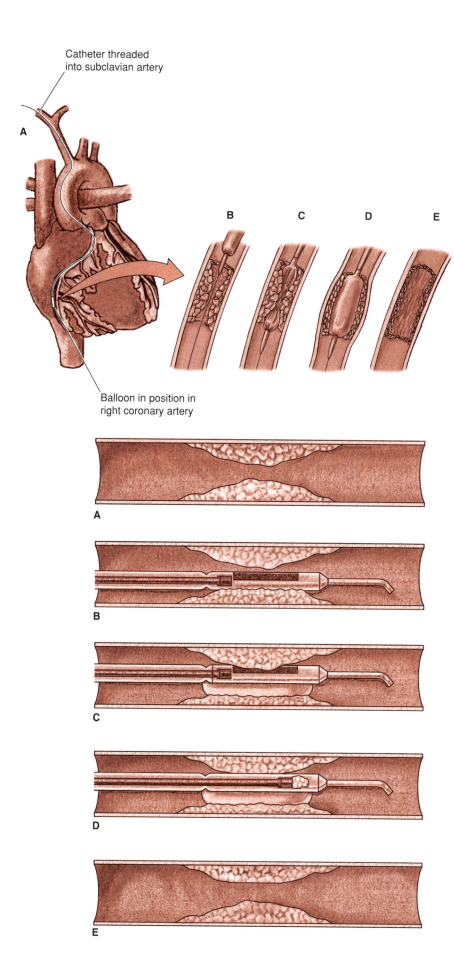

Catheter threaded
into subclavian artery

A

B   C   D   E

Balloon in position in
right coronary artery

A

B

C

D

E

FIGURE 4-5

Percutaneous transluminal coronary angioplasty (PTCA). *A*, balloon-tipped catheter is threaded into a blocked coronary artery. *B*, The balloon is threaded into the blockage. *C*, The balloon expands (*D*) to compress the blockage. *E*, Arterial diameter is restored. (NOTE: From *Medical-Surgical Nursing: Clinical Management for Continuity of Care* [5th ed., pp. 1245–1246], 1996, by J. M. Black & E. Matassain-Jacobs, Philadelphia: W. B. Saunders. Reprinted with permission.)

FIGURE 4-6

Atherectomy. *A*, Arterial blockage. *B*, The catheter is threaded into the artery, and the cutting device is placed over the blockage. *C*, The balloon is inflated. *D*, The blockage is cut away and trapped in the cylindrical housing. The balloon is then deflated, and the catheter is removed. *E*, The results of the procedure. (NOTE: From *Medical-Surgical Nursing: Clinical Management for Continuity of Care* [5th ed., pp. 1245–1246], 1996, by J. M. Black & E. Matassain-Jacobs, Philadelphia: W. B. Saunders. Reprinted with permission.)

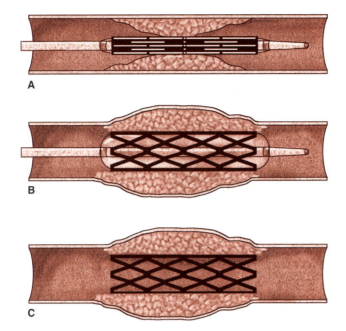

FIGURE 4-7

Placement of a coronary artery stent. *A,* The stent is advanced to the blockage. *B,* The balloon is inflated, causing the stent to expand. The balloon is deflated and removed. *C,* The stent is left in place. (NOTE: From *Medical-Surgical Nursing: Clinical Management for Continuity of Care* [5th ed., pp. 1245–1246], 1996, by J. M. Black & E. Matassain-Jacobs, Philadelphia: W. B. Saunders. Reprinted with permission.)

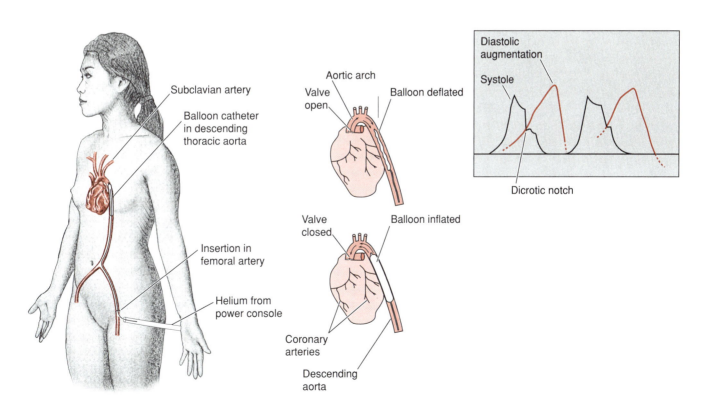

FIGURE 4-8 Placement of intra-aortic balloon pump (IABP), its action and wave-forms. (NOTE: From *Medical-Surgical Nursing: Clinical Management for Continuity of Care* [5th ed., p. 1360], 1996, by J. M. Black & E. Matassain-Jacobs, Philadelphia: W. B. Saunders. Reprinted with permission.)

FIGURE 4-9

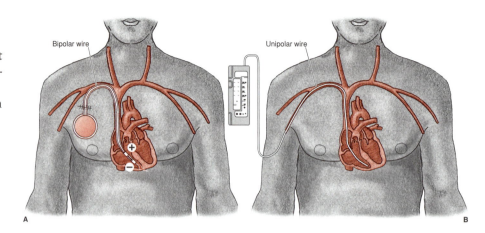

A, Transvenous catheter placement for dual-chamber pacing. The dual-chamber pacing action allows for synchronized contractions between the atrium and ventricle. This improves stroke volume. *B,* A temporary endocardial pacemaker. (NOTE: From *Medical-Surgical Nursing: Clinical Management for Continuity of Care* [5th ed., pp. 1316, 1318], 1996, by J. M. Black & E. Matassain-Jacobs, Philadelphia: W. B. Saunders. Reprinted with permission.)

Signs of **pacemaker failure** include bradycardia, dizziness, syncope, and the resurgence of symptoms that preceded the insertion of the pacemaker.

the pacing wires carry the electrical stimulation to the heart. Pacemakers are either temporary or permanent. Therapeutic signs of improved perfusion will be evident. **Pacemaker failure** is common: the pacemaker may fail to sense or fail to capture. A failure to sense means that the pacemaker fails to recognize spontaneous cardiac activity and fires inappropriately. A failure to capture is when the electrical stimulation is not sufficient to elicit a ventricular response. Signs of pacemaker failure include dizziness, dysrhythmias (especially bradycardia), and a resurgence of the symptoms that preceded the insertion of the pacemaker. After the pacemaker is inserted, clients should be encouraged to seek follow-up care with a physician to assess pacemaker function with a magnet and an ECG. The client should also be taught to keep the incision site clean and dry and to watch for signs of infection. The client must carry a card with information on the pacemaker type and function. The client should not undergo MRI, as the intensity of the magnet can reprogram the pacemaker. The client should also learn how to assess his or her heart rate.

Catheter Ablations   Catheter ablations are performed to disrupt pathways that cause tachydysrhythmias. During this procedure, radio frequency energy or laser energy is used to "burn" the accessory pathways or ectopic sites of the sinoatrial node, atrioventricular node, or ventricles to control ventricular response (Johns, 1996). The risks of this procedure include causing new symptomatic dysrhythmias and failing to stop the aberrant conduction.

Cardioversion is the synchronized electrical stimulation of the heart or a pharmacological agent used to convert the cardiac rhythm to a sinus rhythm.

Defibrillation is the electrical stimulation of the heart used to reverse a life-threatening dysrhythmia.

Defibrillation and Cardioversion   Defibrillation and cardioversion are used to alter the present cardiac rhythm and (ideally) convert it to a sinus rhythm. Cardioversion is synchronized electrical stimulation or pharmaceutical intervention that converts symptomatic atrial fibrillation or atrial flutter to a sinus rhythm. Defibrillation is a type of electrical stimulation that changes a nonperfusing rhythm to a perfusing rhythm. Defibrillation can be an external procedure, such as when the heart is "shocked" during cardiac arrest. It can also be performed by implanting a defibrillator within the body to provide electrical stimulation to correct ventricular dysrhythmias (Fig. 4-10). During times when the client is receiving electrical stimulation from an implanted defibrillator, he or she should lie down and

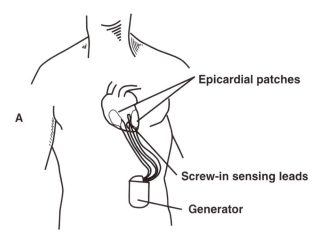

FIGURE 4-10 *A*, Placement of an implantable cardioverter defibrillator (ICD) and epicardial lead system. (NOTE: From Thelan, LA, Davie, JK, Urden, LD & Lough, ME (1994). Cardiovascular Therapeutic Management. In: *Critical Care Nursing: Diagnosis & Management*, Mosby. Reprinted with permission.)

the client's physician should be notified. Clients with these devices must wear a Medic Alert bracelet, carry a card with information on the implanted defibrillator, never undergo MRI, and have the battery checked every two months (Johns, 1996).

Pericardiocentesis and Pericardial Fenestration Pericardiocentesis (Fig. 4-11) and pericardial fenestration are performed in response to a pericardial effusion or cardiac tamponade. Both of these disorders result in fluid accumulation within the pericardial space. The trapped fluid constricts the heart. These two procedures are performed to drain the fluid from the pericardial space. Pericardiocentesis, the intermittent drainage of fluid, is commonly termed pericardial tap. Pericardial fenestration is the continuous drainage of fluid, termed a pericardial window. Atelectasis and infection are two risks these procedures carry.

Surgical Procedures

Several surgical procedures are performed to treat cardiovascular disease. These include coronary artery bypass graft (CABG), cardiac valve replacement, cardiomyoplasty, cardiac transplantation, and peripheral vascular surgeries (see below). Among the complications from these surgeries are infections, atelectasis, graft failures, hemodynamic instability including symptomatic dysrhythmias, pneumothorax, poor wound healing, and cardiac and circulatory dysfunction. The nurse can prevent these complications by frequently monitoring clients for hemodynamic and circulatory stability and intervening when their condition deteriorates. Pharmacological agents, oxygen, incentive spirometers and mechanical circulatory aids such as compression stockings are used to prevent complications. Client education can also help in prevention.

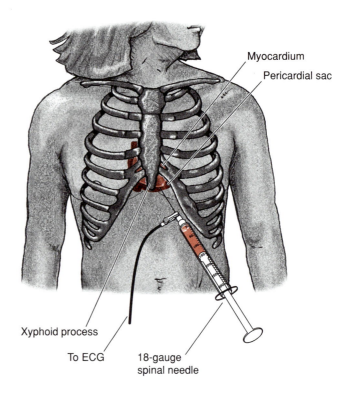

Myocardium

Pericardial sac

Xyphoid process

To ECG

18-gauge
spinal needle

FIGURE 4-11

☒

Percardiocentesis.

CABG In CABG, the surgeon bypasses blocked coronary arteries by connecting one end of a graft vessel above the blockage and another end below. The saphenous vein or internal mammary artery is used to bypass the blocked area within the coronary artery (Fig. 4-12). The radial artery is occasionally used when the client has more coronary vessels to bypass than the internal mammary can supply. When the internal mammary artery is used, the proximal end of the artery remains attached to the subclavian artery, while the distal end is severed and reattached distal to the coronary artery occlusion. When the saphenous vein or radial artery is used, the vessel is removed and one end is sutured proximal to the occlusion, while the other is sutured distal to it. Each of these procedures forms a vessel loop so that blood bypasses, or flows around, the occlusion. Since the chest is opened during the procedure, it is often termed open heart surgery. This is actually a misnomer, as the heart is never opened during the surgery. The heart is often stopped while the surgeon performs the procedure. This is termed cardioplegia. Presently, the most common means of cardioplegia is by a potassium infusion into the coronary arteries. While the heart is stopped, the body is perfused by means of a cardiopulmonary bypass machine.

Cardiopulmonary bypass mechanically circulates and oxygenates the client's blood while the heart is stopped. The blood is drained from the body, chilled, mixed with heparin, diluted with an isotonic crystalloid solution, and returned to the body. This process lowers the body's oxygen needs, which improves perfusion to the organs and tissues. Cardiopulmonary bypass has many adverse effects, including fluid deficits, third spacing,

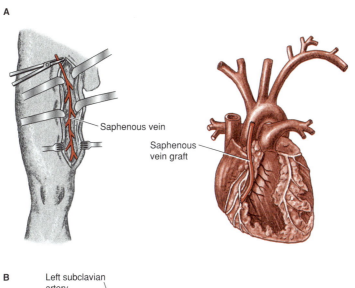

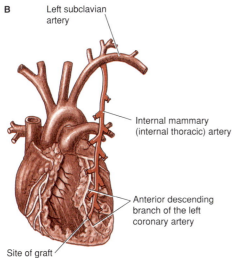

FIGURE 4-12

A, Saphenous vein graft. *B*, Internal mammary artery graft.

decreased cardiac output, bleeding, impaired gas exchange, hemolysis, hyperglycemia, hypokalemia, hypomagnesemia, neurological dysfunction, and hypertension (Thelan, Davie, Urden, & Lough, 1994; see Table 4-4).

Cardiac Valve Replacement Cardiac valve replacement is true open heart surgery. It involves removing damaged valves within the heart and replacing them with prosthetic valves. The prosthetic valves are generally made of synthetic materials. The client needs to remain on an anticoagulant agent such as warfarin (Coumadin) after surgery.

Cardiomyoplasty Cardiomyoplasty is a surgical procedure in which the latissimus dorsi muscle is wrapped around the heart and electrically stimulated to contract with each heart beat. It is used to treat CHF and cardiomyopathy. The implanted electrical stimulator must be replaced every 3–5 years. The procedure is still experimental, and the prognosis for clients who undergo cardiomyoplasty is not good. When a suitable donor heart is not available, cardiomyoplasty is performed instead of heart transplantation.

◙

TABLE 4-4

ADVERSE PHYSIOLOGICAL EFFECTS OF CARDIOPULMONARY BYPASS

Bleeding
Decreased cardiac output
Hemolysis
Hyperglycemia
Transient hypertension
Hypokalemia
Hypomagnesemia
Hypotension resulting from hypovolemia
Hypovolemia resulting from intravascular fluid deficit
Neurological dysfunction resulting from depressed central nervous system
Pulmonary dysfunction
Third-spacing of body fluids

Cardiac Transplantation Cardiac transplantation is another type of cardiac surgery. This procedure involves human lymphocyte antigen (HLA) matching of donor heart tissues with recipient tissues. The recipient's transplanted heart comes from a person who has been determined to be brain dead. The client is required to take immunosuppressant agents for the rest of his or her life to prevent rejection once a transplant has been performed. The availability of suitable donor hearts and the physical and psychosocial demands on the client who receives a cardiac transplant limit the use of this treatment.

Peripheral Vascular Surgery Several types of peripheral vascular surgery are performed, including femoral-popliteal and aortic-femoral bypass endarterectomy, embolectomy, and amputation. In bypass surgery, one end of a graft vessel is connected proximal to the peripheral vascular occlusion, and the other end distal to it. An endarterectomy involves removing plaque from a vessel using a scalpel or laser. During an embolectomy, an embolus is removed. Amputation is the surgical removal of a limb. It is generally performed when gangrene has developed as a result of impaired peripheral perfusion.

For any client who undergoes surgery to correct a cardiac disease state, the nursing care goals are to improve tissue perfusion and to prevent complications. The degree of improvement of tissue perfusion correlates with the amount of collateral circulation that reaches the tissues. The nurse must assess the client's level of perfusion by measuring blood pressure, pulse, and cardiac output. The client's skin color and temperature must be monitored as well. The nurse must assess capillary refill, breath sounds, heart sounds, and perfusion of the kidneys. The capillary refill time should be less than 3 seconds. The client should have palpable peripheral pulses. The skin should be warm and dry. If the kidneys are being perfused, urine output should balance fluid intake, fluid output should be greater than or equal to 30 mL/hr, and the BUN and creatinine levels should stay within normal limits. The client should maintain a normal sinus rhythm or at least not progress to a symptomatic dysrhythmia. The client's vital signs should remain within normal limits. Cardiac output can be determined as being either adequate or inadequate based on the perfusion assessment. It can also be measured using a pulmonary artery catheter (normal cardiac output, 4–6 L/min). Breath sounds should remain clear without adventitious sounds.

Adequate kidney perfusion is urinary output of at least 30 mL per hour and BUN and creatinine levels within normal limits.

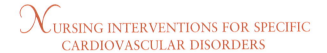

NURSING INTERVENTIONS FOR SPECIFIC CARDIOVASCULAR DISORDERS

The common cardiovascular disorders are angina, myocardial infarction, coronary artery disease, CHF, inflammatory and infectious heart disease, hypertension, and peripheral vascular disorders. There are a variety of cardiovascular emergency conditions as well, including pulmonary edema, cardiac tamponade, cardiogenic shock, and peripheral circulatory occlusions. Nursing care for clients with these disorders includes improving cardiac output, improving tissue perfusion, and preventing complications.

Angina

Angina is chest pain related to reversible myocardial ischemia. It is treated with nitrates, and occasionally, inotropic agents. **Nursing responsibilities** for clients with angina include assessing the pain by taking a thorough history of previous episodes, their location, onset, duration, and relieving factors, whether the pain is activity related, and its intensity (Fig. 4-13). The nurse is responsible for evaluating the client's response to treatment. The nurse also assists with rehabilitation and teaches the client how to prevent anginal pain and the use of pharmacological agents to treat it. A common prescription for angina is sublingual and transdermal nitroglycerin. Clients require specific information concerning the storage and use of this medication.

Myocardial Infarction

Myocardial infarction is the necrosis of cardiac tissue resulting from irreversible cardiac ischemia. It is referred to as a heart attack. Many clients erroneously describe a heart attack as the heart blowing up or exploding. Clients should be taught the actual etiology of myocardial infarctions. When caring for these clients, the nurse should frequently monitor vital signs, including hemodynamic values and heart sounds. The nurse should assess for causative factors such as hyperlipidemia or a history of coronary artery disease. Telemetry monitoring should also be performed to monitor

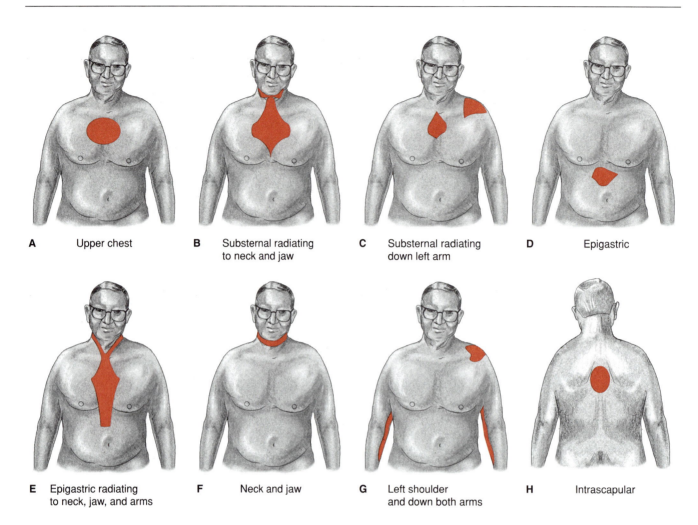

A   Upper chest

B   Substernal radiating to neck and jaw

C   Substernal radiating down left arm

D   Epigastric

E   Epigastric radiating to neck, jaw, and arms

F   Neck and jaw

G   Left shoulder and down both arms

H   Intrascapular

FIGURE 4-13 Common sites of discomfort associated with angina or myocardial infarction. (NOTE: From *Assessment and Management of Clinical Problems* [4th ed., p. 902], by S. L. Lewis, I. C. Collier, & M. M. Heitkemper, 1996, St. Louis: C. V. Mosby. Reprinted with permission.)

Cardiac rehabilitation is a program of risk factor modification that includes a gradual increase in exercise tolerance.

the heart's electrical activity continuously. During the acute phase of the infarction, the nurse should provide a quiet atmosphere for the client. The nurse should assess for the presence of chest pain, noting precipitating factors and measures that provide relief. The client's arterial blood gas (ABG), electrolytes, and cardiac enzymes should be monitored. The nurse also should monitor the client's response to therapy. Postinfarction risk factor modification and **cardiac rehabilitation** are indicated. The client should be instructed to increase activity levels slowly under the care of a physician, and should progress gradually to aerobic activity 30 min/d, three times per week. Isometric exercise is not recommended. Many clients have concerns about resuming sexual activity. However, this subject is rarely broached with their health care providers. The nurse should be sensitive to this concern. Clients should be told that, generally, they may resume sexual activity when they are able to climb two flights of stairs without experiencing undue shortness of breath or chest pain. It is helpful to discuss alternative methods of maintaining intimacy until they reach this goal.

Coronary Artery Disease

In this disease, commonly referred to as hardening of the arteries, the arteries show decreased elasticity as a result of plaque deposits which have hardened onto the vessel walls. Plaque formation can progress to artery occlusion, which contributes to tissue ischemia and, ultimately, necrosis. The CABG procedure is commonly used to treat coronary artery occlusion. Preoperative **nursing responsibilities** include determining if the client understands the operative procedure and postoperative care. Clients must learn about the tubes and medical equipment that are used in the postoperative period, and pain management is a major concern. Most clients receive pain medication intravenously until they are able to tolerate oral pain medications. **Nursing care** goals include restoring physiological stability, maintaining adequate ventilation, preventing complications, and providing psychological support. Prior to discharging the client, he or she should be taught about tolerance to activity, risk factor modification, diet, medications, wound care, cardiac rehabilitation, and resumption of sexual activity.

Congestive Heart Failure

Cardiovascular disorders such as coronary artery disease, hypertension, myocardial infarction, COPD, and rheumatic heart disease can lead to CHF, a mechanical malfunction in which the heart's contractility is not sufficient to eject blood against afterload. It is, simply, pump failure. Since the heart has two separate pumping actions, failure can occur on the right side, left side, or both sides. The clinical manifestations of left-sided heart failure include anxiety, air hunger, dyspnea, diaphoresis, crackles, cyanosis, increased pulmonary artery pressures, and a S3 gallop rhythm. Left-sided heart failure is the most common and often contributes to right-sided failure. The clinical manifestations of right-sided failure include dependent edema, jugular vein distention, bounding pulses, oliguria, dysrhythmias, and increased central venous pressure.

Nursing responsibilities for clients in CHF include assisting them to rest and reduce anxiety. The client is usually prescribed inotropic agents, nitrates, and, frequently, diuretics and antihypertensive agents. ACE inhibitors are the antihypertensive agents of choice, and beta-blockers are contraindicated. The nurse is responsible for monitoring the client's response to treatment. A client in CHF who responds positively to medication should have less shortness of breath, less dependent edema, and an increased tolerance to activity. The client's skin should be warm and dry, and oxygen saturation levels should increase. Breath sounds should be clear without evidence of adventitious sounds. The nurse should teach the client how to recognize the symptoms of an approaching episode of CHF.

Inflammatory and Infectious Heart Disease

Pericarditis and *endocarditis* are inflammatory disease processes. Pericarditis is inflammation and possible infection of the pericardium. Endocarditis is inflammation and possible infection of the inner heart and valves. The clinical manifestations are the typical symptoms of infection: increased body temperature, an elevated WBC count, chills, malaise, and sometimes chest pain and dyspnea. These symptoms are treated with antimicrobial agents. Analgesics and steroids also may be prescribed. The nurse is responsible for treating the fever with antipyretics and cooling measures. The nurse should also encourage fluids, help the client to balance rest and activity periods, and provide analgesics and other comfort measures. Cardiovascular or respiratory system changes should be assessed, and the physician should be notified if any occur. Endocarditis often results from bacterial contamination of the heart following routine dental work, if the client has a history of cardiac valvular disease. To prevent this, clients are prescribed antibiotic therapy whenever dental work must be done. Endocarditis can also occur following rheumatic fever or **staphylococcal infection**. It is therefore important that staphylococcal infections be treated promptly. Intravenous drug users, elderly clients with valve replacements, and clients with central venous access devices are susceptible to developing endocarditis.

> Due to the risk of the development of infectious heart disease, **staphylococcal infections** must be treated early.

Hypertension

Hypertension is a persistent elevation of blood pressure above normal levels. Normal blood pressure is 140/90 mm Hg. Hypertension is the product of peripheral vascular resistance and cardiac output. The risk factors include a family history of hypertension, stress, obesity, and hypernatremia. Smoking increases the risk of developing hypertension. The incidence of hypertension is higher in the elderly and in certain ethnic groups such as African Americans. Elevated blood pressure in serial assessments may be the only clinical manifestation of the disease. Left untreated, hypertension leads to cerebral vascular accidents, coronary artery disease, and renal failure. Other clinical manifestations that may occur include fatigue, dizziness, palpitations, blurred vision, and epistaxis. Hypertension is treated with a low-fat, low-sodium diet, exercise, and weight- and stress-reduction techniques. The client should avoid alcohol and caffeine. Other risk factor modifications, such as quitting smoking, may be useful as well. If nonpharmacological treatments are ineffective, antihypertensive agents are prescribed.

The nurse should monitor the client's blood pressure, body weight, intake and output, electrolyte concentrations, and BUN and creatinine levels. The client should be informed of the devastating effects of untreated hypertension and encouraged to schedule regular follow-up visits. He or she also needs to learn the effects of the medications. Behavioral modification to reduce risk factors may be indicated, and the client should have help to establish a regular exercise program.

> **Hypertension** is a life-long disease process. The nurse assists the client in controlling the disease by encouraging frequent blood pressure checks, routine health provider visits, and medication education.

Peripheral Vascular Disorders

Peripheral vascular disorders result from arterial or venous pathological conditions that inhibit perfusion to the tissues. They usually occur in the lower extremities. The clinical manifestations of arterial perfusion insufficiency differ from those of venous perfusion insufficiency.

Arterial Insufficiency Arterial insufficiency is characterized by two types of pain. The first type, intermittent claudication, occurs during activity and is relieved by rest. The second type, termed rest pain, occurs at rest and is relieved when the extremity is placed in a dependent position. Pulses may be diminished or absent. The skin of the affected extremity often reddens when placed in a dependent position and pales when elevated. The skin is dry, shiny, and cool to the touch, and the nails are thickened.

Peripheral **arterial insufficiency** manifests as intermittent claudication; pain at rest; diminished pulses; reddened skin; skin pallor on elevation of extremity; dry, cool, shiny skin; and thickened nails.

Venous Insufficiency Venous insufficiency is characterized by an aching or cramping sensation that is relieved by elevating the extremity. Pulses are present. The skin is thick and tough with a brawny pigmentation. Dermatitis is often present as well.

Peripheral **venous insufficiency** manifests as aching or cramping pain and thick, tough skin with a brawny pigmentation.

Complications of Vascular Insufficiency

Leg Ulcers Vascular insufficiency can be complicated by the development of leg ulcers. The therapeutic management of leg ulcers depends on the etiology. For arterial ulcers, reconstructive vascular surgery is normally indicated. Compression therapy is generally used for clients with venous ulcers. Compression therapy consists of applying compression daily to the lower extremities. If the venous ulcer is open, continuous compression wraps such as the Unna boot are applied. Since most forms of vascular insufficiency have a mixed etiology, compression can be detrimental to arterial circulation. Thus, compression should be used with caution in the elderly. The client's perfusion to the lower extremities needs to be assessed periodically. The color of the skin, movement of the toes, temperature of the extremity, sensations within the extremity such as numbness and tingling, pulses, and capillary refill time need to be assessed. This is generally referred to as an assessment of CMTS, pulses, and capillary refill. The extremity should have a pink tone, the client should be able to move the toes, the skin should be warm, and the client should be able to distinguish between sharp and dull sensations without numbness and tingling. The pulses should be palpable, and capillary refill time should be less than 3 seconds. **Compression hose** should be applied when the client wakes up in the morning, and they should be removed at bedtime. If these hose are not removed daily, the posterior popliteal fossa may be damaged. The continuous compression wraps are generally changed once a week depending on the amount of drainage from the wound.

Compression hose must be removed daily to prevent damage to the posterior popliteal fossa.

Deep Vein Thrombosis (DVT) DVT is a common complication of venous insufficiency. It is associated with venous stasis that commonly occurs after surgery, obesity, pregnancy, CHF, or when the calf is immobilized for any reason. Hypercoagulability and injury to a vein wall are other possible causes. DVT is the development of thrombosis as a result of platelet adherence to the vein wall. As the thrombosis becomes larger, it obstructs the vein. This condition can lead to a pulmonary embolism and venous stasis ulcers. Preventive measures are the best treatment. These include the use of active and passive range-of-motion exercises if immobilization of a limb is required. Anti-embolic stockings or sequential compression devices can prevent venous stasis from occurring. Early and frequent ambulation following surgery are other preventive measures. Occasionally, the client is treated with platelet aggregate inhibitors and anticoagulants if venous stasis is likely to occur. The clinical manifestations of DVT include pain in the extremity, unilateral swelling distal to the site, low-grade fever, and a positive Homans' sign. Treatment includes anticoagulant therapy; elevation of the affected extremity; applying warm, moist heat to it; and immobilizing it. **Nursing responsibilities** include administering anticoagulants and monitoring for therapeutic and adverse effects. If the client is receiving heparin, the nurse must monitor the APTT, which should be 1.5–2.0 times the normal value. If the client is receiving warfarin, the prothrombin time should be within an INR of 2.0–3.0. The nurse should assess for abnormal bleeding that indicates excess anticoagulation. The nurse should provide excellent skin care and assist in exercising all extremities except the affected one. The client needs to be taught safety measures to prevent bleeding, especially while taking an anticoagulant medication, and blood levels should be tested frequently. The nurse should teach clients how to prevent DVT by instructing them to avoid sitting or standing for long periods of time, to avoid crossing their legs, and to avoid wearing clothing that constricts their legs. The client may need to wear anti-embolic stockings.

Early and **frequent ambulation** are good methods for preventing DVT in postoperative clients.

CARDIOVASCULAR EMERGENCIES

Pulmonary Embolism

A pulmonary embolism is caused by an embolus that travels to the lungs and lodges in the pulmonary vasculature. Perfusion is obstructed by the embolus, causing hypoxemia. Most emboli develop from a DVT. The clinical manifestations include abrupt onset, dyspnea, chest pain, anxiety, crackles, and tachycardia. This condition is treated with anticoagulants and embolectomies. A filter can be inserted to prevent emboli reaching vital organs.

Pulmonary Edema

Pulmonary edema is caused by pulmonary artery congestion often as a result of untreated CHF. The clinical manifestations include acute anxiety, pale and cyanotic skin, diaphoresis, dyspnea, increased heart rate, and pink and frothy sputum. Pulmonary edema has a sudden onset and is treated as a medical emergency. The client should be transferred to an intensive care unit immediately. Treatment generally consists of loop diuretics, morphine sulfate, and oxygen.

Cardiac Tamponade

Cardiac tamponade is a life-threatening condition that occurs when the pericardial sac restricts ventricular filling as a result of a pericardial effusion. It can occur after cardiac surgery or as the result of an inflammatory process. Cardiac tamponade must be treated immediately. A **paradoxical pulse**, in which the pulse loses intensity during inspiration, is the hallmark sign of this condition. A paradoxical pulse is assessed by placing a blood pressure cuff on the client's arm and inflating the cuff until no heart sounds are heard. The cuff is then slowly deflated until sounds are heard during expiration. The pressure is then noted, and the cuff is deflated until sounds are also heard during inspiration. A difference in pressure of more than 10 mm Hg indicates cardiac tamponade. Other clinical manifestations of cardiac tamponade include a narrowed pulse pressure, hypotension, tachycardia, jugular venous distention, muffled heart sounds, diaphoresis, dyspnea, and cyanosis of the lips and nails. Medical management consists of performing pericardiocentesis.

A **paradoxical pulse** is the classic sign of cardiac tamponade.

Cardiogenic Shock

Cardiogenic shock occurs when the heart is unable to maintain adequate cardiac output for tissue perfusion. This usually occurs following a myocardial infarction. Circulatory failure follows, and clients with this condition have a poor prognosis. The clinical manifestations include cool, pale skin; decreased pedal pulses; hypotension; chest pain; increased heart rate; oliguria; metabolic acidosis; and hyperkalemia. Medical management for clients in cardiogenic shock includes administering α-adrenergic agonists, α- and β-adrenergic agonists, vasodilators, and diuretics. **Nursing responsibilities** include administering oxygen by face mask, starting intravenous infusions, and inserting a Foley catheter. This is a life-threatening condition, and the client should be transferred to an intensive care unit immediately.

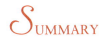

SUMMARY

Many physiological and technical advances have been made that help health care providers diagnose and treat cardiovascular disorders. There are a number of screening and detection procedures that can be performed to help prevent and manage cardiovascular disease. Assessing for risk factors of cardiovascular illness should be routine practice for the nurse. Factors such as a high-fat content diet, a sedentary life style, obesity, stress, smoking, chemical pollutants, family history of heart disease, and underserved populations contribute to the current rate of heart disease. Health-risk questionnaires, community health fairs, blood pressure screenings, and cholesterol measurement help to make people aware of the risk for cardiovascular disease. Clients who are at risk or who have compromised cardiovascular systems are encouraged to see a primary care provider regularly.

Dynamic studies examine the electrical activity of the heart. ECG, telemetry monitoring devices, and the Holter monitor, which records the electrical activity of the heart for a day or two, are commonly used. These devices visualize the electrical activity of the heart, which allows the health care provider to make reasonable deductions concerning the mechanical activity of the client's heart. The technology is efficient, portable, and convenient.

Ultrasonic and radiological studies help the health care provider identify disorders that affect tissue perfusion, vascular circulation, and hemodynamic stability. The structure of the cardiovascular system can be assessed using ultrasonic studies. A number of laboratory tests assist in identifying cardiovascular disorders. Much emphasis has been placed on LDL cholesterol control. HDL is considered to be the "beneficial" lipid within the body. CBC, BUN and creatinine, electrolytes, bleeding factors, and the cardiac enzymes laboratory values help to distinguish cardiovascular disease from other disorders.

Risk factor modification, pharmacotherapy, implantable and external regulatory devices, and invasive and noninvasive interventions are available treatment options for the client with, or at risk for, cardiovascular disease. Risk factor modification to improve dietary habits, stop harmful habits, control weight and stress, and increase physical activity is a proactive treatment of cardiovascular disease. Many pharmacological agents are used to treat cardiovascular disease. The types of drugs used include nitrates, antilipid agents, anticoagulant agents, platelet aggregate inhibitors, thrombolytic agents, inotropic agents. and antihypertensives. The nurse needs to be aware of the client's prescribed drug therapy and monitor therapeutic as well as adverse effects of these agents.

Hemodynamic monitoring and augmentation allow the nurse to care for clients who require frequent if not constant intervention. Central venous catheters, arterial lines, and pulmonary artery catheters facilitate measuring the client's hemodynamic state at bedside. Augmentation therapies such as IABP, pacing, cardioversion, and defibrillation enhance cardiac functioning.

A number of surgical interventions are utilized in the treatment of cardiovascular disorders. They include CABG, cardiomyoplasty, cardiac transplantation, peripheral vascular bypass surgery, endarterectomy, embolectomy, and amputation. Improvement of tissue perfusion following these procedures depends on the amount of collateral circulation that remains in the tissues.

Common cardiovascular disorders are angina, coronary artery disease, myocardial infarction, inflammatory heart disease, and the peripheral vascular diseases of venous and arterial insufficiency. It is the nurse's responsibility to improve tissue perfusion, vascular circulation, and hemodynamic stability. Pulmonary embolism, pulmonary edema, cardiac tamponade, and cardiogenic shock are life-threatening emergencies that the nurse must be able to recognize and respond to with quick and appropriate intervention.

KEY WORDS

Cardiac enzymes	Infarction
Cardiac rehabilitation	International normal ratio
Cardioversion	Isometric
Collateral circulation	Low-density lipoproteins
Continuous compression therapy	Orthostatic hypotension
Defibrillation	Pacemaker
Dysrhythmia	Pericentesis
Hematoma	Risk factors
High-density lipoproteins	Sinus rhythm
Homan's sign	Stress testing
Hyperlipidemia	Telemetry
Hypertension	

QUESTIONS

1. A 65-year-old man in congestive heart failure (CHF) receives the inotropic agent digoxin (Lanoxin). Which of the following symptoms indicates that the medication is effective for this client?

   A. Absence of chest pain
   B. Ambulation without shortness of breath
   C. Blood pressure of 138/88 mm Hg
   D. Bounding, full pulse

2. A nurse assesses the ECG rhythm strip obtained from a client who had a myocardial infarction three days previously. She finds that the PR interval is 0.24 seconds. This indicates that the PR interval is

   A. essentially absent.
   B. normal.
   C. prolonged.
   D. shortened.

3. A 48-year-old woman is admitted with a diagnosis of deep vein thrombosis (DVT) of the right calf. Which of the following nursing actions is appropriate?

   A. Ambulate the client three times a day.
   B. Apply warm, moist heat to the right calf.
   C. Position the client with the knees bent.
   D. Massage the right calf every 4–6 hours as needed.

4. A 78-year-old patient who has recently had an aortic valve replacement begins to complain of tightness in the chest and anxiety. On assessment the nurse discovers the patient has a paradoxical pulse. Which of the following cardiovascular emergencies is this patient likely exhibiting?

    A. Cardiac tamponade
    B. Cardiogenic shock
    C. Myocardial infarction
    D. Pulmonary edema

5. A 67-year-old female has developed venous stasis ulcers to her left leg. The nurse has applied a Unna boot. The boot will need to be changed:

    A. Daily.
    B. Every three days.
    C. Monthly depending on comfort.
    D. Weekly depending on drainage.

6. A 62-year-old male patient following cardiac surgery experiences hypotension, tachycardia, cool clammy skin, and a sense of impending doom. What should be considered before initiating an order to administer dopamine to raise the blood pressure?

    A. Fluid volume status.
    B. Heart rate and rhythm.
    C. Peripheral circulation.
    D. Respiratory status.

ANSWERS TO QUESTIONS

1. *The answer is B.* The inotropic agents are used to strengthen contractility of the heart. This relieves the back pressure of the blood on the pulmonary system, reducing the shortness of breath. The peripheral pulse intensity does not increase from these agents. The inotropic agents do not directly affect blood pressure, nor do they relieve or prevent chest pain. However, patients in CHF are often given a nitrate agent for that purpose.

2. *The answer is C.* The normal PR interval is 0.12–0.20 seconds. The 0.24-second interval is prolonged. If it is measurable, it is present and not shortened, indicating that it is less than 0.12 seconds.

3. *The answer is B.* Warm, moist heat is applied to a thrombotic extremity to increase blood flow to the area. The client should not walk as this may dislodge the thrombus, causing an embolus. The knees should not be bent, as that may impede blood flow to the lower leg. The leg should, however, be elevated higher than heart level. The calf should

not be massaged because of the risk of thrombus dislocation and resultant embolus formation.

4. *The answer is A.* A paradoxical pulse, which means that the pulse fades on inspiration, is a hallmark of cardiac tamponade. If this sign occurs during myocardial infarction, cardiogenic shock, or pulmonary edema, it indicates a developing cardiac tamponade.

5. *The answer is D.* The continuous compression dressing (Unna boot) is kept in place for a week unless drainage is excessive or discomfort occurs. Daily or every three days is not necessary unless drainage is excessive. Monthly is too long.

6. *The answer is A.* These are the clinical manifestations of impending or actual shock. Dopamine is a first-line drug for shock, but the patient must be normovolemic before initiating the drug because it causes severe vasoconstriction.

ANNOTATED REFERENCES

Fischbach, F. (1996). *A manual of laboratory and diagnostic tests* (5th ed.). Philadelphia: J. B. Lippincott.

This laboratory manual provides the tests and their normal values and explains what is likely to elevate or decrease the values. It also instructs how to draw the specimen for the test. The manual provides nursing implications concerning client preparation and interfering factors.

Grossman, E., Messerli, F. H., Grodzicki, T., & Kowey, P. (1996). Should a moratorium be placed on sublingual nifedipine capsules given for hypertensive emergencies and pseudoemergencies? *Journal of the American Medical Association, 276* (16), 1328–1331.

This article reviews the research findings concerning the efficacy of fast-acting calcium channel blockers in hypertensive emergencies and details the risks involved in using these agents. The article discusses the incidence of sudden death from fast-acting calcium channel blockers that were used to decrease blood pressure.

Haak, S. W., Richardson, S. J., Davey, S. S., & Parker-Cohen, P. D. (1994). Alterations in cardiovascular function. In K. L. McCance & S. E. Huether (Eds.), Pathophysiology: A biologic base for disease in adults and children (2nd ed., pp. 1000–1084). St. Louis: C. V. Mosby.

This chapter discusses the development of cardiovascular disease. It describes the pathophysiology at the cellular level and incorporates research findings.

Hancock, E. W. (1991). Coronary artery disease: Epidemiology and pre-vention. Scientific American Medicine, 1, (I–VIII), 1–10.

This article discusses the pathophysiology and danger level of the risk factors associated with coronary artery disease, as well as the physiology of prevention.

Johns, C. I. (1996). Nursing role in the management of dysrhythmias. In S. L. Lewis, I. C. Collier, & M. M. Heitkemper (Eds.), *Medical surgical nursing: Assessment and management of clinical problems* (4th ed., pp. 965–1003). St. Louis: C. V. Mosby.

This textbook is a current, standard resource for medical-surgical nursing. This chapter discusses dysrhythmias and the variety of treatments used to care for clients experiencing a cardiac dysrhythmia.

Stanley, M. (1995). The cardiovascular system and its problems in the elderly. In M. Stanley, & P. G. Beare (Eds.), *Gerontological nursing* (pp. 189–200). Philadelphia: F. A. Davis.

This insightful book describes the pathophysiology of age-related changes. The thorough but succinct text gives the nursing perspective of caring for elderly clients. The chapter concludes with documentation and discharge planning.

Thelan, L. A., Davie, J. K., Urden L. D., & Lough, M. E. (1994a). Cardiovascular therapeutic management. In Thelan, L. A. et al: (Eds.) *Critical care nursing: Diagnosis and management* (2nd ed., pp. 313–352). St. Louis: C. V. Mosby.

This chapter in a critical care nursing textbook describes the treatment of clients with cardiac disease. This highly esteemed text is written for the critical care environment.

Thelan, L. A., Davie, J. K., Urden L. D., & Lough, M. E. (1994b). Cardiovascular diagnostic procedures. In Thelan, L. A. et al: (Eds.) *Critical care nursing: Diagnosis and management* (2nd ed., pp. 182–276). St. Louis: C. V. Mosby.

This chapter is an accessible guide to the procedures used to monitor cardiovascular disorders. It describes both common and complex procedures and demonstrates the basic dysrhythmias clearly.

Thompson, E. J., Detwiler, D. S., & Nelson, C. M. (1996). Dobutamine stress echocardiography: A new noninvasive method for detecting ischemic heart disease. *Heart and Lung, 25* (2), 87–97.

This article discusses the advantages and disadvantages of dobutamine use during exercise tolerance testing. A dobutamine reaction within the body closely mimics the graduated effects of exercise on the myocardium.

INTERNET SITES FOR ADDITIONAL INFORMATION

American Heart Association
http://aztec.asu.edu/medical/azse/amheart.html

Cardiac Health Web
http://www.bev.net/health/cardiac/treatment.html

Cardiac Rehabilitation
http://www.crittenton.com/RESP2HTM

AHA Cardiovascular Risk Assessment
http://11207.211.141.25/risk/index.html

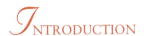

CHAPTER 5

GASTROINTESTINAL SYSTEM: ALTERATIONS IN DIGESTION AND ELIMINATION

INTRODUCTION

The gastrointestinal (GI) system converts ingested nutrients and fluids into a form that can be used by the cells of the body and then excretes the waste products. This is accomplished by four physiologic processes:

1. **Ingestion** is the intake of food and fluid. These ingested sources contain carbohydrates, proteins, fats, water, vitamins, minerals, and trace elements.
2. **Digestion** is the physical and chemical breakdown of food into an absorbable form.
3. **Absorption** is the transfer of food products into the circulation.
4. **Elimination** is the excretion of solid waste products.

The GI system is divided into two tracts, the upper and lower GI tracts. The upper GI (UGI) tract consists of structures that aid in the ingestion and digestion of food. It includes the mouth, esophagus, stomach, duodenum, and related organs of the biliary system and exocrine pancreas. The lower GI (LGI) tract consists of the small and large intestines. The functions or actions of the small intestine promote mixing of the digestive juices for digestion to take place. Peristaltic movement of the small intestine maintains the forward progress of the intestinal content, termed **chyme**. The breakdown of food groups and the absorption of nutrients begin in the small intestine.

Chyme. Chyme is the intestinal content, a semisolid fluid mass of food mixed with gastric juices. The breakdown, mixing, and absorption of food takes place primarily in the small intestine.

Valsalva Maneuver. This process is defined as forced exhalation against a closed glottis, resulting in increased intrathoracic pressure, which impedes venous return to the heart.

The function of the large intestine is primarily storage and excretion of solid waste products in the form of feces. While the small intestine is the primary site of nutrient absorption, water is absorbed in the large intestine. The process of defecation occurs when the rectum and colon contract, accompanied by a voluntary contraction of the diaphragm and abdominal wall (**Valsalva maneuver**). This, in turn, increases pressure in the rectum, and contraction of the external anal sphincter causes defecation. This Valsalva process increases intrathoracic pressure and impedes venous return to the heart. When the pressure or strain is released, there is an increase in venous return to the heart. This explains why constipation or straining may precipitate angina or problems in cardiac patients and thus should be avoided.

𝒜GE-RELATED CHANGES IN THE GI SYSTEM

The elderly are the fastest-growing segment of the population, making it important for nurses to understand the physiological changes of aging in the GI system. The most common age-related changes in the GI system are as follows: The teeth darken, loosen, or fracture, and gums recede, exposing the nerve roots. As salivary gland output decreases, less saliva is produced, which results in a dry mouth and an increased susceptibility to infection and breakdown. A weakening of the lower esophageal sphincter may increase the frequency of esophageal reflux. In addition, there is decreased gastric motility and emptying and decreased secretion of gastric acid, especially hydrochloric acid (HCl). Peristaltic action is also decreased.

These changes can lead to GI difficulties. In the biliary system, the increased cholesterol content of bile contributes to the high incidence of gallstones, which increases with each decade of life. In the pancreas, hyperplasia and fibrosis leads to decreased secretion of pancreatic enzymes. Age-related changes in the small intestine impair the absorption of nutrients, especially carbohydrates. Defective vitamin D absorption in the elderly exacerbates osteoporosis, and there is an impairment of calcium active transport; these changes necessitate supplemental calcium and vitamin D replacement to prevent osteoporosis in perimenopausal and postmenopausal women. In addition, the decrease in production of immunoglobulins with age can lead to increased frequency and severity of infections.

Frequently, elderly individuals report an increased incidence of constipation. This is most often attributed to a decreased intake of water or high-fiber foods, a lack of exercise, or medications (Tables 5-1 and 5-2). Health education of aging clients should emphasize the need to drink 6 to 8 glasses of water a day and to stay as active as possible. Polyps and diverticula can cause changes in stool patterns, and the rectum may have decreased elasticity. When constipation occurs, the stools are small, hard, and difficult to pass.

☒

TABLE 5-1
COMMON DRUGS THAT CAUSE CONSTIPATION

- Haloperidol (Haldol)
- Iron Sulfate (Feo-Sol, Niferex)
- Morphine sulfate (Morphine)
- Vincristine (Oncovin)

It is essential for the nurse to take a thorough health history of the client's elimination habits. Constipation or other stool abnormalities should be defined by a change in that client's normal stool pattern. Abnormalities in stool patterns are often indicative of an underlying health problem. Diarrhea or stools with mucus can indicate enteritis, parasitic invasion, or a response to medication. Severe constipation can cause watery stools to pass around a hard, impacted fecal mass. *Steatorrhea*, characterized by the bulky, foul-smelling, fatty stools seen with poor fat absorption, can occur in clients with cystic fibrosis. Clay-colored stools may be a sign of biliary obstruction. *Melena* is characterized by black, tarry stools, which usually indicate chronic or old bleeding, especially in the UGI tract. When the stool is mixed with bright red blood, active bleeding is indicated. Active bleeding may be from sites such as internal or external hemorrhoids, polyps, diverticula, or cancerous tumors. Clients who have changes in stool patterns require a thorough history and physical along with further diagnostic testing to establish the diagnosis and treatment plan.

Laboratory tests for clients with elimination problems frequently include stool examination. Stool specimens are collected to:

- Identify a specific organism.
- Determine the fat content (in biliary or pancreatic obstruction and malabsorption disorders).
- Determine the presence of and identify ova and parasites.
- Determine the presence of fresh or occult blood (guaiac test).
- Perform a **clostridial toxin assay** to identify bacterial (*Clostridium difficile*) infection of the intestine.

Clostridial Toxin Assay. Clostridial infection results from destruction of the normal flora by antibiotics, which increases the amount of *C. difficile* in the intestines (superinfection). This clostridial bacterium releases a toxin that damages the colonic epithelium, and the presence of this toxin in the stool specimen is diagnostic of clostridial enterocolitis.

☒

TABLE 5-2
HIGH-FIBER FOODS TO DECREASE CONSTIPATION

Fruit	Apples, bananas, berries, oranges, pears
Vegetables	Beans, cabbage, carrots, cauliflower, celery, dried peas, tomatoes, zucchini
Snacks	Bran muffin, popcorn, whole-wheat crackers
Grains	Bran cereal, brown rice, whole-wheat bread

Nursing responsibilities include collecting the stool specimen according to protocol or giving verbal and written instructions to the client who collects the specimen at home. In general, the stool specimen needs to be warm, fresh, and in the appropriate collection device (Pagana & Pagana, 1995).

RADIOLOGICAL TESTS AND PROCEDURES FOR GI CONDITIONS

Radiological tests and procedures are frequently used to establish a diagnosis in a client with a GI condition. With the need to decrease health costs, ordering the diagnostic test that will give the most accurate diagnosis at the lowest expense and risk to the client becomes a challenge for practitioners. Changes in the health care delivery system have brought changes in nursing responsibilities regarding diagnostic tests. Nurses need to view care of the client undergoing diagnostic testing and procedures as a shared responsibility with other members of the health care team, including the physician, radiologist, radiology technician, nuclear medicine staff, and gastroenterologist. Since many procedures are done in an outpatient setting, nurses working in an ambulatory clinic or physician's office often have the responsibility of explaining the purpose of a test or procedure and giving specific instructions to the client before it is performed. Nurses work collaboratively with the radiology and nuclear medicine departments to ensure that written instruction sheets are available for clients. In addition, nursing specialties have evolved where nurses assist in radiology and endoscopy procedures, creating new nursing roles and areas of expertise. Moreover, as they expand into advanced practice roles, nurses themselves are ordering diagnostic tests and procedures for clients. These are only a few examples of the shared roles of nurses and other health care team members in the care of clients undergoing diagnostic testing. Nursing responsibilities for clients having radiologic tests for suspected GI conditions are discussed below.

UGI Series or Barium Swallow

Visualization of the GI tract using a radiopaque substance (barium) and fluoroscopy or x-rays include the UGI and LGI series. The UGI series visualizes the esophagus, stomach, duodenum, and upper jejunum. It is termed a barium swallow if the function of the esophagus alone is examined. The contrast medium is a barium suspension with the consistency of a milkshake. **Nursing interventions** include following the protocol of the radiology department and giving clients undergoing the procedure as outpatients verbal and written instructions. Generally, before the UGI procedure, no preparation is necessary except for instructions and an explanation. The client is given nothing by mouth 6 hours prior to the test. After the UGI test, a laxative is administered and fluids are encouraged to aid in expelling the barium.

LGI Series or Barium Enema

The LGI series, or barium enema, evaluates the large intestine. The contrast medium is administered as a retention-type enema. In many instances, air is inserted into the colon after the barium (air-contrast barium enema). With air contrast, the colonic mucosa can be visualized more accurately. Barium enemas are used to detect polyps, tumors, diverticula, and chronic inflammatory bowel disease. **Nursing interventions** before the test involve bowel preparation with laxatives or enemas to cleanse the colon thoroughly. One day prior to the test, the client is limited to a liquid diet with no dairy products. The client is given nothing by mouth after midnight prior to the test. After the test, laxatives and increased fluids are required to facilitate removal of the barium. Instructions to clients should explain that bowel movements will be white until the barium is expelled. The barium enema procedure may be unpleasant or exhausting, especially for the elderly; therefore rest should be encouraged for elderly clients. The nurse should monitor clients for signs of complications such as abdominal pain or persistent constipation with failure to expel the barium (Pagana & Pagana, 1995.)

Ultrasonography

Ultrasonography involves the use of high-frequency sound waves transmitted into the abdomen, which create echoes that vary with tissue density. Echoes bounce back to a transducer and are electronically converted to x-ray–like pictures of the organs (without exposure to radiation). Ultrasound is useful as a diagnostic tool to identify organ size, shape, and position; it is a noninvasive, low-risk method to diagnose cysts, tumors, and stones. Ultrasound procedures are painless and safe. **Nursing interventions** may include verbal and written instructions for the client to be given nothing by mouth for at least 8–12 hours prior to the test; after ultrasound, the client may return to a normal diet and activity.

Computed Tomography (CT) Scan

CT scan is a noninvasive yet very accurate radiology procedure. Unfortunately, it is also a very expensive one, costing approximately $1000. After x-rays are passed through the tissue, the computer reconstructs the data into two-dimensional images on the monitor, and serial photographs are then taken. The CT scan may be done with or without contrast media, or the image may be enhanced by repeating the scan with the intravenous administration of iodine-containing contrast dye (Pagana & Pagana, 1995). CT scan of the abdomen is useful to identify the gallbladder, biliary ductal system, pancreatic problems, liver tumors, abscesses, bleeding, and the abdominal aorta and its branches for evaluation of dilation indicating an aneurysm. **Nursing interventions** include the following: The client is to be given nothing by mouth 8–12 hours prior to the CT scan. The nurse should assess the client for iodine allergies in case contrast media are used.

If the client has a known allergy to iodine or shellfish, the radiologist must be notified. The allergy should be documented on the front of the client's chart, on the client's name band and medication administration record, and any other location required by the hospital policy. Retained barium from previous studies may obscure visualization; therefore, a CT scan should be performed before any barium studies.

GI Scintigraphy

GI scintigraphy (GI bleeding scan) is a nuclear scan used to localize the site of GI bleeding. The procedure is performed with the intravenous administration of a radionuclide that pools at the site of the bleeding. No pretest preparation is required. The scan takes approximately 30 minutes, and clients experience no discomfort. This scan localizes the site of the bleeding, but does not indicate the exact pathologic condition causing it. If surgery is required, the scan indicates the area to be explored by the surgeon in the hope of detecting and resecting the bleeding source (Pagana & Pagana, 1995).

Cholangiography

Cholangiography is an x-ray with contrast dye to visualize the hepatic and common bile ducts and to look for the presence of stones, strictures, or tumors. Radiopaque dye is administered intravenously or directly into the bile duct during surgery. In recent years, since the introduction of endoscopic retrograde cholangiopancreatography (ERCP) and the use of the HIDA (hepatobiliary iminodiacetic acid analogues) gallbladder scan, the indications for cholangiography have almost ceased. After intravenous administration of a technetium 99m (^{99m}Tc)-labeled IDA (Choletec), the right upper quadrant (RUQ) and biliary tract are scanned. **Nursing interventions** include giving the client nothing by mouth 8 hours prior to the test. After the test, clients are monitored closely for bleeding and for reactions to the contrast media. The client is maintained on bed rest on the right side for 6 hours after the test.

Esophageal Function Tests

Esophageal function tests are used to evaluate functioning of the esophagus and to diagnose esophageal reflux or motility problems. Manometry measures pressure and peristaltic movements within the esophagus as the patient swallows and thus is used to diagnose esophageal reflux. A pH test, measured by an electrode connected to a manometry catheter (pH probe), indicates if acid reflux into the esophagus is occurring. Normally, the pH of the esophagus is greater than 6.0, and a drop in pH occurs with regurgitation of gastric acid into the esophagus. Esophageal tests are usually performed in the endoscopy room. The client is asked to swallow two or three tiny tubes to obtain the measurements.

Nursing interventions for esophageal studies include giving the client nothing by mouth 8 hours prior to the tests. GI medications such as antacids, histamine (H_2)-receptor antagonists, cholinergics, and anticholinergics may be withheld according to the physician's orders. The client should be instructed to avoid alcohol and smoking the day before the test. After testing, the client can resume normal activities and diet. The client may have a mild sore throat after removal of the tubes.

Tests of Gastric Function and Endoscopic Procedures

Gastric Analysis

Gastric analysis examines the fasting contents of the stomach for the diagnosis of organic gastric disease. This procedure involves a basal gastric secretion and gastric acid stimulation test. A nasogastric (NG) tube is inserted, and gastric contents are aspirated. Subcutaneous histamine is administered, and the NG tube is aspirated every 15 minutes for 1.5 hours to evaluate the stimulated flow of gastric acid. With the advent of more advanced diagnostic procedures and treatments for peptic ulcer disease (PUD), the only present use for gastric analysis is to determine the efficacy of the medical or surgical treatment of PUD. Effective therapy is indicated when the acid output of the stomach is reduced by 50% from the pretreatment baseline value (Pagana & Pagana, 1995).

Schilling Test

The Schilling test evaluates vitamin B_{12} absorption and is used to diagnose pernicious anemia. The client is given vitamin B_{12} orally and intramuscularly, and vitamin B_{12} levels are measured 24–48 hours later. Normally, the ileum absorbs more vitamin B_{12} than the body needs and excretes the excess into the urine. Malabsorption is indicated when there is little vitamin B_{12} excreted into the urine.

Biopsy

Biopsy is frequently needed to evaluate lesions of the GI tract. Lesions of the oral cavity or tongue may be biopsied under local anesthesia. Biopsy of the stomach and intestines is typically done by endoscopy. Biopsies of tumors, polyps, or ulcers in the anus, rectum, and sigmoid colon can be performed with a sigmoidoscope. **Nursing interventions** include instructions on preprocedure bowel preparation and postprocedure expectations.

Endoscopy

Endoscopy allows for direct visualization of portions of the GI tract. A long, flexible, illuminated fiberoptic scope provides images that can be viewed through an eyepiece or on a video screen. Endoscopy is used for direct inspection to determine a diagnosis, for biopsy and removal of polyps or stones, and to control bleeding using laser, photocoagulation, or injection of sclerosing agents. It may include visualization of the entire UGI tract (esophagogastroduodenoscopy, EGD) or may be limited to the esophagus (esophagoscopy), the stomach (gastroscopy), or the duodenum (duodenoscopy). The role of endoscopic surgery is expanding and is a good example of technology providing improved treatment with lower risks than the previous standard surgical procedures. While endoscopic procedures are costly, they are less expensive than traditional surgery, hospitalization, or prolonged and less successful medical treatments.

The various types of endoscopy are useful for both the diagnosis and treatment of conditions in the UGI tract. Endoscopy is used for UGI bleeds, gastric cancer, ulcers, esophageal varices, tumors, hiatal hernias, and biopsy with removal of gastric polyps. The procedure involves insertion of the scope through the oropharynx. This may be uncomfortable to the client and cause some choking and gagging despite topical anesthetics and sedation. The throat is topically anesthetized with viscous lidocaine (Xylocaine) to decrease the gag reflex. Intravenous sedation is given with midazolam (Versed) or diazepam (Valium). Midazolam (Versed) is effective as an amnestic agent, so the client will not have unpleasant memories of the procedure. The analgesic narcotic meperidine (Demerol) is usually given as a premedication. This leaves the client conscious but sedated. The procedure is performed by a gastroenterologist and lasts approximately 30 minutes unless additional treatments are required.

Nursing responsibilities include making the client aware as to what to expect. The procedure is frequently performed on an outpatient basis, and the client is given nothing by mouth 8 hours prior to the procedure. After the procedure, the client is monitored according to the standards and policies for a client undergoing conscious sedation. Vital signs and the status of the client are assessed for 3–4 hours before the client is discharged. The client is monitored for signs and symptoms of dyspnea, pain, bleeding, or dysphagia. The nurse should ascertain that the client's gag reflex is intact and then have the client resume fluids and diet.

Endoscopic Retrograde Cholangiopancreatography (ERCP)

In this procedure, the endoscope is inserted orally, and dye is injected into the ampulla of Vater to outline the pancreatic and biliary ducts. Since only ERCP can visualize the pancreatic and biliary ducts directly, this test has become extremely useful for clients with tumors, strictures, cysts, or stones. The procedure is performed in the endoscopy room by a gastroenterologist and lasts approximately 1 hour. Precautions are similar to those taken with a client who has had an EGD; the client can usually be discharged after recovery. After the procedure, the nurse must watch for signs of abdominal pain and nausea or vomiting, which might indicate ERCP-induced pancreatitis. When this is suspected, serum amylase and lipase levels should be monitored, and hospitalization for observation is usually required.

Colonoscopy

Colonoscopy is an endoscopic examination of the entire colon, used to evaluate benign versus malignant growths, remove polyps, take biopsy specimens, and localize sites of bleeding. A thorough bowel preparation that includes a clear liquid diet and strong laxatives is required 2–3 days before the procedure; enemas are required the day of the test. The bowel is also prepared the day before the procedure using an oral osmotic solution such as a gallon of polyethylene glycol (Golytely, Colyte). This induces watery diarrhea to cleanse the bowel thoroughly for visualization. The client is given nothing by mouth 8 hours before the test. Premedications include midazolam (Versed), diazepam (Valium), and meperidine (Demerol). Medications are augmented as needed during the procedure to maintain conscious sedation. The procedure lasts 20–60 minutes. Air is injected with the scope to improve visualization, causing some abdominal cramping. After the procedure, the client is monitored for changes in vital signs and for abdominal pain, rectal bleeding, or fever.

Sigmoidoscopy

Sigmoidoscopy allows for visualization of the anus, rectum (proctoscopy), and distal sigmoid colon. It is performed using either a rigid or flexible sigmoidoscope (scope with larger diameter). The client is limited to clear liquids for 24 hours and then given nothing by mouth for 8 hours before the procedure. Sodium phosphate enemas (Fleet) are usually sufficient for bowel preparation. After the procedure, the nurse should monitor for distention, increased abdominal tenderness, or rectal bleeding.

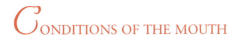

Conditions of the Mouth

Dental Disorders

Problems of the mouth commonly include dental disorders. Dental health is essential for good nutrition, prevention of weight loss, and maintenance of the digestive process. Dental caries (tooth decay) and gum disease can be prevented by good oral hygiene, flossing, fluoridation of the water, restricting simple sugars in the diet, daily doses of vitamin C, and regular dental examinations with cleanings every 6 months. Fillings and dental work should be performed as needed. Periodontal (gum) disease, most often due to bacterial plaque buildup, is the most common cause of tooth loss after 50 years of age. *Gingivitis,* the earliest form of periodontal disease, is characterized by swollen, discolored gums that bleed easily. Inflamed pockets collect debris, which results in receding gums, bone resorption, and loose teeth. The cost of dental care may be a barrier for many clients. To refer clients, nurses should be aware of community resources such as university dental clinics or other agencies that provide need-based dental care.

Mouth Infections

Infections of the mouth may be primary infections or may result from other systemic diseases, drug treatments, or vitamin deficiencies. Types of mouth infections are discussed below.

Aphthous Stomatitis (Canker Sores) These are painful ulcers on the soft tissues of the mouth, lips, tongue, inner cheeks, pharynx, and soft palate. This type of stomatitis is noncontagious. The ulcers are possibly associated with stress, vitamin deficiency, or a localized reaction to food. Palliative treatment includes oral steroid solutions or ointments, topical analgesics, and antibiotics if the ulcers become infected.

Herpes Simplex Virus (Cold Sores; Fever Blisters) These are fluid-filled blisters caused by the herpes simplex type I virus; they are usually seen as a vesicle on the mucocutaneous border of the lip. The blisters occur as an initial outbreak with reactivation after stress, fever, or exposure to cold or ultraviolet light. While these lesions are extremely common and require no treatment in most healthy adults, the virus is communicable and may be a problem in immunosuppressed clients, newborns, and clients with acquired immunodeficiency syndrome (AIDS). The lesions are contagious until crusted, which usually takes 7–10 days. Body fluid precautions should be maintained, and procedures should be followed to prevent exposure of newborns and immunosuppressed clients. Topical acyclovir (Zovirax) provides palliative relief.

Vincent's Angina (Trench Mouth) This is an acute inflammatory gum disease with proliferation of normal mouth flora that is caused by poor oral hygiene, nutritional deficiencies, alcohol abuse, infection, and immunosuppression. Signs and symptoms include painful lesions, bleeding gums, tonsillitis, fever, foul halitosis, and swollen lymph nodes. It is treated with a regimen of analgesics, antibiotics, mouthwash, and frequent brushing with a soft toothbrush. The client usually requires a comprehensive health education plan to improve general health habits, dental hygiene, and access to and utilization of affordable health services.

Candidiasis Candidiasis (oral thrush) is an overgrowth of *Candida albicans*, a yeast-like fungus, which is normally found on the skin and in the GI tract, vagina, and mouth. Overgrowth may result from antibiotics destroying the balance of the normal flora, immunosuppression due to chemotherapy, prolonged steroid use, human immunodeficiency virus (HIV) infection, or hyperglycemia. Oral thrush is also common in newborns and infants and may be communicated to the nipple and breast of the breast-feeding mother. Symptoms are distinctive, with creamy white patches of exudate lying over a reddened tissue base. Women with vaginal thrush complain of creamy white, curdlike vaginal discharge. Thrush, whether in the mouth, GI tract, vulva, or breast of the breast-feeding mother, is extremely painful.

Treatment of candidiasis is aimed at reducing the quantity of the fungus and restoring the balance of normal flora. For oral thrush, medications include clotrimazole (Mycelex) lozenges, and nystatin (Myostatin, Nilstat) tabs, or the more traditional swish and swallow. Ketoconazole (Nizoral) is another option. For vulvovaginal candidiasis, topical azole drugs are more effective (Allen & Phillips, 1997). Breast-feeding infants and mothers must both be treated to prevent continued cross-infection. Buttermilk, yogurt, or lactobacillus tablets should be encouraged to repopulate the GI tract with flora. In severe or recurrent thrush, systemic illnesses such as diabetes or HIV should be ruled out.

Parotitis Parotitis is an inflammation of the parotid glands, the largest salivary glands. Mumps is a viral parotitis, but nonviral parotitis can occur in clients debilitated from dehydration, poor oral fluid intake, or immunosuppression. Signs and symptoms are abrupt and include fever, swelling, and pain in the parotid glands and surrounding lymph nodes. Treatment includes antibiotics. Other comfort measures include local hot or cold compresses, frequent oral hygiene, hydration, and hard candies or lozenges to stimulate salivary gland secretion.

Cancer of the Mouth

Cancer of the mouth is clearly linked to tobacco and alcohol use and is most common in people over 45 years of age. Most oral cancers arise from squamous cells, but epithelial, basal cell, and other carcinomas also occur. Metastases to adjacent areas or the neck may be rapid, and the client is usually asymptomatic, making oral cancer difficult to detect in the early stages. Any oral or neck lesion requires careful evaluation with biopsy. Premalignant lesions (leukoplakia, erythroplasia, erythroplakia) are treated by biopsy, and the client is instructed to eliminate the use of tobacco and alcohol. Good oral hygiene and frequent dental and oral examinations are required as follow-up for high-risk clients.

Ultrasound is useful to evaluate superficial masses, but CT and magnetic resonance imaging (MRI) are needed for deeper lesions. The diagnostic workup must include a tissue biopsy for diagnosis and staging. A CT scan or MRI evaluates the deeper structure of the tumor and shows whether metastases are present. Treatment of cancer of the mouth depends on the location and stage of the tumor. Early stage tumors are usually treated by radiation or surgery. More invasive cancers require both radiation and surgery, and advanced stage tumors are treated by palliative means.

Surgical resection for oral cancers includes partial mandibulectomy, hemiglossectomy or total glossectomy, and resections of the floor of the mouth with buccal mucosa. Oral cancers frequently metastasize early to the cervical lymph nodes. Surgical procedures include neck dissections with removal of nodes and their channels and, in advanced cases, removal of the sternocleidomastoid muscle or other neck muscles, internal jugular vein, thyroid gland, submandibular gland, and spinal accessory nerve.

Treatment of clients with oral cancer is managed by an entire health team. Referrals to a speech therapist, occupational therapist, psychologist, and dietitian are necessary due to difficulties that may arise with verbal communication, chewing, and swallowing, as well as changes in body image and self-esteem.

Nursing requirements for preoperative care include thorough oral hygiene to reduce bacteria. The nurse should carefully explain the procedure, along with the realistic postoperative expectations such as planned treatments and feeding and communication adaptations. Emotional support should also be given as changes in facial features may be extensive.

Postoperative care should focus on facilitating verbal communication. The nurse must phrase questions in a yes or no format so that the client can respond by gestures and nods. Answers should be repeated before acting on perceived requests. The nurse should be calm and reassure the client frequently, encouraging slow speech. The client should be referred to speech therapy early in the postoperative period.

In addition to communication difficulties, the client may experience chewing and swallowing difficulties, as sensation in the mouth is decreased. The client often needs assistance with feeding; no hot or very cold foods or forks are allowed. To ensure good oral hygiene, the nurse uses only sterile equipment for gentle mouth irrigation with peroxide and saline. Toothbrushes are not sterile.

Another focus of care is respiration and airway maintenance. To assist with respiration and to maintain the airway, the head of the bed is elevated. The nurse suctions the oral cavity and teaches the clients how to perform the task themselves. The lungs should be auscultated frequently. The nurse should expect persistent drooling. Finally, the client and family are included in all self-care and discharge planning.

Trauma of the Mouth and Jaw

Trauma can be due to soft tissue injury (bruises, lacerations, edema) or bony injury (fractures). Trauma frequently occurs in sports injuries, motor vehicle accidents, or fighting. Treatment includes emergency assessment and x-rays to establish the diagnosis. Analgesics are administered for pain. Ice decreases swelling, and antibiotics are prescribed to prevent infection.

A fracture of the jaw is treated with open or closed reduction and inter-maxillary fixation. The teeth are wired or banded for 5–8 weeks to immobilize the jaw until the bone has healed.

Nursing management focuses on maintaining the airway. Frequently, edema occurs in the face and neck. Elevating the head of the bed promotes drainage and decreases edema. If the jaw is wired, the nurse monitors the client for nausea and vomiting and prevents aspiration. Wire cutters are kept at the bedside or with the client at all times. Suction may be needed. A liquid diet is necessary while the jaw is wired. Referral to a dietitian is essential. The nurse should encourage good oral hygiene. The client should be taught to rinse with gentle water swishes.

CONDITIONS OF THE ESOPHAGUS, STOMACH, AND DUODENUM

Gastroesophageal Reflux Disease (GERD)

GERD occurs when gastric contents move back into the distal esophagus due to inappropriate relaxation of the lower esophageal sphincter (LES). Many variables contribute to decreased LES pressure. Frequent causes include fatty foods, chocolate, xanthine, nicotine, ganglionic stimulants, β-adrenergic drugs, elevated levels of estrogen and progesterone, delayed gastric emptying, and the elevated intra-abdominal pressure commonly associated with pregnancy, obesity, and heavy lifting.

Reflux may be accompanied by an inflammatory response when the mucosal barrier breaks down. Repeated reflux episodes cause esophageal irritation, and fibrotic tissue changes can result in esophageal stricture and impaired swallowing. Signs and symptoms vary in severity. Heartburn 20–120 minutes after eating, regurgitation with a sour or bitter taste, water brash (reflex hypersecretion without a bitter taste), frequent belching, and gas are common complaints.

Complications of GERD include esophageal ulceration, hemorrhage, and adenocarcinoma. Repeated scarring can permanently damage esophageal tissue and produce stricture and dysphagia. Chronic nighttime reflux places clients at risk for aspiration, which can lead to aspiration pneumonia, especially in the elderly. A diagnosis of GERD is made primarily by endoscopy. Esophageal pH and LES function should be monitored.

Treatment of GERD is primarily pharmacologic. Drug categories for GERD are as follows:

1. **Antacids.** Maalox and Mylanta are well tolerated and inexpensive. However, they may not control GERD without the use of other drugs.
2. **H$_2$-receptor antagonists** such as cimetidine (Tagamet), ranitidine (Zantac), famotidine (Pepcid), or nizatidine (Axid) are effective for more severe GERD, to reduce gastric acid secretion and support tissue healing.

3. **Cholinergic drugs.** In severe cases, bethanechol (Urecholine) or metoclopramide (Reglan) may be added to H$_2$-receptor antagonists.
4. **Proton pump inhibitors.** These potent drugs, which are now being researched, reduce acid secretion by 90% within 24 hours after a single dose, but relapse is common when the drug is discontinued.

Anticholinergics, calcium channel blockers, xanthine derivatives, and diazepam (Valium) lower the LES pressure and should be avoided. In addition, clients should be cautioned about drug interactions when taking H$_2$-receptor antagonists.

Surgical intervention is reserved for clients with severe GERD who do not respond to aggressive medical management. Early diagnosis and treatment and the newer drug therapies have decreased the need for surgery. When necessary, a fundoplication may be performed. This involves wrapping and suturing the gastric fundus around the esophagus, which reinforces the LES area and anchors it to the diaphragm. The Angelchik prosthesis is an L-shaped silicone prosthesis that is placed around the distal esophagus. The prosthesis anchors the sphincter in the abdomen and reinforces the LES (Phipps, et al., 1995).

Nursing interventions include the following health education points: Clients should be informed of the medication regimen and side effects. They will need to eliminate foods known to lower LES pressure from their diet. The nurse should encourage a low-fat diet and limited caffeine intake. The client should eat 4–6 small meals per day, avoiding evening snacks. A weight reduction diet should be initiated if the client is overweight. Eating slowly and chewing thoroughly to reduce belching must be emphasized. Since smoking causes a rapid drop in LES pressure, the nurse should encourage clients who smoke to quit. Finally, the client needs to avoid straining or heavy lifting.

Hiatal Hernia

A hiatal hernia (diaphragmatic hernia) is the herniation of the upper portion of the stomach through the diaphragm into the thoracic cavity. The two major types of hiatal hernias are the *sliding hernia* (90%), in which the distal esophagus, gastroesophageal junction, and a portion of the stomach herniate upward into the thorax, creating a freely movable structure that slides back and forth in response to changes in position or intra-abdominal pressure, and the *rolling (paraesophageal) hernia*, in which the gastroesophageal junction remains anchored, but the fundus of the stomach rolls into the thorax, causing herniation next to the esophagus.

Hiatal hernias usually occur in middle-aged and older clients and are seen more often in women. Conditions that cause increased intra-abdominal pressure may be precipitating factors. Clinical manifestations include symptoms of reflux such as heartburn and indigestion. The reflux is precipitated by large, fatty meals, alcohol, or stress. Other symptoms include nocturnal attacks of pain, regurgitation, and dysphagia. Diagnostic tests are the same as for a reflux workup, with the addition of a barium swallow with fluoroscopy. Treatment includes antacids 1 hour before and 2–3 hours after meals. Cholinergic medications (Urecholine) and H_2-receptor antagonists such as famotidine (Pepcid), ranitidine (Zantac), and cimetidine (Tagamet) are effective.

Nursing interventions for hiatal hernia include administering antacids, elevating the head of the bed 4–6 inches, discouraging highly seasoned foods, and encouraging clients to eat frequent small meals to prevent gastric dilation. Dietary instructions are to avoid carbonated beverages, fats, caffeine, chocolate, and nicotine. Clients who smoke need to stop, and overweight clients need to lose weight.

When surgical correction is required, preoperative teaching should include explaining the use of the inspirometer and splinting of the incision for effective coughing. If a thoracic approach is planned, explanations should be given concerning chest tubes.

Postoperative care includes facilitating airway clearance by keeping the head of the bed elevated. The client should turn, cough, and breathe deeply every 2 hours and, when able, should begin to use the inspirometer and initiate early ambulation. Medications for pain management and prevention of nausea and vomiting should be offered. A NG tube remains in place until peristalsis returns. NG-tube output should be recorded (color and amount). Parenteral fluids and electrolyte replacement are required. Serum electrolytes from any client with an NG tube should be monitored daily. Once the client can begin to eat, the nurse should encourage small frequent feedings with the head of the bed elevated. The client should avoid carbonated beverages and not drink through a straw.

Esophageal Carcinoma

Benign tumors of the esophagus are extremely rare, asymptomatic, and generally require no care. Malignant tumors, while not common, are very virulent and are almost always fatal. Contributing factors include heavy use of tobacco and alcohol, contaminants in soil and foods, especially nitrosamines, and diets chronically inadequate in fresh fruits, vegetables, vitamins, and certain proteins. Long-term effects of other esophageal problems such as stricture, achalasia, or GERD can be risk factors for esophageal cancer. Diagnosis is made by barium swallow with fluoroscopy and endoscopy with biopsy. CT scan may be required.

Treatment includes antineoplastic agents cisplatin (Platinol) combined with radiation therapy or surgery. Radiation therapy for 6–8 weeks reduces tumor size, but side effects of radiation may cause esophageal stricture. If this occurs, dilation may be performed. As dysphagia worsens, gastrostomy feedings or short-term total parenteral nutrition (TPN) may be required to meet nutritional needs, taking into account the desires of the client and his or her family.

Extensive surgical procedures are associated with a high mortality rate. Subtotal and total esophagectomy involve removal of the esophagus. Esophagastrostomy involves removal of the diseased portion of the esophagus, and the stump is then attached to the stomach. Clients undergoing these procedures require intensive postoperative monitoring for shock, hemorrhage, infection, leakage at the anastomotic site, and aspiration due to the removal of the LES. These clients need assistance in dealing with a terminal illness. The nurse should encourage the client and family to talk about their concerns and needs and to use support offered through cancer groups, counseling, and their religious affiliation.

Gastritis

Gastritis is a diffuse or localized inflammation of the gastric mucosa, which develops when the protective mechanism of the mucosa is overwhelmed by bacteria or other irritating substances. Acute gastritis is a short-term inflammatory process that may be related to ingestion of chemical agents or foods that irritate and erode the gastric mucosa. Agents can include seasonings, spices, alcohol, medications, radiation, chemotherapy, and infective microorganisms.

Chronic gastritis is subdivided into types A and B. *Type A gastritis* is autoimmune in nature. It is associated with atrophy of the gastric glands and deterioration of the mucosa. The eventual decrease in gastric secretion may affect antibody production. Pernicious anemia develops by this process. *Type B gastritis* is more common. It is associated with infection with *Helicobacter pylori* bacteria, which causes ulcers in the lining of the stomach.

Clinical manifestations of chronic gastritis include anorexia, nausea, vomiting, abdominal cramps, diarrhea, epigastric pain, and fever. Painless GI bleeding may occur with the use of **aspirin (ASA)** or nonsteroidal anti-inflammatory drugs (NSAIDs). In acute stages, clients are treated symptomatically with antacids and by the avoidance of known irritants. For type A chronic gastritis, vitamin B_{12} injections are given for pernicious anemia. For type B, drug therapy with antacids, sucralfate (Carafate), H_2-receptor antagonists, or antimicrobial agents to eradicate *H. pylori* is administered. **Nursing interventions** include preventive health teaching to discourage alcohol, smoking, or other known gastric irritants, such as any ASA-containing products.

Aspirin as an Ulcerogenic Drug. Aspirin is an acid and therefore can be very irritating to the gastric mucosa. Clients should be instructed to read all labels of the over-the-counter (OTC) medications for the presence of aspirin. Many OTC drugs contain aspirin.

Peptic Ulcer Disease (PUD)

PUD refers to gastric, duodenal, and stress ulcers. Ulcerations of the mucosa of the UGI tract are caused by an imbalance of gastric acid and pepsin secretion and alterations of the mucosa. In PUD, ulcers appear as "craters" in the mucosa of the stomach, duodenum, or jejunum (Fig. 5-1). Patterns of exacerbation and remission frequently occur in the same clients.

PUD has multiple causes. Genetics plays a role in the incidence of PUD. Environmental factors include smoking, which interferes with gastric mucosal protection and healing, and alcohol, which can cause mucosal damage and bleeding. Caffeine acts as a strong acid secretor, while chronic stressors are more likely to cause ulcers than acute stressors. Drugs such as NSAIDs, ASA, and corticosteroids are considered ulcerogenic (ulcer causing). Bacterial infection (*H. pylori*) makes the gastric mucosa more vulnerable to damage due to impaired mucosal defenses, thus allowing chronic ulcers to form. Gastrin-producing tumors found in the islet cells of the pancreas massively overstimulate gastric acid secretion, causing erosion of the gastric mucosa. Duodenal ulcers are generally more common than gastric ulcers in young adults. Gastric ulcers are on the rise due to the use of NSAIDs for arthritis management in the elderly.

Clinical manifestations seen with duodenal ulcers include burning, cramping, and midepigastric pain, especially 2–4 hours after meals. Eating generally relieves the pain, which is episodic. It may occur at night and be relieved in the morning. Clients experience nausea and have a tendency to gain weight as they eat more in an attempt to decrease the pain.

Symptoms seen with gastric ulcers include a burning pain in the epigastric area that may radiate to the back. This usually occurs 1–2 hours after meals. Food may relieve the pain but frequently aggravates it. Pain generally does not occur at night, and clients have a tendency to lose weight.

UGI series and endoscopic examination (gastroscopy) are performed to diagnose PUD. The presence of *H. pylori* can be detected by blood analysis. Treatments include antacids such as aluminum hydroxide preparations administered 1–3 hours after meals and at bedtime. Antacids should not be given concurrently with other ulcer drugs as they interfere with drug absorption. H_2-receptor antagonists aid healing, resulting in the resolution of most ulcers after 4 weeks of therapy. Medications in current use include cimetidine (Tagamet), ranitidine (Zantac), famotidine (Pepcid), and nizatidine (Axid). These drugs, which suppress gastric acid production, are given in divided doses throughout the day and at bedtime.

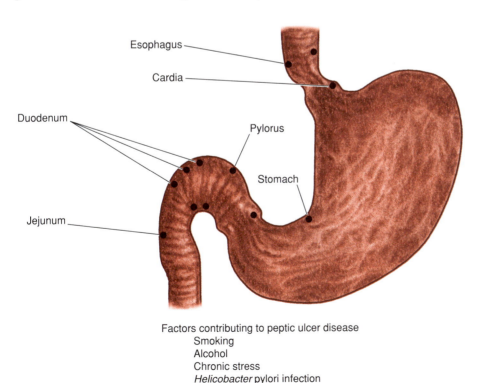

Factors contributing to peptic ulcer disease
Smoking
Alcohol
Chronic stress
Helicobacter pylori infection
Drug effects

FIGURE 5-1 Common locations of peptic ulcer disease.

An additional medication, sucralfate (Carafate), coats the ulcer, sealing it against acid irritation, which promotes healing. Misoprostol (Cytotec) enhances mucosal defenses to prevent the development of ulcerations. Omeprazole (Prilosec) and lansoprazole (Prevacid) decrease acid secretion and improve the rate of ulcer healing. Various preparations exist for antimicrobial treatment of *H. pylori*. One treatment consists of a triple-drug regimen for a minimum of 3 weeks, using bismuth subsalicylate (Pepto-Bismol), amoxicillin or tetracycline, and metronidazole (Flagyl). Tritec is a newer antibiotic specific for *H. pylori* that may be used alone or in combination with another antibiotic. Tritec is often given in combination with H_2-receptor antagonists. Helidac is a combination of bismuth, metronidazole, and tetracycline, packaged in one medication. **Nursing education** should include encouraging the client to eliminate foods that cause discomfort, to rest, seek stress management activities, and avoid smoking, persistent alcohol use, and ASA.

With early diagnosis and improved pharmacologic treatment of PUD, surgical interventions are used only for the management of complications (e.g., hemorrhage, perforation into the peritoneal cavity, gastric obstruction) or the failure to respond to aggressive medical treatment. Surgical procedures are as follows:

1. **Vagotomy** reduces acid production by decreasing cholinergic stimulation of parietal cells and limiting the response to gastrin.
2. **Pyloroplasty** widens the pyloric valve to enhance gastric emptying. This procedure may be done with a vagotomy.
3. **Antrectomy** involves removal of the lower part of the stomach to reduce acid secretion. This technique may be performed with a vagotomy.
4. **Gastric resection** involves removal of portions of the distal stomach, which may include the gastrin-producing antrum and parietal cells (includes Bilroth I and II; partial gastric resection; gastrectomy).

Stress Ulcers

Stress ulcers are less common than duodenal or gastric ulcers. Inflammation, erosion, and bleeding of the mucosa can develop rapidly following a major physical trauma or illness. Lesions can occur within hours of injury in critically ill clients. The classic presentation is painless UGI bleeding within 3–7 days of physiologic stress. There are two major types of stress ulcers: *Curling's ulcers*, which involve multiple sites in the superficial mucosa of the duodenum and are associated with burns, trauma, hemorrhage, sepsis, and respiratory and renal failure, and *Cushing's ulcers*, which manifest as a single, deep lesion and are associated with central nervous system (CNS) injury or surgery.

Medical management of stress ulcers requires aggressive prevention. Continuous intravenous administration of H_2-receptor antagonists to all intensive care unit (ICU) or critically ill clients neutralizes gastric secretions (reduces gastric acidity) and thus prevents ulceration. If bleeding does occur, endoscopy with cauterization or laser photocoagulation usually controls the bleeding.

Cancer of the Stomach

Cancer of the stomach is thought to involve environmental, genetic, and possibly cultural factors. The incidence of stomach cancer is related to the presence of chronic achlorhydria (absence of HCl in the stomach), pernicious anemia, and villous adenoma (tumor of the mucosa of the large intestine). Most of the lesions are in the pyloric area. Gastric cancers are primary adenocarcinomas. Because of the ability of the stomach to accommodate the growing tumor, signs and symptoms may not be evident until metastases have already occurred. Pain usually does not appear until very late in the disease. Tumors metastasize into adjacent organs and structures (i.e., esophagus, spleen, pancreas, regional lymph nodes). Primary prevention aims at cessation of cigarette smoking and a diet high in vegetables, fruits, and vitamin C. Heavily cured or processed foods should be avoided.

Cancer of the Stomach, Esophagus, and Liver. Cancer of the stomach, esophagus, and liver occurs more frequently among Japanese Americans (Giger & Davidhizar, 1995). It is thought that dried salted fish, salt-cured food, nitrites, and poor vitamin C intake are associated with a greater incidence of stomach cancer.

Signs and Symptoms Signs and symptoms include vague, persistent gastric distress, gas, loss of appetite, nausea without vomiting, indigestion, traces of occult blood in the stool, gradual weight loss, loss of strength, and anemia. The presence of a palpable mass in the stomach, ascites, or bone pain from metastases may be the first symptoms. Gastroscopy and biopsy are the procedures of choice for definitive diagnosis. CT scanning and ultrasound determine the presence of metastases.

Treatment consists of chemotherapy, alone or in combination with radiation therapy, for clients with nonresectable or recurrent tumors. Surgical resection is the only potentially curative treatment. The procedure of choice depends on the location and extent of the tumor. Partial or subtotal gastrectomy is performed in an attempt to remove all of the tumor. Because a gastric tumor is usually not diagnosed until it is at an advanced stage, the 5-year survival rate is only 5–15%.

Nausea and vomiting are such common presenting symptoms that the nurse is required to use astute history, assessment, and diagnostic skills to determine the problem. Nausea and vomiting are part of the body's protective mechanisms and are usually a response to chemical or infectious insults. Nausea is an unpleasant sensation signalling that vomiting is imminent. Vomiting is an involuntary act in which the stomach contracts and forcefully expels gastric contents. Loss of fluid and electrolytes are the primary consequences of repeated vomiting. Metabolic alkalosis is associated with prolonged vomiting due to the loss of HCl. Metabolic acidosis occurs with severe prolonged vomiting of contents of the small intestines, resulting in loss of bicarbonate.

Causes of nausea and vomiting are classified as pathogenic, iatrogenic, or psychogenic. *Pathogenic causes,* which are related to a disease process, include intestinal obstruction, pregnancy, increased intracranial pressure (ICP), ingestion of toxic substances, allergies and hypersensitivity reactions, and streptococcal pharyngitis or tonsillitis. *Iatrogenic causes,* which result from disease treatment, include chemotherapy, radiation, and medications. *Psychogenic causes* include psychosis or neurosis and reaction to psychological trauma.

Nurses need to assess and document the frequency, amount, and type of vomiting and the contents of the vomitus. An assessment of the vomitus includes noting the presence of blood in the vomitus, termed hematemesis. Bright-red blood is indicative of hemorrhage. Dark-brown "coffee ground" material is indicative of blood retained in the stomach or "old" blood. Projectile vomiting is vomiting not preceded by nausea, which is expelled by excessive force. This occurs in infants with pyloric stenosis and severely increased ICP. The presence of fecal odor and bile in the vomitus indicates backflow of intestinal contents into the stomach and intestinal obstruction.

Treatment Treatment includes diagnosing and eliminating the precipitating cause, administering antiemetics, and restoring fluid and electrolyte balance. Antiemetics are administered orally, rectally, intramuscularly, or intravenously to block the stimulus that triggers nausea and vomiting. Clear liquids and Gatorade are suggested to provide hydration, and parenteral replacement of fluid and electrolytes is necessary if the loss is excessive.

Mint tea or aromatherapy with extract of peppermint are natural remedies useful to alleviate nausea.

Conditions of the Liver, Gallbladder, and Exocrine Pancreas

The liver has a unique spectrum of functions, and is intricately linked to the other organs. Therefore, an abnormality of the liver has great impact on every system of the body. Liver functions include: converting glucose to glycogen and storing it until needed; lipid (fat) metabolism, in which fatty acids are broken down to provide a source of body energy; protein metabolism, in which the liver synthesizes plasma proteins; and synthesis of prothrombin, which is needed for normal clotting of the blood. Vitamin K is necessary for adequate prothrombin production. The liver produces and stores vitamins A and D and stores vitamin B_{12} and iron. Barbiturates, amphetamines, and alcohol are metabolized, bile and bile salts are produced (600–1200 mL/day) and bilirubin, a bile pigment, is excreted by the liver. Blood flow is dependent on the portal vein and hepatic artery. The portal vein carries venous blood rich in nutrients absorbed from the GI system into the liver. The hepatic artery provides oxygenated blood to the liver.

Bile Salts. Bile salts emulsify fat for digestion and absorption in the intestine. The fat globules are broken into smaller particles, which increases the surface area on which pancreatic lipase can work.

Disorders of the Liver

Jaundice Jaundice is a strong indicator of a disorder of the liver. Increased levels of retained bilirubin cause a yellowish discoloration of mucous membranes, sclera, and skin. The yellow color may be noted first in the sclera of the eyes or in the mucous membranes of the hard palate. The type of jaundice indicates the primary pathology.

Hemolytic jaundice occurs as a result of an increase in the breakdown of red blood cells (RBCs), which produce an increased amount of unconjugated bilirubin in the blood. The liver cannot handle this increased level. The bilirubin is not water soluble, therefore it cannot be excreted. Unconjugated bilirubin is lipid soluble and is capable of entering nerve cells, causing brain damage. Hemolytic jaundice is caused by blood transfusion reactions, sickle cell crisis, hemolytic anemias, and hemolytic disease of the newborn.

Hepatocellular jaundice results from the inability of the liver to clear normal amounts of bilirubin from the blood. The causes of hepatocellular jaundice include hepatitis, cirrhosis, and hepatic cancer.

Obstructive jaundice results from impeded bile flow through the liver and biliary system. Obstruction may be within or outside the liver. Causes of obstructive jaundice include hepatitis, liver tumors, cirrhosis, and common bile duct obstruction by a stone.

Hepatitis Hepatitis is the widespread inflammation of liver tissue, which causes hepatic cell degeneration and necrosis. The different types of hepatitis are discussed below.

1. **Hepatitis A (HAV; infectious hepatitis).** HAV is transmitted by fecal–oral contamination, generally through contaminated food and water. Carriers are most contagious just prior to the onset of signs and symptoms, especially jaundice. Administration of intramuscular immune globulin (gamma globulin) to people who have been exposed may decrease the severity of the illness. People who travel to high-risk areas should be immunized. HAV is associated with permanent immunity after illness.

2. **Hepatitis B (HBV; serum hepatitis).** HBV is transmitted by percutaneous inoculation with contaminated needles or instruments, contact with body fluids contaminated with hepatitis B surface antigen (HBsAg) (e.g., during sexual contact), and cross-transmission of the virus from mothers with HBV to infants. Cross-transmission between newborn and mother may occur in utero, at birth, or during the postnatal period. An infected host can be an asymptomatic carrier. Laboratory assays identify the virus by the presence of HBsAg (Australian antigen). All units of donor blood are screened for HBsAg, and high-risk individuals are asked not to donate blood. Postexposure prophylaxis is available with the administration of HBIG (hepatitis B immunoglobulin), which provides temporary immunity. HBV is an occupational hazard for health care workers, reinforcing the need for blood and body fluid precautions with all clients and compliance with HBV immunization.

    The only real hope of combating the HBV epidemic is through immunization. HBV vaccine is available as long-term protection. To be effective, it must be given as a series of three injections at 1,

2, and 6 months. In addition, a titer must be screened 1–2 months after completion of the series. In some individuals with a low titer, an additional booster (fourth injection) is required to obtain protection. Universal HBV immunization at birth and during infancy is recommended to prevent perinatal transmission and to combat the HBV epidemic in general.

3. **Hepatitis C (HCV; non-A, non-B).** HCV is parenterally transmitted, especially through contaminated blood transfusions (before 1990), contaminated needles of drug users, and through body fluid contact such as sexual contact. It is diagnosed by the presence of the HCV antibody.

4. **Hepatitis D (HDV; delta hepatitis).** HDV is transmitted by the same routes as HBV and requires the presence of HBV infection to occur. HDV is thought to be either a coinfection with HBV or a superinfection in a HBV carrier. It is diagnosed by identifying the antibody to HDV and by determining the presence of hepatitis D antigen (HDAg).

5. **Hepatitis E (HEV).** HEV occurs through fecal–oral transmission. Its clinical presentation is similar to HAV. HEV is diagnosed by determining the presence of antibody to HEV (anti-HEV).

6. **Toxic and drug-induced hepatitis.** This hepatitis can be caused by toxic levels of drugs, alcohol, industrial toxins, or plant poisons.

HAV and HEV are found primarily in older children and young adults. An increased incidence occurs in crowded living conditions and in areas of poor hygiene. HBV, HCV, and HDV affect all ages when the person comes in contact with the blood or body fluid of an infected person. The virus is transmitted in the blood and all body fluids (e.g., saliva, semen, vaginal fluids).

In all types of hepatitis, the following phases occur:

1. **Preicteric phase (prior to jaundice).** Clinical manifestations include anorexia, nausea, RUQ discomfort, metallic taste, malaise, headache, fatigue, low-grade fever, and hepatomegaly.

2. **Icteric phase (jaundice).** Clinical manifestations include dark, tea-colored urine due to increased excretion of bilirubin; pruritus (itching); light, clay-colored stools if conjugated bilirubin does not flow out of the liver into the intestine; and a tender, enlarged liver.

3. **Posticteric phase (after jaundice).** Clinical manifestations include malaise, easy fatigability, and hepatomegaly that remains for several weeks or months.

Anicteric hepatitis (without jaundice) can occur in children. Also, many clients with HAV and HCV may not show clinical jaundice. Thus, the absence of jaundice does not rule out hepatitis. The onset of HAV is acute. The signs and symptoms generally are less severe than HBV. Clients may think they have the flu. The onset of HBV is more insidious, and the signs and symptoms are more severe.

Serum laboratory tests required to diagnose hepatitis include antibody and antigen tests specific for each type of hepatitis, and liver function tests

(LFTs). Increased LFTs (aminotransferase [AST], alanine aminotransferase [ALT], and bilirubin) are seen with a positive diagnosis. Prothrombin time (PT) is also tested. A prolonged PT occurs with hepatitis.

Nursing interventions include the following: Blood and body fluid isolation should be maintained for *all* clients. Bed rest with bathroom privileges is advised. Activity can be advanced as LFTs improve. Frequent rest periods and naps are recommended. The nurse should promote psychological and emotional rest. Diet should be low in fat with small frequent feedings and snacks. Rest and nutrition are continued until liver function returns to normal. Alcohol consumption is avoided for at least 1 year after liver function normalizes. Clients with HBV and HCV are taught safer sex practices. Clients should avoid intimate and sexual contact until laboratory tests are normal. These clients should *always* use latex condoms with intercourse. Regular follow-up is continued for at least 1 year or as long as indicated. Clients should be advised that they are not eligible blood donors and educated to recognize the signs and symptoms of recurrence.

Cirrhosis Cirrhosis is defined as a chronic, progressive disease of the liver characterized by degeneration and destruction of hepatic cells and tissue. The liver undergoes drastic structural changes (tissue fibrosis) and loss of function. Liver regeneration is disorganized and results in the formation of malfunctioning scar tissue, which in time exceeds the amount of normal liver tissue. Types of cirrhosis include the following:

1. **Laennec's cirrhosis.** Laennec's cirrhosis is usually associated with alcohol abuse and malnutrition. A buildup of fat in the liver cells results in widespread scar formation.
2. **Postnecrotic cirrhosis.** Massive necrosis results from hepatotoxins, usually after hepatitis.
3. **Biliary cirrhosis.** This type of cirrhosis involves diffuse tissue fibrosis and scarring as a result of chronic biliary obstruction and infection.
4. **Cardiac cirrhosis.** Right-sided congestive heart failure (CHF) causes edema in the liver. It is reversible if treated promptly.
5. **Nonspecific, metabolic cirrhosis.** This type is caused by metabolic problems, infectious diseases, infiltrative diseases, and GI diseases.

Early signs and symptoms of cirrhosis include GI disturbances such as anorexia, indigestion, changes in bowel elimination, malaise, and RUQ discomfort due to the enlarging liver. Later signs include jaundice; spider angiomas on the face, neck, and shoulders; reddened palms; anemia; thrombocytopenia; clotting disorders; peripheral neuropathy; and hepatosplenomegaly. The presence of portal hypertension is characterized by bleeding esophageal varices, hemorrhoids, collateral veins on the abdominal wall, peripheral edema (swollen feet, ankles, presacral area), and ascites. Hepatic encephalopathy is characterized by changes in mental responsiveness, an altered level of concentration, and poor memory.

Diagnosis is established by a combination of history, symptomatology, laboratory findings, and liver biopsy. Laboratory tests reveal increased liver enzymes (AST, ALT, lactate dehydrogenase [LDH]), a decrease in total protein and hypoalbuminemia, prolonged PT, altered bilirubin metabolism, and increased serum ammonia.

There are several complications of cirrhosis. Portal hypertension, an obstruction to normal hepatic blood flow, results in increased pressure in the portal circulation. Collateral circulation compensates as the body attempts to reduce portal pressure. Common areas for collateral channels include the lower esophagus at the area of the gastric vein (esophageal varices), the anterior abdominal wall (caput medusa), the parietal peritoneum, and hemorrhoids.

Peripheral edema and ascites are characterized by the accumulation of serous fluid in the peritoneal cavity, which results from increased pressure in the liver. This, in turn, causes excess protein and water to leak out of the liver into the abdomen (Fig. 5-2). Hypoalbuminemia causes decreased osmotic pressure, which facilitates the movement of fluid and protein into the abdominal cavity. Increased amounts of sodium and water are retained as a result of hyperaldosteronism (see Fig. 5-2).

FIGURE 5-2

☒

Development of ascites in liver disease.

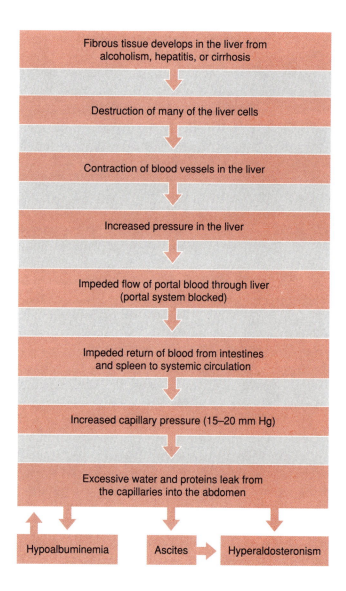

Hepatic encephalopathy (coma) results from the inability of the liver to detoxify ammonia, a by-product of protein metabolism. If high levels of ammonia stay in the systemic circulation and cross the blood-brain barrier, toxic neurological effects may develop. Coma and death can result.

Cirrhosis is a chronic, comprehensive disease. Holistic nursing care focuses on managing the illness and decreasing the complications as much as possible. Nursing care cannot halt the progression of cirrhosis, but it can improve comfort, emotional and spiritual well-being, and the quality of life. Depending on economic and other factors, clients with cirrhosis are seen in all health care settings, including ICUs, home care, homeless shelters, and hospices.

Chronic alcohol abuse is the most common, although certainly not the only cause of cirrhosis. Approximately half of all alcoholics in the United States develop cirrhosis. A comprehensive health history and assessment of the client's social situation are required to develop a nursing plan of care for clients with cirrhosis. Management of these clients is complex and constantly changing. However, many clients with deteriorating cirrhosis are now managed at home. In these situations, there is a support system of people trained in the necessary care and supervised by home health nurses.

Highlights of **nursing care** for a client with cirrhosis include diet modification. Protein intake is based on ammonia levels and the client's condition. A protein-restricted diet is given when the liver cannot process the end products of protein metabolism. As the client improves, protein can sometimes be added to aid in liver regeneration. Carbohydrates and vitamins, especially B-complex vitamins, are supplemented to ensure adequate intake.

It is also important to avoid hepatotoxins. The client should avoid ASA and acetaminophen (Tylenol) and abstain from alcohol. A rest and activity schedule is created, based on signs and symptoms and laboratory data. Complications of immobility are prevented. The nurse assists with activities of daily living (ADL) to prevent undue fatigue. Good skin care prevents skin breakdown. Pruritus is a common problem. A circulating air bed is useful to maintain skin integrity. Trauma to the mucous membranes should be avoided, as this can result in bleeding. Stool softeners may be needed. Stools should also be monitored for blood. Family involvement should be promoted by referring the family to community support services and counseling. The nurse should monitor the client for complications and treat them when they occur.

When esophageal varices are present, soft, nonirritating foods should be given. The client should be discouraged from drinking coffee and told to avoid straining during bowel movements. The nurse should evaluate the client for active bleeding by monitoring vital signs, assessing for melena or hematemesis, and reporting these findings to the physician immediately. When bleeding from varices is evident, treatment is initiated to prevent associated complications. The physician may order a gastric lavage or esophageal tamponade tube. More often, the gastroenterologist performs an endoscopy to assess the varices and treat them by sclerotherapy injection. The nurse must assess complications associated with ascites, and prevent them by decreasing sodium intake and administering diuretics and potassium supplements as ordered. When hypoalbuminemia is severe, plasma expanders may be given. Serum electrolyte, ammonia, and albumin concentrations must be monitored. Abdominal girth and weight must be measured daily. Paracentesis may be necessary to drain the abdominal fluid. The client should be maintained in semi-Fowler's position to decrease pressure on the diaphragm.

Hepatic encephalopathy is common in clients with advanced cirrhosis. Responsiveness and any sensory and motor abnormalities must be assessed. Serum ammonia levels and decreased protein in the diet must be monitored. Any electrolyte imbalances such as hypokalemia must be treated promptly. The client's condition may be complicated by seizures or delirium tremens (DTs).

Cancer of the Liver Cancer of the liver is most often due to metastatic disease as opposed to primary hepatocellular carcinoma. In either instance, prognosis for clients with liver cancer is poor, and death may occur within 4–7 months of the diagnosis. Clinical manifestations include anorexia, weight loss, fatigue, anemia, abdominal pain as a result of rapid liver enlargement, ascites, and jaundice. Radioisotope and CT scans or MRI may reveal lesions or masses in the liver. A liver biopsy is necessary to establish a definitive diagnosis. A hepatic arteriogram may be performed. Treatment includes surgical excision of the tumor if it is localized. Clients respond poorly to chemotherapy. **Nursing interventions** focus on maintaining comfort and quality of life. The nursing care is the same as for a client with advanced cirrhosis.

Reye's Syndrome Reye's syndrome is an acute childhood illness that causes fatty infiltration of the liver and subsequent liver degeneration. The damaged liver cells can no longer convert ammonia to urea for excretion from the body, causing an alarming rise in the concentration of serum ammonia. Circulating ammonia crosses the blood-brain barrier to produce acute neurological effects. Reye's syndrome is frequently preceded by an acute viral illness, and it has been associated with the administration of ASA to control fever in children from 6 months of age to adolescence. For this reason, no pediatric clients should be given ASA. Acetaminophen (Tylenol) is the antipyretic of choice.

Children with Reye's syndrome often exhibit a brief recovery after a viral illness followed by the onset of a rapidly deteriorating illness. Initial signs and symptoms, which are severe, include persistent vomiting, lethargy, and listlessness. Progressive CNS involvement (encephalopathy) is characterized by hyperventilation, tachycardia, a decreased level of consciousness, seizures, and pupillary changes. The child is generally afebrile without jaundice. Serum laboratory tests demonstrate elevated AST and ALT, prolonged PTT, and elevated serum ammonia concentrations. Treatment includes admission to an ICU or pediatric ICU, as intensive treatment is required to provide respiratory support, decrease ICP, and prevent complications such as bleeding.

Nursing interventions for clients with Reye's syndrome include monitoring serum LFTs, ammonia, PTT, and electrolytes; maintaining respiratory status often with mechanical ventilation; and assessing the client for problems of impaired coagulation.

Nursing care includes neurological assessment. It is important to monitor for increased ICP when it is detected. Signs and symptoms of increased ICP include an altered level of consciousness (LOC) (irritability, restlessness), changes in vital signs (decreased pulse, increased blood pressure), changes in pupils (sluggish reactions to light or change in size), papilledema, doll's eyes phenomenon (involuntary rolling movements of the eyes), a decrease in sensory and motor function, headache, and vomiting.

General nursing care for clients with increased ICP includes placing the client in a semi-Fowler's position, maintaining a quiet environment, strictly monitoring fluid intake and output, and fluid restriction. The client must avoid straining. The nurse supports respiratory function and provides suction as needed. A special air bed may be required to prevent injury and protect pressure points on the skin. Along with physical health, psychological equilibrium is maintained. The nurse must talk to the client and give simple explanations.

Disorders of the Gallbladder

The gallbladder is a sac located under the liver that concentrates and stores bile until it is released into the intestine. The three common disorders of the gallbladder are cholelithiasis, **choledocholithiasis**, and cholecystitis.

Cholelithiasis Cholelithiasis is the presence of gallstones. Formation of stones in the gallbladder occurs when bile supersaturated with cholesterol or bilirubin precipitates. Stone growth may also be due to infection or disturbances in cholesterol metabolism. An increased incidence of cholelithiasis may be seen in the high-risk group termed the "5 Fs": female, fertile (especially during pregnancy), fat, fair, and forty. *Escherichia coli* is the most common source of bacterial infection in the gallbladder. This causes inflammation, ischemia, and eventually can result in perforation of the wall of the gallbladder, causing peritonitis (Fig. 5-3).

Clinical manifestations of cholelithiasis vary in nature and severity, depending on the mobility of the stone and whether obstruction occurs. Common signs and symptoms of obstruction include epigastric distress such as indigestion after a fatty meal, a feeling of fullness and abdominal distention, and dull, nondescript pain in the RUQ after eating a high-fat meal.

If the cystic ducts become obstructed by a stone, the client may also experience gallstone or biliary colic, which presents as severe abdominal pain radiating to the back or shoulder. This may occur several hours after eating a heavy meal. Obstruction also causes nausea and vomiting, tachycardia, and diaphoresis. Jaundice may occur. The urine may become dark and stools clay-colored, as in hepatitis.

Cholelithiasis may be treated medically by dissolution therapy or lithotripsy or surgically by cholecystectomy. Lithotripsy causes disintegration of the stones by ultrasonic shock waves. Stone particles are then excreted through the common bile duct into the small intestine. Today,

Choledocholithiasis. This condition is characterized by calculi in the common bile duct. It usually occurs in conjunction with cholelithiasis and cholecystitis.

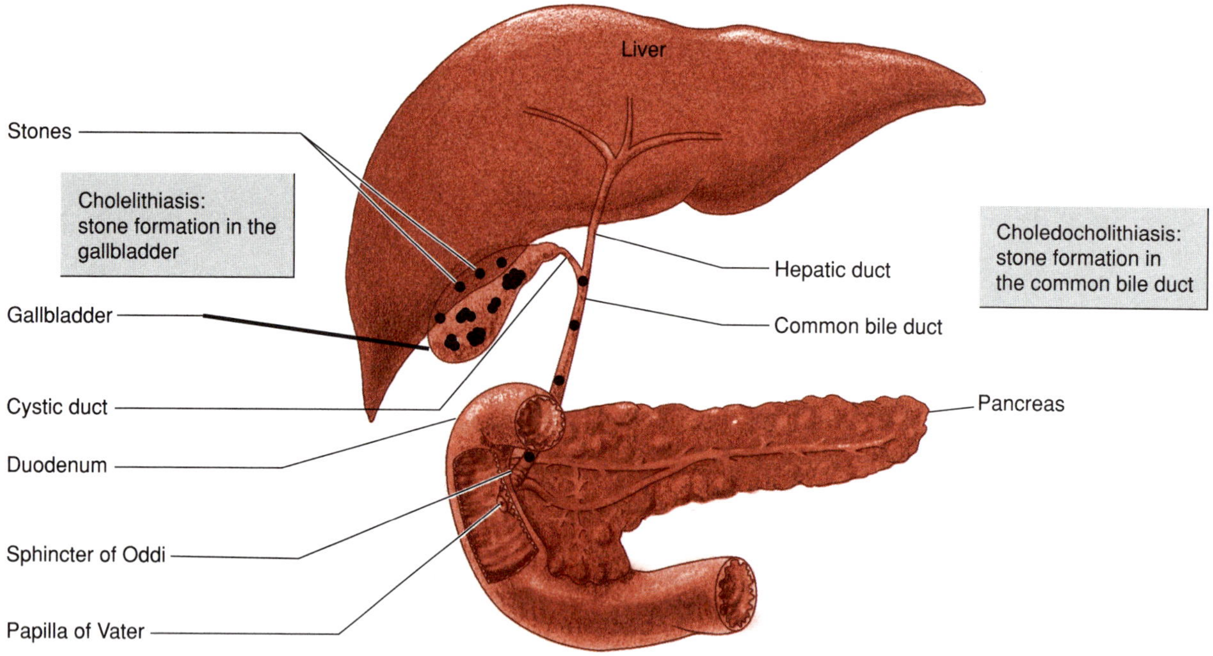

FIGURE 5-3 Formation of stones in the gallbladder (cholelithiasis) and formation of stones in the common bile duct (choledocholithiasis).

laparoscopic cholecystectomy is the method of choice for surgical resection of the gallbladder. Four small incisions are made, and a laser or cautery is used to remove the gallbladder. This procedure is less invasive and less expensive (less or no hospitalization is required) than an abdominal cholecystectomy, and the client has a shorter recovery time. There is earlier ambulation, decreased pain, and fewer complications with laparoscopic cholecystectomy. Abdominal cholecystectomy is performed when the situation requires surgical access to a larger operative field, such as when complications exist, multiple stones are present, or extensive surgery to the duct system is needed. A large, high abdominal scar is required, making deep breathing and coughing uncomfortable. A long postoperative hospitalization (3–4 days) and recuperation time are required. Abdominal cholecystectomy is also associated with more postoperative complications.

For clients having a laparoscopic cholecystectomy, **nursing care** is usually managed in outpatient surgery because the client is usually discharged the day of the procedure. The client should recover from anesthesia without respiratory or cardiac complications, be able to tolerate liquids, and be able to walk before discharge. Instructions and a prescription for oral analgesia are given before discharge. The client can return to work in 3 days, and a follow-up appointment is scheduled in 2 weeks.

If abdominal cholecystectomy is required, postoperative care is more detailed, focusing on care that is needed for a client having abdominal surgery. The dressing is monitored for bleeding or drainage. Respiratory status is maintained by having the client turn, cough, and breathe deeply every 2 hours. When able, the client should use the inspirometer and change positions frequently. Intravenous fluids for fluid and electrolyte replacement are necessary for 1–2 days until bowel sounds return. Urine output and the passage of gas or stools should be documented. The nurse should promote activity and early ambulation with assistance immediately after surgery to decrease the incidence of respiratory and circulatory complications.

Occasionally, the surgeon will place a drainage tube (T-tube) to maintain patency of the bile duct and drain bile until postoperative edema subsides. Care of the client necessitates maintaining gravity drainage through the T-tube, observing and recording the amount and color of bile drainage, observing for bile leaking from around the T-tube insertion site, and maintaining skin integrity around the T-tube site. The tube should not be irrigated or clamped. Typical drainage is approximately 55 mL a day for several days after which it gradually decreases. The surgeon removes the T-tube when most of the drainage has subsided.

Cholecystitis Cholecystitis is an inflammation of the gallbladder. It may be an acute or chronic condition and may or may not be associated with stones. It is often linked with stones that block the cystic duct and is classically characterized by severe pain in the RUQ. The pain may appear suddenly and be aggravated by deep breathing. Palpation of the RUQ may elicit a positive **Murphy's sign**. This inflammation also causes chills, fever, anorexia, nausea, and vomiting. Bowel sounds may be absent.

Diagnostic testing usually includes a gallbladder and biliary ultrasound or a nuclear medicine scan of the gallbladder and ducts, termed cholescintigraphy or HIDA scanning (Pagana & Pagana, 1995). Serum laboratory tests include a white blood cell (WBC) count to detect signs of infection, and serum transaminase, alkaline phosphatase, serum amylase, and direct and indirect bilirubin levels to monitor gallbladder, liver, and pancreatic function.

The following medications are used to provide comfort and alleviate colic at the time of an episode of cholecystitis: Anticholinergics decrease secretions and promote relaxation of the gallbladder. Analgesics, usually meperidine (Demerol), alleviate pain. Antibiotics eradicate the organism causing the inflammatory process, and atropine sulfate (Atropine) and propantheline (Probanthine) relieve spasms and decrease pain. Surgical options for cholecystitis are the same as those described above for cholelithiasis.

Nursing interventions include giving the client nothing by mouth or a low-fat liquid diet during an acute attack and adding low-fat solids as tolerated. Intravenous fluids and gastric decompression (NG to suction) are provided if nausea and vomiting are severe and persistent. The nurse must administer antibiotics and analgesics as prescribed, assess for indications of infection, and prepare the client for tests to confirm the diagnosis.

Murphy's Sign. Murphy's sign is severe pain in the RUQ with palpation. Clients hold their breath as a result of the sudden increase in the intensity of pain.

Pancreatic Disorders

Pancreatitis Pancreatitis is a serious inflammatory disorder that can be either acute or chronic. Pancreatitis refers to inflammation, edema, and necrosis that occur as a result of the "self-digestion" of the pancreas by enzymes it normally secretes.

Acute pancreatitis is characterized by a single episode or recurrent attacks of inflammation and edema. Except in cases of alcohol-induced pancreatitis, the pancreas returns to normal after successful treatment, and the client has no irreversible sequelae. Alcoholism is the most common cause of pancreatitis. Biliary tract disease caused by cholelithiasis or chole-cystitis and viral infections can also precipitate acute pancreatitis.

Chronic pancreatitis causes permanent and progressive destruction of the pancreas as normal tissue is replaced by fibrous tissue. The chronic condition may follow acute pancreatitis or occur alone. The most common cause in adults is alcoholism. In children, cystic fibrosis is the primary cause. This condition leads to chronic insufficiency of pancreatic enzymes.

Clinical manifestations include abdominal pain that radiates to the back or flank area and is aggravated by eating. Acute pancreatitis causes nausea and vomiting, dehydration, low-grade fever, tachycardia, hypotension, jaundice, and a decrease in bowel sounds and abdominal distention. Chronic pancreatitis is marked by severe and constant pain and general signs and symptoms of acute illness, along with weight loss, mild jaundice, diarrhea, steatorrhea, and abdominal tenderness.

Measurement of serum pancreatic enzyme levels, the primary laboratory test to diagnose pancreatitis, demonstrates an increase in serum amylase (> 300 IU/L) and lipase. An increase in urine amylase and elevated serum bilirubin and alkaline phosphatase may occur in clients with chronic pancreatitis. Hyperglycemia may also occur. Ultrasonography and ERCP confirm the diagnosis. Ultrasound rules out an edematous pancreas or pseudocyst. ECRP identifies an obstructed pancreatic or bile duct.

Treatment of pancreatitis focuses on alleviating pain and avoiding pancreatic stimulation by analgesics such as meperidine (Demerol). Morphine is contraindicated. Smooth muscle relaxants, anticholinergics such as propantheline (Probanthine), antacids, and antibiotics are also used. Nothing is given by mouth initially. A NG tube attached to low suction may be required. Intravenous fluids and TPN may be needed if episodes are prolonged. A bland, low-fat, high-carbohydrate diet is gradually added, and stimulants (spices, alcohol, tea, coffee, caffeinated drinks) are decreased. Midchain triglyceride (MCT) oil, which is easy to absorb, may replace the usual dietary fats. Diet counseling is provided (Moore, 1997). Pancreatic enzyme replacement may be needed in chronic cases. If insulin secretion is impaired, the client is treated as a diabetic.

Pancreatic Cancer Pancreatic cancer is an insidious condition that has a very poor prognosis. The tumor may result in chronic pancreatitis, jaundice, and chronic pain. Pancreatoduodenal resection (Whipple's procedure) is the only surgical procedure and is curative in only a small percentage of cases.

Conditions of the Intestines (LGI Tract)

Common Bowel Dysfunctions

Flatulence Flatulence occurs with a sensation of bloating and abdominal distention accompanied by flatus (gas) or belching. It is a condition that can be both uncomfortable and embarrassing. Assessment of the GI system always includes auscultation for bowel sounds in all four quadrants, as flatulence sometimes heralds an underlying bowel disorder such as an ileus when peristalsis decreases or is absent.

Nursing care and client education for flatulence include encouraging clients to avoid chewing gum or drinking carbonated beverages, especially through a straw. The client should avoid gas-forming foods (e.g., legumes, onions, cucumbers) and eat a high-fiber and low-fat diet. Increased exercise reduces flatulence. The client should also be told to maintain an erect posture after eating, and when lying down, to lie on the right side.

Appendicitis Obstruction of the blind sac of the appendix precipitates inflammation, ulceration, and necrosis. If necrosis causes the appendix to rupture, intestinal contents spill into the peritoneal cavity, resulting in peritonitis. Appendicitis is most common in clients who are 10–30 years of age. When it occurs in elderly individuals, it can be extremely serious.

Clinical manifestations begin with vague abdominal pain coming in waves and typically starting in the epigastric/umbilical region. The pain becomes more intense at McBurney's point, which is located at the corner of the right lower quadrant (RLQ). On examination, tenderness in the RLQ may be characterized as rebound tenderness, which occurs when the nurse or physician palpates the RLQ and then releases pressure by the hand. Nausea, anorexia, vomiting, and low-grade temperature (100.5–101.5°F) are often present. The most comfortable position for the client is lying on the side with knees flexed. Sudden relief of pain may indicate a ruptured appendix.

Appendicitis is not always easy to diagnose as clients do not always present with the classic signs and symptoms. Diagnostic laboratory tests for appendicitis include a complete blood count (CBC) with WBC differential. A leukocytosis (elevated WBC > 10,000 mm^3) as well as a neutrophil count greater than 75% aid in the diagnosis. Laboratory findings in combination with a client history and abdominal assessment determine the diagnosis. Rigidity over the entire abdomen can indicate rupture with peritonitis.

The treatment of appendicitis is the surgical removal of the appendix, termed an appendectomy. This is performed if the inflammatory condition is localized without rupture. More extensive abdominal surgery (abdominal laparotomy) must be performed if the appendix has ruptured. Abscess formation is a serious complication of a ruptured appendix.

Nursing interventions for a client with suspected or known appendicitis include the following: Nothing by mouth is ordered until otherwise indicated. Bed rest in a comfortable position is advised. Heat should not be applied to the abdomen. Cold applications may provide some comfort.

Enemas are contraindicated. Any unnecessary palpation of the abdomen should be avoided, and intravenous fluids and antibiotic therapy should be started.

Postoperatively, the client should be monitored for abdominal distention and the return of bowel sounds, which indicate the restoration of peristalsis. Analgesics are offered frequently. Vital signs are monitored for any indication of infection, especially temperature elevation. The wound must be evaluated for healing and the presence of drainage. The diet can be advanced as peristalsis returns. In an uncomplicated appendectomy, the client is usually discharged in 3 days.

Peritonitis Peritonitis is a local or generalized inflammation of the peritoneum. Intestinal motility is decreased, and fluid accumulates in the peritoneal cavity, precipitating fluid, electrolyte, and protein loss. Peritonitis can be classified as primary (due to an infection) or secondary (trauma, surgery), aseptic (noninfectious) or septic (infectious), as well as acute (isolated incident) or chronic (smouldering and persistent condition). Chemical peritonitis results from gastric ulcer perforation or a ruptured ectopic pregnancy. Chemical peritonitis is rapidly followed by bacterial peritonitis. Bacterial peritonitis results from abdominal trauma or a ruptured appendix.

Clinical manifestations include pain and tenderness over the involved area, abdominal distention, abdominal muscle guarding and rigidity, fever, anorexia, nausea, and vomiting. Symptoms accompanying sepsis, hypovolemia, and shock include increased pulse; decreased blood pressure; rapid, shallow respirations; oliguria; restlessness; weakness; and pallor. Decreased or absent bowel sounds indicate accompanying paralytic ileus.

Diagnostic tests supportive of peritonitis include a CBC with an elevated WBC count and an x-ray of the abdomen that shows abnormal gas and air patterns. Paracentesis may be required to evaluate abdominal fluid and obtain specimens for cell culture.

Nursing interventions include the administration of broad-spectrum intravenous antibiotics, intravenous fluid replacement, and monitoring electrolytes and renal function closely. Depending on the age and condition of the client, treatment in the ICU is frequently required. If the client is hypovolemic, colloids such as plasma proteins for fluid and electrolyte balance are administered. The client is given nothing by mouth with a NG tube attached to low suction until the condition improves and peristalsis returns. TPN may be needed for caloric and electrolyte replacement. Vital signs, urinary output, and abdominal girth are all monitored closely.

Diverticular Disease Diverticula are small outpouchings or herniations of the mucosal lining of the LGI tract, especially the colon. *Diverticulosis* is the presence of asymptomatic multiple diverticula. It is a progressive disorder of aging. *Diverticulitis* is the process by which circulation to the diverticulum is compromised, allowing trapped food, fecal matter, and bacteria to combine and produce inflammation and infection of the diverticula. Edema accompanying the inflammation results in further bowel irritation. This is a symptomatic condition (Fig. 5-4).

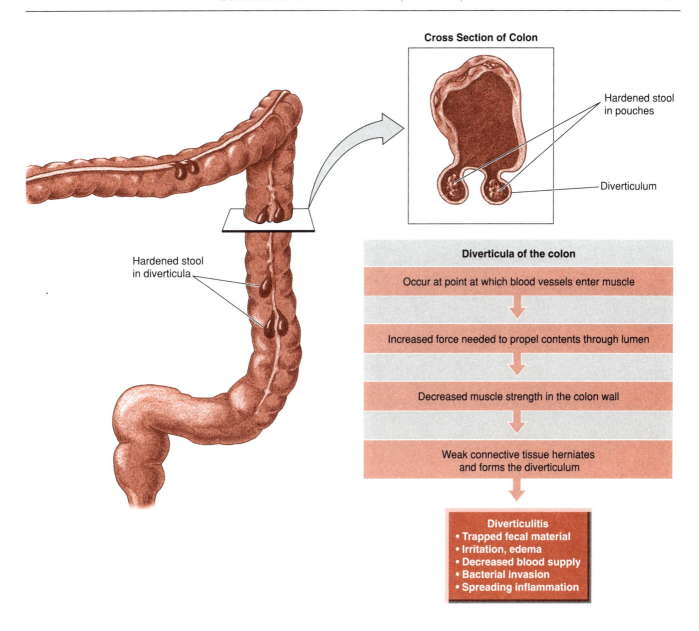

Cross Section of Colon

Hardened stool in pouches

Diverticulum

Hardened stool in diverticula

Diverticula of the colon

Occur at point at which blood vessels enter muscle

Increased force needed to propel contents through lumen

Decreased muscle strength in the colon wall

Weak connective tissue herniates and forms the diverticulum

Diverticulitis
- **Trapped fecal material**
- **Irritation, edema**
- **Decreased blood supply**
- **Bacterial invasion**
- **Spreading inflammation**

FIGURE 5-4 Pathophysiology of diverticulitis.

There is an increased incidence of diverticulosis in clients over 40 years of age. The client may have a congenital weakness of the intestinal wall (*Meckel's diverticulum*), which occurs in approximately 2% of the population, especially in men who have a history of chronic constipation. Clinical manifestations of diverticulitis include occult blood in the stool; low-grade fever; left lower quadrant pain (LLQ), usually accompanied by nausea and vomiting; abdominal distention and cramping; and constipation or alternating diarrhea. The symptoms may progress to intestinal obstruction, blood in the stool (melena), microperforation, or abscess.

Diagnostic testing includes obtaining a stool specimen for occult blood, barium enema, sigmoidoscopy or colonoscopy, and CT scan or ultrasound.

Nursing interventions include health education to reduce the risk of constipation and diverticulosis by advising the client to consume 25–30 g of dietary fiber every day. Rice, oatmeal, fruits, and vegetables are good food choices for increased fiber (Moore, 1997). The client should exercise 20–30 minutes at least 3–4 times a week. Bulk laxatives such as Metamucil (psyllium hydrophilic mucilloid) may be helpful. Otherwise, the regular use of laxative medications should be avoided. A high-fluid intake of at least 3000 mL/day should be maintained. Nursing care at the time a client presents with acute diverticulitis includes administering anticholinergics such as propantheline (Probanthine) to decrease bowel spasms, as well as stool softeners and antibiotics. Nothing is given by mouth initially, to give the bowel a chance to recover; the client is then advanced to clear liquids. The client may require a NG tube for abdominal distention or severe nausea and vomiting. Analgesics such as meperidine (Demerol) are given; morphine is contraindicated.

If bowel obstruction or perforation occurs, surgery is necessary. This may include a bowel resection with an end-to-end anastomosis. At a later date a temporary colostomy with reanastomosis may be performed.

A diet high in fiber is recommended both to prevent and to treat diverticulosis. Once diverticula develop, a high-fiber diet cannot make them disappear, but it can decrease the incidence of inflammation by producing soft, bulky stools that are easily passed. Foods such as nuts, popcorn, cucumbers, corn, tomatoes, and raspberries that contain indigestible roughage should be avoided because they become trapped in the diverticula and cause disease (Dudek, 1997). A low-residue diet may be ordered during an acute phase of diverticulitis or when complications of perforation or abscess occur. Nurses need to give explanations to clients, particularly the elderly, that help them understand the rationale for a high-fiber diet for the long-term treatment of diverticulosis and to prevent diverticulitis. The clients' willingness and motivation to follow the diet improve if they understand the reason for it.

Parasitic Intestinal Infections

Parasites enter the GI tract and cause infections, usually by the fecal–oral route as a result of contaminated food or water. Diagnosis is made by examining a stool specimen for ova and parasites and culturing the stool specimen for bacteria. The goal of treatment is to provide symptomatic relief, eradicate the parasite, and prevent further spread. Fluids and electrolytes need to be replaced and nutritional support maintained. **Nursing interventions** include monitoring the client during the acute phase for dehydration and electrolyte imbalance and providing comfort with opiates and analgesics. Stool precautions and proper hygiene practices, especially hand washing, must be taught. The nurse must also promote health education and public health measures for prevention. There are three common types of parasitic infections: amebiasis, giardiasis, and trichinosis.

Amebiasis Amebiasis primarily affects the large intestine, causing amebic dysentery. Infected persons with mild disease may have abdominal cramping, intermittent diarrhea, and flatulence. In severe cases, clients have copious diarrhea with blood and mucus, colicky abdominal pain, rectal spasms (tenesmus), and fever. Amebiasis is transmitted by person-to-person contact, by insects, and through contaminated water, milk, and food. Liver abscess is the most common complication, due to the parasite's migration to the liver via the portal vein.

Giardiasis Giardiasis is a protozoan infection of the small intestine. It is a common cause of traveler's diarrhea. Clinical manifestations include persistent watery diarrhea with abdominal cramping and weight loss. In mild cases, clients complain of a constant bloated feeling with abdominal discomfort. Severe cases are associated with malabsorption of fats and vitamins.

Trichinosis Trichinosis is caused by larvae of the roundworm, which live in the intestine of humans, pigs, and rats. It is usually transmitted by ingestion of undercooked pork. Clinical presentations include nausea, anorexia, abdominal cramping, and diarrhea. After 2–8 weeks, clients experience fever, weakness, and muscle pain with movement.

Irritable Bowel Syndrome (IBS)

IBS is also known as spastic colon or mucous colitis. Clients complain of abdominal pain and altered bowel habits, usually diarrhea. The symptoms occur intermittently and vary among clients. The syndrome may be precipitated by stress, anxiety, or dietary factors. Symptoms generally appear in two major patterns. The *spastic colon type* is characterized by colicky abdominal pain that is relieved by the passage of stool. There is periodic constipation and diarrhea. The *painless diarrhea type* consists of urgent diarrhea occurring during or after meals. Radiography and endoscopy are performed to diagnose IBS.

Nursing care includes educating the client regarding a low-fat diet. The client should avoid gas-producing foods and carbonated beverages, eat a well-balanced diet, and follow a regular schedule for meals. In addition, the client should avoid alcohol, smoking, and any other irritants. The client must use bulk-forming laxatives (psyllium hydrophilic mucilloid [Metamucil]) and antidiarrheal agents (loperamide [Imodium], diaphenoxylate hydrochloride with atropine sulfate [Lomotil]) when needed. Regular exercise, relaxation techniques, support groups, and counseling are also helpful.

Inflammatory Bowel Diseases

The diagnosis and management of Crohn's disease and ulcerative colitis, the two classic forms of inflammatory bowel disease, are discussed below. While they are distinct diseases, they share many features.

Diagnostic testing for inflammatory bowel disease includes a stool culture to rule out bacterial or parasitic infection and stool analysis to determine the presence of blood and leukocytes. A barium enema and lower endoscopy are frequently performed. Crohn's disease is identified by a characteristic cobblestone pattern of deep longitudinal fissures and erosions. Ulcerative colitis has a different ulcerative pattern. During endoscopy, a biopsy specimen is taken to confirm the diagnosis. A CBC is obtained to assess severe leukocytosis (WBC greater than 15,000/uL). Laboratory tests often reveal an elevated erythrocyte sedimentation rate (ESR) and decreased albumin and potasssium levels.

Complications of inflammatory bowel disease include perirectal and intra-abdominal fistulas, strictures, and abscesses. Inflammation of the intestine can lead to perforation and generalized peritonitis. Fat malabsorption results in a deficiency in fat-soluble vitamins (A, D, E, K). With ulcerative colitis, pseudocyst development may pose an increased risk of bowel cancer.

Nursing interventions focus on dietary and other life-style modifications needed to control symptoms and avoid complications and hospitalizations. Diet therapy includes decreased residue, roughage, and fat intake with increased calories and vitamin supplements. A diet high in protein and calories and low in fat and fiber is best to reduce inflammation and promote bowel regeneration (Moore, 1997). During an exacerbation, hospitalization with intense treatment may be required. Intravenous fluids and a clear liquid diet are provided. TPN may be necessary to ensure essential nutrients.

Pharmacological treatment of inflammatory bowel disease includes corticosteroids to reduce the inflammation. Antibiotics are also administered. Sulfasalazine (Azulfidine) is the drug of choice to prevent exacerbation because of its combined bacteriostatic and anti-inflammatory action. Metronidazole (Flagyl) may also be prescribed. Antidiarrheal agents such as Lomotil and antocholinergics such as propantheline (Probanthine) are given, as well as vitamin replacement. Iron replacement may be needed.

Surgical intervention is necessary if fistulas, perforation, bleeding, or intestinal obstruction occur. Segmental resection with reanastomosis is frequently successful, but a temporary ileostomy may be required until healing takes place. Strictureplasty is useful to open strictures. If ulcerative colitis does not respond to aggressive medical treatment, removal of the colon, rectum, and anus with permanent closure of the anus may be performed. To create a permanent ileostomy, the end of the terminal ileum is brought through the abdominal wall to form a stoma. An ileostomy drains liquid to very soft stool continuously, and unlike a colostomy, does not allow the client to establish a bowel pattern.

Nursing care during an exacerbation or following surgery includes giving nothing by mouth to decrease bowel activity. Intravenous fluids with electrolyte replacement are administered, and TPN may be required. Fluids are introduced gradually into the diet. Good skin hygiene around the anal area or ileostomy is practiced, and the nurse must assess stool patterns and characteristics. A quiet atmosphere is provided. The client should avoid lactose (dairy products). Appropriate measures are taken to decrease stress in the client's life style. Open communication to express concerns as well as support groups are encouraged.

Crohn's Disease (Regional Enteritis) Crohn's disease is a chronic, inflammatory disease of the GI tract. It most commonly affects the small bowel, especially the terminal ileum. Lesions may also arise in the cecum and ascending colon. Edema, inflammation, and fibrosis occur, involving all layers of the bowel wall. The inflammation occurs in patchy segments separated by normal tissue. The client may experience periods of complete remission that alternate with exacerbations. Crohn's disease may begin in adolescence. The peak incidence is between 20–40 years of age. Familial tendencies exist, and autoimmune factors may also contribute to its origin.

Clinical manifestations include colicky abdominal pain that is relieved by bowel movements and three to five large semisolid stools a day with mucus or pus but no blood. Pain and symptoms may be more severe with emotional upset or poorly tolerated foods. Steatorrhea occurs due to inefficient bile salt resorption and poor absorption of fat-soluble vitamins (A, D, E, K). Borborygmi (abnormally loud bowel sounds) and RLQ tenderness, which may mimic appendicitis, occur, as well as nausea, vomiting, anorexia, weakness, and malaise. As the disease progresses, melena (dark, tarry stools due to old blood), weight loss, dehydration, electrolyte imbalance, and iron deficiency anemia occur.

Ulcerative Colitis Ulcerative colitis, another common inflammatory bowel disease, is characterized by an inflammation and ulceration of the colon and rectum. The area of inflammation is diffuse, involving the mucosa and submucosa of the intestinal wall. The inflammatory process leads to scar formation. The problem frequently begins in the rectum and spreads continuously throughout the colon. Ulcerated areas develop and can precipitate hemorrhage. As with Crohn's disease, the client experiences periods of exacerbation and remission.

There are three types of ulcerative colitis. *Recurrent ulcerative colitis* is characterized by a gradual onset. The diarrhea is generally not disabling. Exacerbation usually occurs with a gradual decline in health. *Chronic intermittent ulcerative colitis* is characterized by persistent signs of colon edema and inflammation. The onset is abrupt. *Acute fulminating ulcerative colitis* has an abrupt onset with a rapid course. It is uncommon but more dangerous, and perforation of the intestinal wall and hemorrhage may occur.

Clinical manifestations of ulcerative colitis include profuse diarrhea that frequently contains blood, mucus, or pus (15–20 stools a day). Rectal bleeding, abdominal pain, tenderness and cramps before a bowel movement, fever, and rapid depletion of fluid and electrolytes also occur during exacerbations. Anorexia, weakness, malaise, weight loss, growth retardation in children, and anemia are seen in chronic conditions. The client often loses the feeling of the urge to defecate, and suffers from involuntary leakage of stool.

CASE STUDY: INFLAMMATORY BOWEL DISEASE

Mr. L. is a 40-year-old client with a history of inflammatory bowel disease. He presents to the emergency room with severe abdominal pain, inability to pass gas, and no bowel movement for the past 3 days. Upon examination, the nurse notes abdominal distension associated with firmness of the abdomen. Bowel sounds are absent in three quadrants.

The emergency room nurse proceeds to admit the client from the triage area and reports the history and physical examination findings to the physician. The nurse documents these findings on the client's record.

The physician orders an abdominal x-ray and laboratory tests for blood chemistry. The abdominal x-ray demonstrates a complete small bowel obstruction. A diagnosis of inflammatory bowel disease with small bowel obstruction is made on the basis of the history and the x-ray findings.

The nurse assesses the client for nausea and vomiting. A basin and washcloth are placed with the client, and mouth rinse is provided. The client will require surgery to relieve the obstruction, so the nurse administers nothing by mouth. The nurse checks the physician's orders regarding the need to place a NG tube and to initiate intravenous fluids. The nurse performs a venipuncture to initiate intravenous fluids and inserts the tube as ordered. The operative procedure is explained to the client and family, and once informed consent is obtained, the nurse administers the preoperative medication as ordered by the anesthesiologist or surgeon.

Postoperatively, the nurse realizes that a diet will not be ordered until bowel sounds and function return. Until then, the NG tube remains at low intermittent suction to keep the stomach decompressed. The nurse documents an accurate intake and output, especially noting the amount and color of the gastric drainage. Vital signs are checked every 4 hours. The nurse provides analgesia as ordered, which is often administered via a patient-controlled analgesia (PCA) intravenous pump. Frequent physical assessments include auscultation for bowel sounds and questions to the client concerning flatus. When flatus is noted, bowel sounds should be auscultated and the physician notified when they are present. The nurse also encourages the client to increase ambulation and activity. If bowel function does not return within 3 days, it is very likely that the physician will order TPN to provide for the nutrition of the client. The nurse is also concerned about the abdominal incision line and observes and documents whether the line is well approximated, noting the presence of any drainage. Any incisional redness or drainage and fever should be reported to the physician as infection is possible. A client who undergoes bowel surgery is usually given prophylactic antibiotics, and the nurse administers these as ordered.

Frequently a client will have a family physician, a surgeon, the nursing staff, and a dietitian involved in the therapeutic plan of care. An open dialogue between the physicians, nurses, and dietitian is critical for the continuity of client care and to encourage a successful outcome.

Intestinal Obstruction

Obstruction takes place when interference with normal peristalsis and impairment of forward flow of the intestinal contents occurs. Intestinal obstruction is generally classified as mechanical or nonmechanical (Fig. 5-5).

Mechanical intestinal obstruction affects the patency of the intestinal lumen and is caused by the following:

- **Adhesions.** Scar tissue loops over the bowel segments, causing it to kink or compress.
- **Strangulated hernia.** This is a defect in the abdominal wall through which the bowel becomes tangled and strangulates.
- **Tumor.** This gradually restricts the lumen of the bowel. Cancer accounts for 80% of large bowel obstructions.
- **Volvulus.** The bowel twists upon itself, obstructing the intestinal lumen proximally and distally. It is a common bowel obstruction in infants that can be life-threatening as a result of necrosis, perforation, or peritonitis.
- **Intussusception.** This is a telescoping or invagination of the bowel upon itself. This occurs in infants as well as adults.

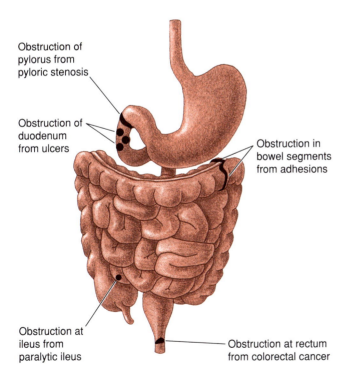

Obstruction of pylorus from pyloric stenosis

Obstruction of duodenum from ulcers

Obstruction in bowel segments from adhesions

Obstruction at ileus from paralytic ileus

Obstruction at rectum from colorectal cancer

FIGURE 5-5

Common causes and locations of intestinal obstructions.

Nonmechanical intestinal obstruction is related to dysfunction of GI motility as a result of an abnormality in peristalsis. A paralytic ileus occurs following abdominal surgery or an inflammatory process (*neurogenic*). An ileus can also be due to mesenteric vascular occlusion precipitated by atherosclerosis and thrombosis of the mesenteric arteries, which provide the vascular supply to the intestine (*vascular*). Obstructions related to intestinal ischemia may occur rapidly and be life-threatening.

The pathophysiology of bowel obstruction is related to the location of the obstruction and the accompanying physiologic changes. In general, the higher in the intestine the obstruction occurs, the more severe the signs and symptoms. Fluid, gas, and intestinal contents accumulate proximal to the obstruction, causing proximal distention and distal bowel collapse. This precipitates extravasation of fluids and electrolytes into the peritoneal cavity, which causes increased pressure. Rupture may occur as an accompanying complication. The higher the obstruction, the more rapidly dehydration occurs. Dehydration and electrolyte imbalance do not occur rapidly if the obstruction is in the large intestine. If there is persistent vomiting, the client develops metabolic alkalosis due to the dramatic loss of HCl from the stomach. Clinical manifestations of intestinal obstruction include vomiting (occurs early if the obstruction is high), abdominal distention, colicky-type abdominal pain, and bowel sounds. The bowel sounds initially may be hyperactive proximal to the obstruction, and decreased or absent distal to the obstruction. Eventually, all bowel sounds are absent.

Diagnostic testing includes radiographs of the abdomen (flat plate) to look for air or fluid entrapment in the obstructed area and laboratory tests to identify an electrolyte imbalance or dehydration. Hyponatremia (low sodium) and hypokalemia (low potassium) may be present. Leukocytosis may occur with strangulation. Finally, elevated hemoglobin and hematocrit levels may result from hemoconcentration resulting from hypovolemia.

Bowel obstructions are treated to correct the fluid and electrolyte imbalances and to address the underlying cause. Analgesics are rarely used as they decrease peristalsis. Once diagnostic testing is completed, a treatment plan is developed to correct the underlying condition. Emergency surgery may be necessary.

Nursing interventions for clients with bowel obstruction include initiating intravenous fluids and reviewing laboratory values to maintain fluid and electrolyte balance. Neurogenic obstructions (due to paralytic ileus) are treated by giving the patients nothing by mouth and a tube or intestinal intubation and decompression. Allowing the bowel to rest helps relieve the obstruction and also alleviates such symptoms as nausea, vomiting, and abdominal pain. Mechanical and vascular obstructions are usually treated surgically, and an ileostomy or colostomy may be necessary. Normal saline or lactated Ringer's solutions are given. Electrolyte values are monitored. Potassium supplements are administered with caution because of complications of decreased renal function. Urine output, serum creatinine, and blood urea nitrogen are monitored. The nurse should monitor intake, output, weight patterns, bowel sounds, and vital signs. The client must be assessed for dehydration or hypovolemia. If in shock, the client should be monitored in the ICU. Insertion of central lines such as a Swan-Ganz for pulmonary pressure monitoring may be needed. Abdominal girth is measured to determine if distention is decreasing or increasing. Intravenous antibiotics are usually administered. When surgery is performed, the drainage from the abdominal drains (Penrose drain) and the incision area is evaluated. Finally, the client should be placed in a comfortable position (typically lying on the side).

Abdominal Hernias Abdominal hernias are a protrusion of the intestine through an abnormal opening or weakened area of the abdominal wall. Types of hernias include the following:

1. **Inguinal hernia.** In this type, a weakness exists where the spermatic cord in men and the round ligament in women pass through the abdominal wall in the groin area (more common in men). These are further classified as indirect or direct. In *indirect inguinal hernias*, the weakness in the abdominal wall emerges during fetal development. The hernia passes through the inguinal ring. In *direct inguinal hernias*, the weakness is caused by increased intra-abdominal pressure. The hernia passes through an area of weak muscle.
2. **Femoral hernia.** This is a protrusion of the intestine through the femoral ring. It is more common in women and is often related to changes during pregnancy.
3. **Umbilical hernia.** This occurs most often in children whose umbilical opening fails to close adequately and in adults with weak rectus muscles.
4. **Incisional hernia.** The abdominal wall is weak due to a previous incision.

Anatomic characteristics of hernias include the following:

1. **Sliding hernia.** This hernia moves freely in and out of the hernia sac.
2. **Reducible hernia.** This hernia may be placed back into the abdominal cavity by manual manipulation.
3. **Incarcerated or irreducible hernia.** This hernia cannot be placed back into the abdominal cavity with manipulation.
4. **Strangulated hernia.** The blood supply and intestinal flow in the herniated area are obstructed. A strangulated hernia leads to intestinal obstruction.

Clinical manifestations include visible protrusion of the hernia in the involved area when the client stands or strains. A strangulated hernia occurs with signs and symptoms of intestinal obstruction and severe pain. It is treated with a surgical repair termed herniorrhaphy. A strangulated hernia requires resection of the involved bowel.

Nursing care for the client following herniorrhaphy includes the following: advancing the diet and giving fluids as tolerated once peristalsis returns; assessing male clients for the development of scrotal edema and providing scrotal support if necessary; encouraging deep breathing and turning, but not coughing; discouraging the Valsalva maneuver immediately postoperatively; administering stool softeners; and advising restraint from heavy lifting for 6–8 weeks postoperatively.

Colorectal Cancer

Cancer of the Colon. In recent years, Japanese Americans have experienced an increased incidence of colorectal cancer, which is thought to be related to the adoption of the Western diet and life style (Giger & Davidhizar, 1995).

Incidence and Mortality of Colorectal Cancer. Both the incidence and mortality of colon cancer have decreased among Caucasians. Unfortunately, this is not true for African Americans and Hispanics, who are also more likely to have advanced cancer at the time of presentation (Giger & Davidhizar, 1995).

Colorectal cancer is the most prevalent internal cancer in this country. The most common sites include the rectosigmoid area, rectum, and cecum. The peak incidence of colorectal cancer occurs in clients from 50–60 years of age. Colorectal cancer may be associated with ulcerative colitis, granulomas, adenomas, and polyps. A diet high in fat, protein, and carbohydrates and low in residue or fiber is a risk factor. Colon cancer is also familial, and research studies are following clients with the genetic markers for colon cancer. For high-risk clients, a sigmoidoscopy is suggested, either once a year or as ordered by the physician.

Clinical manifestations include changes in bowel habits, a change in the shape of stool (pencil or ribbon-shaped as in sigmoid or rectal cancer), weakness, rectal bleeding, nausea and vomiting, and signs and symptoms of bowel obstruction. Pain is a late symptom.

A rectal examination and hemoccult stool test to assess for occult blood should be done in the office. Diagnosis is confirmed by a sigmoidoscopy with biopsy.

Treatment involves surgical resection of the tumor. If the tumor is located in the ascending, transverse, or descending colon, a resection with end-to-end anastomosis is possible. This preserves the natural process of defecation. Tumors of the rectum are treated with abdominoperineal resection, which necessitates a permanent colostomy. Types of colostomy procedures include the following:

1. **Ascending colostomy.** This is performed for right-sided tumors.
2. **Transverse (double-barreled) colostomy.** This is for emergency repair of intestinal obstruction from perforation and results in two stomas.
3. **Transverse loop colostomy.** This has two openings in the transverse colon but only one stoma.
4. **Descending colostomy.** This is a colostomy done for tumors in the descending colon.
5. **Sigmoid colostomy.** This is a colostomy located in the sigmoid colon.

Radiation therapy is an important component of therapy for rectal cancer, but it has minimal value in the management of colon cancer located elsewhere in the body. Chemotherapy is generally combined with radiation therapy postoperatively. **Nursing interventions** include referrals to and consultations with an enterostomal therapist to educate the client concerning self-care of the colostomy and acceptance of change in body image. A referral to a dietitian is also valuable to assess caloric requirements and plan scheduled meals and supplements. Nurses should encourage the client and family to be involved in preoperative explanations and to take an active role in the postoperative instructions and care. A low-residue diet to decrease intestinal contents is usually recommended. The enterostomal therapist assists with stoma care and appliances for home care.

When an abdominal perineal resection is performed, the client will frequently have three incisions: an abdominal incision, an incision for the colostomy, and a perineal incision. The perineal wound may be closed after insertion of a Penrose drain, or it may be left open to heal by secondary intention. Generally, the perineal wound is irrigated with saline or peroxide solution and then repacked with a sterile dressing. Warm sitz baths promote debridement and increased circulation to the area. The abdominal wound may need frequent dressing changes due to profuse serosanguineous drainage immediately postoperatively. The nurse should monitor the stoma closely for color, edema, quality and quantity of drainage, and flatus. For these clients, mastering self-care of the colostomy as well as emotional recovery may be prolonged. The nurse must assist the client in identifying community resources and arranging home care follow-up upon discharge.

Key points must be addressed when teaching a client and his or her family colostomy care. The nurse must assess for characteristics of a healthy stoma. Pink to red color, no sensation of touch or pain, and a shape that changes slightly in response to peristalsis all indicate a healthy stoma. A pouch system is selected that is most appropriate for each individual. The system protects the skin, contains stool and odor, molds to the body's contours, allows for movement, and is inconspicuous under clothing. The products come in a variety of styles, shapes, and sizes. Peristomal skin care is performed by cleansing the area with warm soapy water during each pouch change to prevent skin irritation from stool. Skin barriers are used to protect the peristomal skin. The skin must be allowed to dry completely prior to attaching the stoma drainage bag. The nurse performs colostomy irrigation through the stoma to stimulate bowel emptying only if needed (with sigmoid colostomies).

The client must learn to manage odor by correctly using leak-proof pouches. They are emptied frequently to prevent overfilling, and pouch deodorizers are used. A balanced diet is encouraged, and odor- and gas-producing foods are avoided. Dairy products, highly seasoned foods, fish, and many vegetables produce odor in stool. Beans, cabbage, and brussels sprouts cause gas.

The nurse must also provide the client and partner with specific suggestions for dealing with sexual concerns. Positions that minimize pressure and stress on the pouch should be discussed. The client must be instructed to empty and clean the pouch before sexual activity. A small-sized pouch or pouch cover can be used during sexual activity. In addition, special underwear on a binder to hold the pouch securely can be used.

Anorectal Disorders

Hemorrhoids Hemorrhoids are dilated varicose veins of the anus and rectum. Common causes include pregnancy, chronic constipation, prolonged standing or sitting, heavy lifting, and portal hypertension. Clinical manifestations depend on the location and condition of the varicosities. *External hemorrhoids* occur below the anal sphincter and appear as reddish protrusions at the anus. *Internal hemorrhoids* occur above the anal sphincter. They may be enlarged from strenuous activity and eventually prolapse through the anus, causing itching or painless rectal bleeding. *Thrombosed hemorrhoids* are blood clots in hemorrhoids that cause inflammation, edema, and pain.

Diagnostic tests include a rectal examination and digital palpation. Proctoscopy or colonoscopy are performed to visualize internal hemorrhoids.

Comprehensive treatment plans provide comfort; diet therapy prevents constipation, and surgical correction is performed when necessary. **Nursing care** includes administering ointments and suppositories to shrink the mucous membranes (dibucaine [Nupercainal]). A high-fiber diet and stool softeners (bulk laxatives) as well as increased fluid intake help to avoid aggravating the hemorrhoids. Warm sitz baths provide comfort and gentle cleansing and decrease swelling. Sclerotherapy, cryosurgery, and rubber-band ligation are the preferred options for internal hemorrhoids.

The surgical excision of a hemorrhoid is termed a hemorrhoidectomy. Both internal and external hemorrhoids may be removed. This surgery is frequently done on an outpatient basis. Following hemorrhoidectomy, the client should be offered analgesics every 3–4 hours. Sitz baths to promote cleanliness, decrease pain, and increase healing should be taken daily and after each bowel movement. The nurse must promote passage of normal stool 2–3 days postoperatively by encouraging the client to walk, eat a high-fiber diet, and take stool softeners.

Anal Fissure, Abscess, and Fistula An *anal fissure* is an elongated laceration between the anal canal and the perianal skin. It may be primary (idiopathic) or secondary (associated with chronic constipation or trauma). Most fissures are superficial and heal spontaneously. A fissure may cause significant bleeding. An *anal abscess* results from feces obstructing gland ducts in the anorectal region. Infection may occur, and sepsis can result, especially in immunosuppressed clients. An *anal fistula* is an abnormal passage between the anal canal and the skin outside the anus, frequently caused by rupture and drainage of an abscess. A fistula may need to be repaired surgically. Clinical manifestations include pain from the abscess due to pressure on somatic nerves in the perianal area; constipation; local swelling, erythema, and acute tenderness; pruritus; and purulent drainage.

Treatment for anorectal disorders is as follows. Fissures are treated with stool softeners, analgesic ointments, and sitz baths. They are surgically repaired if medical therapy is ineffective. Abscesses are treated with incision and drainage, and antibiotics. Fistulas are surgically repaired (fistulotomy or fistulectomy).

Nursing care for clients with anorectal conditions involves analgesics, sitz baths, local applications of hot or cold compresses, and topical applications of soothing products (witch hazel pads). Good perianal hygiene should be maintained after every bowel movement. Constipation should be avoided with a high-fiber diet, fluids, and regular exercise. Stool softeners and bulk laxatives are used.

Malnutrition

Protein and Caloric Malnutrition Malnutrition may occur in up to 20–50% of hospitalized clients. If a diet is adequate in carbohydrates and fats, the body uses protein to meet its energy and tissue-building needs (positive nitrogen balance). Ongoing severe protein loss (negative nitrogen balance) results in decreased muscle and visceral mass as well as decreased cardiac output and weakened respiratory muscles. Malabsorption occurs in the GI tract. Immunocompetence is impaired, and a high risk of infection exists. In addition, weight loss, decreased muscle mass, and weakness are common signs of severe protein loss. Hypoalbuminemia is present, and edema occurs due to the loss of osmotic pressure.

Nursing management includes monitoring calorie count, weight, intake, and output in ill, elderly, or high-risk clients. Serum albumin and transferrin levels in clients at risk are also monitored. Intervention with oral supplements, tube feedings, and TPN may be required. The client should be given a high-calorie, high-protein diet with oral supplements. Small frequent meals are required, and a dietitian should be consulted.

$\mathcal{E}$NTERAL AND PARENTERAL NUTRITION

Nutritional supplements administered enterally or parenterally may be necessary for a client who is incapable of adequate oral dietary intake. This situation can arise in anyone from a premature infant to an elderly client. In general, the utilization of enteral and parenteral fluids has become commonplace in the treatment plan of clients with a variety of conditions. In many instances, it has dramatically contributed to the recovery of the client. However, each client situation requires individual evaluation and attention regarding care.

Before enteral or parenteral nutrition is initiated, the following **nursing care** is required: The client must be weighed, as the consulting dietitian calculates body requirements based on body surface mass (height and weight). A calorie count requirement is essential, and the dietitian also recommends the type of solution to use. (Many commercial products are available.) The client's electrolytes, glucose, iron, and albumin are monitored. The client and family are educated, and informed consent should be obtained. There must be sensitivity and awareness of the ethical dilemmas involved. The client, or person with the power of attorney when the client is incompetent, may choose not to initiate enteral or parenteral nutrition or intravenous fluids if a client is terminally ill.

Enteral Nutrition

Enteral nutrition is defined as the delivery of nutrients directly into the GI tract. This method is used only in patients who have normal GI motility and absorption. Types of enteral administration include short-term and long-term tube feedings.

Enteral tube feedings for short-term need may be given if the client has an intact swallow reflex, or a special weighted feeding tube (Dobbhoff) may be used. Nasogastric access delivers nutrition to the stomach, whereas nasointestinal access delivers nutrition to the distal duodenum or proximal jejunum.

Enteral feedings over the long-term generally require permanent access. For a gastrostomy, the tube enters through the abdominal wall into the stomach (by surgical or endoscopic insertion), and for a jejunostomy, the tube is inserted similarly but is placed directly into the jejunum.

Parenteral Nutrition

Parenteral nutrition consists of giving highly concentrated solutions intravenously to maintain the client's nutritional balance when oral or enteral nutrition is not possible. Indications for parenteral nutrition include major GI diseases, IBD, severe trauma or burns, or severe GI side effects from radiation or chemotherapy. Parenteral nutrition is almost always administered through a central venous route, not a peripheral vein. Any solution containing more than or equal to 10% dextrose must be given via a central venous line. The client must be monitored for high blood glucose levels every 6 hours during a 24-hour TPN administration. The client receiving TPN should be monitored daily, and the solution of electrolytes and glucose changed according to the physician's orders.

$\mathcal{S}$UMMARY

The digestive system is composed of the UGI and LGI tracts and the accessory organs (liver, gallbladder, and pancreas). A variety of conditions affect the GI system, both primary diseases and those secondary to other disorders. Impaired nutrition, fluid and electrolyte imbalance, abnormalities in bowel patterns, and discomfort frequently accompany diseased conditions of the GI system. The nurse must be skilled in history taking, assessment, and common diagnostic testing to evaluate the GI status of the client.

Diagnostic testing such as ultrasound, endoscopy, ERCP, and CT and gall-bladder scans have improved the rapid diagnosis and treatment of clients with GI disorders. Nutritional and pharmacological therapies are often used to control GI disorders. Nursing care should focus on health education in terms of diet, medications, and life-style factors to promote or restore GI function. With many conditions such as HBV, PUD, Crohn's disease, ulcerative colitis, and hemorrhoids, the therapies often aim at palliating symptoms rather than long-term cures. Malignancies of the GI system remain a major health concern. Health education to decrease colon cancer focuses on diet therapy and preventive screening for high-risk clients.

KEY WORDS

Abdominal perineal resection
Appendicitis
Ascites
Cholecystitis
Cholelithiasis
Cirrhosis
Crohn's disease
Esophageal varices
Gastroesophageal reflux disease
Hemorrhoids

Hepatitis
Hernia
Jaundice
Pancreatitis
Parotitis
Peptic ulcer disease
Peritonitis
Portal hypertension
Ulcerative colitis

QUESTIONS

DIRECTIONS: Choose the one **best** response to each of the following questions.

1. All of the following conditions can be indicators of gastrointestinal (GI) hemorrhage *except*

   A. vertigo and nausea
   B. occult blood in the stools
   C. decreasing abdominal girth
   D. hypotension and tachycardia

2. Mrs. J. has had a partial gastrectomy with a vagotomy and pyloroplasty today. She has a nasogastric (NG) tube in her right nares connected to low intermittent suction. The nurse should take which of the following precautions?

   A. Do not irrigate or reposition the NG tube because the stomach sutures can be ruptured
   B. Always use wrist restraints to assure placement of the NG tube
   C. The NG tube should not be taped to the nose
   D. Expect copious amounts of bright red blood from the NG tube postoperatively

3. Mrs. E. J.'s physician suspects she has a liver tumor. the nurse should expect all of the following diagnostic tests to be ordered *except*

   A. endoscopy
   B. abdominal ultrasound
   C. abdominal computed tomography (CT) scan
   D. liver biopsy

4. Mr. J. R. complains of cramping abdominal pain. He has been diagnosed with acute diverticulitis. What nursing interventions are likely to be ordered?

   A. Increase activity and regular diet as tolerated
   B. Advise bed rest, clear liquids, and meperidine (Demerol), 50 mg intramuscularly every 3–4 hours as needed
   C. Use ice packs on the abdomen and place the client in the Trendelenberg position
   D. Use a K-pad (a temperature-controlled heating pad) on the abdomen and allow regular diet as tolerated

5. Mrs. C. J. undergoes an abdominal cholecystectomy. She is returned to her room, and the nurse notices she has a T-tube sutured to her abdomen. The most likely reason for the T-tube is

   A. it empties all the gallstones from the gallbladder after surgery
   B. it allows the pancreatic enzymes to drain
   C. it prevents the common bile duct from closing as a result of scarring
   D. it allows for splenic drainage

6. Mrs. L. M. has a small bowel obstruction and has a nasogastric (NG) tube in her right nares. The nurse notes there has been no drainage in the past hour. What should the nurse do **first** to facilitate the drainage?

   A. Have the client change positions in bed
   B. Irrigate the NG tube with 60 mL normal saline
   C. Turn the suction to high for 20 minutes
   D. Take the NG tube out and reinsert it

7. Mrs. H. T. has been diagnosed with esophageal varices. The physician notes there is active bleeding and orders the nurse to insert a nasogastric (NG) tube. The nurse should do which of the following?

   A. Insert the NG tube immediately
   B. Question the order because a varix might be perforated during insertion
   C. Use copious amounts of K-Y jelly to insert the NG tube
   D. Refuse the order because a varix might be perforated during insertion

ANSWERS

1. *The answer is* C. Indicators of GI hemorrhage include vertigo and nausea, occult blood loss in the stools, and changes in vital signs such as hypotension and tahcycardia. Abdominal distension and an increase in abdominal girth might occur; a decrease in abdominal girth would not.

2. *The answer is* A. The nurse should not irrigate or move the NG tube because this might disrupt the internal stomach sutures. The tube should be taped to the nose. Copious amounts of bright red blood would indicate postoperative bleeding, and the nurse should report this to the surgeon immediately. Wrist restraints, when ordered by the physician, are only used if the client is confused and is likely to pull on the tube. Wrist restraints will not assure placement of the tube.

3. *The answer is* A. Endoscopy allows for direct visualization of the GI tract but not the liver. Abdominal ultrasound and CT scan indicate the presence of a lesion or mass in the liver. The diagnosis can be confirmed only by a liver biopsy. The pathology report gives the specifics on the presence and cell type of the cancer.

4. *The answer is* B. The client should rest and decrease stimulation and irritation to the bowel by limiting the diet to clear liquids. A regular diet is contraindicated during an acute episode of diverticulitis; the client should either have nothing by mouth or clear liquids. Acute diverticulitis is very painful, and the client should be offered analgesia such as meperidine (Demerol) every 3–4 hours. Neither an ice pack nor a K-pad would provide adequate pain relief for acute diverticulitis.

5. *The answer is* C. The T-tube maintains patency of the common bile duct during the healing process. The tube acts as a stint to prevent the duct from closing as a result of scarring. The diameter of the duct is small, so even scarring could occlude the patency of the common bile duct.

6. *The answer is* A. The drainage pores of the NG tube might not be in a position to access the gastric fluid (i.e., it could be along the side of the stomach). The first action, as it is the least invasive, is to have the client change positions. Sometimes a side-lying position on the right side facilitates drainage of the tube. The suction should never be placed on high; it should be maintained on a low, intermittent suction. If repositioning the client is not successful, the physician should be notified. Depending on further orders, the tube could be irrigated or replaced.

7. *The answer is* D. The nurse is legally and ethically responsible to question and refuse an order that is unsafe. Inserting a NG tube in a client with esophageal varices that are bleeding could cause rupture of varices and life-threatening hemorrhage. When a nurse refuses a physician's order, it is best to briefly and calmly explain your concerns to the physician. The nursing supervisor, or immediate supervisor in your unit, should then be notified immediately of the situation. When a nurse carries

out an order that is known to be life-threatening to the client, the nurse is not legally protected by the fact that "The physician ordered it." A nurse is judged by the "usual standard of care by a nurse in that situation." In this case, the nurse should know that inserting a nasogastric tube in a client with bleeding varices could cause rupture of varices, resulting in hemorrhage and death.

ANNOTATED REFERENCES

Allen, K., & Phillips, J. (1997). *Women's health across the lifespan.* Philadelphia: J. B. Lippincott.

This text covers health promotion, systems-related disorders, and cultural and social issues of women from childhood to advanced age.

Dudek, S. G. (1997). Nutrition handbook for nursing practice. Philadelphia: J. B. Lippincott.

Sample diets and menus with emphasis on the role of nutrition in nursing care are given in this text. The format of systems-related diets and disorders makes the information easy to access.

Giger, J., & Davidhizar, R. E. (1995). Transcultural nursing assessment and intervention. St. Louis: C. V. Mosby.

This text gives a framework for cultural assessment. Individual chapters include details on cultural beliefs of various ethnic groups common in the United States.

Moore, M. C. (1997). Nutritional care. St. Louis: C. V. Mosby.

A pocket guide series for quick reference, this text includes sections on obesity and eating disorders, enteral and parenteral nutrition, and specific clinical conditions.

Pagana, K., & Pagana, T. (1995). Diagnostic and laboratory test reference. St. Louis: C. V. Mosby.

This text presents tests alphabetically for quick reference. It includes normal and abnormal findings. There is patient education segment for each test.

Phipps, W., Cassemeyer, V., Sands, J., & Lehman, M. K. (1995). Medical-surgical nursing concepts and clinical practice. St. Louis: C. V. Mosby.

This text is an extensive treatment of alterations in the body systems and the nursing care for common problems in ill adults. It is useful for a detailed review.

INTERNET SITES FOR ADDITIONAL INFORMATION

American Liver Foundation
  http://sadieo.ucsf.edu/alf/alffinal/homepagealf.html

Colon Cancer
  listserv@sjuvm.stjohns.edu
  Subscribe COLON Firstname Lastname

Safer Sex Pages
  http://www.safersex.org/

International Food Information Council
  http://ificinfo.health.org/

Food and Nutrition Information Center
  http://www.nalusda.gov/fnic

Antibiotic Subscribing Guide
  http://www.intmed.mcw.edu/ AntibioticGuide.html

ℋEMATOLOGICAL SYSTEM

𝒥NTRODUCTION

The hematological system consists of the blood and the sites of blood production, the bone marrow, and the lymph nodes. Blood comprises three major cell types, the red blood cells (RBC), white blood cells (WBC), and platelets. Each blood cell type undergoes complex stages of maturation and differentiation when developing from the original stem cell to the mature cell. In the adult, blood cell formation occurs primarily in the bone marrow. Blood consists of cellular components suspended in plasma (the "watery" portion of the blood). This chapter covers the function of blood cells and the diseases that result from overdestruction, underproduction, or massive loss of cells.

Erythrocytes (RBCs)

RBCs are the most abundant cells in the body and are necessary for the delivery of oxygen to the tissues. Mature RBCs consist primarily of hemoglobin, which transports oxygen between lungs and tissues. After birth, RBCs are produced exclusively in the bone marrow. Almost all of the bone marrow produces RBCs until 5 years of age, but by early adulthood most RBCs are produced in the marrow of membranous bones, such as the vertebrae, the sternum, ribs, and ilia. In the bone marrow, RBCs undergo a sophisticated process of differentiation from initial to the mature cells. *Erythropoiesis* describes the stages of differentiation in the production of

Normocyte is an erythrocyte (RBC) that is normal in size, shape, and color.

erythrocytes. Erythropoiesis requires vitamin B_{12}, folic acid, and a hormone called erythropoietin, among other substances. *Erythroblasts* and *reticulocytes* are immature erythrocytes attached to hemoglobin. The average life span of a RBC is 120 days.

Two vitamins, vitamin B_{12} and folic acid, are especially important for the final maturation of RBCs. Either vitamin B_{12} or folic acid deficiency cause failure of normal cell maturation and division. With these deficiencies, the RBC becomes larger than normal, developing into *megaloblasts*. These poorly formed cells are capable of carrying oxygen normally, but their fragility shortens their life span from one-half to one-third of normal. Therefore, vitamin B_{12} and folic acid deficiencies both prevent maturation so the mature RBCs are decreased in number. This condition is called megaloblastic anemia.

Anemia Anemia is defined as a significant reduction in RBC mass and a corresponding decrease in the oxygen-carrying capacity of the blood (Fenstermacher & Hudson, 1997). Anemia is caused by many different types of diseases, but all of the disorders significantly decrease the amount of oxygen available to the tissues. During the life cycle of the RBC, aged RBCs are broken down by the liver and spleen and converted to bilirubin. Disturbances in the RBC life span from destruction, underproduction, or hemorrhage can result in anemia. Hemoglobin (the oxygen-carrying molecule in RBC) and hematocrit (the percent of RBCs per volume of whole blood) values demonstrate the presence of anemia. Massive blood loss causes the body to release reticulocytes; the hemoglobin, hematocrit, and RBC values are initially within normal limits and then dramatically decrease within 6–24 hours.

Nurses should know the laboratory indices of RBCs in order to classify the anemia and plan care for the client. Anemia should be classified according to the RBC indices for size, color, and volume. Cell size is classified as *normocytic* (normal size), *microcytic* (small size), and *macrocytic* (large size). Hemoglobin content and color are indicated by the terms *normochromic* (normal color), *hypochromic* (decreased hemoglobin content and color), and *hyperchromic* (increased hemoglobin content and color). Mean corpuscular volume (MCV) is a measure of the average volume, or size, of a RBC (Pagana & Pagana, 1995). The MCV of a single RBC decreases as the RBC ages (normal = $80–100\mu^3$). An increased MCV and abnormally large, or macrocytic, RBCs indicate megaloblastic anemia. This condition can result from vitamin B_{12} or folic acid deficiency. A decrease in MCV and microcytic RBCs indicate iron deficiency anemia and thalassemia.

Mean corpuscular hemoglobin (MCH) is the average weight of hemoglobin in a single RBC (normal = 32.34pg). Increases in MCH occur with macrocytic anemia, and decreases occur with microcytic anemia, closely resembling those for the MCV values (normal = 32–36g/dL). The MCH concentration (MCHC) is the average concentration of hemoglobin in each RBC. MCHC decreases occur in iron deficiency anemia and thalassemia. When values are normal, the anemia is said to be normocytic (e.g., hemolytic anemia). RBC distribution width (RDW) indicates variations in

Normochromia. This term describes the normal color of erythrocytes.

Hypochromia. This term describes how decreased hemoglobin in the erythrocytes causes them to look abnormally pale.

Hyperchromia. This term describes how an abnormal increase in the hemoglobin content of the erythrocytes makes them excessively pigmented.

RBC size (normal = 11–14.5%). This value is important when classifying certain types of anemia. The RDW is normal in aplastic anemia and increased in leukemia, vitamin B_{12} deficiency, and hemolytic anemia. Erythrocyte sedimentation rate (ESR) is increased in clients with inflammatory diseases, cancer, and conditions causing elevated albumin levels. The ESR is decreased in clients with sickle cell anemia.

Leukocytes (WBCs)

The WBC count is the concentration of WBCs (i.e., the number of WBCs in 1 mm³ of venous blood) and differential count, which measures the percentage of each type of WBC in the same specimen. The differential count, in descending frequency, includes neutrophils, lymphocytes, monocytes, eosinophils, and basophils. WBCs protect the body from invasion from bacteria and react against foreign bodies or tissues. The WBC count screens for leukocytic disorders. A decreased WBC count indicates *leukopenia* and leaves the client prone to infection. An increased WBC count, or *leukocytosis*, indicates the presence of an infection, inflammation, or leukemic neoplasia. Trauma or stress may increase the WBC count as well.

Neutrophils, basophils, and eosinophils are granulocytes, a category of WBCs. Granulocytes live 10–14 days in blood or 4–5 days in tissue. Granulocyte levels are increased in clients with anemia, fever and elevated blood sugar and decreased in clients who are malnourished. Cells shrink as they age. The primary function of **neutrophils** is phagocytosis, the killing and ingesting of bacterial microorganisms. When bacteria or foreign material are ingested, these cells are activated within 1 hour for phagocytosis. Bands, or immature neutrophils, are often present at an infection site when neutrophil production is stimulated. The increase in the number of bands that occurs with acute infections is termed a "shift to the left." This left shift is frequently used as a parameter of diagnosis for an ongoing bacterial infection (Pagana & Pagana, 1995). Basophils mobilize bodily defenses, and their level increases during allergic reactions, the healing phase, parasitic infestation, and leukemia. Eosinophil levels may also be increased during allergic reactions, inflammatory conditions, and parasitic infestation, as well as pernicious anemia. An increased number of eosinophils is termed a "right shift" and aids in the diagnosis of an inflammatory or allergic condition.

Agranulocytes are monocytes and lymphocytes. Monocytes are activated for phagocytosis in the later phases of infection. Lymphocytes, which live 100 days, are essential for antibody production. Lymphocytes further differentiate into T cells and B cells. T cells increase phagocytosis and provide thymus cell–based immunity (delayed hypersensitivity). B cells are responsible for antibody production. The primary function of the T cells and B cells is to fight bacterial and acute viral infections. The normal differential count does not separate the T and B cells, but it counts the combination of the two as lymphocytes. When a separate T-cell count is desired, such as in human immunodeficiency virus (HIV)–positive clients, this laboratory value is ordered specifically.

The total WBC count and differential count have important diagnostic value in the three phases of generalized infection. The changes occur as follows:

Neutrophils are granular leukocytes having a nucleus with three to five lobes, also called polymorphonuclear leukocytes. Bands, basophils and eosinophils are types of neutrophils, or granulocytic leukocytes.

Neutrophilia is an increased number of neutrophils in the blood.

1. **Acute.** The total WBC count increases above 10,000 mm^3. During the acute phase of infection, the number of bands (left shift) increases. If the WBC count is above 100,000 mm^3, the blood becomes viscous and circulation decreases.
2. **Recovery.** During the recovery period, the total WBC count drops, the number of bands decrease, and the monocytes and eosinophils increase.
3. **Convalescence.** The number of lymphocytes increase during the convalescent phase.

Blood Plasma and Platelets

The two other blood components are the blood plasma and the platelets. Platelets aggregate and induce the release of coagulation factors to control bleeding. Blood plasma is the cell-free liquid portion of the blood. If the plasma is clotted, the remaining fluid is serum. Plasma is part of the extracellular fluid and communicates continually through pores in the capillaries. The plasma volume averages 3 L in the adult (Guyton & Hall, 1996). Plasma proteins include albumin and globulins. Gamma globulins consist of antibodies called immunoglobulins that are produced by lymphocytes and plasma cells. Albumin maintains fluid volume in the vascular system by creating an osmotic force that holds fluid in the vascular space. It is produced by the liver and transports fatty acids, bilirubin, and medications. Fibrinogen clotting factors are other important constituents of the blood plasma.

$\mathcal{A}$NEMIAS

Anemias have several etiologies and multiple types exist, but they all result in decreased oxygen availability to the tissues (Fig. 6-1). A discussion of some of the common classifications of anemias follows.

Aplastic Anemia

Cytopenia is a deficiency of any of the blood cell elements.

In aplastic anemia, fat replaces bone marrow, resulting in a decrease of precursor cells of all blood cells in the bone marrow. This decreases the amount of RBCs, WBCs, and platelets. Aplastic anemia may be congenital, acquired, or idiopathic. Infections, medications, and heavy metals can also cause this condition. Adolescent males with hepatitis are at risk for a severe form of the disease that has a 90% mortality rate within 1 year. A definitive diagnosis is made by bone marrow biopsy. Clinical manifestations include a gradual onset of weakness, pallor, and shortness of breath on exertion. The client may have abnormal bleeding as a result of thrombocytopenia (a decrease in platelets). Treatment consists of bone marrow transplant or immunosuppressive therapy with antithymocyte globulin (ATG) administered through a central line for 7–10 days. The prognosis is poor without a

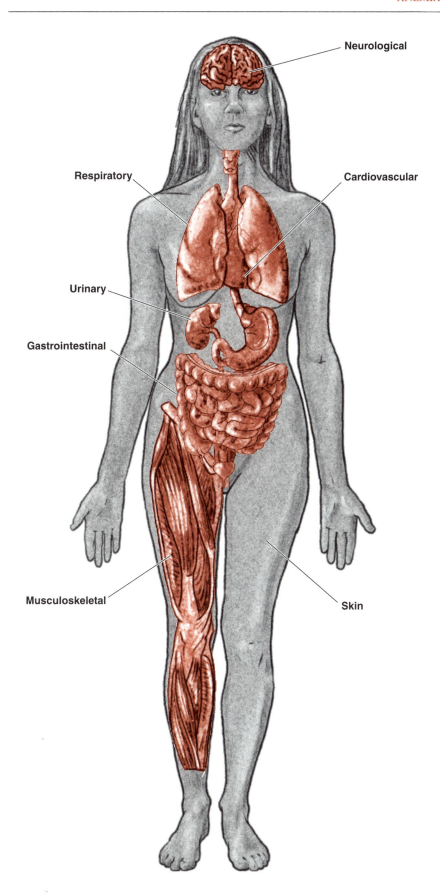

FIGURE 6-1

Clinical manifestations of anemia as the hypoxia affects various tissues and organs.

successful bone marrow transplant. If mature blood cell production stops, death can result from fulminating infection or hemorrhage. Transplant centers report survival rates of 60–80%. Clients have the best chance for survival if the transplant is performed as early as possible and blood products are avoided. When RBC and platelet transfusions are needed to manage symptoms, leukocyte-poor RBCs and platelets should be used (Phipps, Cassmeyer, Sands, & Lehman, 1995). Nursing care includes assessing for signs and symptoms of infection, tissue hypoxia, and bleeding. Clients must preserve energy with frequent rest periods. Stool softeners and high-fiber diet are given to promote regular bowel movements, as constipation may cause hemorrhage of the rectal mucosa. The nurse must also take precautions with the oral mucosa; only soft swabs are used for mouth care.

Iron Deficiency Anemia

Iron deficiency anemia is the most common type of anemia. In this type, the amount of body iron is decreased. Iron deficiency anemia may be caused by bleeding, malabsorption, dietary deficiencies, excessive menstruation, and pregnancy. Clinical manifestations include decreased hemoglobin and RBCs. The hallmark symptom is small, hypochromic RBCs. Symptoms may vary depending on slow or rapid onset. Symptoms can be slow to manifest or be noticed by the client. Clients with anemia may exhibit smooth, sore tongues; irritability; dizziness; difficulty concentrating; lack of energy; syncope; pallor; and pica (behavioral disturbance from neurological symptoms manifesting as cravings for non-food items such as clay, laundry starch, or ice). When hemoglobin falls below 7.5 g/dL, clients often experience cardiovascular symptoms such as tachycardia, chest pain, congestive heart failure (CHF), and shortness of breath (see Fig. 6-1). Iron deficiency anemia is managed by (1) treating the underlying cause, and (2) pharmacologically replacing the iron for 1 year. Medications include ferrous sulfate (most economical), ferrous gluconate, and ferrous fumarate. The nurse may need to perform other diagnostic tests or make referrals to identify and treat the cause of the anemia. The nurse should provide nutritional counseling, teaching clients about foods rich in iron such as organ meats, beans, leafy vegetables, raisins, and molasses. Vitamin C increases iron absorption. Clients are encouraged to take iron preparations with orange juice, not milk or antacids, as these block iron absorption. Iron dextran (Imferon) may be given when malabsorption in the gastric mucosa is a problem. It is usually given intravenously or intramuscularly (Z-Track) because it stains the skin. Iron salts change the color of the stool to dark green or black, and clients should be instructed beforehand that this is normal.

Megaloblastic Anemias

In megaloblastic anemia, the RBCs are enlarged or megaloblastic. This condition is caused by vitamin B_{12} and/or folate deficiency.

High iron foods include organ and lean meats, egg yolks, apricots, raisins, green-leafy vegetables, breads and cereals enriched with iron, and other foods fortified with iron.

Iron requirements. Men require 10 mg/day. Menstruating women require 15 mg/day, but postmenopausal women require only 10 mg/day. A constant although small intake of iron in food is needed to replace erythrocytes that are destroyed in the natural body processes. Iron is very important because it is a major constituent of hemoglobin.

Pernicious Anemia Pernicious anemia is a type of megaloblastic anemia caused by vitamin B_{12} deficiency. An absence of intrinsic factor in the gastric mucosal cells prevents ileal absorption of vitamin B_{12}. Vitamin B_{12} is essential for deoxyribonucleic acid (DNA) synthesis. Clients with a partial or complete gastrectomy or severe Crohn's disease are at high risk for developing pernicious anemia. Clinical manifestations include weakness, listlessness, and pallor. The hallmark symptom is a "beefy," red, inflamed tongue (glossitis). Neurological symptoms such as confusion, lack of balance, peripheral paresthesias, and loss of sense of position can occur. If left untreated, after several years these clients will die from CHF. The definitive diagnosis is made with the Schilling test, which detects the absence of intrinsic factor in the gastric mucosa. Other general laboratory values include low hemoglobin and hematocrit, normal total iron binding capacity, and a low serum B_{12} level. Treatment consists of vitamin B_{12} replacement (100 mg/month) for the rest of the client's life. As a result of gastric mucosal atrophy, these clients are at risk for gastric cancer.

Folate Deficiency Folate deficiency, the inadequate intake of folic acid, is more commonly seen than vitamin B_{12} deficiency. This deficiency is seen in clients who rarely eat uncooked (raw) vegetables or fruits. Clients with poor dietary intake, alcoholics, and chronically malnourished persons are at high risk. The rapid growth experienced during adolescence and pregnancy place these clients at particular risk of developing folate deficiency. Folate deficiency in pregnant women is associated with neural tubal defects in the fetus. Folate deficiency also may occur with clients on prolonged intravenous or total parenteral nutrition (TPN) over several months. This condition may co-exist with vitamin B_{12} deficiency. Clinical manifestations are the same as those with vitamin B_{12} deficiency. The differential diagnosis is established by a low serum folate level. A normal level of folic acid is 5–20 µg/mL. Decreased levels may be seen in conditions such as malnutrition, malignancy, pregnancy, alcoholism, anorexia nervosa, malabsorption, and hemolytic anemia as well as folic acid deficiency anemia (Pagana & Pagana, 1995). Management includes administration of 1 mg/day of folic acid and a well-balanced diet. Any other underlying conditions such as alcoholism or anorexia must also be treated.

Sickle Cell Anemia (SCA)

SCA is caused by defective hemoglobin molecules shaped like "sickles," hence the classification of this anemia (Fig. 6-2). The sickle-shaped cells cause vascular occlusion in the capillaries, and this is associated with attacks of severe pain. SCA is a genetic disorder and is seen predominantly in clients of African heritage. It is a recessive, hereditary hemolytic anemia. A laboratory test can determine if the client is a carrier. As many as 10% of African Americans in North America have the sickle cell trait, but less than 1% have SCA (Wong & Perry, 1998)

The pathophysiology of SCA results from the vascular obstruction caused by the sickled RBC and the rapid destruction of the RBC (hemolysis). The

Sickle cell anemias are hemolytic anemias caused by the genetically transmitted sickled hemoglobin.

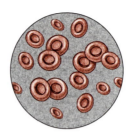

A   Normal red blood cells

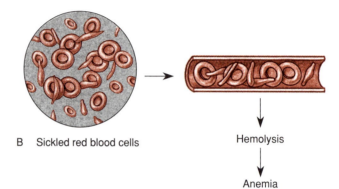

B   Sickled red blood cells

Hemolysis

Anemia

FIGURE 6-2

The sickle-cell
hemoglobinopathy.

Electrophoresis is the movement
of charged particles suspended in
liquid under the influence of an
applied electrical field. **Hemoglobin electrophoresis** is performed to diagnose sickle cell
hemoglobinopathies.

Hemoglobinopathy is any
hemolytic disorder resulting
from alterations in the
genetically determined molecular
structure of hemoglobin, with
characteristic laboratory and
clinical abnormalities that define
the anemia.

cells containing defective hemoglobin molecules become deformed, rigid,
and sickle-shaped as they circulate through the veins. The cells lodge in
small vessels and slow the circulation of blood to the organs. Ischemia, pain,
swelling, fever, and infarction can occur. Sickled RBCs live only 15–25 days,
and clients usually have a hemoglobin level of 7–10 g/dL. As a result of the
rapid destruction of sickled RBCs, jaundice is often evident in the sclera.
The rapid hemolysis of the RBCs causes marked viscosity of the blood.

The diagnosis is obtained by a **hemoglobin electrophoresis.** SCA is one
of a group of diseases termed hemoglobinopathies in which normal hemoglobin is replaced by abnormal sickled hemoglobin (HbS). Newborns are
screened for SCA in most states in the United States so that the disorder is
identified before symptoms can occur. The first sickle cell crisis usually
occurs at 1–3 years of age and often follows a respiratory or gastrointestinal infection. Many clients die in the first years of life; the life expectancy
for clients with SCA is around 40 years. Although the prognosis does vary,
SCA is a chronic, potentially fatal illness. A bone marrow transplant
may provide a possible cure. Siblings should be tested as possible donors.
Preventive genetic counseling and screening of African Americans may
decrease the incidence of SCA in the future. When both parents are carriers of the sickle cell trait, their offspring have a 25% chance of having
sickle cell anemia (Wong & Perry, 1998).

There is no cure for SCA. The goals of treatment are to prevent conditions that trigger the sickling phenomenon and to alleviate the symptoms
during the sickle cell crisis. Hydroxyurea (Hydrea) is given to increase fetal
hemoglobin and prolong hemoglobin survival. Pentoxifylline (Trental)
decreases blood viscosity and peripheral vascular resistance and decreases

the length of the sickle cell crisis. Vanillin, a food additive, has anti-sickling properties. Precautions should be taken to prevent infections, such as immunizing infants at 2 months of age against *Haemophilus influenzae* and prescribing prophylactic penicillin at the earliest signs of respiratory infection. Administration of pneumococcal and meningococcal vaccines beginning at age 2 years is also recommended because of the susceptibility to infection from decreased or absent splenic function (Wong & Perry, 1998). These precautions against infections have improved morbidity and mortality rates of children with SCA. Infection seems to predispose clients to the onset of sickle cell crisis; thus, all clients with SCA should be treated promptly for infections. The prevention of dehydration and hypoxia is crucial as well. Folic acid is given to stimulate the bone marrow production.

When a sickle cell crisis occurs, clients are hospitalized for intravenous hydration and analgesia. Since water decreases blood viscosity, 3–5 L/day are administered intravenously in adults. Small-gauge angiocatheters are used to decrease trauma to the vessels. Oxygen may be given to treat tissue hypoxia and ischemia, and pulse oximetry should be monitored for evidence of adequate oxygenation. Analgesia, typically morphine sulfate (Morphine), is usually administered via patient controlled analgesia (PCA) pump. Meperidine (Demerol) is not recommended as clients with SCA are particularly at risk for meperidine-induced seizures (American Pain Society, 1992, as cited in Wong & Perry, 1998). Renal failure is a major cause of death for adults with this disease. Intake and output should always be recorded. Electrolytes and renal function (blood urea nitrogen [BUN] and creatinine) laboratory values should be monitored closely. Cerebrovascular accident (CVA) is another potentially fatal complication that the nurse should monitor, and any abnormalities in neurological signs should be reported to the physician immediately.

Polycythemia Vera

Polycythemia vera is a bone marrow disorder characterized by an overproduction of RBCs, called erythrocytosis. It is usually accompanied by increased WBCs (leukocytosis) and platelets (thrombocytosis). The etiology is unknown. Laboratory results reveal an increased RBC volume and a hematocrit that is greater than 53% (Phipps et al, 1995). The increased production of RBCs causes increased blood viscosity, and platelet dysfunctions also may occur, leading to bleeding. Clinical manifestations include a ruddy complexion, hepatosplenomegaly, headache, dizziness, and fatigue with blurred vision as a result of increased blood volume. Increased blood viscosity may cause angina, claudication, thrombophlebitis, and pruritus. Thrombosis and embolization may result from increased blood viscosity and hypovolemia.

Treatment consists of periodically removing blood from a vein (therapeutic phlebotomy) to maintain hemoglobin and hematocrit within normal limits. Antihistamines may be used to decrease pruritus. Nurses must teach clients and their families about this anemia and stress the importance and purpose of continued care, therapeutic phlebotomy, and periodic laboratory tests. Client education should emphasize the importance of maintaining hydration to decrease blood viscosity. The signs and symptoms of extremity thrombosis such as calf pain, swelling, and redness should be taken seriously, and the client should seek care immediately.

Agranulocytosis

Agranulocytosis is an acute disease in which there is a dramatic decrease in the production of granulocytes. Therefore, a severe neutropenia develops, and the body is defenseless against any bacterial invasion. Agranulocytosis is potentially fatal. This disorder is most commonly caused by medication toxicity or chemical sensitization that depresses the formation of bone marrow cells. Laboratory values reveal severe leukopenia (<2000 granulocytes/mm^3 of blood). Clients often present with high fever, severe sore throat, and ulcerations of the mucous membranes. Bacteremia may develop or may already be present when the client seeks care. Treatment consists of immediate withdrawal of the medication, and eradication of the infection. Septic workup includes a culture and sensitivity of the blood, nose, throat, and urine. Broad-spectrum antibiotics are given until the results of the culture and sensitivity are available. Saline gargles and ice collars effectively comfort clients with a sore throat. Analgesics, antipyretics, and sedatives are also frequently prescribed. Common medications that can cause an adverse reaction or toxic effect resulting in agranulocytosis include: chemotherapy drugs, nonsteroidal anti-inflammatory drugs (NSAIDs) such as ketorolac (Toradol) and naproxen (Naprosyn), and sulfa drugs such as trimethoprim/sulfamethoxazole (Bactrim), and mafenide acetate (Sulfamylon) topical ointment for burns.

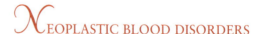

$\mathcal{N}$EOPLASTIC BLOOD DISORDERS

Leukemia

Leukemia is a chronic or acute neoplasm of blood-forming cells in the bone marrow and lymph nodes. It is marked by diffuse replacement of mature leukocytes in the bone marrow with immature WBCs. Laboratory values demonstrate a marked increase in WBCs, which are of an immature differentiation. The diagnosis is confirmed by a bone marrow aspiration with differentiation of cells types. Following differentiation of the cells from the bone marrow aspirate, leukemia is classified as acute or chronic based on the type of predominant proliferating cells that are present (myelocytic, granulocytic, lymphocytic) and number of abnormal cells in the blood at the time of diagnosis. The etiology of leukemia is unknown, but it is thought to be viral or genetic. (See Chap. 14 for details on neoplastic disorders.)

Acute Myelogenous Leukemia (AML)

AML is a malignant disorder that affects monocytes, granulocytes, erythrocytes, and platelets. The proliferation of immature myeloblasts interferes with the normal production of other blood cells, thus decreasing the number of erythrocytes and platelets. In all types of leukemias, normal cell production in the bone marrow is literally crowded out by the malignant proliferation of WBCs (Fig. 6-3). The diagnosis is confirmed by bone marrow aspiration, revealing a marked increase in immature myeloblasts. The presence of Auer rods in the blood is also indicative of AML. AML can occur at any age but is seen more frequently in adolescence and those over age 55 (Wong & Perry, 1998). Clinical manifestations include decreased levels of mature granulocytes, weakness, fatigue, bleeding tendencies, lymphadenopathy, hepatosplenomegaly, headache, vomiting, and bone pain. Symptoms may appear 1–6 months after developing the disorder.

Treatment involves a protocol of chemotherapy, including cytarabine (Cytosar-U), 6-thioguanine (Thioguanine or TG), doxorubicin (Adriamycin), and daunomycin (Cerubinine). While some clients achieve complete remission with chemotherapy, bone marrow transplants with allogenic bone

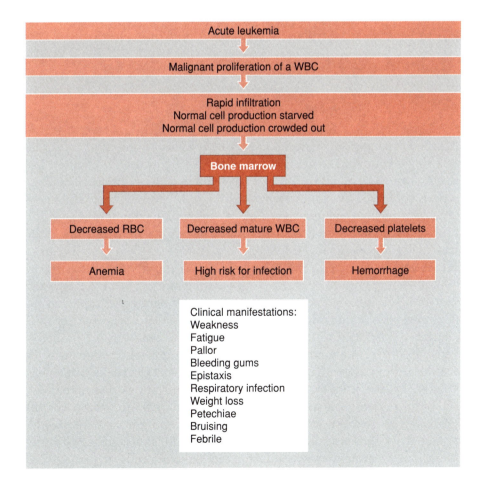

FIGURE 6-3

The development of cellular pathology and clinical manifestations in leukemia.

marrow are performed more frequently (see Chap. 14). Another transplant option is an autologous bone marrow transplant, in which the client's own marrow is transplanted after remission is achieved with chemotherapy (Wong & Perry, 1998). In general, the prognosis varies, but clients receiving chemotherapy may survive 1–3 years without a bone marrow transplant. Death may occur from infection or hemorrhage. If left untreated, the survival time is only 2–5 months.

Chronic Myelogenous Leukemia (CML)

CML is a malignancy of the myeloid stem cells that causes the uncontrolled proliferation of granulocytes. The onset is insidious, and the disorder, long-term. CML is seen most frequently between the ages of 50–70 years and is more common in men. Signs and symptoms are less severe than those of AML. Laboratory tests reveal an increase in leukocytes and splenomegaly. Clients present with weakness, fatigue, anorexia, and weight loss and may have anemia and thrombocytopenia. As with other leukemias, treatment consists of a regimen of chemotherapy, including busulfan (Myleran). However, long-term survival is possible only with a bone marrow transplant. The pathophysiology of leukemias vary, but the prognosis of clients with CML who do not receive a transplant may be only 3–5 years. As with all leukemias, death usually results from infection or hemorrhage.

Acute Lymphocytic Leukemia (ALL)

Neutropenia is the diminished number of neutrophils in the blood, which puts the client prone to infection.

Leukopenia is the reduction of the number of leukocytes in the blood, with a total WBC count of less than 5000 mm^3, which puts the client at risk for infection.

ALL is the malignant proliferation of lymphoblasts arising from a disorder of a single lymphoid stem cell. It occurs most frequently in children 2–4 years of age. The incidence drops sharply after 10 years of age. The diagnosis is confirmed by bone marrow aspiration or biopsy. The clinical manifestations include anemia, bleeding of the mucous membranes, pallor, bruising, lymphadenopathy, hepatosplenomegaly, vomiting, bone pain, and a predisposition to infection. Laboratory values demonstrate a decrease in erythrocytes and platelet counts, and abnormalities in the WBCs. Perhaps more than any other malignancy, chemotherapy and radiation research on specific protocols of treatment have improved the prognosis of children with ALL. Most children survive 5 years with chemotherapy and irradiation, and approximately 50% can be cured (Wong & Perry, 1998). To maintain remission, chemotherapy and treatment of the central nervous system (CNS) to prevent recurrences in the cerebrospinal fluid (CSF) are necessary. The intrathecal administration (via a spinal tap) of methotrexate with or without craniospinal radiation improves the survival rate. Because chemotherapeutic agents do not cross the blood-brain barrier, the leukemic cells migrate to the CSF as a sanctuary for proliferation. Treatment that eradicates the leukemic cells in the CSF has greatly improved the prognosis of those with ALL.

Chronic Lymphocytic Leukemia (CLL)

CLL is caused by a proliferation of small, abnormal B lymphocytes. It primarily affects people 50–70 years of age and is three times more common in men. Clinical manifestations include anemia, infection, lymphadenopathy, weakness, and fatigue. Laboratory values demonstrate a decreased number of erythrocytes, and either a decreased or normal number of platelets. A decreased mature lymphocyte count is always present, and the total WBC count is elevated from 20,000 mm^3 to 100,000 mm^3. A bone marrow biopsy demonstrates the infiltration of lymphocytes. Treatment involves a chemotherapy protocol and corticosteroids. The prognosis is typically 5–7 years.

Malignant Lymphomas

Malignant lymphomas are neoplasms of the lymphatic system. Lymph node enlargement results from an increase in the size of lymphoid tissue along with the proliferation of lymphocytes (as in infection), or leukemic cells and cancer cells (as in malignancies). In lymphoma, the actual node structure is eventually destroyed by malignant cells. Normally, lymph nodes should be barely palpable or nonpalpable. During the physical examination, the major chains of lymph node tissue in the face, neck, chest, axilla, and groin, should always be palpated to detect possible infection or malignancy.

Hodgkin's Disease

Hodgkin's lymphoma is a common malignancy of the lymph nodes. It is seen more often in men in their early 20s or older than 50 years of age. A biopsy and histopathological examination of the lymph nodes confirm the diagnosis. The presence of malignant cells (Reed-Steinberg cells) remains the pathological hallmark of Hodgkin's disease. However, pathological differentiation is important, as there are various types of Hodgkin's lymphomas.

The etiology of Hodgkin's disease is unknown. Clinical manifestations include painless lymphadenopathy on one side of the neck. On palpation, the nodes feel "rubbery." Eventually the cervical nodes on the other side of the neck swell, or node enlargement in the axilla or the groin occurs. Progressive anemia develops, the leukocyte count increases, and eosinophil levels increase. Unexplained fever with temperatures reaching 101°F or night sweats often occurs. Diagnostic tests include a lymph node biopsy, complete blood count (CBC), ESR, and chest x-rays to identify the presence of any mediastinal mass. Treatment includes radiation and chemotherapy, depending on the staging of the disease. Nursing care includes encouraging the client to eat bland, soft foods to maintain adequate nutritional intake and prevent weight loss. Anesthetic throat lozenges are often effective for sore throats, and good dental hygiene is required. Antiemetics such as ondansetron hydrochloride (Zofran) have proven helpful in the prevention and treatment of the nausea and vomiting that accompany chemotherapy. The nurse should help clients and their families to cope with the hair loss by providing resources for caps and wigs.

Non-Hodgkin's Lymphoma

Non-Hodgkin's lymphoma includes a variety of lymphoid malignancies with different cell pathologies. The etiology of this disorder may be viral. These lymphoid malignancies are common in clients with acquired immunodeficiency syndrome (AIDS). The median age is 50–60 years. Clients often present with nontender lymphadenopathy, hepatomegaly, splenomegaly, fever, and night sweats. Histological classification is important, and the pathology slides are often sent to major cancer centers for consultation. Once the cell type is identified, the staging is determined. As with Hodgkin's disease, the staging workup is similar, and it is a crucial factor in determining the course of treatment. The options for treatment should always be discussed in detail with the client and his or her family. The nurse needs to provide support and explanations during this diagnostic period to help the client make informed decisions. Treatment usually includes **radiation therapy** when the disease has a localized presentation. Chemotherapy is the mainstay of treatment when the lymphomas are not localized.

Multiple Myeloma

Multiple myeloma is a malignancy of the plasma cells of bone, lymph nodes, liver, spleen, and kidneys. Signs and symptoms include back pain, bone pain, increased calcium levels, and fractures. Laboratory values demonstrate decreased platelets, decreased leukocytes, and RBCs within normal limits. The diagnosis is made by bone marrow biopsy. Treatment consists of a chemotherapy regimen, corticosteroids, and radiation. These patients must be kept hydrated to prevent increased blood viscosity. Clients with this disorder survive approximately 2–5 years, and death often occurs from infection or renal failure.

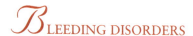

$\mathcal{B}$LEEDING DISORDERS

Conditions that cause an underproduction or destruction of platelets result in platelet deficits, which trigger the onset of petechiae, an increase in bruising and bleeding from the nasal or oropharyngeal mucosa. *Thrombocytopenia* is the term used to describe a deficit in platelets. These clients are at high risk for abnormal bleeding. When the platelet count decreases below 20,000/mm³, petechiae appear, and epistaxis often occurs. Platelet counts below 5000/mm3 can result in fatal CNS or gastrointestinal (GI) hemorrhages. Treatment is aimed at the underlying cause and administering platelet transfusions (Table 6-1).

Radiation therapy includes treatment by x-rays and gamma rays and may be used to destroy the abnormal cells that form tumors. Gonads, blood cells, and cancer cells are especially sensitive to radiation, particularly x-rays and gamma rays. Leukemias and lymphomas are frequently treated with radiation.

TABLE 6-1

SUMMARY OF BLOOD COMPONENTS

Component	Major Indications	Action	Condition for Which Not Indicated	Special Precautions	Hazards	Rate of Infusion
Whole blood	Symptomatic anemia with large volume deficit	Restoration of oxygen-carrying capacity; restoration of blood volume	Condition responsive to specific component	Must be ABO-identical Labile coagulation factors deteriorate within 24 hours after collection	Infectious diseases; septic/toxic, allergic, febrile reactions; circulatory overload	For massive loss; fast as patient can tolerate
Red blood cells	Symptomatic anemia	Restoration of oxygen-carrying capacity	Pharmacologically treatable anemia Coagulation deficiency	Must be ABO-compatible	Infectious diseases; septic/toxic, allergic, febrile reactions	As patient can tolerate but less than 4 hours
Red blood cells Leukocytes removed	Symptomatic anemia; febrile reactions from leukocyte antibodies	Restoration of oxygen-carrying capacity	Pharmacologically treatable anemia Coagulation deficiency	Must be ABO-compatible	Infectious diseases; septic/toxic, allergic reaction (unless plasma also removed by washing)	As patient can tolerate but less than 4 hours
Adenine–saline added	Symptomatic anemia with volume deficit	Restoration of oxygen-carrying capacity	Pharmacologically treatable anemia Coagulation deficiency	Must be ABO-compatible	Infectious diseases; septic/toxic, allergic, febrile reactions; circulatory overload	As patient can tolerate but less than 4 hours
Fresh frozen plasma	Deficit of labile and stable plasma coagulation factors and increased PTT	Source of labile and nonlabile plasma factors	Condition responsive to volume replacement	Should be ABO-compatible	Infectious diseases; allergic reactions; circulatory overload	Less than 4 hours
Liquid plasma and plasma	Deficit of stable plasma coagulation factors	Source of non-labile factors	Deficit of labile coagulation factors or volume replacement	Should be ABO-compatible	Infectious diseases, allergic reactions	Less than 4 hours

TABLE 6-1 (*continued*)

SUMMARY OF BLOOD COMPONENTS

Component	Major Indications	Action	Condition for Which Not Indicated	Special Precautions	Hazards	Rate of Infusion
Cryo-precipitated AHF	Hemophilia A; von Willebrand's disease; hypo-fibrinogenemia; factor VIII or XIII deficiency	Provides factor VIII, fibrinogen, vWF, factor XIII	Conditions not deficient in contained factors	Frequent repeat doses may be necessary	Infectious diseases, allergic reactions	Less than 4 hours
Platelets: platelets, pheresis	Bleeding from thrombocytopenia or platelet function abnormality	Improves hemostasis	Plasma coagulation deficits and some conditions with rapid platelet destruction (e.g., ITP)	Should not use some microaggregate filters (check manufacturer's instructions)	Infectious diseases; septic/toxic, allergic, febrile reactions	Lesss than 4 hours
Granulocytes	Neutropenia with infection	Provides granulocytes	Infection responsive to antibiotics	Must be ABO-compatible, do not use depth-type microaggregate filters	Infectious diseases, allergic reactions, febrile reactions	One pheresis unit over 2–4-hour period—closely observe for reactions

NOTE: From American Association of Blood Banks. PTT = prolonged thromboplastin time; AHF = antihemophilic factor; vWF = von Willebrand's factor; ITP = idiopathic thrombocytopenic purpura.

Idiopathic Thrombocytopenia Purpura (ITP)

ITP is a type of platelet deficiency that occurs more commonly in women and children. A viral disease usually precedes the incidence of ITP in children. The life span of the RBC is also decreased. Signs and symptoms include petechiae, mucosal bleeding, and heavy menses in women. Laboratory tests reveal a decreased platelet count (below 20,000/mm^3). Treatment involves corticosteroids or intravenous immunoglobulin. A splenectomy may be performed in severe cases.

Clotting Factor Defects

Hemophilia A is caused by a deficiency of factor VIII. It is an inherited blood disorder and is much more common in men. Clinical manifestations include large, spreading bruises and bleeding in muscles, joints, and soft tissue after minimal trauma. The joint pain, swelling, and limited range of motion that occurs can lead to permanent joint problems. Treatment includes periodic factor VIII transfusions (see Table 6-1). These clients are never given intramuscular injections, and all venipunctures and injections are kept to a minimum. Aspirin and other drugs that affect clotting time are contraindicated. Nurses need to educate the client and family about good dental hygiene and prevention of bleeding from sports or trauma.

CASE STUDY: MAN WITH EPISTAXIS AND HEMOPHILIA

Mr. J, a 20-year-old man, was admitted to the emergency room (ER) with the diagnosis of epistaxis. He reports a football hit his nose during a touch football game with his friends. He also states that he has hemophilia.

An icebag and manual pressure are applied over the bridge of the client's nose. The ER physician orders the administration of factor VIII cryoprecipitate. An assessment is performed and recorded by the nurse. The vital signs are: temperature, 98°F; blood pressure, 116/82 mm Hg; pulse, 100 beats/min; and respirations, 18 breaths/min. The skin is warm, but pallor is present. Venipuncture is performed for laboratory tests and administration of the cryoprecipitate. The same venipuncture is used for both procedures to avoid excessive bruising and bleeding as much as possible. Laboratory tests reveal a prolonged partial thromboplastin time (PTT) and normal prothrombin time (PT). Following treatment, the bleeding subsides. The nurse realizes that the following complications might have occurred without prompt treatment: hypovolemic shock as a result of fluid loss and hemorrhage and aspiration as a result of the nose bleed. The nurse cautions the client to seek prompt medical attention for any injury, no matter how slight, and to wear the Medical Alert bracelet at all times. As part of the continuing education process for this client's chronic condition, the nurse should stress the importance of participating in less dangerous sports, such as golf or swimming. It is important that the client be allowed to participate in mutual goal planning; this facilitates compliance and improves the quality of life. Family members should participate in the goal planning, and the nurse can discuss how to treat a bleeding emergency until help arrives. The nurse should stress that the client can have a normal life with a few precautions. The nurse should allow the family members and the client to express their concerns and should answer their questions to promote self-management skills.

Disseminated Intravascular Coagulopathy (DIC)

DIC causes widespread clotting in small vessels, which uses up clotting factors and platelets. This leads to bleeding, decreased fibrinogen levels, increased PT, increased PTT and decreased platelets. Life-threatening hemorrhages can occur. Predisposing factors to DIC include septicemia, premature separation of the placenta, metastatic cancer, hemolytic transfusion reactions, massive tissue trauma or burns, and shock. Clients with DIC develop purpura, hypoxemia, hypovolemia, and signs of renal damage. Treatment includes hospitalization in an intensive care unit. Nursing management of DIC involves controlling the hemorrhage, restoring the acid-base balance, and maintaining life support measures. Packed red blood cells (PRBCs), platelets, and albumin are administered. If blood products with clotting factors are used, heparin is usually administered first to decrease intravascular clotting.

SUMMARY

Normal blood cell production and good nutrition are essential to maintain the health of the hematological system. Anemias develop due to blood loss, destruction of blood cells by hemolysis, and problems with production due to either a deficiency in nutrients such as iron, vitamin B_{12}, or folic acid, or a problem in production in the bone marrow such as in leukemia or aplastic anemia. The leukemias result from a malignant proliferation of leukocytes that impairs normal hematopoiesis of all blood cells. Nursing care for clients with anemia, neoplastic blood disorders, or bleeding includes astute assessment, frequent monitoring of laboratory values, administering chemotherapy or other pharmacological agents, assisting the client and family to cope, and educating them regarding treatment options. Bone marrow transplantation is becoming a far more common therapeutic option for clients with hematological disorders. While further research is needed to follow client outcomes comparing the success of bone marrow transplantation against other conventional treatment options, bone marrow transplantation is an exciting possibility with promise for many clients.

KEY WORDS

Acute lymphocytic leukemia
Acute myelogenous leukemia
Agranulocytosis
Aplastic anemia
Chronic lymphocytic leukemia
Chronic myelogenous leukemia
Disseminated intravascular
   coagulopathy
Erythrocytes
Folate deficiency
Hemophilia
Hodgkin's disease
Idiopathic thrombocytopenia
   purpura

Iron deficiency anemia
Leukemia
Leukocytes
Megaloblastic anemia
Multiple myeloma
Non-Hodgkin's lymphoma
Pernicious anemia
Polycythemia vera
Thrombocytes
Thrombocytopenia
Sickle cell anemia

QUESTIONS

1. Mrs. J. has been diagnosed with folic acid deficiency. The client asks the nurse which foods are high in folic acid, and nurse correctly responds

   A. green leafy vegetables, organ meats, nuts, and eggs
   B. fresh shrimp and oysters
   C. dried fruits and oatmeal
   D. tofu and tuna

2. Mrs. F. has been diagnosed with full-thickness burns and disseminated intravascular coagulopathy (DIC). Which of the following products could be administered?

   A. Vitamin B_{12}
   B. Frozen plasma, platelets, or cryoprecipitate
   C. Acetylsalicylic acid (ASA, aspirin)
   D. Naproxen (Naprosyn)

3. Mrs. R. has been diagnosed with pernicious anemia. The nurse practitioner has ordered 100 μg of vitamin B_{12} intramuscularly. The nurse correctly states that

   A. this drug only has to be given once since the duration is extended.
   B. vitamin B_{12} can be given orally from now on.
   C. the client must take vitamin B_{12} injections monthly for the rest of his or her life.
   D. vitamin B_{12} can be administered by superficial subcutaneous injection.

4. Mrs. P. has been diagnosed with acute myelogenous leukemia, and the physician cautions her to avoid infection. The nurse's educational training should include all of the following EXCEPT
   A. seek medical attention for every break in skin integrity or respiratory infection.
   B. practice good hand-washing technique.
   C. avoid crowds and people who are ill.
   D. keep weekly appointments with the physician to practice good preventive screening

5. Which of the following is an example of pica?
   A. A craving for sweets
   B. A craving for laundry starch and ice
   C. A craving for shellfish
   D. A craving for pickles

ANSWERS

1. *The answer is A.* The nurse should encourage foods rich in B vitamins and stress proper ways to cook vegetables to preserve potency by using the microwave or boiling them in small amounts of water.

2. *The answer is B.* Once the underlying cause of DIC is treated, the goal is to control bleeding and restore normal clotting factors. Blood products may be replaced to restore depleted factors.

3. *The answer is C.* The client with pernicious anemia lacks the intrinsic factor in the gastric mucosa to absorb vitamin B_{12}. Monthly intramuscular injections for life are necessary to manage this anemia.

4. *The answer is D.* All of the other strategies assist the client in the early prevention and treatment of infections. Weekly follow-up appointments are not necessary.

5. *The answer is B.* Pica is a craving for a nonfood item. This behavioral disturbance can result from a change in the neurological system altered by anemia.

ANNOTATED REFERENCES

Fenstermacher, K., & Hudson, B. T. (1998). *Practice guidelines for family nurse practitioners*. Philadelphia: W. B. Saunders.

This is a good resource for quick review of assessments, laboratory values, and treatment regimens. It is useful for nurses at all levels of practice.

Guyton, A., & Hall, J. (1996). *Textbook of medical physiology.* Philadelphia: W.B. Saunders.

This text is a classic source for explanations of pathophysiology. It is a recommended addition to the nurse's library to continue to advance understanding of pathophysiology.

Pagana, K., & Pagana, T. (1995). *Mosby's diagnostic and laboratory test reference.* St. Louis: C. V. Mosby.

This is a clinical handbook that features laboratory and diagnostic tests. Normal and abnormal findings and patient education content are included.

Phipps, W., Cassmeyer, V., Sands, J., & Lehman, M. (1995). *Medical-surgical nursing concepts and clinical practice.* St. Louis: C. V. Mosby.

This text is a very comprehensive book of alterations of health in adults and nursing management.

Wong, D., & Perry, S. (1998). *Maternal child nursing care.* St. Louis: C. V. Mosby.

This text includes comprehensive information on both maternity and pediatric care. Anemias in pregnancy and neoplastic blood disorders in childhood are covered extensively.

INTERNET SITES FOR ADDITIONAL INFORMATION

Hodgkin's disease
    http://www.xnet.com/~ladyhawk/health.html

Hem-onc
    listserv@sjuvm.stjohns.edu
    Subscribe HEM-ONC Firstname Lastname

Hodgkin's
    listserv@solar.org
    Subscribe HODGKINS
    (do not follow by typing name)

ONCOLINK
    http://www.oncolink.upenn.edu

ℱLUID REGULATION AND RENAL DISORDERS

ℐNTRODUCTION

Fluid regulation in the body involves the interrelationship of numerous components, including body water and other fluids, fluid compartments, fluid spacing, membranes, transport systems, enzymes, and tonicity. An understanding of these components is necessary to determine therapeutic care interventions for the client.

Fluid and Electrolyte Regulation

Body fluids consist of water (the major fluid of the body) and dissolved substances called solutes. The body must maintain homeostasis, a balance between the water and the solutes. The solutes within the body fluids contain some cations (positively charged electrolytes), anions (negatively charged electrolytes), and other substances such as glucose.

Fluids and solutes shift between fluid compartments. The fluid compartments are generally categorized as either intracellular or extracellular. **Intracellular fluid** (ICF) is contained within the cells and makes up approximately 40% of total body weight (Lemone & Burke, 1996). The **extracellular fluid** (ECF), including interstitial and intravascular fluids, is located out of the cells. Interstitial fluid is found between the cells; intravascular fluid is within the blood vessels. The ECF makes up approximately 20% of total body weight (Lemone & Burke, 1996). Therefore, 60% of total body weight can be attributed to body fluids.

Intracellular fluids are found within the cells. **Extracellular fluids** are found in intravascular and interstitial spaces.

Osmosis is the transport of water across a semipermeable membrane from an area of lower concentration to one of higher concentration.

The cell wall membrane separates intracellular fluid from interstitial fluid. The capillary wall membrane separates intravascular fluid from interstitial fluid. The fluid and solutes move across these membranes by way of three processes: osmosis, diffusion, and active transport.

Osmosis is the transport of water across a semipermeable membrane from an area of lower solute concentration to one of higher solute concentration. The solutes of greater concentration in one compartment pull the water of the other compartment across the membrane, which is permeable to water but not to solutes. The movement of water between the intracellular and extracellular fluid compartments generally occurs due to osmosis. This force also balances fluid between the interstitial and intravascular spaces. The intravascular space has a higher concentration of plasma proteins, particularly albumin, than the interstitial space. Due to these proteins and the sodium within the intravascular fluid, water is normally held within the intravascular space. When the body's level of albumin is decreased, vessel leakage occurs, and the fluids leave the intravascular space and move into the interstitial space, causing edema. The albumin acts like a magnet in preventing water from leaving the intravascular space and entering the interstitial space.

Diffusion is the movement of particles from an area of higher concentration to one of lower concentration so that the particles are evenly distributed between the two compartments.

Diffusion is a process in which particles move from an area of higher concentration to one of lower concentration so that they are evenly distributed between the two concentrations. Water, oxygen, carbon dioxide, and solutes diffuse between the intravascular and interstitial spaces through the capillary membrane (Lemone & Burke, 1996). The kidney filtration process is an example of the diffusion process. Diffusion occurs with the help of a carrier substance that assists in the movement of solutes. For example, when glucose moves into the cell from the plasma, proteins within the cell membrane help "carry" the glucose across the cell membrane.

Active transport is the movement of particles from one concentration to another without regard to concentration gradients.

Active transport is a carrier process by which molecules are moved across cell membranes without regard to concentration gradients. A higher concentration of the substance is maintained by use of an energy source, adenosine triphosphate (ATP). For example, insulin binds with glucose to allow entry of the glucose into the cell.

The concentration of solutes and water in a solution is called *tonicity*. Tonicity exerts osmotic pressure on cells causing a change in cell size (Lemone & Burke, 1996) (Fig. 7-1). Fluid tonicity is classified as isotonic, hypotonic, or hypertonic. Isotonic fluids have essentially the same tonicity as plasma. Hypotonic fluids have lower effective osmotic pressure, and hypertonic fluids have higher osmotic pressure. Osmolarity is the osmotic concentration of a solution expressed as number of osmoles found in a liter of solution. The osmolarity of an isotonic solution is 275–295 mOsm/L; that of a hypotonic solution is less than 275 mOsm/L; and that of a hypertonic solution is more than 295 mOsm/L (Fig. 7-2).

Osmolarity and the tonicity of intravenous fluids is important to know in determining their appropriateness for specific clients. For example, a client experiencing cellular edema requires a different tonicity of fluid than a client with cellular dehydration. In determining fluid type requirements, it is necessary to know the client's serum osmolality. This can be calculated using the following formula.

Serum osmolality = 2 sodium (Na$^+$) + blood urea nitrogen (BUN) / 2.4 + glucose/18

If the value is between 275 and 295 mOsm/L, the intravascular fluid is isotonic. It is very possible for a client to have an isotonic plasma and be dehydrated. This condition of isotonic fluid deficit is termed *hypovolemia*. If a client has a normal serum osmolality but exhibits signs of weakness, syncope, orthostatic hypotension, dry skin, poor skin turgor, nausea, vomiting, and decreased urine output, then an isotonic fluid is the most appropriate replacement fluid. If hemorrhage is the cause of the hypovolemia, a plasma expander such as plasma, hetastarch (Hespan) or dextran (Gentran 70) is used to replace lost fluids. A blood transfusion may also

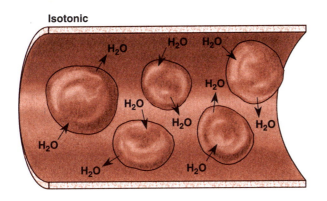
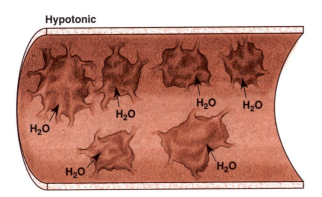
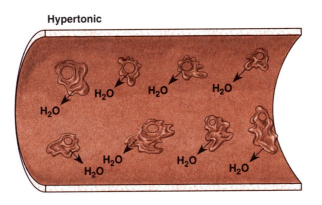

FIGURE 7-1

Effect of tonicity on cell size.

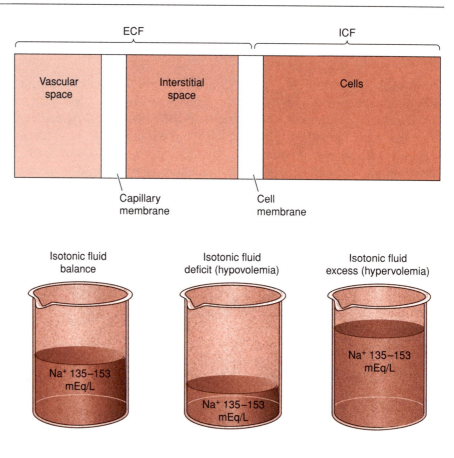

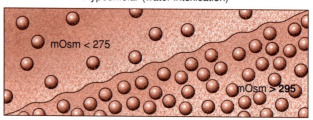

FIGURE 7-2

◈

Fluid and electrolyte balance and imbalance. ECF = extracellular fluid; ICF = intracellular fluid.

be administered. Because synthetic plasma expanders do not carry oxygen to the cells, plasma or packed cells are generally used to replace the cell's ability to transport oxygen.

A client with normal serum osmolality who exhibits hypertension, bounding pulse, jugular vein distention, weight gain, edema, cough, frothy or pink sputum, rales, or dyspnea may be experiencing an isotonic fluid volume excess. In this case, the intravenous fluids should be withheld, and diuretics should be used to pull fluid out of the body. Edema is an indicator of fluid overload, but the fluid overload is sometimes only in the interstitial and intracellular tissues. This condition is termed *intravascular dehydration* with interstitial and intracellular overhydration. In that case, a hypertonic solution should be used to move the fluid from the interstitial and intracellular tissues back into the intravascular space. The clinical manifestations of intravascular dehydration include edema caused by third-spacing, dyspnea, abdominal distention, oliguria, positive intake and output, hypertension, and weakness. This generally occurs with a loss of albumin within the intravascular space. It is common following surgery due to the shift of plasma to the incision site (Bove, 1994). It is occasionally necessary to replace albumin in the intravascular space as well.

A hypotonic solution is used when a client is experiencing cellular dehydration. These fluids are not commonly used, but clients with diabetic ketoacidosis, for example, should receive a hypotonic solution during recovery. Hypotonic solutions are indicated when intravascular fluids become hypertonic, (i.e., have an abnormally high serum osmolality). Contributing factors include excessive administration of hypertonic fluids, hyperaldosteronism, Cushing's syndrome, diabetes mellitus, diabetes insipidus, polyuria, profuse sweating, and diarrhea (Huether, 1994). Administering insufficient fluids to clients receiving enteral feedings can also cause this condition.

Hypo-osmolar excess, known as water intoxication, results from the excessive use of hypotonic fluids. This condition is usually seen in persons who drink excessive amounts of water following heat intolerance or strenuous exercise or those undergoing an excessive number of tap water enemas. Water intoxication causes an abnormally low serum osmolality, resulting in polyuria or oliguria, edema, twitching, headache, hyperirritability, disorientation, and possibly coma.

Sodium depletion can cause water intoxication as well. Hypertonic fluids are administered to clients experiencing sodium depletion. The administration of hypertonic saline requires close observation of the client and is performed for a limited time only. Metheny (1990), a respected fluid and electrolyte expert, recommends that hypertonic saline be administered only in intensive care units (ICUs). It is administered slowly and with constant monitoring of the client's blood pressure, central venous pressure, lung sounds, and serum sodium level (Metheny, 1990). The nurse needs to watch for signs of developing fluid overload that occurs as the fluid shifts out of the intracellular space into the extracellular space to dilute the hypertonic solution. To prevent fluid overload, the client usually receives a loop diuretic. It is important to monitor the sodium levels carefully because an increase greater than 2 mEq/L per hour can damage the cells (Bove, 1996).

Sodium depletion with resulting hyponatremic encephalopathy is a life-threatening disorder that occurs most often in young women, following the overuse of 5% dextrose in water (D5W). Typically, these clients receive D5W following a simple surgical procedure. Hyponatremia then develops as intravascular sodium becomes diluted. Researchers believe that women of childbearing age are more at risk for this disorder due to higher levels of estrogen. Estrogen stimulates the release of antidiuretic hormone (ADH), which impedes the brain's ability to adapt to the swelling (Metheny, 1997). Clinical manifestations include nausea following the infusion of

⌘

TABLE 7-1

CLASSIFICATION OF FLUIDS BY TONICITY

	Isotonic	Hypotonic	Hypertonic
Fluids	D5W, 0.9% NS, RL	0.45% NS, 0.20% NS, 0.33% NS, D2.5W	D5RL, D5NS, D5½NS, D5¼NS, D10W, D50W
Osmolarity	275–295 mOsm/L	< 275 mOsm/L	> 295 mOsm/L
Fluid compartment effect	Infused fluid initially stays in the intravascular space	Infused fluid shifts from the intravascular space to the intracellular space	Solutes in the infused fluids pull fluids from the intracellular space into the intravascular space
Indications	Intravascular dehydration	Cellular dehydration	Intravascular dehydration with intracellular or interstitial overload

NOTE: D5W = 5% dextrose in water; NS = normal saline; RL = Ringer's lactate; D5RL = 5% dextrose in Ringer's lactate; D5NS = 5% dextrose in normal saline.

D5W, decreased urine output, positive fluid intake to output, hyponatremia, vomiting, headache, and lethargy. If left untreated, the client will develop seizures, become comatose, and die. The best treatment for hyponatremic encephalopathy is prevention. Clients returning from surgery should receive isotonic or slightly hypertonic saline fluid replacement such as normal saline (NS), Ringer's lactate (RL), 5% dextrose in half normal saline (D5½NS) or 5% dextrose in Ringer's lactate (D5RL). Any order for D5W or 0.45% NS following surgery should be questioned. The nurse must monitor the client's intake and output and electrolyte levels and monitor for the signs and symptoms of hyponatremia (Table 7-1).

CASE STUDY: HYPOVOLEMIA RELATED TO THIRD-SPACING OF FLUIDS

A 72-year-old man was admitted with a fractured left hip. He underwent open reduction internal fixation of the left hip. His vital signs were blood pressure, 110/52 mm Hg; pulse, 92 beats/min; respiration, 28 breaths/min; and temperature, 100.4°F. He currently complains of shortness of breath. His respirations are moist and labored. Anasarca is present and he has a positive intake to output. His urine is caramel colored and the output via the indwelling catheter is 100 mL for the last 5 hours. He is receiving D5½NS with 30 mEq/KCL at 75 mL/h. His abdomen is distended with hypoactive bowel sounds. His laboratory and arterial blood gas (ABG) values are as follows:

SMA 7		ABG	
Glucose	126 mg/dL	pH	7.42
Sodium (Na^+)	134 mEq/dL	PaO_2	82 mm Hg
Potassium (K^+)	3.4 mEq/dL	$PaCO_2$	36 mm Hg
Carbon dioxide (CO_2)	25 mEq/dL	Bicarbonate (HCO_3^-)	24 mEq/L
Chloride (Cl^-)	98 mEq/dL	O_2 saturation	97% on 3 L/min via nasal cannula
BUN	24 mg/dL	Base excess	0.0
Creatinine	0.7 mg/dL		

The nurse must determine whether this client is experiencing fluid overload, as suggested by the presence of gross anasarca or relative hypovolemia related to third-spacing of fluids. The first thing the nurse should do is calculate this client's serum osmolality, using the formula

$$2(134) + 24/2.4 + 126/18 = 268 + 10 + 7 = 285 \text{ mOsm/L}$$

This client's serum osmolality is normal. Since this client has recently undergone surgery, is elderly, has anasarca including abdominal distention, and has normal serum osmolality, the nurse should suspect hypovolemia related to third-spacing of fluids. The client's wife further confirms this when she states that blisters began to form on his arms late yesterday after the surgery. The client's BUN and creatinine levels are normal, however, the output is much less than the intake. Renal insufficiency has not yet occurred, but since the urine output is only 20 mL/h, it is likely that the BUN and creatinine levels may be elevated when next measured.

Treatment of this client consists of administering a hypertonic saline solution with added potassium, since both the sodium and potassium levels are slightly low. The client needs the hypertonic solution to help pull the fluids out of the intracellular and interstitial tissues back into the intravascular space. Albumin may be indicated to help maintain fluid in the intravascular space. The physician should change the intravenous order to D5NS with 30 mEq KCl/L to raise the low sodium and potassium levels. D5½NS is hypertonic with an osmolarity of 447 mOsm/L; however, the D5NS is more hypertonic with an osmolarity of 560 mOsm/L. Since the client's sodium concentration is already low before the intravascular fluid is diluted and he is extremely edematous, the physician decides that

D5NS is the appropriate fluid for this client. D5RL is not appropriate because the client has decreased renal function and would be unable to excrete the bicarbonate that results from the metabolism of the lactate in the solution.

Anatomy and Physiology of the Kidneys

The kidneys are two small, lima bean–shaped organs that lie on each side of the abdomen between the twelfth thoracic and third lumbar vertebrae. The right kidney lies a little lower than the left one because the liver pushes it down. The kidney is made up of the renal capsule; the renal cortex, medulla, and sinus; the nephron; the renal corpuscles; the renal tubules; the collecting duct; and the ureters.

The renal capsule is a tough fibrous coat that encapsulates the kidney. Surrounding this capsule is a mass of fat. This fat and the renal capsule protect the kidney structures from traumatic damage. Within the renal capsule are the renal cortex, the renal medulla, and the renal sinus. The renal cortex is the outer section of the interior of the renal capsule. It is pale and has a granular surface. The nephrons lie within this section. The renal medulla is the center section and is commonly called the renal pyramids. The pyramids within this section are striated matter with the bases facing the cortex and the apexes facing the center of the kidney. Portions of the nephron and the renal tubules lie in these spaces. The renal sinus is the interior section, a cavity filled with blood vessels, which is connected to a notch in the kidney called the hilum.

The nephrons are the functional units of the kidney. Each kidney contains approximately 1 million nephrons (Bartucci, 1995). The nephrons are involved in urine formation. They contain the renal corpuscle, renal tubules, and the collecting duct. The renal corpuscles contain the glomerulus and Bowman's capsule. The renal tubules consist of the proximal convoluted tubule, the loop of Henle, and the distal convoluted tubule. The collecting duct is located within the nephron.

The ureters are extensions of the renal pelvis at the hilum and connect the kidney to the bladder. The ureters use peristaltic smooth muscle action that is activated by the sympathetic nervous system. There is a ureterovesical junction within the ureters that prevents the reflux of urine back into the kidneys.

As blood passes through the capillary bed of the glomerulus, plasma filtration occurs. The kidney receives approximately 20% of the cardiac output, approximately 1200 mL/min of blood flow. This filtration process is called ultrafiltration. The volume of glomerular filtrate approximates 180 mL/day, and 99% of it is reabsorbed by the kidney. The glomerular filtration rate (GFR) is the measurement of this process; the average adult GFR is 125 mL/hr (Bartucci, 1995).

When the filtered blood enters the Bowman's capsule of the glomeruli, primitive urine is formed. As this ultrafiltrate passes through the rest of the nephron, reabsorption and secretion occur to produce the urine that we excrete. The proximal convoluted tubule reabsorbs most of the filtered water and electrolytes. The loop of Henle reabsorbs sodium. The distal convoluted tubule and collecting duct form the urine, which is passed into the ureters. The ureters transport the urine to the bladder by peristaltic waves of smooth muscle.

The bladder collects the urine until it has a volume of 150–300 mL of fluid. Then the urge to urinate occurs. The bladder has the capacity to hold substantially more than 300 mL of fluid. During urination, the bladder is completely emptied of urine. Normal urine output is approximately 1500 mL/day.

Fluid Regulation

Decreased blood volume or increased serum osmolality stimulates the release of ADH (antidiuretic hormone). The kidneys reabsorb water and decrease the loss of water from urination, which increases the circulating volume of water and sodium and inhibits the production of ADH. As arterial blood pressure drops, renal perfusion decreases. Less water and sodium are filtered by the kidneys, and renin, angiotensin I and II, and aldosterone are released, resulting in less sodium and water excretion (Fig. 7-3).

Blood Pressure Regulation and Erythrocyte Production
The nephrons of the kidneys regulate blood pressure by secreting renin in response to hypotension, sodium depletion, or renal nerve stimulation. Renin is converted to angiotensin I and II, which are potent vasoconstrictors. In addition to this process, the nephrons secrete erythropoietin in response to decreased oxygen delivery to the cells of the kidney. Erythropoietin stimulates the bone marrow to produce erythrocytes (red blood cells, RBCs).

The kidneys produce prostaglandin. Prostaglandin is promoted by the presence of angiotensin II, bradykinin, ADH, sympathetic nervous system stimulation, and renal ischemia (Bartucci, 1995). Circulating prostaglandins use vasodilation to increase renal blood flow and promote sodium excretion by the kidneys. The kidneys also metabolize vitamin D, which controls calcium and phosphate metabolism.

The kidneys are vital to our survival. Death inevitably follows within 2–3 weeks if the kidneys fail without intervention to resolve the condition. Therefore, it is important to protect and maintain a functional urinary system. Renal disorders are classified as infectious, immunological, obstructive, and neurological. All of these disorders decrease the renal system's ability to regulate fluid volume and excrete metabolic wastes.

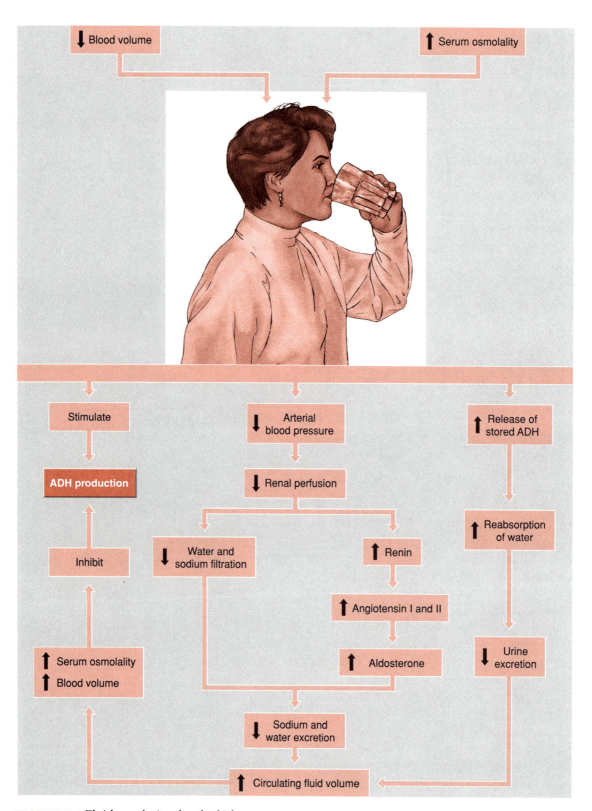

FIGURE 7-3 Fluid regulation by the kidneys.

ASSESSMENT OF THE URINARY SYSTEM

The nurse must take a thorough health history and perform a complete physical examination of a client who may have a urinary system dysfunction. There are a number of noninvasive and invasive diagnostic procedures that can be used to detect urological problems. By using these, the health care providers can provide early diagnosis and intervention.

Health History

The nurse assesses the client's usual voiding pattern. Does the client urinate frequently in relatively small amounts or hold urine for a long period of time? It is important to explore how often and how much urine is produced. Sometimes clients develop changes so slowly that they may not recognize the abnormality of their condition. Evidence of difficulty in starting or maintaining a stream of urine is one sign of urinary difficulty that tends to have an insidious onset. Changes in the voiding pattern such as frequency or nocturia could be a sign of an urinary disorder. Asking about frequency, urgency, burning, or incontinence is also important. Urine characteristics are assessed by asking about its color, odor, and whether or not it is cloudy or clear.

It is important to elicit a history of urinary tract disease, surgery, trauma, or renal disease. Conditions such as gout, diabetes mellitus, connective tissue disorders, recent streptococcal upper respiratory infections, and hypertension adversely affect the kidneys.

The client's social and personal histories are also pertinent. The nurse needs to assess for occupational exposures to chemicals or radiation. The client's use of diuretics, antibiotics, narcotics, nephrotoxins, and cholinergics is pertinent, as is water intake, calcium intake, and mineral content. Smoking can cause bladder irritation and may lead to bladder cancer. The client's exercise regimen and fluid intake patterns are also significant.

Objective Data

The structure of the genital system should be assessed for surgically created urinary tract diversions. The nurse should assess urine color, odor, and clarity. The client's abdomen should be palpated for bladder distention. As people age, blood flow to the kidneys decreases. This affects the GFR and the body's ability to dilute or concentrate urine. It is important to assess for clinical manifestations of acidosis, because aging affects the body's ability to excrete the acid load. The client's blood pressure may fluctuate as the body attempts to improve renal perfusion.

Diagnostic Studies

When diagnostic studies are performed to detect urinary disease, general nursing responsibilities include ensuring that the client is hydrated and receives correct nourishment between studies, explaining the procedures, and monitoring for adverse effects. Monitoring the results and reporting abnormalities to the physician are very important; early detection and intervention are the best way to reduce kidney damage arising from a urinary system disorder.

Urinalysis A urinalysis is the most common test performed to detect urinary system disorders. It is best to collect the first voided urine of the day as a clean-catch or midstream specimen. To accomplish this, the urethral meatus is cleaned with a soap and water solution, and the client is instructed to begin voiding and then catch the urine midstream in a sterile specimen cup. This is done to limit bacterial cross-contamination from the structures surrounding the urethra. Catheterization for a urine specimen may be done, but this is not a routine method because of the risk of contaminating the urinary system with environmental pathogens.

Once the urine specimen is obtained, it should be examined within 1 hour or refrigerated, as room temperature causes bacteria to multiply rapidly, RBCs to hemolyze, casts to disintegrate, and the urine to become alkaline. Composite samples can be kept for 2–24 hours. When these are done, the urine is collected in a large jug that either has an added preservative or is placed on ice. These samples are used to measure electrolytes, glucose, protein, 17-ketosteroids, catecholamines, and creatinine. For a 24-hour creatinine clearance, serum creatinine is measured within the 24-hour time frame. In this procedure the nurse disposes of the first voided specimen and documents the time as the beginning of the test. The subsequent specimens are collected in the container. If a urine specimen is missed, the test can still be performed, but the nurse should notify the laboratory and follow their instructions.

Intravenous Pyelogram (IVP) An IVP is a radiological examination done to visualize the urinary tract using a radiopaque dye. Clients are often allergic to this dye and must be assessed for allergies to iodine, seafood, and radiopaque dyes. If the client is allergic to any of these, the test is usually not performed. IVP is also contraindicated for clients with decreased renal function. There is no preparation for this test, but some departments prefer that the client receive nothing by mouth 8 hours prior to the examination.

Retrograde Pyelography Retrograde pyelography, another commonly used test, examines the same structures as the IVP. The urologist uses cystoscopy to visualize the ureteral orifice in the bladder. An injection dye is instilled into a urethral catheter, and then x-rays are taken. The procedure is done under local or general anesthesia and requires informed consent. Possible complications include infection and the effects of anesthesia.

Renal Angiography Renal angiography is used to visualize the renal blood vessels. It involves the use of an arterial catheter inserted into the femoral artery, and a dye is instilled into the catheter. The structures are then visualized using radiographic or computerization techniques. Using digital technology, the structures can be visualized on a computer terminal. The procedure requires informed consent. The client must be given nothing by mouth for 6–8 hours prior to the examination, and a mild preprocedure sedative may be ordered. Possible complications include thrombus and embolus formation, local inflammation, and hematoma. When the client returns from this procedure, the nurse is responsible for assessing for hematoma formation at the insertion site, applying pressure to the site if a hematoma occurs, and frequently assessing vital signs and peripheral circulation, including pulses and capillary refill. The client is generally kept on bed rest for approximately 6 hours to prevent trauma to the femoral artery.

Renal Radionuclide Imaging Renal radionuclide imaging is generally done to evaluate the anatomical structures, functions, and perfusion of the kidneys. The radioisotope is injected into an intravenous line, and radiation detector probes are placed over the kidneys. This test reveals differences between the two kidneys. No dietary or activity restrictions are necessary.

Renal Biopsy A renal biopsy is performed to detect the presence of malignancy. There are a number of absolute contraindications and some relative contraindications. The *absolute contraindications* include bleeding disorders, the presence of only one kidney, and uncontrolled hypertension. The *relative contraindications* include suspected renal infection, hydronephrons, and possible vascular lesions. Possible complications include hemorrhage, hematoma, and infection. The client must give informed consent. A complete blood count (CBC), hemoglobin, hematocrit, prothrombin time (PT), activated partial thromboplastin time (PTT), and bleeding times need to be assessed prior to the biopsy. The biopsy is performed with either computed tomography (CT) or ultrasound guidance. Postprocedure, the client should remain prone for 30–60 minutes and kept on bed rest for 3–4 hours. The client's vital signs should be checked frequently, and the site should be assessed for signs of bleeding. Urinalysis and hematuria assessments need to be done. The client should not lift anything heavier than 5 lbs for 1 week. Flank pain should be reported to the physician.

Cystoscopy Cystoscopy is used to inspect the bladder, insert urethral catheters, remove calculi, obtain biopsies, and treat bleeding. Preprocedure sedation and local or general anesthesia are administered. The client must give informed consent. The client needs to be well hydrated to keep urine flowing. Expected complications include pain from bladder spasms, burning on urination, hematuria (but not frank bleeding), and urinary frequency. Other possible complications include urinary retention, urinary tract hemorrhage, bladder infection, and perforation of the bladder. The nurse must assess for signs of bleeding, prevent postural hypotension through the adequate hydration, and make the client comfortable. Analgesics, sitz baths, and local heat may be indicated for pain control.

Cystogram   A cystogram outlines and visualizes the bladder and evaluates the ureterovesical valves for reflux. A radiopaque dye is instilled into the bladder through a urethral catheter or a cystoscope. This examination detects diverticula, calculi, and tumors. A voiding cystogram is performed to study the bladder opening and the urethra.

Cystometrogram   A cystometrogram evaluates bladder tone. It involves a catheter inserted into the bladder, a liter of water, and a cystometer. The pressure is measured by the cystometer; then fluid is instilled into the bladder until the client feels an urge to urinate, and pressure is measured again. After voiding, the amount of residual urine is determined.

Portable ultrasonic bladder scan is a noninvasive technique used to assess for the presence of urinary retention.

Portable Bladder Scan   A portable bladder scan is performed to assess for the presence of postvoiding residual urine (Wagner & Schmid, 1997). This ultrasonic device, housed on the nursing unit, provides a noninvasive technique for evaluating urinary retention. It is believed that the portable bladder scan lowers the incidence of nosocomial urinary tract infections (UTIs) and decreases the number of catheterizations required to assess for urinary retention (Wagner & Schmid, 1997) (Fig. 7-4).

FIGURE 7-4

⬛

Bladder Scan BVI 2500+. (NOTE: From Diagnostic Ultrasound Corporation, San Diego, CA. Reprinted with permission.)

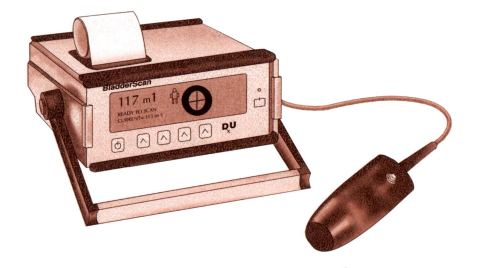

UROLOGICAL DISORDERS

Urological disorders are classified as infectious, immunological, obstructive, and neurological in nature. Each classification has specific manifestations and sequelae that the nurse must recognize in order to intervene promptly to prevent damage to the kidneys.

Infectious Disorders

Urinary Tract Infections (UTIs) UTIs are the second most common bacterial disease. *Escherichia coli, Klebsiella aerobacter, Proteus mirabilis, Enterobacter cloacae, Pseudomonas aeruginosa, Staphylococcus saprophyticus,* and *Streptococcus pyogenes* are the most common etiological pathogens. Upper UTIs involve the kidneys (pyelonephritis) and ureters. Lower UTIs involve the bladder (cystitis) and urethra (urethritis). Cystitis is commonly called a bladder infection, and pyelonephritis is called a kidney infection.

The clinical manifestations of a UTI include fever, pain or burning on urination, frequency, urgency, incontinence, cloudy urine, and hematuria. The urine turns dark and has a strong odor. The client may complain of flank pain or tenderness over the kidneys or bladder. The presence of a UTI is detected when urinalysis shows increased white blood cells (WBCs). Urine culture and sensitivity are performed, and a Gram stain is done. Kidney infections show an antibody-coated bacteria in the urine. IVP is contraindicated to prevent spread of the infection. The infection is generally treated with a sulfonamide such as sulfamethoxazole/trimethoprim (Bactrim). Clients who are allergic to sulfa drugs are given ciprofloxacin (Cipro). Phenazopyridine hydrochloride (Pyridium) is often used to treat the symptom of burning on urination.

Clinical manifestations of urinary tract infections (UTIs) include burning on urination, frequency, urgency, cloudy urine, hematuria, and incontinence.

Clients taking a sulfonamide or ciprofloxacin (Cipro) need to be aware that direct sunlight causes a sensitivity reaction that results in a severe rash. The client should be instructed to keep well hydrated to avoid crystallization in the kidneys. Clients receiving ciprofloxacin (Cipro) need to avoid calcium-containing foods, antacids, and sodium bicarbonate as these decrease absorption of the drug. Clients receiving phenazopyridine hydrochloride (Pyridium) must be warned that the medication will turn their urine a bright red-orange color.

Clients receiving sulfonamide or ciprofloxacin (Cipro) need to be aware that direct sunlight can cause a severe rash to skin that is exposed to sunlight.

Factors that predispose a person to UTIs include renal scarring from previous infections, urinary retention, neurogenic bladder, and diminished ureteral peristalsis during pregnancy. Because of the shortened urethra and the proximity of the urethra to the rectum, women are predisposed to UTIs. It is important for women to learn to wipe from front to back following urination and defecation. Any artificial entry into the bladder such as an indwelling catheter puts the client at risk for a UTI as well. Immune deficiencies and any disorder that causes retrograde reflux puts the client at risk for developing a UTI.

Nursing interventions for these clients include teaching the client proper hygiene methods, encouraging fluids, and teaching clients to urinate when they feel the urge. The client needs to be taught not to discontinue antibiotics when the symptoms disappear but to complete the full 10–14-day course of treatment. If the client is catheterized, it is important to clean around the meatus several times a day with soap and water. The nurse should monitor for the clinical manifestations of UTI and teach the client to do the same.

CASE STUDY: ELDERLY WOMAN WITH A UTI

An 88-year-old woman with an indwelling urethral catheter lives in an extended care facility. She is being treated with warfarin (Coumadin) for a recent cerebrovascular accident (CVA). Ten days after the catheter was inserted the client's urine is cloudy and concentrated with a strong odor.

The nurse should immediately assess for other manifestations of a UTI by obtaining an order for a urinalysis with culture and sensitivity and possibly an order for antibiotics. The nurse should also encourage fluids.

The client is started on trimethoprim/sulfamethoxazol (Bactrim), one tablet twice daily for 7 days. Five days later, the nurse finds the client in the bathroom with blood on the floor; the water in the toilet is bright red.

The nurse should assist the client back to bed and take her vital signs. Her perineal area must be examined to determine the origin of bleeding. The nurse should assess for abdominal pain, tenderness, or rigidity, and obtain a recent urinary elimination history including 24-hour intake and output, frequency of urination, and any manifestations of a UTI. The findings should be reported to the physician. Likely causes for the bleeding include insufficient response to the antibiotic therapy, drug interaction between the trimethoprim/sulfamethoxazol (Bactrim) and the warfarin (Coumadin), possibly causing hypothrombinemia, or prolonged anticoagulation times due to the warfarin (Coumadin).

Culture and sensitivity analyses determine that the client has not been responding to the therapy. The client is placed on ciprofloxacin (Cipro) and begins to improve. The daughter asks how her mother could prevent a UTI from developing.

The nurse should instruct the client and her daughter on proper hygiene methods. This includes wearing 100% cotton panties and drinking more fluids. Both women need to understand the special risk women have of developing a UTI because of their anatomical structure.

Immunological Disorders

Immunological disorders of the kidney affect the glomeruli. They occur as the result of circulating antibodies that damage the glomerular basement membrane. The accumulation of antigen, antibody, and complement in the glomeruli causes injury and the injury leads to an inflammatory process. The client often presents with a recent history of treatment with nephrotoxic drugs, immunizations, and microbial or viral infections. Immunological disorders such as systemic lupus erythematosus (SLE) and scleroderma also contribute to kidney disorders. Types of immunological kidney disorders include acute poststreptococcal glomerulonephritis, Goodpasture's syndrome, rapid progressive glomerulonephritis, and chronic glomerulonephritis.

Poststreptococcal Glomerulonephritis
Acute poststreptococcal glomerulonephritis can occur following a streptococcal respiratory infection. For this reason, it is essential to treat streptococcal infections promptly and to take a full course of antibiotics. The clinical manifestations of this type of glomerulonephritis include hematuria, dark-colored urine, urinary excretion of WBC, and granular casts. Proteinuria and elevated BUN and creatinine levels are also common manifestations.

Treatment includes bed rest, sodium and fluid restriction, and a low-protein diet to decrease stress on the kidneys. The dietary intake of protein is generally reduced to 0.5–1 g/kg/day. Loop diuretics may be required to lower circulating fluid volume. Antihypertensive agents may be used to lower blood pressure and decrease the blood volume filtered by the kidneys.

Nephrotic Syndrome
Nephrotic syndrome can develop from a number of diseases, including chronic glomerulonephritis, diabetes mellitus, amyloidosis of the kidney, SLE, and renal vein thrombosis. The clinical manifestations are edema including periorbital edema, malaise, headache, irritability, fatigue, massive proteinuria, hyperlipidemia, hypoalbuminemia, skeletal abnormalities, and hypercoagulability. Loop diuretics control the edema, and corticosteroids treat the underlying conditions and reduce the proteinuria. Antineoplastic and immunosuppressant agents also may be used. **Nursing interventions** include weighing the client daily, measuring intake and output accurately, and preventing skin breakdown, bleeding, and infections. The nurse should measure the abdominal girth and report any enlargement. The client loses a lot of protein; therefore, a high-protein, low-sodium diet should be given. The diet should be low in cholesterol and triglycerides as well. Bed rest is recommended to promote diuresis and reduce edema.

Clients with nephrotic syndrome often complain of a loss of appetite and a bad taste in the mouth. This can be relieved with good oral hygiene three times a day and at bedtime.

Obstructive Disorders

Renal calculi and structural deformities can obstruct urine flow. Renal calculi are stones that form from body substances. Abnormal amounts of these substances or external conditions can contribute to the formation of stones. Tissue deformities, such as scar formation and the resultant stricture, can obstruct the flow of urine. Benign prostatic hypertrophy (BPH) causes the prostate to grow and obstruct the bladder outlet. Certain drugs and conditions that stimulate the sympathetic pathway of the autonomic nervous system cause sphincter constriction that blocks the flow of urine from the bladder. In each of these conditions, the kidneys produce normal urine flow, but because of an obstruction, the urine is not eliminated effectively. This can result in backflow and damage to the urinary system.

Renal Calculi Metabolic conditions such as increased urine levels of calcium, oxaluric acid, citric acid, and uric acid can contribute to the formation of renal calculi. People who live in warm climates are often at risk for the development of renal calculi because warm weather contributes to increased fluid loss, resulting in low urine volume and increased solute concentration in the urine. A family history of gout, cystinuria, renal acidosis, or stone formation is a risk factor for the development of renal calculi. Large amounts of protein in the diet increase uric acid secretion and contribute to the development of renal calculi. Excessive amounts of tea, fruit juices, or foods that contain oxalate and excessive amounts of calcium can lead to the development of renal calculi. A sedentary life style and immobility are also contributing factors.

Several types of renal calculi can form, including calcium oxalate, calcium phosphate, struvite, uric acid, and cystine stones. Each type has its own characteristics and precipitating factors. Both calcium oxalate and calcium phosphate stones are related to the intake of dietary calcium. Calcium stones account for approximately 50% of all renal calculi. Clients experiencing a calcium stone of either composition need to limit dietary calcium intake and follow an **acid ash diet** to acidify their urine. Foods that acidify urine include meats, whole grains, eggs, cranberries, prunes, and plums. Foods high in calcium include milk, cheese, dairy products, beans (except green beans), lentils, fish with fine bones, dried fruits, nuts, and chocolate. Clients experiencing calcium oxalate stones need to limit the oxalate in their diets. Foods that are high in oxalate include spinach, beets, rhubarb, asparagus, cabbage, tomatoes, beets, celery, beans, chocolate, nuts, parsley, and tea. Clients with either type of stone need to increase their fluid intake.

Cholestyramine (Questran) may be ordered for the treatment of oxalate stones. This antilipidemic drug binds with oxalate so that the oxalate is not absorbed by the body. Cholestyramine (Questran) is a difficult drug for clients to tolerate. They frequently complain of headaches, joint pain, and gastrointestinal (GI) distress. The drug comes in a powder form and must be mixed with a beverage or applesauce; it should be taken before meals to improve absorption. It should not be abruptly discontinued.

Both uric acid and cystine stones occur in acidic urine; therefore, the client needs to eat an **alkaline ash diet**. Foods that lower urine acidity include milk, green vegetables, and fruits, except cranberries, prunes, and plums. Clients with uric acid stones must decrease their intake of foods containing purine. These are organ meats, seafood, cured meats such as

Acid ash diet consists of foods that acidify the urine, such as meats, whole grains, eggs, cranberries, prunes, and plums.

An **alkali ash diet** consists of foods that alkalyze urine, such as milk, green vegetables, and all fruits except cranberries, prunes, and plums.

ham and bacon, and luncheon meats. Allopurinol (Zyloprim) may be ordered to lower the client's serum uric acid concentration.

Cystine stones are caused by an autosomal recessive defect. These stones are treated by increasing fluid intake and maintaining an alkaline urine. Sodium bicarbonate may be given to maintain an alkaline urine. α-Penicillamine helps to prevent cystine crystallization in the urine.

Struvite stones can occur as a result of UTI. These are often very large kidney stones (staghorn calculi). These stones commonly appear in the bladder around Foley catheters that have been in place for an extended period of time. At times a stone becomes so large that it must be removed surgically from the bladder. Clients should follow an acid ash diet. Antibiotics are given to treat the UTI that caused the stone (Table 7-2).

TABLE 7-2
TYPES OF URINARY TRACT CALCULI

Type	Characteristics	Causative Factors	Treatment Diet	Treatment
Calcium oxalate	Small, often get trapped in the ureters. Seen more frequently in men	High calcium and oxalate diets	Acid ash (helps prevent calcium stone formation but not necessarily oxalate stones)	Increase hydration; administer diuretics and cholestyramine (Questran); and decrease dietary calcium and oxalates
Calcium phosphate	Generally mixed stones with struvite or oxalate	Alkaline urine and primary hyperparathyroidism	Acid ash	Increase hydration; treat underlying causes; decrease calcium in diet
Uric acid	Seen predominantly in men	Gout, acid urine, and familial history	Alkaline ash	Allopurinol (Zyloprim); decrease purines in diet
Cystine	Autosomal recessive	Defective absorption of cystine in the gastrointestinal tract, acid urine	Alkaline ash	Increase hydration; administer sodium bicarbonate and α-penicillamine
Struvite	Large, horny stones that often form around Foley catheters. More common in women	Urinary tract infection and alkaline urine	Acid ash	Antibiotics, surgical removal of stone

Treatment for any type of renal calculi includes encouraging the client to increase fluid intake. If the stone is lodged in a ureter, it will cause a great deal of pain; therefore, pain control is an important aspect of care. Narcotics are often given to treat the pain. The client should be encouraged to ambulate to improve peristalsis. (This is important especially for the client who has a stone lodged in the ureter.) The nurse should carefully monitor intake and output. All urine should be strained to capture any stones passed from the urinary tract. The nurse should monitor for hematuria and report any obvious bleeding to the physician.

Surgery may be necessary to remove or to facilitate removal of a stone if the stone is too large to pass through the urinary tract. Stones associated with bacteriuria, such as struvite stones, are generally removed surgically, as are stones that impair renal function or cause persistent pain.

Lithotripsy and lithotomy are the surgical procedures most commonly used. The client is anesthetized with either general or spinal anesthesia before any of these procedures. Lithotripsy techniques include percutaneous ultrasonic lithotripsy, electrohydraulic lithotripsy, laser lithotripsy, and extracorporeal shock-wave lithotripsy. Percutaneous ultrasonic lithotripsy (Fig. 7-5) involves using an endoscope and placing an ultrasonic probe on the renal pelvis. The scope is inserted through a small opening made in the flank. The probe emits ultrasonic waves that break the stone into sandlike particles. The particles are then flushed with continuous normal saline and removed with suction. Electrohydraulic lithotripsy involves placing a probe directly on the stone to crush it. Laser lithotripsy is similar to electrohydraulic lithotripsy except that laser waves are used to break up the stone.

FIGURE 7-5

⬛

Percutaneous ultrasonic lithotripsy.

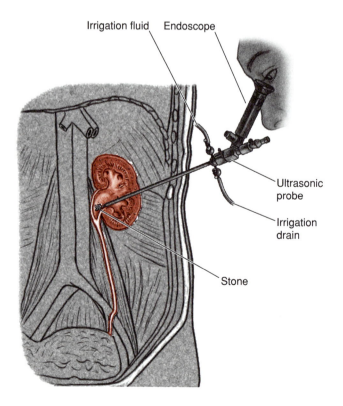

Extracorporeal shock-wave lithotripsy is the most commonly used technique. For this noninvasive procedure, the client is first anesthetized with either spinal or general anesthesia and then immersed in a water bath where shock waves are used to fragment the stone. With some of the newer technology, immersion and anesthesia are unnecessary because less power is used (Bates & Lewis, 1996). Clients generally require a mild sedative (Fig. 7-6).

All types of lithotripsy require the client's informed consent. Because the kidneys are very vascular structures, there is a risk of postprocedure bleeding. Therefore, the nurse should assess the client's vital signs often. The client may experience hematuria, but it should subside in 2–3 days. Clients who have undergone a lithotripsy procedure generally complain of mild-to-moderate achy pain and tenderness in the flank area. Mild analgesics are usually ordered to provide comfort. The client should ambulate frequently and increase fluid intake to facilitate removal of any stone fragments. The client's intake and output must be carefully monitored. The client must be instructed to report any signs of infection, frank bleeding, and increased pain.

Lithotomy involves making an incision and removing the stone from the renal pelvis or ureter. It is performed most commonly when the lithotripsy procedure has been unsuccessful. The care of the client after this surgery is similar to the care of the client following a nephrectomy (discussed below). Recovery time, however, is much shorter. The client does not undergo the severe shifts in electrolytes as experienced after nephrectomy. The goals of client care postoperatively are to relieve pain, prevent atelectasis, ensure adequate protein and calorie intake for healing, and restore adequate urinary elimination.

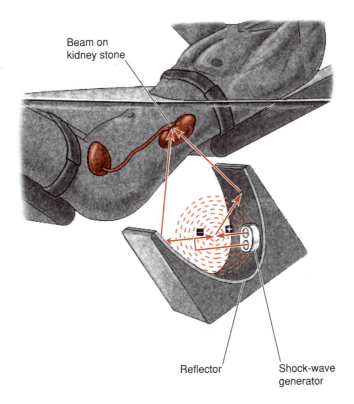

Beam on kidney stone

Reflector

Shock-wave generator

FIGURE 7-6

Extracorporeal shock-wave lithotripsy.

Tumors Tumors may also obstruct urinary flow. Bladder cancer is the most common urinary tract malignancy. The two etiological factors associated with the development of bladder cancer are chronic inflammation of the bladder and the presence of carcinogens in the urine. Smoking is a major risk factor for bladder cancer. Surgery is commonly required to treat bladder cancer. In a cystectomy, the bladder is removed, and a urinary diversion is created. The two most common types of urinary diversions are ileal conduits and continent urinary diversion. Chemotherapy or radiation therapy is used in addition to the surgery.

An ileal conduit procedure involves using part of the ileum to form a pouch. The ureters are attached to the pouch, and part of the ileum pouch is brought to the skin, creating a stoma. Since the diversion constantly drains urine, a continuous urine drainage device must be applied. A continent urinary diversion involves constructing valves into a pouch formed from the ileum. This device, often called a Koch's pouch, must be catheterized intermittently (Fig. 7-7).

The stomas created by these procedures and the surrounding skin must be watched and protected (Table 7-3). Following surgery, the stoma should be a bright pink-red color. A dark red stoma indicates ischemia, and a pale stoma or one that blanches when touched indicates compromised circulation. As the stoma heals, it should turn a healthy pink color. After surgery the client will have nephrostomy stents and tubes in place. It is extremely important for the nurse to maintain the patency of the tubes. The kidney has the capacity to store only 3–5 mL of fluid. If the tubing becomes kinked, the kidney can be irreparably damaged by urine reflux.

FIGURE 7-7 Ileal conduit and continent urinary diversion.

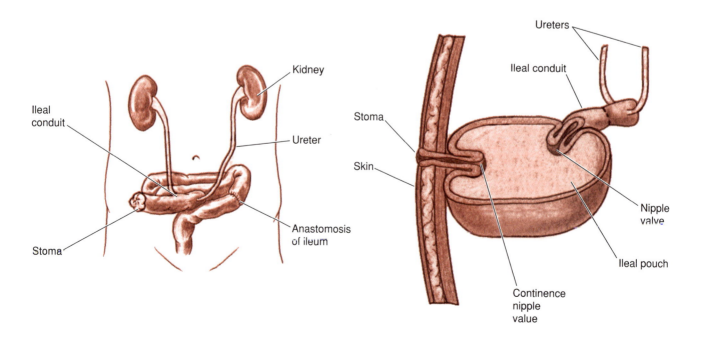

⌖

TABLE 7-3
CARE OF A URINARY STOMA

Supplies:

Clean, disposable pouch
4 × 4 gauze
Skin barrier (liquid or ring)
Stoma guide
Adhesive solvent
Stoma paste
Clean gloves
Washcloth
Soap
Water

Procedure:

1. Wash hands and put on gloves.
2. Remove the pouch, using warm water or adhesive remover if necessary.
3. Assess the stoma and the surrounding skin.
4. Place a rolled up 4 × 4 gauze into the stoma to prevent urine leakage.
5. Gently clean the stoma and the surrounding skin with soap and water; then rinse and pat or air dry.
6. Cut the bag opening, using the stoma guide to measure and determine the correct size for the stoma.
7. Apply the skin barrier and allow it to dry.
8. Apply a ring of stoma paste to the bag and around the stoma.
9. Attach the bag allowing an opening no more than 1–2 mm wider than the stoma. Be sure there are no creases or wrinkles where the bag connects to the skin.
10. Connect the bag to the urine collection device.

The client's vital signs should be monitored carefully and intake and output measured accurately. The nurse must monitor the client's electrolytes, BUN, creatinine levels, and renal function. The nurse must also observe for signs of acid–base imbalance as well. Abnormal test results may occur as the result of the reabsorption of electrolytes from the reservoirs created by the ileum. The color and character of the urine should also be monitored. Bleeding and infection are two complications of this urinary diversion.

The nurse must teach the client about stoma and urinary diversion care. The client should be taught how to irrigate the urinary diversion catheter. Since the intestine is used to construct the stoma, mucous production can block the conduit. The conduit is irrigated using 30–60 mL of normal saline. Clients with continent urinary diversions must be taught how to self-catheterize every 2–4 hours and to report signs of infection to the physician.

Urinary Retention Urinary retention is another problem associated with obstructive urinary tract disorders. This condition may be caused by certain medications, tumors, and neurogenic bladder. Clients with urinary retention are unable to empty the bladder completely. The client may complain of a full feeling in the bladder, bladder distention, or voiding frequently in small amounts. Catheterization is the usual treatment of urinary retention. Intermittent catheterization has been used commonly to diagnosis urinary retention, but with the development of portable ultrasonic scans, catheterization is being used less often for diagnosis. The cholinergic medication bethanechol chloride (Urecholine) is often used to relax the bladder sphincter to promote urination. The nurse needs to review the client's list of medications and determine if they are contributing to the problem. If the client is taking certain anticholinergic medications, including some over-the-counter antihistamines, the nurse should obtain a physician's order to replace these medications with drugs without anticholinergic action.

Nursing measures to promote urination include positioning the client in a normal position for voiding and providing privacy. Some clients report that it is helpful to hear water running or to have their hands in warm water. Nurses can pour warm water over the perineum or use a sitz bath to promote voiding.

Incontinence

Urinary incontinence is the involuntary loss of urine in amounts large enough to be perceived as a problem for the person. It is often thought to be a condition of aging but should not be thought of as inevitable. Most clients who experience incontinence significantly improve with treatment. The clinical manifestations of urinary incontinence are urgency, frequency, retention, and involuntary leakage of urine. Incontinence is frequently caused by temporary conditions such as infection or confusion. Neurogenic bladder, a central nervous system (CNS) dysfunction in which the bladder either fails to store urine or fails to empty urine, is another cause of incontinence. Conditions such as diabetic neuropathy and CVA can lead to the development of a neurogenic bladder.

Urinary incontinence is generally classified as urge incontinence, stress incontinence, or overflow incontinence. *Urge incontinence* is the involuntary release of urine following a short warning of a need to urinate. It is caused by overactivity of the detrusor muscle or uncontrolled contractions of the bladder. Urge incontinence occurs with CNS disorders, urinary system tumors, spinal cord disorders, and bladder outlet obstructions. The condition is treated with vaginal estrogen creams, anticholinergic medications, and imipramine (Tofranil) at night. The client should make an effort to urinate more frequently.

Stress incontinence is the involuntary release of urine during activities that increase the pressure in the intra-abdominal cavity. Coughing, sneezing, and lifting are activities that commonly cause stress incontinence. This type of incontinence is most frequently seen in women and occurs with relaxed musculature. Treatment includes consistently performing pelvic muscle exercises (Kegel exercises), applying vaginal estrogen creams, and losing weight if the client is obese. Kegel exercises strengthen the pubococcygeal muscle. The nurse should teach the female client to urinate and stop the flow of urine midstream. The muscle that stops the flow of urine is the pubococcygeal muscle; thus, the woman contracts that muscle for a few seconds at a time and then releases it. She may also be instructed to contract the muscle, release it, and then immediately contract it again. The third exercise consists of slowly contracting the muscle, holding it for a few seconds, and then slowly releasing the muscle. The last exercise involves bearing down with the muscle. After performing the exercise three times per day for approximately 6 weeks, clients should notice a difference in their ability to hold urine.

Overflow incontinence occurs when retention causes the bladder to become too full and some of the urine is involuntarily released. This is generally caused by a neurogenic bladder or a bladder outlet obstruction. It is treated with catheterization to decompress the bladder. Pharmacological agents such as prazocin (Minipress) and bethanecol chloride (Urecholine) are given to decrease outlet resistance and enhance bladder contraction. Surgery may be required to correct the underlying problem. Some clients have to be catheterized intermittently to resolve the urinary retention.

The elderly often accept incontinence. This is especially true if the clients are confused or unable to tell someone of their need to urinate. Current research has shown that incontinence in the elderly need not be inevitable. In most cases, prompted voiding schedules in which clients are assisted to void every 2–3 hours can reduce incontinent episodes. Other measures such as adult protective devices and water-resistant padding should be used only after trying to solve the problem with prompted voiding schedules. It is not appropriate to insert an indwelling urinary catheter as a solution to urinary incontinence for the convenience of the caregiver.

Catheterization

Urinary catheterization is a major cause of UTIs. The insertion of a catheter should be performed using strict aseptic technique and only when absolutely necessary. Urinary catheterization is generally accomplished using a catheter inserted through the urethra into the bladder, although suprapubic catheterization is also an option. If an indwelling catheter is in place, the system should stay closed as much as possible. The catheter should be irrigated only when necessary to restore or maintain patency. There are eight indications for a catheter: (1) to relieve urinary retention, (2) to decompress the bladder, (3) to facilitate surgical repair, (4) to facilitate tissue healing following surgery, (5) to instill medication into the bladder, (6) to accurately measure urinary output, (7) to measure residual output, and (8) to visualize anatomic structures radiographically (Fig. 7-8).

Intermittent catheterization is an alternative to long-term catheterization with some clients. This involves either the caregiver inserting the catheter using aseptic technique or the client inserting the catheter using

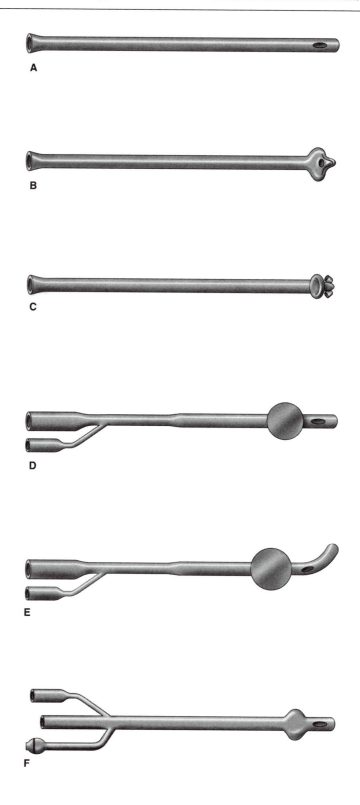

FIGURE 7-8

⬚

Various types of urinary
catheters.

clean technique every 4–6 hours as needed. When trauma has occurred to
the urinary tract catheterization is often necessary until the resulting
edema resolves. Intermittent catheterization is also useful for clients with
neurogenic bladders, who need to be taught to perform self-catheteriza-
tion. The nurse helps the client locate the urethra. Sometimes a mirror can

help women visualize the urethra. The client does not need to wear gloves but should use equipment that has been cleaned with soap and water. The nurse teaches the client to insert the catheter until urine freely returns. The urine is drained, the catheter is removed, and the equipment is cleaned and stored. The client may need to self-catheterize every 4–6 hours or when they feel the need to urinate. The nurse can also teach the client how to palpate the bladder for fullness.

RENAL CELL CARCINOMA

Renal cell carcinoma is the major malignant neoplasm of the kidney. Neoplasms occur most frequently in the epithelium of the proximal convoluted tubules. The clinical manifestations may be inconsistent and insidious. The presentation of symptoms occurs in a triad pattern: hematuria is the most consistent presentation, followed by flank pain and a palpable abdominal mass. These symptoms occur in only approximately 15% of clients. Other clinical manifestations include fever, anemia or polycythemia, and weight loss. Renal tumors produce hormone-like substances that can lead to hypertension, hypercalcemia, and hyperglycemia (Lemone & Burke, 1996).

Renal carcinoma occurs more often in men. Risk factors include family history, gender, smoking, and exposure to cadmium. Cadmium is a metallic element used primarily for plating and in transistors and solar batteries because of its light sensitivity. Persons who work in factories who use this substance should be aware of the risk for renal cell carcinoma. Renal carcinoma is more prevalent after the age of 55.

The malignancy is generally confirmed using renal ultrasonography and CT scan. A renal biopsy is the definitive test for malignancy. Percutaneous needle aspiration is used to obtain a renal biopsy. This is usually performed in the radiology department following an IVP to locate the kidney. Some absolute contraindications for a renal biopsy include: having a single kidney, bleeding disorders, uncontrolled hypertension, and kidney infection. Renal biopsy is an invasive procedure and therefore requires informed consent. Bleeding and coagulation times are assessed prior to the procedure.

Postprocedure care includes applying a pressure dressing to the injection site. The client is kept prone for approximately 30–60 minutes. Bed rest is generally ordered for 12–24 hours. Vital signs should be assessed frequently. The nurse also should assess the client for possible complications: bleeding (including hemorrhage) from the site, hematoma, and infection.

Renal cell carcinoma has a very poor prognosis. Chemotherapy and radiation therapy have not been found to be effective in treating renal carcinoma. Treatment is usually a radical nephrectomy. Radiation is used to help control tumors that are inoperable or metastatic. If chemotherapy is administered, actinomycin D and vincristine are the agents generally used (Bates & Lewis, 1996). When radiation or chemotherapy is used, it is to control tumor growth rather than to cure the client.

Nephrectomy

Renal cell carcinoma, polycystic renal disease, a severely infected kidney, and renal trauma are indications for a partial or radical nephrectomy (Bates & Lewis, 1996). A partial nephrectomy involves removal of the kidney or a portion of the kidney. In a radical nephrectomy, the kidney, the adrenal gland, perirenal fat, upper ureter, and fascia surrounding the kidney are all removed (Lemone & Burke, 1996). A nephrectomy is performed on only one kidney; therefore, if the renal malignancy is bilateral, nephrectomy is not an option for treatment.

Preoperatively, the client should be well hydrated. The nurse must teach the client how the body functions with only one kidney. The client is positioned in a hyperextended, side-lying position during surgery, which causes muscle aches following the procedure (Bates & Lewis, 1996). The client also needs to be informed that there will be postoperative flank pain and told what measures can be taken to relieve the pain. The kidneys are located high in the abdomen; therefore, there is a risk for developing postoperative atelectastasis. To help prevent this, the client should be taught about pulmonary hygiene, which entails turning, coughing, deep breathing, and early ambulation. Incentive spirometry performed every 2 hours is a common intervention used to prevent postoperative atelectastasis.

Postoperative care includes ensuring adequate urine output. Urinary output should be assessed every 1–2 hours. Two priorities of care include ensuring that drainage tubes remain patent and that urine output of at least 30 mL/hr is maintained. The color of the urine should be monitored, and any frank bleeding should be reported to the physician. The presence of mucous in the urine should also be reported. The client's urinary output should be essentially equivalent to the client's intake; severe imbalances should be reported to the physician.

The client will have pain and may be reluctant to ambulate and to perform pulmonary hygiene measures if the pain is severe; therefore, it is very important that the pain be controlled with narcotic analgesics. Renal sufficiency should be monitored to ensure adequacy but also to ensure excretion of the analgesics. The nurse should monitor the client's BUN and creatinine levels. An elevated BUN level indicates protein metabolism and possible dehydration. An elevated creatinine level indicates renal insufficiency.

The client's nutritional status must be monitored. In order for the kidney to heal, the client must have sufficient protein and carbohydrates. If the client's appetite is diminished, high protein supplements should be encouraged. Packaged supplements have been designed specifically for clients with renal disease. The client should receive at least 1.2–2.0 g/kg of body weight in protein per day to counteract the stress that the surgery has placed on the body. If renal failure occurs, protein intake may be restricted. The client should ingest total calories of at least 35–40 kcal/kg of body weight per day.

The client is at risk for developing paralytic ileus as a result of manipulation of the bowel during surgery. Therefore, the client should be monitored for the presence of bowel sounds, abdominal distention, and nausea. Clients with paralytic ileus typically have absent bowel sounds; abdominal distention; nausea; and vomiting of a green, bile-like emesis. As the pressure increases, the client may develop a whispered speech pattern from compression on the diaphragm. Paralytic ileus is best prevented by early ambulation. Treatment consists of withholding oral intake until peristalsis returns. A nasogastric tube is inserted and connected to suction to remove excess gastric secretions. The client should be administered parenteral nutrition until oral intake can be resumed.

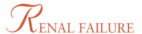RENAL FAILURE

Renal failure, the impairment of kidney function, is classified as either acute or chronic. Acute renal failure is a potentially reversible condition. Chronic renal failure is irreversible and often leads to a complete loss of kidney function. Acute renal failure usually has a rapid onset, whereas chronic renal failure is insidious in nature. Both are potentially life-threatening conditions.

Acute Renal Failure

Acute renal failure has three etiological factors: prerenal, intrarenal, and postrenal. Prerenal factors interfere with perfusion and result in decreasing blood flow and glomerular filtration, ischemia, and oliguria. Examples of these factors include congestive heart failure (CHF), cardiogenic shock, acute vasoconstriction, hemorrhage, burns, septicemia, and hypotension. Intrarenal factors cause damage to the nephrons. Some examples include acute tubular necrosis, endocarditis, diabetes mellitus, malignant hypertension, acute glomerulonephritis, tumors, blood transfusion reactions, hypercalcemia, and nephrotoxins. Postrenal factors include conditions in which mechanical obstruction occurs anywhere from the tubules to the urethra. Examples of mechanical obstruction are renal calculi, BPH, tumors, strictures, blood clots, trauma, and anatomical malformations. Regardless of the etiology, the result of these factors is renal insufficiency.

Oliguric Phase Acute renal failure occurs in three phases. The first phase, the oliguric phase, is caused by a reduction in the GFR. The clinical manifestation of this phase is urine output less than 400 mL/day that lasts for 1–2 weeks. During this phase, the client is at risk for hyponatremia, hyperkalemia, hyperphosphatemia, hypocalcemia, hypermagnesemia, and metabolic acidosis. Clients in the first phase have elevated BUN and creatinine levels. The oliguric phase comes on suddenly, usually occurring within 1–7 days of the causative agent (McCarley & Lewis, 1996). The longer this phase lasts, the poorer the prognosis for the client.

It is important to distinguish prerenal oliguria from intrarenal oliguria. With prerenal oliguria, the client's urine has a high specific gravity and a low sodium concentration (McCarley & Lewis, 1996). Prerenal oliguria can sometimes be reversed by treating the underlying problem. Intrarenal oliguria manifests with a low specific gravity and a high sodium concentration (McCarley & Lewis, 1996).

A urinalysis may show hematuria with a specific gravity and urine osmolality that is equivalent to plasma. This reflects the kidney's inability to concentrate urine as a result of the tubular damage (McCarley & Lewis, 1996). The client is at risk for fluid volume excess during the oliguric phase. The client is also at risk for electrolyte disturbances; therefore, it is necessary to monitor the client's electrolyte levels.

Diuretic Phase The second phase of acute renal failure is the diuretic phase. This phase occurs gradually. Clients have a urine output of 3–5 L/day as a result of the partially regenerated tubules' inability to concentrate urine. The duration of this phase is 2–3 weeks. It is manifested by hyponatremia, hypokalemia, and hypovolemia. Clients in the second phase have elevated BUN and creatinine levels and low creatinine clearances. Clients are at risk for fluid volume deficit and should be monitored for hyponatremia, hypokalemia, and dehydration. As the diuretic phase ends, the client's acid–base balance, electrolytes, BUN, and creatinine levels return to normal.

> Clients experiencing the second phase of acute renal failure, the **diuretic phase,** are at great risk for developing severe hyponatremia, hypokalemia, and dehydration.

Convalescent Phase The third phase of acute renal failure is the recovery or convalescent phase. This occurs when the GFR increases and the BUN and creatinine levels begin to stabilize and return to normal. This phase can last from 3–12 months.

The mortality rate of acute renal failure is high. The outcomes are influenced by the client's overall health, the severity of renal failure, and the number and types of complications (McCarley & Lewis, 1996).

Nursing care includes monitoring the client's intake and output on an hourly basis and reporting excessive gains and losses. The client may require the administration of intravenous fluids and electrolyte supplements. The client should be weighed daily: a gain or loss of 1 kg of body weight equals the gain or loss of 1 L of fluid. The client's electrolytes and ABG values should be monitored frequently. The client's electrocardiogram (ECG) must be monitored because of the alterations that occur with hyperkalemia and hypokalemia. The nurse must monitor the client's urine, serum osmolality, serum osmolarity, urine specific gravity, and vital signs.

> Fluid gains or losses can be estimated using this formula: 1 kg of body weight equals 1 L of fluid.

The client's protein concentration should be maintained at a level that is sufficient to replace metabolized protein but prevents excessive metabolism. Protein restriction is usually 1–1.5 g/kg of ideal body weight per day. The intake of adequate protein is determined by a BUN to creatinine ratio of 10:1. The client's protein level may be high as well. The client's diet should be high in carbohydrates, and he or she may require a multivitamin supplement.

> The intake of adequate protein in clients with renal failure is achieved when the BUN to creatinine ratio is 10:1.

CASE STUDY: WOMAN IN ACUTE RENAL FAILURE

A 49-year-old woman presents with right lower lobe pneumonia and diabetes mellitus. Her vital signs are: blood pressure, 162/94 mm Hg; pulse, 80 beats/min; respirations, 16 breaths/min; and temperature,

100.2°F. Her CBC shows a WBC count of 20,000/μL, RBC count of 3.2/μL, hemoglobin of 10.4 g/dL, and hematocrit of 37%. Her urine output for the last 24 hours is 450 mL. She is receiving regular and NPH insulin and ceftriaxone (Rocephin), 2 g every 12 hours, intravenous bolus push. Her SMA on days one and two are listed below.

SMA 7	Day One	Day Two
Glucose	150 mg/dL	182 mg/dL
Sodium (Na^+)	131 mEq/L	132 mEq/L
Potassium (K^+)	5.3 mEq/L	6.4 mEq/L
BUN	73 mg/dL	95 mg/dL
Creatinine	3.1 mg/dL	6.2 mg/dL
Carbon dioxide (CO_2)	22 mEq/L	21 mEq/L

NOTE: SMA 7 = [Sequential Multiple Analyzer] trademark for an automated chemistry system that determines the concentration of serum substances in 60 minutes.

This client is in phase one of acute renal failure. Her BUN and creatinine levels are elevated, and she is oliguric. The creatinine level, the most sensitive indicator of renal insufficiency, has doubled within 24 hours. The factors that have led to this condition are impaired renal perfusion related to the effect diabetes has on blood vessels and the cephalosporin antibiotic she is receiving. Prior to her hospitalization, the client most likely experienced a nonsymptomatic decrease in renal functioning as a result of the diabetes. Cephalosporins, such as ceftriaxone, are not nephrotoxic but can contribute to the development of renal failure. Other agents such as analgesics, sedative, antihypertensives, antiarrhythmics, diuretics, anticoagulants, and hypoglycemic agents can also damage the kidneys. Anti-infectives such as antifungals, penicillins, and sulfonamides are other factors contributing to renal disease, and the aminoglycosides are nephrotoxic antibiotics.

The first priority is to lower the client's potassium level as hyperkalemia can lead to cardiac dysrhythmias and cardiac arrest. The client should be treated with intravenous calcium gluconate to decrease the effect the potassium has on the cardiac muscle. The client should then receive intravenous D50W followed immediately by regular insulin. This moves the potassium from the plasma back into the intracellular tissues. The client may also receive a kayexelate and sorbital enema that binds with the potassium in the GI tract and promotes potassium excretion through bowel movements. The client may also receive a loop diuretic such as furosemide (Lasix) to promote urination and sodium bicarbonate to treat the metabolic acidosis that occurs with renal failure. Cardiac monitoring should be performed until the client is stabilized and maintains a normal serum potassium level.

Treatment of hyperkalemia

- Calcium gluconate decreases the effect of the potassium on the heart.
- Infusion of D50W and regular insulin intravenously moves the potassium into the cells.
- Kayexelate and sorbital bind with and facilitate the excretion of potassium.
- Dialysis is performed if necessary.

Chronic Renal Failure

Chronic renal failure is the irreversible and progressive destruction of the kidneys. It is caused by a number of conditions and leads to multisystem failure. The disease can be characterized by three stages: diminished renal reserve, renal insufficiency, and end-stage renal disease (ESRD).

Diminished Renal Reserve The first phase is characterized by normal BUN and creatinine levels and an absence of symptoms. This phase occurs due to diminished blood flow to the kidneys or from conditions that damage the kidneys, such as untreated acute renal failure, or as a progression of acute renal failure. Its onset and duration are frequently undetected because of the absence of symptoms.

Renal Insufficiency The second phase of chronic renal failure is renal insufficiency. This occurs when the GFR is 25% of normal (McCarley & Lewis, 1996), and the BUN and creatinine levels are increased. The clinical manifestations are fatigue, weakness, headaches, nausea, and pruritus. The client may experience nocturia and polyuria as a result of the kidneys' loss of ability to concentrate urine (McCarley & Lewis, 1996).

ESRD The third phase is ESRD or uremia. This occurs when the GFR is less than 5–10% of normal or when the creatinine clearance is less than 5–10 mL/min (McCarley & Lewis, 1996). As chronic renal failure progresses, the retained substances cause the body's organs to deteriorate, leading to multisystem failure. The clinical manifestations of ESRD are neurological deficits, hematological deficits, GI distress, respiratory distress, fluid and electrolyte disturbances, acid–base imbalance, and skin integrity impairment.

The client may require phosphate binding agents such as aluminum hydroxide gels to treat hyperphosphatemia as a result of decreased excretion of phosphorus by the kidneys. The signs and symptoms of hyperphosphatemia are paresthesias, muscle cramps, seizures, and abnormal reflexes. The client may also need antihypertensives to treat hypertension. If the client experiences acute anemia, a colony-stimulating agent such as epoetin alfa (Procrit) is administered to stimulate the production of RBC. The client's platelet level may be decreased as well.

Clients in chronic renal failure are susceptible to infection because of the renal failure–induced leukocytosis. Infection is a leading cause of death in chronic renal failure. The nurse must use strict aseptic technique when caring for these clients, and they should be protected from others who may be infectious. The nurse must monitor the client for signs of infection, including edema, pain, redness, anorexia, malaise, and leukocytosis. The client may not exhibit a fever in response to the infection because of the effect of renal failure on the immune system. If antibiotics are ordered, the client should be monitored for signs of antibiotic toxicity because some antibiotics are excreted by the kidneys.

Clients experience neurological complications as well. The nurse should assess the client every hour for signs of uremia, fatigue, loss of appetite, decreased urinary output, apathy, confusion, elevated blood pressure, edema of the face and feet, dry itchy skin, restlessness, and seizures. The nurse should also monitor for changes in mental function. The confused client requires orientation and safety precautions.

The client also experiences GI distress resulting from the inflammation of the mucosa caused by excessive urea. The nurse should assess for the presence of stomatitis, which is treated with warm saline gargles and topical anesthetics such as viscous lidocaine. The client may experience nausea and vomiting, which can be treated with antiemetics. The client also should be assessed for signs of GI bleeding.

The client may experience Kussmaul's respirations as a result of metabolic acidosis. Kussmaul's respirations are deep, gasping, labored breaths. Dyspnea from CHF, pulmonary edema, pleurisy, pleural effusion, and pneumonia is common in clients with chronic renal failure, and the cough reflex is often depressed (McCauley & Lewis, 1996). Diuretics and dialysis are the treatments for the interstitial edema that occurs.

Nurses must care for the client's skin, including assessment for pruritus. The skin appears yellowish and is dry and scaly. The client should be bathed in plain water to wash off the urea crystals on the skin. This can help to decrease severe pruritus. Petechiae and ecchymoses may be present.

Treatment of chronic renal failure includes restricting fluid, phosphate, and protein intake. These clients also receive diuretics to promote urination. As the disease progresses, the client needs dialysis and eventually kidney transplantation.

Dialysis

Dialysis, both hemodialysis and peritoneal dialysis, filters waste products from the blood.

Hemodialysis
An external dialysis machine contains a coil that acts as a semipermeable membrane. The client's blood is removed from the body and passed alongside the coil and then returned to the body. On the other side of the coil, a hypertonic solution called dialysate pulls the waste products from the blood across the semipermeable membrane.

During hemodialysis, blood is moved through a vascular access device, an arteriovenous shunt, arteriovenous fistula, or a subclavian or femoral catheter. These devices are necessary to provide the high blood flow required for hemodialysis.

Successful dialysis involves properly caring for the venous access devices and peritoneal shunts. If the client has an arteriovenous shunt or arteriovenous fistula, the nurse should auscultate to detect a bruit and palpate to detect a thrill over the access site, which indicate that the access device is patent. The nurse should assess arteriovenous devices for signs of clotting such as color change of blood and the absence of pulsations in the tubing during dialysis. The access sites should be assessed for bleeding, hematoma formation, skin discoloration, drainage, and pain. The dressing over the site should be changed frequently. The vessels must not become constricted as this may lead to clotting of the device; therefore, it is necessary to avoid restrictive dressings and clothing over the site. The nurse should avoid taking blood pressure and laboratory specimens from the extremity on which the access device is located. Intravenous infusions and injections should not be administered in the extremity with the access device.

If the client has a femoral or subclavian venous access device, the nurse should palpate the pulses in the cannulized area or extremity and monitor for hematoma formation and bleeding. The catheter must be securely positioned to prevent dislodgement. If dislodged, a tremendous amount of blood can be lost as a result of the high flow through of these devices. These catheters require site care and fresh dressings every 24–72 hours. The device must be flushed with heparinized saline after every treatment.

Prior to hemodialysis, the client should urinate, and the nurse should assess the client's vital signs. The client should be weighed and the weight communicated to the dialysis nurse. The physician usually withholds antihypertensive agents, sedatives, and vasodilators prior to the treatment. This is necessary because of the cardiovascular changes that occur during dialysis.

During hemodialysis, the client's vital signs should be assessed every 30 minutes. The client must remain on bed rest but should change position frequently. The client needs to know that headache and nausea may occur and to report these to the nurse. The client should receive meals during dialysis, but this may not prevent anorexia.

Following hemodialysis, the nurse should weigh the client using the same scale used before dialysis. There should be a reduction in weight after the dialysis treatment. The nurse should assess the client for complications such as hypovolemic shock and disequilibrium syndrome. Disequilibrium syndrome is a life-threatening condition that occurs when urea of the blood is removed more rapidly than urea from the brain. The clinical manifestations are nausea and vomiting, hypertension, disorientation, leg cramps, and peripheral paresthesias. The physician should be notified of any signs of disequilibrium syndrome. Nursing treatment includes keeping the client quiet in a calm environment and administering mild analgesics to control headache pain.

The client may experience chronic leg cramps due to fluid and electrolyte imbalances and uremia. Treatment includes adding a little sodium to the client's plasma and quinine sulfate (Quinaglute) at bedtime. Applying warm moist heat and massage may also be helpful.

Peritoneal Dialysis As with hemodialysis, the client should be weighed prior to peritoneal dialysis. The client's vital signs should be assessed before and 15 minutes after the first exchange. The client should urinate before the treatment. The nurse should warm the dialysate to body temperature by wrapping the solution in a warm, moist heating pad or soaking it in warm water. The dialysate is weighed prior to infusion into the peritoneal cavity.

The client's peritoneum is used as the semipermeable membrane. The dialysate is infused into the peritoneal cavity for 10–20 minutes. The dialysate is connected to the peritoneal catheter using aseptic technique.

Chronic leg cramps are common with clients undergoing hemodialysis. Quinine sulfate and sodium are used to treat the cramps. The client may experience some relief with stretching exercises, warm moist packs, and massage.

Some clients use an infrared ultraviolet light to "sterilize" the connections between the dialysate and the peritoneal catheter. The dialysate is left in the peritoneal cavity for 30–45 minutes. During this time, the body's waste products are pulled into the hypotonic solution. The dialysate bag is then lowered below body level, and the dialysate is allowed to run back into the bag. Waste is removed by draining the dialysate. The returned dialysate is then weighed; it should be heavier after dialysis. The client should also be weighed and his or her weight should be reduced after dialysis. The physician determines the number of exchanges performed per day.

The returned dialysate should be observed for color and consistency. Normally, returned dialysate is a clear, pale yellow color. The returned dialysate from the first few exchanges after the peritoneal catheter is inserted may be slightly bloody. However, it would be abnormal for the returned dialysate to be bloody with an established catheter. Returned dialysate that is cloudy or has sediment may indicate an infection. Peritonitis is very common with peritoneal dialysis. If the returned dialysate is cloudy, the nurse should take the client's temperature and alert the physician. If the returned dialysis is brownish, this may indicate a bowel perforation. The physician should be notified immediately if this occurs.

Clients receiving peritoneal dialysis may experience severe protein loss. If this occurs, the nurse must increase the protein in the diet. The client should receive enough protein for nutritional need to prevent stored protein metabolism. The protein level is best monitored by assessing for a BUN to creatinine ratio of 10:1.

Kidney Transplantation

Successful transplantation of donor kidneys has enabled many clients with renal disease to lead a normal life. Dialysis is very hard on the body, and clients who receive dialysis complain that it limits their lives. Hemodialysis must be done in a dialysis center several times a week for hours at a time. Peritoneal dialysis can be performed at home but is done 2–4 times a day. When the client receives and is able to maintain a transplanted kidney, the limitations of renal disease are greatly reduced.

In order for a client to receive a donor kidney, it is necessary to find a suitable match. This is done by testing human leukocyte antigen (HLA) markers and ABO blood types from the donor's and the recipient's tissues. Generally, a close relative, in particular a sibling, has the greatest chance for a match. Since people can have normal kidney function with only one kidney, live-donor kidney transplantation is possible. Once the kidney is transplanted, the recipient must take antirejection agents for the rest of his or her life. The costs of transplantation and antirejection drugs are covered currently under Medicare. All chronic renal failure clients are eligible for Medicare coverage. Since antirejection medicines have numerous adverse effects including suppression of the immune system, clients must learn how to prevent infections.

Transplant Rejection The clinical manifestations of transplant rejection is flank pain on the affected side, fever, generalized edema including periorbital edema, oliguria or anuria, malaise, hypertension, elevated BUN and creatinine levels, and decreased creatinine clearance. Rejections can be accelerated, acute, or chronic. An accelerated rejection occurs 3–5 days after the transplant. An acute rejection occurs within 2 weeks of the transplant. Chronic rejections can occur anytime after the transplant. All are treated with corticosteroids and increased dosages of antirejection or immunosuppressive agents. Nurses must teach clients to recognize the clinical manifestations of a rejection and to report them to their physician immediately.

Summary

Nurses must have a working knowledge of fluid regulation and urinary elimination to care properly for clients with a variety of disease processes. Fluid regulation is vital as 90% of body weight is composed of fluid. The concepts of volume, osmolarity, osmolality, and tonicity are important in understanding fluid and electrolyte balance. These concepts are applied to clinical situations. Surgery and other medical interventions affect fluid balance, and fluid replacement therapy is often required.

Urinary tract disorders are treated by monitoring fluid intake and output and assessing for the clinical manifestations of obstruction or loss of bladder tone. The client with a urinary disorder may need medication adjustments, surgery, or education on management of the disorder.

Nurses should monitor the client's creatinine level and creatinine clearance for the development of renal insufficiency. The treatment for ESRD is usually hemodialysis or peritoneal dialysis. Renal transplantation may be necessary for those in ESRD. Clients are eligible for a transplanted kidney if their HLA markers and ABO blood types match those of the donors. Clients who receive a transplanted kidney must take antirejection agents for the rest of their lives. Organ rejection can occur anytime after transplantation.

KEY WORDS

Acid ash diet	Hypotonic
Active transport	Ileal conduit
Alkali ash diet	Incontinence
Cystine stones	Intracellular
Cystoscopy	Isotonic
Dialysis	Lithotripsy
Diffusion	Nephrostomy
Extracellular	Nephrotic syndrome
Glomerulonephritis	Neurogenic bladder
Hypertonic	Oliguria

Osmolality   Residual urine
Osmolarity   Struvite stones
Osmosis   Urinary retention
Pyelonephritis

QUESTIONS

1. An 82-year-old woman living in a long-term care facility develops urinary incontinence. After ruling out the presence of urinary retention or a urinary tract infection (UTI), the nurse should

   A. establish a 3-hour prompted voiding schedule.
   B. insert a Foley catheter or teach the client to self-catheterize.
   C. restrict her fluid intake to 1500 mL per day.
   D. use adult diapers and change them frequently.

2. A client with a serum potassium level of 6.8 mEq/L receives intravenous glucose and insulin. This therapy will cause the potassium to

   A. be absorbed by the pancreas.
   B. be excreted in the stool.
   C. bind with the calcium.
   D. enter the cell.

3. A client diagnosed with struvite-type renal calculi should be assessed for

   A. an excessive calcium intake.
   B. high serum uric acid level.
   C. a poor nutritional status.
   D. a possible urinary tract infection.

4. In which one of the following cases should a portable bladder scan be used?

   A. To assist in placing a suprapubic catheter to avoid bladder trauma
   B. To detect the presence of bacteria in the urinary tract
   C. To assess postvoid residual bladder volume
   D. To verify the accuracy of urinary output obtained from intermittent catheterization

5. A 22-year-old woman is admitted following a breast reduction. She received 1000 mL of 5% dextrose in Ringer's lactate (D5RL) during surgery and in the recovery room and 1000 mL of 5% dextrose in water (D5W) since she returned to the unit 5 hours ago. Which of the following clinical manifestations, if exhibited by the client, could be related to the development of hyponatremic encephalopathy?

   A. Anxiety, hyperactivity, and hyperventilation
   B. Excessive thirst
   C. Headache following the D5RL infusion
   D. Nausea following the D5W infusion

ANSWERS

1. *The answer is A.* Research has shown that urinary incontinence can be decreased using a 3-hour prompted voiding schedule. Catheterization for the convenience of the staff is not indicated. Restricting the client's fluids and using adult diapers can cause complications such as dehydration and impaired skin integrity.

2. *The answer is D.* Intravenous dextrose and insulin move the potassium from the extracellular fluid to the intercellular fluid.

3. *The answer is D.* Struvite renal calculi are associated with urinary tract infections. They are often seen with long-term indwelling catheters. Excessive calcium intake and high serum uric acid levels are associated with calcium stones and uric acid stones, respectively.

4. *The answer is C.* A portable bladder scan is primarily used to prevent intermittent catheterization for postvoid assessment of urinary retention. The portable bladder scan uses ultrasound to show urine volume in the bladder.

5. *The answer is D.* Nausea is a classic sign of hyponatremic encephalopathy caused by the rapid infusion of a large amount of D5W. The client does not experience excessive thirst or hyperactivity.

ANNOTATED REFERENCES

Bartucci, M. R. (1995). Assessment of the renal system. In W. J. Phipps, V. L. Cassmeyer, J. K. Sands, & M. K. Lehman (Eds.), *Medical-surgical nursing: Concepts and clinical practice* (4th ed., pp. 1592–1610), St Louis: C. V. Mosby.

This chapter gives a brief but comprehensive summary of the anatomy and physiology of the renal system.

Bates, P., & Lewis, S. L. (1996). Nursing role in management: Renal and urologic problems. In S. L. Lewis, I. C. Collier, & M. M. Heitkemper (Eds.), *Medical-surgical nursing: Assessment and management of clinical problems* (4th ed., pp. 1332–1370), St. Louis: C. V. Mosby.

This textbook is recognized in the nursing literature as an excellent comprehensive medical-surgical reference. The chapter on urological problems explains the procedures for various surgical techniques in urology.

Bove, L. A. (1994). How fluids and electrolytes shift after surgery. *Nursing 94* (August), 34–39.

This article uses a case study approach to provide a comprehensive overview of fluid and electrolyte shifts following surgery. It discusses kidney and gastrointestinal regulation of fluids, third-spacing, and the differentiation of relational hypovolemia versus fluid overload in clients with edema.

Bove, L. A. (1996). Restoring electrolyte balance: Sodium chloride. *RN* (January), 25–28.

This article gives a clear description of the changes that occur due to hypernatremia and hyponatremia. It also discusses the role chloride plays in the balance of sodium. Bove has written numerous articles on the physiology and pathophysiology of fluid and electrolyte shifts.

Huether, S. E. (1994). The cellular environment: Fluids and electrolytes, acids and bases. In K. L. McCance & S. E. Huether (Eds.), *Pathophysiology: The biologic basis for disease in adults and children* (2nd ed., pp. 91–123), St. Louis: C. V. Mosby.

This chapter gives a comprehensive description of the pathophysiology that affects the body's fluid and electrolyte balance. It describes these phenomena down to the cellular level.

Lemone, P., & Burke, K. M. (1996). Nursing care of clients with alterations in fluid, electrolyte, or acid–base balance. In *Medical-surgical nursing: Critical thinking in client care* (pp. 96–158), Menlo Park: Addison-Wesley.

This chapter discusses fluid shifts and the principles that cause them. It deals with the concepts of osmosis, diffusion, and active transport in relation to client fluid and electrolyte balance.

McCarley, T., & Lewis, S. L. (1996). Nursing role in management: Acute and chronic renal failure. In S. L. Lewis, I. C. Collier, & M. M. Heitkemper (Eds.), *Medical-surgical nursing: Assessment and management of clinical problems* (4th ed., pp. 1371–1412), St. Louis: C. V. Mosby.

This chapter in this well-known textbook gives comprehensive information concerning the care of clients with acute and chronic renal failure. It covers the pathophysiology as well as nursing care.

Metheny, N. M. (1990). Why worry about IV fluids? *American Journal of Nursing* (June), 50–55.

Norma Metheny is a noted expert in the principles of fluid regulation. This article explains the uses of intravenous fluids. She writes about the clinical manifestations of altered fluid and electrolyte regulation.

Metheny, N. M. (1997). Focusing on the dangers of D5W. *Nursing 97, 27* (10), 55–59.

This article warns nurses of the life-threatening risk young women take in receiving D5W. It is a seemingly harmless fluid but can cause severe hyponatremia. This article gives the clinical manifestations and discusses why young women are most at risk. Many young healthy women have died following minor surgeries due to hyponatremic encephalopathy that developed from the use of D5W.

Wagner, M. L., & Schmid, M. M. (1997). Exploring the research base and outcome measures for portable bladder ultrasound technology. *MED-SURG Nursing, 6* (5), 1–11.

This article discusses new technology available for urinary retention. It gives the indications and describes how to use the technology. It also discusses the clinical outcomes measured to date using this equipment.

DISORDERS OF THE MUSCULOSKELETAL SYSTEM

ANATOMY AND PHYSIOLOGY

The musculoskeletal system works in harmony to produce motion and actions that allow human beings independence and discovery. The musculoskeletal system is comprised of the skeleton, joints, muscles, ligaments, and bursae. The skeleton provides shape and support to the body, protects the vital organs, and serves as a reservoir for minerals such as calcium, magnesium, and phosphate. The medullary cavity of the bones is the primary site for the production of blood cells. The muscles provide the force to move the body, close the external orifices of the gastrointestinal and urinary tracts, and increase heat production to maintain temperature control.

Bone

Bone is made up of a matrix of fibers and protein that is ossified with calcium, magnesium phosphate, and carbonate. There are 206 bones in the body, classified as long, short, flat, and irregular, according to their shape. The hard outer bone surface, the periosteum, is made up of fibrous connective tissue. The periosteum contains blood vessels that supply oxygen and nutrients to the bone cells. The inner cavity of the bone is filled with yellow marrow and red marrow. Red bone marrow is the site of hematopoiesis—the manufacture of red and white blood cells (RBCs; WBCs) and platelets.

Bone Density and Ethnicity. Bone density is greater in African Americans and Polynesians than in age-matched white Americans. In contrast, Asian Americans have lower bone density values than other racial groups (Giger & Davidhizar, 1995).

The bony structures consist of the axial and appendicular skeletons. The axial skeleton is made up of the cranium, the vertebrae, the ribs, and the sternum. The girdles that transfer weight of the axial structure to the limbs and the limbs themselves make up the appendicular skeleton (Fig. 8-1).

FIGURE 8-1 Anterior and posterior views of a skeleton.

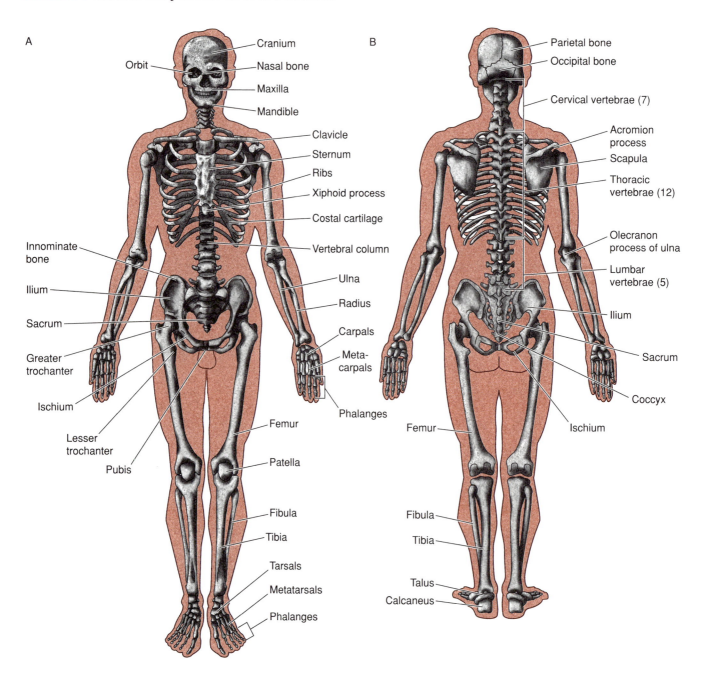

There are two types of bony tissue involved in the construction of the appendicular skeleton—the diaphysis and the epiphysis. The hard, compact diaphysis, or the shaft of the long bone, is fused with the epiphysis, the sponge-like ends, once full growth is achieved.

Accessory Structures Bones attach to each other at points called joints or articulations. There are three types of joints, which are classified by the degree of movement they allow. The *fibrous joints*, or synarthroses, are immovable and are found between the bones of the cranium, the distal ends of the radius and ulna, and between the teeth and jaw bones. The freely movable joints are known as diarthroses, or *synovial joints*. Typically, a synovial joint has articulating surfaces covered by hyaline cartilage and a capsule filled with fluid (the bursa) to lubricate and reduce friction. Hinge, ball and socket, and pivot joints are synovial joints. The third type are the *amphiarthroses*, which allow only slight movement. They are cartilaginous in construction and are located between the vertebrae, pubic bones, and where the first 10 ribs connect to the sternum.

Muscle

Skeletal muscles are striated; that is, they are made up of fibers consisting of many myofibrils that are enclosed in a network of endoplasmic reticulum. Muscle fibers are wrapped in bundles, and together the bundles form a muscle. Each muscle is covered by a sheath of connective tissue called *fascia*. Tendons are the ends of the fascia that are lengthened into tough cords where they attach muscles to bones. Skeletal muscles usually join two bones and cross at least one joint (Fig. 8-2).

Muscle tissue has the unique characteristics of contractility, extensibility, elasticity, and irritability. Because muscles are elastic, they work in pairs having opposite actions; when one muscle contracts (the prime mover), the other relaxes (the antagonist). The strength of each movement or contraction depends on the original length of the fibers, the number of fibers activated by the nervous system, and the metabolic condition of the muscles. Some muscles (synergists) contract at the same time as the prime movers to help stabilize the body.

Assessment

Nursing assessment of the musculoskeletal system begins with gathering subjective information. The nurse uses knowledge of pathophysiology to guide the *subjective assessment* in a relevant and complete manner. A focused health history of a client with a suspected or previously diagnosed musculoskeletal disorder should include major illnesses, surgeries, injuries, hospitalizations, immunizations, allergies, current medications, significant family medical history, participation in physical activities and exercise, and occupation. Possible symptoms to review with the client are listed in Table 8-1.

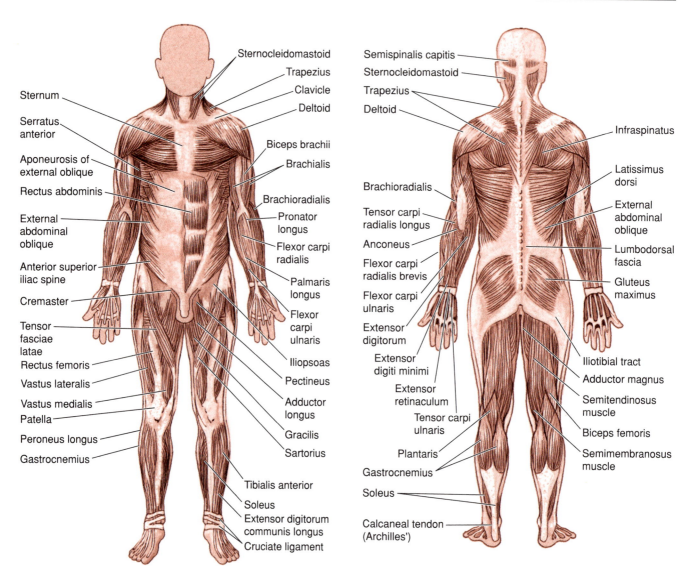

FIGURE 8-2 Anterior and posterior views of the superficial muscles.

Joint Crepitus is the grating sensation caused by dry synovial surfaces rubbing together.

The *objective assessment* includes a general assessment, inspection, palpation, range of motion (Fig. 8-3), and muscle strength. The general assessment includes height, weight, vital signs, apparent age relative to chronological age, nutritional status, general appearance, and stature. Inspection includes observation for posture, symmetry, size, gait, involuntary movements, and gross deformities. Palpate to assess muscle tone, temperature variations, tenderness, swelling, masses, tremors, and **joint crepitus**. Assessment of active and passive range of motion (ROM) can determine any limitation of movement. Muscle strength is assessed on a gradation of 0–5 and is compared for symmetry (Table 8-2).

🔯

TABLE 8-1
POSSIBLE SYMPTOMS RELATED TO MUSCULOSKELETAL DISORDERS

Muscles
  Atrophy
  Hypertrophy
  Pain
  Cramping
  Weakness

Bones and Joints
  Inability to bear weight
  Pain
  Stiffness
  Swelling
  Redness
  Increased local temperature (heat)
  Decreased range of motion (ROM)
  Fractures
  Clicking, clunking
  Locking or catching
  Giving way (buckling)

Other
  "Pins and needles" or numbness (paresthesias)
  Skin changes such as pale, cyanotic, dusky, butterfly rash

NOTE: From *Principles and practice of adult health nursing* (3rd ed., p. 1192), by P. G. Beare and J. L. Myers, 1998, St. Louis, MO: Mosby. Reprinted with permission.

Diagnostic Tests

X-rays Standard x-rays reveal structural or functional changes in bones and joints and are commonly used to assess musculoskeletal disorders. Usually at least two views, the anteroposterior and lateral views, are obtained.

Arthrography Arthrography provides radiographic visualization after a contrast medium or air has been injected into the joint. It is particularly useful for viewing ligaments or cartilage, which are not well visualized by x-ray alone.

Myelography This test is used to evaluate spinal cord or nerve root damage. It involves fluoroscopic examination of a subarachnoid space after injection with contrast medium.

Bone Scan A bone scan provides imaging of the skeletal system after injection of a radioactive tracer. It helps identify "hot spots" of increased

Upper extremities

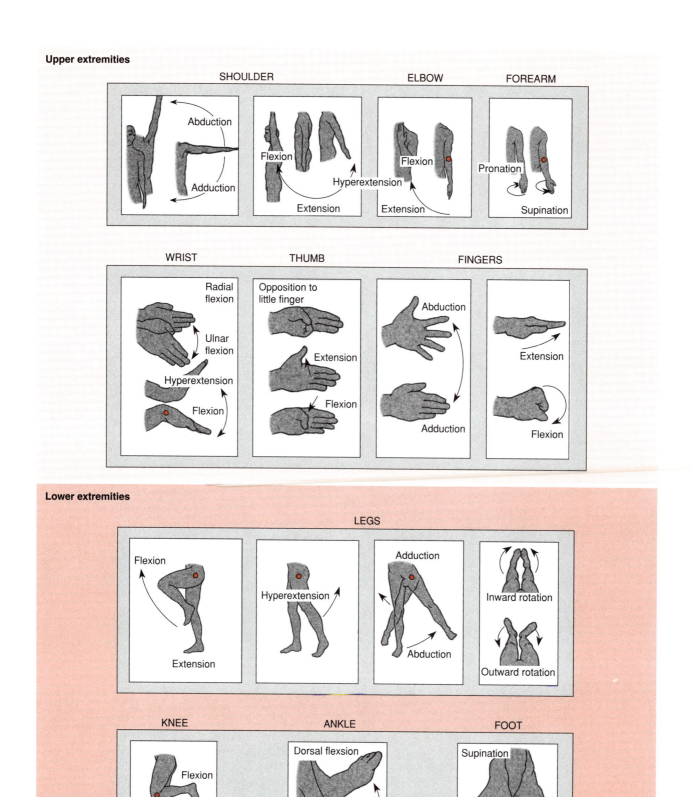

FIGURE 8-3 Range of motion (ROM) standards for mobility for the upper and lower extremities.
NOTE: From *Principles and practice of adult health nursing* (3rd ed., p. 1194), by P. G. Beare and J. L. Myers, 1998, St. Louis, MO: Mosby. Reprinted with permission.

🔀

TABLE 8-2

Muscle Strength Grading

Gradation	Description
5—Normal	Complete range of motion (ROM) against gravity, with full resistance
4—Good	Complete ROM against gravity, with some resistance
3—Fair	Complete ROM against gravity
2—Poor	Complete ROM, with gravity eliminated
1—Trace	Evidence of slight contractility, with no joint motion
0—None	No evidence of contractility

NOTE: From *Principles and practice of adult health nursing* (3rd ed., p. 1195), by P. G. Beare and J. L. Myers, 1998, St. Louis, MO: Mosby. Reprinted with permission.

metabolism and is useful in detecting malignancy, trauma, degenerative disorders, and osteomyelitis.

Computed Tomography (CT) Scan A CT scan provides a cross-sectional picture of bony and soft tissue abnormalities. The CT scan keeps radiation exposure to a minimum and requires no additional manipulation of the client (a consideration for a trauma victim).

Magnetic Resonance Imaging (MRI) MRI provides sensitive images that differentiate between solid tissue, fat, blood, and bone. It is particularly useful in diagnosing demyelinating spinal lesions, tumors, disc disease, and osteomyelitis.

Arthroscopy Arthroscopy directly visualizes a joint through an arthroscope inserted into an incision. It is particularly useful for evaluating and repairing knee disorders.

Electromyography Electromyography provides a measurement of the muscle action potential—the electric currents produced by muscles. It is particularly useful in diagnosing muscular dystrophy and motor neuron disease.

Synovial Fluid Analysis A portion of synovial fluid is removed via a large-bore needle inserted into the joint capsule. It is then analyzed for septic, hemorrhagic, inflammatory, and noninflammatory joint disorders.

Biopsy In a biopsy, a portion of bone or tissue is removed for histological examination. It is usually performed after abnormal or inconclusive results of a CT scan, bone scan, or x-rays. A biopsy can help distinguish between a benign and a malignant lesion.

SOFT TISSUE INJURY

Contusion

A contusion is a soft tissue injury usually caused by some type of blunt trauma resulting in the rupture of small blood vessels and subsequent hemorrhage at the site.

Clinical Manifestations The signs and symptoms of a contusion include pain, swelling, and discoloration at the trauma site. As the blood is reabsorbed, the skin discoloration may progress from a bruised bluish purple color to brown, to yellow, and then back to a normal appearance.

Strain

A strain is an injury to the muscle or tendon due to overuse, excessive stress, or overstretching. The affected muscle tissue often has microscopic, incomplete tears that bleed into the affected site.

Clinical Manifestations The signs and symptoms of a strain include pain, swelling, and muscle spasms. The client may or may not experience any objective symptoms immediately following a strain. Subsequent movement of the affected part may produce pain, which hinders physical activity. In some instances, the client may say that the affected part has a "dead feeling." Discoloration is usually not present unless the client has sustained an injury to the soft tissue.

Sprain

A sprain is an injury to some of the ligamentous structures surrounding a joint. This injury may involve a tear or stretching of the ligament. A sprain is often associated with joint disability and is a more severe injury than a strain.

Clinical Manifestations The typical symptoms of a sprain include rapid swelling at the injury site, pain, and discoloration. Hemorrhage into the soft tissue may occur if blood vessels are also injured. Sprains are classified as mild, moderate, and severe.

Mild Sprain In a mild sprain, there is local tenderness and swelling, but movement is minimally compromised. The ligament is stretched or microscopically torn.

Moderate Sprain In a moderate sprain, the affected part is edematous and tender, with moderate pain on movement, and some ligamentous tearing has occurred.

Severe Sprain In a severe sprain, the affected part is edematous and tender, and flexion and weight bearing are grossly compromised. The ligament is disrupted with definite joint instability.

Assessment The nurse performs a general assessment, as most clients with a soft tissue injury have suffered some type of trauma. A focused assessment should determine the extent of injury and involvement of various structures. An accurate history of the events of the injury should include the activities leading up to the injury, the position of the affected part on injury (inversion or eversion), approximate amount of weight that came to bear on the affected part, and the presence of a cracking, popping, or snapping sensation felt or sound heard during the injury. Make focused observations to ascertain the extent of swelling, discoloration, limitation to normal range of motion, and movements that cause pain. Also examine the unaffected part to use as baseline data for comparison. An x-ray of the affected part can rule out a possible fracture in the case of a suspicious sprain.

Therapeutic Management and Nursing Care Therapeutic management of support tissue trauma is directed toward relief of pain and muscle spasms, reduction of swelling, and restoration of normal weight bearing and mobility. Primary treatment includes rest, ice, compression, and elevation (RICE) of the injured part. Immediately after the injury, the client should stop all weight bearing and keep the affected part immobilized. A cold compress or an ice pack promotes vasoconstriction and is applied to the site to decrease swelling. The nurse should place a cloth between the client's skin and the cold pack to avoid thermal injury, which is similar to frostbite. Cold therapy should begin immediately and continue for the first 24–36 hours after the injury is sustained. Some practitioners prescribe intermittent cold therapy for 20-minute periods every 3–4 hours, while others prefer continuous therapy, as tolerated by the client. Compression is accomplished by wrapping the affected part with an Ace bandage, which can also hold the ice pack in place, and is continued after cold therapy to prevent further swelling. The compression bandage is applied to an extremity by wrapping from distal to proximal to prevent trapping blood and venous engorgement. The compression bandage helps support the injured tissue. The injured part is elevated above the heart for the first 24–36 hours to promote blood return and to decrease swelling.

The nurse should instruct the client to keep the affected part at rest, which at times is accomplished with the use of a splint, brace, or crutches (for injured lower extremities). Braces provide more support than a wrap and allow a gradual increase in weight-bearing activities as the ligaments heal. Readymade splints are available but may be somewhat bulky and restricting for more active and athletic clients.

After the first 36 hours, moist or dry heat may be prescribed. Heat compresses promote vasodilatation, absorption of blood, and subsequently enhance tissue repair. Pharmacological therapy may include analgesics such as acetaminophen (Tylenol) or ibuprofen (Motrin) and occasionally muscle relaxants.

Instructions to the client provided by the nurse are based on RICE. Instruct the client and his or her family about the proper positioning, elevation, and wrapping (if applicable) of the affected part and the proper use of cold and heat therapies. If the client is taking analgesics or muscle relaxants, instruct him or her about proper dosage, frequency, and side effects of the medications. Emphasize limiting activities, as a sprain may take longer than 1 month to heal. In some cases, surgical repair may be necessary. As with all injuries, instruct the client to report increased pain, swelling, discoloration, or muscle spasms to the health care provider, as complications such as a hematoma or compartment syndrome may occur.

CASE STUDY: MODERATE SPRAIN

Jason, a 21-year-old college athlete, presents to the emergency room on a Friday evening reporting severe ankle pain. He states that he was playing basketball in the gymnasium when he landed on his right foot in an abnormal position. Immediately after the injury, he was unable to bear any weight due to pain and instability of the joint. The nurse takes a thorough history of the events relating to the injury and learns that Jason had an ankle sprain 9 months ago, has basketball practice six afternoons each week, and runs track during the off season from basketball. Jason states that he landed with his full weight in an inverted position on his right foot and describes his pain as throbbing. Objective assessment reveals edema, reddened discoloration, limitation of movement on extension and rotation, generalized pain, and point tenderness at the lateral malleolus. The nurse immediately applies a cold pack to the affected part and elevates the limb with pillows on the stretcher. The physician examines Jason and orders ankle x-rays, as the client has tenderness at the tip of the lateral malleolus and was unable to bear weight immediately after the injury. The x-rays ruled out a fracture, and Jason was diagnosed with a moderate ankle sprain and appropriate orders were written.

The nurse wraps the ankle with an Ace bandage from the toes to just above the malleoli about mid-calf and reinforces this with 2-inch tape applied medially and laterally. The nurse provides client education based on RICE. She suggests that Jason use a bag of frozen peas or corn, which can mold around his ankle and be refrozen, for cold therapy whenever necessary. He is discharged with crutches and instructed to refrain from weight bearing for 48 hours. The nurse also gives him instructions for ROM exercises four times daily once he is pain-free and a list of symptoms to report. He is given a prescription for ibuprofen (Motrin), 800 mg every 8 hours for the first 48 hours, then as needed, and the nurse instructs him to take this medication with meals. He is scheduled for a follow-up at the student health clinic in 1 week.

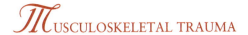USCULOSKELETAL TRAUMA

Dislocation

A dislocation occurs when a ligament gives way to such an extent that a bone is displaced from its normal position in the joint. Dislocations can be caused by congenital or acquired disorders or trauma. Most dislocations in adults result from trauma consisting of a force that dislodges the bone and also may damage the joint structure, ligaments, nerves, and vascular system of the surrounding tissues.

Clinical Manifestations Signs and symptoms include a change in extremity length and joint contour and shape, severe pain, and decreased movement.

Therapeutic Management and Nursing Care Therapeutic management of the client with a dislocation is directed toward relief of pain, immobilization of the affected part to allow for healing, and maintenance of normal neurovascular status. First, the affected part should be immobilized. An affected upper extremity can be placed in a sling, and an affected leg can be placed on a firm board, fracture splint, or taped to the unaffected leg. The diagnosis of dislocation is confirmed by an x-ray, which may also reveal a fracture. Manual reduction is performed by a skilled practitioner to return the bone to its normal position within the joint. Prior to reduction, intravenous sedation or general anesthesia is given. The affected part is immobilized using techniques similar to those used in fractures, such as skin traction or splint.

The nurse should assess the client's neurovascular status as outlined in Table 8-3. Be sure to evaluate not only the site of dislocation but also the dependent distal area and document the findings at regular intervals. Report any signs or symptoms of circulatory or nerve impairment and provide medication for pain relief.

Fracture

A fracture is any break or crack in the continuity of a bone. Although bones may break spontaneously, as occurs in osteomalacia and osteomyelitis, most fractures are caused by a trauma that places excessive stress on a bone. Fractures occur more often in men than women up to the age of 45 and are most often associated with sports, work, and motor vehicle accident injuries. Among the elderly, women suffer more fractures than men due to the increased incidence of osteoporosis associated with the hormonal changes of menopause.

Bones weaken with age because new bone formation does not keep up with the bone resorption. The hormonal changes of menopause cause this process to occur at an earlier age in women; therefore, elderly women have a greater risk of bone fractures than men.

Clinical Manifestations Signs and symptoms of a fracture vary to some degree based on the cause, location, type, classification, and alignment of the affected part. A fracture is classified based on breaks in skin integrity, location, pattern of the break, and alignment status:

- **Closed fracture (simple fracture).** Skin integrity remains intact.
- **Open fracture (compound fracture).** Skin integrity is broken, and ends of bone protrude through the skin.
- **Complete fracture.** Break extends through the entire cross section of bone and is usually associated with displacement.
- **Incomplete fracture.** Only a portion of the cross section of bone is involved.

There are several types of fractures (Fig. 8-4):

- **Oblique.** This fracture is in a slanted direction.
- **Spiral.** This fracture extends around the bone.
- **Transverse.** This fracture extends across the bone.
- **Segmental.** With this fracture, a segment of bone is fractured and detached.
- **Comminuted.** This fracture involves several fragments.

FIGURE 8-4

◪

Types of fractures.
NOTE: From *Principles and practice of adult health nursing* (2nd ed., p. 1518), by P. G. Beare and J. L. Myers, 1994, St. Louis, MO: Mosby: Reprinted with permission.

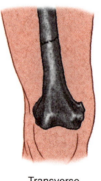 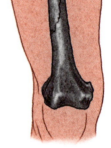
Transverse   Oblique

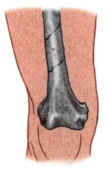 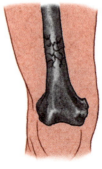 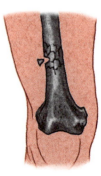
Spiral   Comminuted   Segmental

The most pronounced symptoms of a fracture are pain, swelling, and deformity. Pain often becomes more severe with movement and pressure over the fracture and may be associated with loss of function. Swelling at the site may be the first sign of a fracture; as swelling increases, pain increases. The most specific sign of a fracture is deformity, as the other symptoms may be present with a sprain or strain. Discoloration and crepitus also may be present. Of course, if an open wound exists, bleeding and hemorrhage may be present.

Assessment Initial assessment of a client with a possible bone fracture is similar to the assessment of a client with a soft-tissue injury due to trauma. The nurse assesses the client for the signs and symptoms mentioned in Table 8-1. Once the affected part has been properly immobilized, the nurse assesses the five Ps—pain, pallor, paralysis, paresthesia, and pulselessness—to determine the neurovascular status and motor function in the part distal to the fracture (see Table 8-3). X-rays of the affected part are the definitive diagnostic tools used to determine the presence of a fracture. However, some fractures may be difficult to detect on initial x-ray and may require radiographic evaluation at a later date to detect callus formation. If hemorrhage is suspected, a complete blood count (CBC) is performed to assess the loss of blood. Additionally, the nurse assesses the client for possible complications and determines any risk factors for future complications.

Therapeutic Management and Nursing Care Therapeutic management of fractures is directed toward realignment of bone fragments, immobilization to maintain proper realignment, and restoration of function. Obviously, prior to realignment of the fracture, emergency measures are taken to address any life-threatening injuries. Maintenance of an open airway and control of hemorrhage take priority.

Splinting The affected part should be immoblized with a splint at the injury site before moving the client. Splinting prevents further injury and pain and reduces the possibility of complications such as fat embolism syndrome. Splint an upper extremity with a sling or board placed along the forearm or over a flexed elbow. If no splinting apparatus is available, the arm should be splinted to the torso. Splint a lower extremity by placing a firm object under the leg or by splinting the affected leg to the unaffected one. A cervical collar, rolled towels or clothes, or sandbags can be used to immobilize the neck in the case of a suspected cervical fracture.

Once the client is in a health care facility and a fracture is diagnosed, bone fragments can be realigned (reduced) by the use of manual traction as prescribed or implemented by a skilled practitioner. Following realignment, the affected part may be immobilized by casting, traction, or internal fixation.

Casting Casting is the primary treatment after closed reduction of a fracture and may be used with other treatments. There are two types of casts, plaster and synthetic.

Plaster Cast A plaster cast must dry in the shape it was applied. This can take up to 48 hours. A wet cast is handled with the palms of the hands, not the fingertips, to prevent denting the cast, and creating pressure points. If using a cast dryer, avoid applying intense heat, which can burn the client, crack the cast, or dry the outside of the cast, leaving the inside wet, which can cause mold to develop. Rest the entire length of the cast on cloth covered-pillows to provide support. Help the client turn every 2–3 hours to prevent pressure areas. If the cast's edges are rough, protect the client's skin by covering the edges with tape (petaling) or by folding the edge of the stockinette over the rough cast edge and securing it with tape.

Synthetic Cast Synthetic casts are used for immobilization of nondisplaced fractures with minimal swelling and for long-term wear. They harden in minutes and allow weight-bearing within half an hour; they are not, however, ideal for full weight-bearing extremities. They are lighter (made of fiberglass), which allows easier resumption of activities. Synthetic casts are easily cared for by wiping with mild soap and water. They are water resistant, thus their strength is unaffected if the cast gets wet. Synthetic casts are ideal for elderly clients.

Nursing care for a client with a cast should facilitate fracture healing and prevention of complications. Care includes assessing subjective symptoms, presence of movement, condition of the cast, neurovascular checks, and anticipation of any fall risks. Listen carefully to the client's descriptions of how the affected part feels and any other subjective complaints. A report of pain may signify excessive swelling of the part or tightness of the cast and should be investigated prior to administering any analgesics. Neurovascular checks (the five Ps) are performed every 30 minutes for the first 4 hours, as ordered, and then every 4 hours (see Table 8-3). Use the unaffected extremity for baseline comparison. The casted extremity should be elevated above the level of the heart for the first few days after casting to decrease swelling. Assess movement and sensation of the parts distal to the affected area. Observe the cast for drainage stains, increased heat, or foul odor, and if found, report these promptly. Drainage stains may be marked with a pencil to provide a baseline for evaluation of possible increase. Monitor the client for the following complications: neurovascular compromise, skin maceration, compartment syndrome, and immobility complications. Remember to assess the client's feelings regarding body image and the presence of the cast and provide emotional support and adequate client and family education (Table 8-4).

Traction Traction is the exertion of a pulling force utilized to align and immobilize bone fragments, relieve muscle spasms, and correct flexion contractures, deformities, and dislocations. Effective traction uses weights, pulleys, and counterbalance to provide a force strong enough to counteract the overall pull of the client's muscles. There are two types of traction, skin and skeletal.

Skin Traction. *Buck's traction* is a type of skin traction that is often used before surgery for hip fractures to decrease spasms, reduce dislocations,

The basic principles of **traction** must be maintained for the treatment to be effective. Weights should always hang freely and the pulley, spreader bar, and foot plate should not rest against the foot of the bed. Continuous traction and countertraction must be maintained.

⌧

TABLE 8-3

ASSESSMENT OF CIRCULATORY AND NEUROLOGIC STATUS

---

1. *Pain:* usually the patient will report pain to the nurse. Facial grimace and overprotective behaviors indicate pain. Unrelenting or unusual pain as well as pain on passive motion indicates neurovascular impairment. Questions to ask the patient include the following:
   - Tell me about the pain.
   - Is it constant, or does it come at intervals?
   - Is the pain sharp, dull, or throbbing?
   - What activity causes the pain to occur?
   - When you are still, is the pain present?
   - Show me exactly where the pain is located.

2. *Pallor:* inspection of the dependent part below the injury is one of the most effective methods to determine circulation. The skin is assessed to determine the color and capillary filling. Use an unaffected area to determine if the affected area fills as rapidly as the unaffected area. Capillary refill is considered abnormal if it takes longer than 3 seconds.
   - Check to see if the nail beds blanch when pressed.
   - Check to see if there is a rapid return of color when the pressure is released.
   - Compare the affected part with the patient's unaffected part to determine what the color should be.

3. *Paralysis:* have the patient move the fingers or toes on the affected extremity. Since paralysis is the temporary suspension or permanent loss of function, the nurse must encourage and insist that the patient attempt to demonstrate mobility. Excessive swelling may hinder the patient's ability to voluntarily move a part, so the nurse keeps the dependent part at heart level to prevent and reduce swelling.
   - Instruct the patient to move the affected part. This should not involve any weight-bearing or lifting activity; but rather ask the patient to wiggle the toes or the fingers of the affected part.
   - Many patients will immediately say, "I can't do that," when told to move the part. The nurse may need to do passive motion to the part several times at 15- to 30-minute intervals to enhance the blood supply to the part. (Active or passive exercise will cause the cells to demand an increase in oxygen and nutrients to the tissue. Therefore, movement will enhance the blood supply to the part and also reduce swelling.) It is imperative that the nurse determines the patient's ability to move the part in order to detect any signs of paralysis.

4. *Paresthesia:* defined as an abnormal sensation that may be described by the patient as numbness, prickling, or tingling. When the patient complains of any of these symptoms, the nurse assesses the part to determine any exterior causes. If there is a cast, an immobilizer, or a bandage, this may be constricting or tight and may create a circulatory impairment. If such a circulatory impairment exists, it is also

likely that an impairment to the nerve supply is present. If there is no external cause of impairment the nurse assesses for edema. If edema is present, it is likely that this excess fluid is creating pressure on the nerve supply and thus causing symptoms of paresthesia. When edema is present, the nurse elevates the part above the heart and assesses for the remaining four of the five P's.

- Many patients, especially those who are reluctant to move the affected part, will frequently report numbness and tingling. The nurse encourages these patients to move the affected part so adequate circulatory and neurologic status is restored.

- Be alert to the fact that damage to the nerve supply from the injury or from edema may be present when a patient complains of the symptoms of paresthesia. This damage may become permanent without prompt treatment.

5. *Pulselessness:* it is imperative to establish a baseline presence of a pulse in the location of the injury or distal to the injury. This baseline will serve as a guide for the evaluation of the serial pulses taken at intervals after the injury. The peripheral pulse, color, and temperature are assessed on the *un*affected side to serve as a comparison with the injured part. With circulatory impairment the nurse expects to find a cool to cold skin temperature.

The lack of a pulse when the pulse had previously been present constitutes an emergency situation. Pulselessness may indicate that the affected part is not being supplied with the necessary oxygen and other nutrients to sustain cellular life. The presence of a pulse does not necessarily constitute adequate circulation. Pulselessness may be one of the last findings in neurovascular deficit. Therefore, the nurse manages a diminished pulse in the same manner as pulselessness.

Routine (at least every hour) pulse checks are imperative during the first 24 to 48 hours after an injury occurred or was treated. When the nurse observes a change in the pulse or the inability to locate a pulse occurs, the injured area is immediately repositioned and reassessed for pulse.

NOTE: From *Principles and practice of adult health nursing* (3rd ed., p. 1212), by P. G. Beare and J. L. Myers, 1998, St. Louis, MO: Mosby. Reprinted with permission.

prevent hip flexion contractures, and decrease low back pain. It is applied through a weight attached to a spreader bar below the foot, which is connected to a foam boot or elastic bandage wrapped on the leg.

Cervical-head halter traction is used for neck pain, strain, and whiplash. Weights are connected via a spreader bar to a halter with straps under the chin and around the head at the base of the skull.

Russell's traction is similar to Buck's traction, with the addition of upward lift of suspension provided by a sling under the knee or lower thigh. It is used for hip fractures, femur injuries, and some knee injuries. Russell's traction allows more movement.

There are two types of *pelvic traction*. One uses a belt for lower back pain, and the other uses a sling for pelvic fractures. The belt causes a downward pull on the pelvis and is usually intermittent. The sling suspends the buttocks off the bed and provides continuous stabilization and immobilization of pelvic fractures.

Skeletal Traction A *Steinmann pin* or *Kirschner wire* is a device drilled through the shaft of a bone and attached to a traction apparatus. These skeletal tractions are most often used for leg fractures. They allow visibility of the injury and access for care of the traumatized tissue.

Skull or *head traction* uses Vincke or Crutchfield tongs, which are inserted into the skull and attached to weights. This is usually a temporary means of skeletal traction.

The *halo device* is attached to the skull bone and a vest worn on the torso. This skeletal traction is used for vertebral fractures.

Nursing care for the client in traction should facilitate healing and prevent the hazards of immobility. Skin assessment is performed every 8 hours

---

TABLE 8-4
PATIENT AND FAMILY EDUCATION FOR A PERSON WEARING A CAST

1. Follow the physician's instructions regarding physical activity and limitations.
2. Exercise muscles. Move fingers and toes frequently to reduce swelling, prevent joint stiffness, and maintain muscle strength. Do muscle-setting exercise inside the cast to maintain muscle mass, tone, and strength.
3. Wear cast walking shoes at all times except when sleeping or showering.
4. Do not bump the cast.
5. Do not put anything inside the cast. Itching, infection, or decreased circulation may result.
6. Never trim or cut back the cast.
7. Protect furniture with a pad if the cast is rested on furniture.
8. Contact the physician if you experience any of the following:
   Unrelenting itching
   Pain unrelieved by medication
   Cast feels very tight
   Cast breaks, cracks, or becomes dented
   Cast feels loose
   Painful rubbing or pressure inside the cast, especially if in one place
   Limb constantly feels cold
   Fingers or toes are numb or tingling
   Fingers or toes are white or blue or color does not return

NOTE: From *You and Your Cast* by 3M Health Care, 1993, St. Paul, MN. Reprinted with permission.

with particular attention paid to bony prominences such as the occipital portion of the head, scapulae, elbows, coccyx, malleoli, and heels. Vital signs should be assessed every 4 hours while the client is awake, and temperature elevations over 100°F should be reported. If external fixation traction is used, assess the pin sites at a minimum of every 8 hours and provide skin care as ordered. Monitor for signs and symptoms of infection such as redness, drainage, edema, and warmth. Assess for neurovascular complications (the five Ps) as outlined in Table 8-3 and for the complications of immobility (Table 8-5).

Open Reduction Internal Fixation (ORIF) Open reduction internal fixation (ORIF) immobilizes a fracture by surgically inserting a nail, screw, or pin into the fracture site to fix the fractured bony parts together. Internal fixation is often used to treat hip fractures, a common injury among the elderly. The client is usually hospitalized for 5 days or longer.

Nursing care of the client who has undergone ORIF involves several observations and interventions: Monitor neurovascular checks every 1–2 hours, as ordered. Monitor vital signs hourly for 4 hours, then every 4 hours for 1–3 days, or as ordered. Hematocrit and hemoglobin must also be monitored. Observe the amount and character of drainage on dressings and drains; report drainage greater than 100–150 mL/hr after the first 4 hours. Turn the client every 2 hours, and provide an overhead trapeze for the client to use for repositioning. Place a small pillow between the client's legs to maintain alignment. Encourage deep-breathing exercises, coughing, and use of an incentive spirometer. Administer medications such as analgesics, muscle relaxants, anticoagulants, or antibiotics, as ordered. After assessing the weight-bearing ability of the injured part, the nurse should encourage early mobilization as ordered. This may be after discharge from the hospital.

Rehabilitation

Rehabilitative care of the client with a musculoskeletal injury involves physical therapy, including various types of exercise; cold and heat therapies; and massage. Isometric exercises increase muscle tension without moving the adjacent joints. They are useful when ROM is limited by the injury or a cast. Active and passive ROM exercises help to maintain or increase joint mobility. Isotonic exercise involves movement and change in the length of the muscles. Isokinetic exercises use resistance to strengthen muscles after the injured part is no longer immobilized. The nurse should document the particular therapy and the client's response to it.

Complications

Complications of a musculoskeletal injury include any of the complications of immobility (see Table 8-5), depending on the type and extent of

TABLE 8-5

IMMOBILITY COMPLICATIONS

Complication	Nursing Interventions	Rationale
Discomfort	Assess body area involved to determine cause of pain.	May be caused by external factors such as skin pressure or tight cast or dressing
	Complete a neurovascular assessment.	To determine circulatory status; suspect impairment if any of five P's are present
	Question patient about duration and type of discomfort.	Suspect pressure sore or circulatory impairment if patient continues to complain after pain medication is provided
Skin irritation and pressure sores	Wash skin around cast with warm water.	Remove particles of plaster that may break skin
	Place moleskin or gauze pads over rough edges of the cast or traction equipment (half ring of Thomas splint).	Prevents skin irritation
	Assess skin site at point of pain and at any point where pain occurred previously.	Usually patient can pinpoint a specific area when pain is result of a pressure sore; as sore becomes deep (below skin layers) patient will complain of less pain or offer no complaint of pain
Thrombophlebitis	Encourage leg exercises every 2 to 4 hours while patient is in bed. Some physicians order antiembolic stocking, low-dose heparin, sodium warfarin (Coumadin), or aspirin for patients confined to bed.	Prevents coagulation and venous stasis
	Provide adequate fluid intake.	Decreases blood viscosity
	Assess lower extremities for redness, warmth, and positive Homan's sign. Maintain bed rest in presence of these signs and symptoms.	Indicators of thrombophlebitis
Pulmonary emboli	Monitor for sudden chest pain, hypotension, dyspnea, and anxiety. (Calf pain may have occurred earlier but usually disappears before onset of chest pain.)	Indicators of pulmonary emboli
	Assess vital signs for increased pulse and respirations and decreased blood pressure. (If signs are present, prepare to administer oxygen and anticoagulants as ordered.)	
Postural hypotension	Assess for dizziness on standing. If it occurs, have patient sit down and assess for drop in blood pressure. Place patient on a tilt table four times daily until blood pressure stabilizes.	Usually related to bed rest and lack of activity and will disappear as activity increases

TABLE 8-5 (*continued*)

IMMOBILITY COMPLICATIONS

Complication	Nursing Interventions	Rationale
Postural hypotension (*cont.*)	If dizziness occurs, it is helpful to force fluids if not contraindicated.	Increases blood volume so hypotension is less likely
Muscle wasting	Consult with physician or physical therapist to determine type and frequency of activity that is permitted.	Within 3 weeks, inactive patients can lose muscle mass unless unaffected muscles are exercised
	Assess amounts of liquids and food patient consumes. Allow patient food choices.	Muscle wasting can cause negative nitrogen balance, which causes loss of appetite
	Assist in oral hygiene and hand washing.	Measures to counteract anorexia

NOTE: From *Principles and practice of adult health nursing* (3rd ed., p. 1241), by P. G. Beare and J. L. Myers, 1998, St. Louis, MO: Mosby. Reprinted with permission.

the injury. Complications specifically associated with bone fracture are fat embolis syndrome, compartment syndrome, avascular necrosis, osteomyelitis, and gas gangrene.

Fat Emboli Syndrome   Fat emboli syndrome is an acute pulmonary and potentially fatal condition that results when fat globules are released from bone marrow and surrounding damaged tissue. These fat globules pass through the circulation and eventually can occlude pulmonary vessels, leading to respiratory distress. Symptoms of fat emboli syndrome include dyspnea, changes in mental status (restlessness, agitation, confusion, stupor), tachypnea, tachycardia, fever (>103°F), petechial skin rash, and diffuse rales.

Compartment Syndrome   This complication occurs when a rise in tissue pressure within a closed space in the muscle, often due to fluid accumulation, causes severe interruption of blood flow and subsequent muscle damage. Symptoms include pain that is disproportionate to the injury, pain associated with pressure over the compartment, pain with passive stretching of the involved muscle, and paresthesia. This complication occurs most often with fracture of the tibia or radius and ulna.

Avascular Necrosis (Aseptic Necrosis)   Avascular necrosis can occur whenever blood supply to a bone is compromised. This most often affects intrascapular fractures (i.e., head and neck) of the femur when the head of the femur has been twisted or dislocated from the joint, disrupting the blood supply. Because avascular necrosis involves a process occurring over a period of time, the client may not experience symptoms until after being discharged from the hospital. Therefore, client education is of primary importance. The nurse must instruct the client to report intermittent or constant pain with weight bearing and any limitation of ROM of the affected joint. Joint replacement with a prosthesis is the usual treatment for avascular necrosis.

Osteomyelitis Osteomyelitis—infection of osseous tissue involving bone cortex and/or marrow—can be exogenous (infection enters from outside the body) or hematogenous (infection originates from sites within the body). The pathogen may enter through open fractures, penetrating wounds, or during surgical procedures. Gun shot wounds, long-bone fractures, compound fractures, traumatic amputations, and fractures with compartment syndrome or vascular injury increase the risk of osteomyelitis. Monitor the client for low-grade fever, malaise, pain, local tenderness, increased swelling and warmth, and purulent drainage. Prophylactic antibiotics and early and proper debridement of open fractures to remove necrotic tissue can decrease the incidence of this complication.

Gas Gangrene Gas gangrene results from infection with the anaerobic gram-positive saprophytic bacterium *Clostridium welchii* or *Clostridium perfringens*. *Clostridium* usually grows in deep wounds that have decreased oxygen supply due to muscle trauma. Monitor the client for changes in mental status, fever, chills, decreased blood pressure, increased pulse and respiratory rate, and prostration. As the condition progresses, edema, gas bubbles at the wound site, and profuse drainage having a characteristic fruity odor may occur. Without treatment, this toxic infection can be fatal. The wound should be debrided and irrigated, and antibiotics should be given. Hyperbaric oxygen therapy exposes the client to 100% oxygen in a dive chamber for 1–2 hours, saturates the tissues with oxygen, and kills the anaerobic bacteria. Despite these measures, amputation of the affected limb may still be required.

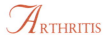

Arthritis

Arthritis is inflammation of the joint and includes more than 100 different types of disease. The two primary classifications of arthritis are noninflammatory and inflammatory. Osteoarthritis (degenerative joint disease [DJD]) is the most common noninflammatory type of arthritis, and rheumatoid arthritis is the most common inflammatory type of disease (Table 8-6). Systemic lupus erythematosus and gout are also types of inflammatory arthritis.

More than 36 million Americans are affected by one of the 100 types of **arthritis**.

A **high prevalence** of rheumatoid arthritis and osteoarthritis has been reported among selected American Indian tribes as compared with non-Indian populations in the United States.

Osteoarthritis

This is a chronic, nonsystemic, noninflammatory, progressive disease of the weight-bearing joints. Osteoarthritis is more prevalent in persons over the age of 35, women over 55 years of age, and Native Americans. Although the cause is unknown, trauma or overuse of particular joints can cause osteoarthritis in a younger person and aging seems to be an important associated factor. Risk factors include repetitive physical tasks (such as in certain occupations or athletics), trauma, joint inflammation and

🔲

TABLE 8-6

RHEUMATOID ARTHRITIS COMPARED TO OSTEOARTHRITIS

Rheumatoid Arthritis	Osteoarthritis (DJD)
Systemic (fatigue, weight loss, anemia)	Nonsystemic (results from wear and tear)
Fever	No fever
Systemic inflammation	Local inflammation (joint only)
Probable autoimmune origin	Most common arthritis
3:1 in women	2:1 in women
Affects young adults (ages 20–30)	Affects older adults (over age 45) Common in women after menopause More common in obese people
Affects small and large joints (symmetrical); most common in fingers, knees, elbows, ankles	Affects primarily large weight-bearing joints and knuckles (knees, hips, knuckles, spine)
May remain the same for life	May be progressive
Causes inflammatory process in other parts of body (lungs, kidneys, eyes)	Sets up local inflammation Can be hereditary
Surgery does not help (condition returns)	May surgically replace or fuse joints (last choice for treatment)
May have painful nodules on joints	Often have nodules, but do not restrict activity and are not painful
Fingers may swell; joints feel cold and moist; bluish color; muscles may weaken	Joints usually do not swell; muscles remain firm
Joints distorted and dislocated	Not as likely to be disabling; may remain localized
Joints may ankylose (fuse)	Joints usually do not ankylose
Abnormal laboratory values (rheumatoid factor, sedimentation rate high; hemoglobin low)	

NOTE: From Arthritis Foundation, 1314 Spring Street NW, Atlanta, GA 30309. Reprinted with permission.

instability, neurological disorders, and congenital or acquired bone deformities. Primary disease may be inherited as an autosomal recessive trait, causing faulty connective tissue formation in joints, degeneration, and bony hypertrophy or overgrowths in the form of bone spurs. Portions of these bone spurs or cartilage break off, move into the synovial fluid, and cause pain. The articular cartilage continues to deteriorate, bone ends rub against one another, and pain and swelling become the predominant symptoms experienced by the client.

Clinical Manifestations Pain, joint swelling, and stiffness are the predominant symptoms of osteoarthritis. The pain is often described as a deep ache associated with use and weight bearing. The pain may lead to limitation of the client's mobility. Stiffness is transient, usually lasting 15–30 minutes. Joint swelling and deformity result from the development of Heberden's nodes (bony proliferations at the distal interphalangeal joint) and Bouchard's nodes (similar deformities at the proximal interphalangeal joint). As the disease progresses, muscle wasting and spasms occur. Many clients have multiple affected joints and associated constant pain.

The diagnosis is based on clinical assessment and radiological examinations. X-ray studies reveal narrowing of joint spaces due to articular cartilage destruction, bone spurs, cysts, and joint deformity. There are no specific laboratory studies for osteoarthritis. CBC and erythrocyte sedimentation rate (ESR) are usually normal, and rheumatoid factor and antinuclear antibodies are negative.

Therapeutic Management and Nursing Care Therapeutic management of osteoarthritis is directed toward pain management and maintenance of joint function and mobility. The nurse should assess pain, stiffness, limitation in range of motion, joint deformity, symmetry, nodules, and crepitus. Because of the chronic nature of the disease, assessment also includes alteration in body image, functional limitations affecting work and physical activities, changes in family and social roles, and the presence of depression and fatigue. Nursing care should involve in-depth client education that helps the individual to assimilate osteoarthritis into his or her life style. It is important for the nurse to help each client find a balance between rest and activity, while maintaining functional independence. Heat therapy applied to the affected joint may increase comfort, and cold packs can produce an anesthetic effect. Diversional activities such as the use of imagery and relaxation techniques are also useful. Isometric and isotonic exercises can strengthen the muscles that provide support to the affected joints. Proper, balanced nutrition can assist the client in maintaining optimal weight to avoid excessive weight-bearing stress on the affected joints. Analgesics and anti-inflammatory medications are also mainstays of treatment (Table 8-7). In some cases, surgical procedures including joint replacement (arthroplasty), arthrodesis, osteotomy, resection, or synovectomy may be the treatment of choice. Long-term nursing care involves coordinating various health care professionals such as physical and occupational therapists and facilitating the safe use of assistive devices. The nurse can encourage the client to participate in arthritis support groups and provide current information from the Arthritis Foundation.

Rheumatoid Arthritis

This systemic, chronically progressive disease of connective tissue involves symmetric inflammation of the synovial joints leading to joint destruction.

(text continues on 259)

Researchers studying osteoarthritis have found that most of the **cost** associated with treatment of osteoarthritis comes from treating the side effects of medications.

The first ever **guidelines** published by the American College of Rheumatology (ACR) for osteoarthritis of the hip and knee can be obtained by request from the ACR, 60 Executive Park South, Suite 150, Atlanta GA 30329.

Mexican-American folk medicine views illness as an imbalance between hot and cold. Rheumatism and paralysis are thought to be caused by cold "aires" entering the body and are treated with the application of heat and "hot" herbs.

✿

TABLE 8-7

Pharmacology Summary: Agents for Musculoskeletal Disorders

Drugs	Disorders	Dosage	Side Effects	Nursing Implications
Salicylate (aspirin)	Rheumatoid arthritis Osteoarthritis Osteoporosis Osteitis deformans Osteomalacia Bursitis Epicondylitis Low back pain	3.2–6 g/day in divided doses	Gastrointestinal irritation including nausea, vomiting, and abdominal pain Mild liver enzyme elevation Tinnitus (frequent and reversible) Mild salicylism (tinnitus, dizziness, difficulty hearing, vomiting or diarrhea, mental confusion, headache, sweating, hyperventilation)	Therapeutic serum level 150–300 µg/mL before morning dose (after 2–3 weeks of therapy) Take with food or milk or use enteric-coated preparations Monitor for signs of bleeding (bruising) or melena (black stools) Large doses may potentiate peptic ulcer Monitor liver function
Nonsteroidal anti-inflammatory drugs (NSAIDs)	Rheumatoid arthritis Osteoarthritis Gout Bursitis Epicondylitis Osteitis deformans Osteomalacia Osteoporosis Low back pain	See specific drug	See specific drug	General considerations NSAIDs must be administered for 2 weeks to evaluate efficacy Administer with food, milk, or antacids to decrease gastrointestinal irritation Compliance may be enhanced with once or twice daily dosages Monitor renal and hepatic function Monitor dosage and enhanced side effects in elderly persons Not recommended during pregnancy NSAIDs may mask infections
Diclofenac (Voltaren)	Rheumatoid arthritis Osteoarthritis	150–200 mg/day in divided doses for rheumatoid arthritis 100–150 mg/day in divided doses for osteoarthritis	Gastrointestinal irritation Headache Dizziness	See General considerations
Etodolac (Lodine)	Osteoarthritis Tissue inflammation associated with fractures	600–1200 mg/day in divided doses	Gastrointestinal irritation, particularly dyspepsia	See General considerations

Drug	Uses	Dosage	Adverse Effects	Considerations
Fenoprofen calcium (Fenoprofen, Nalfon)	Rheumatoid arthritis Osteoarthritis	300–600 mg three or four times daily	Gastrointestinal irritation Headache Genitourinary problems: dysuria, cystitis, hematuria, nephrotic syndrome Somnolence/drowsiness	Contraindicated with renal disease Improvement may be noted in a few days but may require 2–3 weeks
Flurbiprofen (Ansaid)	Rheumatoid arthritis Osteoarthritis	200–300 mg daily in three or four divided doses	Gastrointestinal irritation Dizziness Headache	See General considerations
Ibuprofen (Motrin, Advil, Nuprin)	Rheumatoid arthritis Osteoarthritis Osteoporosis Osteitis deformans Osteomalacia Epicondylitis	1200–3200 mg/day in three or four divided doses; not to exceed 3200 mg	Gastrointestinal irritation Hypersensitivity reaction Rash/dermatitis	Therapeutic responses in a few days to 2 weeks
Indomethacin (Indocin)	Rheumatoid arthritis Osteoarthritis Osteoporosis Bursitis Gout Osteitis deformans Osteomalacia Epicondylitis	25–50 mg three times daily, not to exceed 200 mg/day, for rheumatoid arthritis and osteoarthritis 75–150 mg/day in divided doses for bursitis 50 mg three times daily for gout	Gastrointestinal irritation: Feeling of dissociation (especially in elderly patients) Severe headaches	Contraindicated with active gastric lesions Use with caution in individuals with depressive disorders, epilepsy, and parkinsonism Administer with food, milk, or antacids Adverse effects correlate with dosage, and women may have increased intensity of side effects
Ketoprofen (Orudis)	Rheumatoid arthritis Osteoarthritis	150–300 mg/day, in divided doses, not to exceed 300 mg/day	Gastrointestinal irritation, particularly dyspepsia Headache	See General considerations
Meclofenamate (Meclomen)	Rheumatoid arthritis Osteoarthritis	200–400 mg/day, in three or four divided doses, not to exceed 400 mg/day	Gastrointestinal irritation, particularly dyspepsia Headache Rash/dermatitis Drowsiness/somnolence	Contraindicated in patients with renal disease or active ulceration or inflammation of upper or lower gastrointestinal tract May administer with food or milk Improvement in a few days with optimal

TABLE 8-7 (continued)

PHARMACOLOGY SUMMARY: AGENTS FOR MUSCULOSKELETAL DISORDERS

Drugs	Disorders	Dosage	Side Effects	Nursing Implications
Nabumetone (Relafen)	Rheumatoid arthritis Osteoarthritis	1000–2000 mg/day	Gastrointestinal irritation, particularly diarrhea, dyspepsia, and distress/cramps/pain Drowsiness/somnolence	See General considerations
Naproxen (Naprosyn, Anaprox)	Rheumatoid arthritis Osteoarthritis Bursitis Gout Epicondylitis	250–500 mg twice daily for rheumatoid arthritis and osteoarthritis 750 mg initially, then 250 mg three times daily for gout	Gastrointestinal irritation Headache Tinnitus Pulmonary infiltrates Drowsiness/somnolence	Therapeutic effect generally within 2 weeks Monitor hepatic and renal studies
Piroxicam (Feldene)	Rheumatoid arthritis Osteoarthritis Gout Bursitis	20 mg/day	Gastrointestinal irritation Allergic reaction	Assess therapeutic effects at 2 weeks
Sulindac (Clinoril)	Rheumatoid arthritis Osteoarthritis Gout Bursitis Epicondylitis	150–200 mg twice daily, not to exceed 400 mg	Gastrointestinal irritation Rash/dermatitis Hypersensitivity	Do not administer with active gastro-intestinal lesions Administer with food Therapeutic response in approximately 1 week for 50% of patients
Tolmetin sodium (Tolectin)	Rheumatoid arthritis Osteoarthritis	300–1800 mg/day in divided doses	Gastrointestinal irritation Tinnitus Headache Anaphylactoid reaction	Take on arising and at bedtime Take with antacids other than sodium bicarbonate; bioavailability affected by milk and food
Pyrazoline Derivatives Phenylbutazone (Azolid, Butazolidin)	Rheumatoid arthritis Osteoarthritis Gout Epicondylitis Bursitis	Initial dose 300–600 mg/day in divided doses; maintenance dose not to exceed 400 mg/day Rheumatoid arthritis and osteoarthritis: 400 mg followed by 100 mg every 4 hours	Gastrointestinal irritation, particularly abdominal discomfort and distress Fluid retention Bone marrow depression Agranulocytosis and aplastic anemia Drowsiness	Trial period of 1 week recommended Use with caution in adults older than 40 years Use only after NSAIDs have proven unsatisfactory Monitor hematologic values Take with food or milk

NOTE: From *Principles and practice of adult health nursing* (3rd ed., pp. 1269–1273), by P. G. Beare and J. L. Myers, 1998, St. Louis, MO: Mosby. Reprinted with permission.

Some theories suggest that a triggering mechanism within the body (possibly a virus) causes overactivity in the immune system, resulting in the secretion of excess synovial fluid, swelling within the joints, and inflammation of the synovial lining. As overgrowth of the synovial lining ensues, the joint capsule is invaded, and the cartilage and bone erode. The joint becomes painful as bone rubs against bone (crepitus). Eventually, fibrous connective tissue replaces the cartilage and joint capsule, resulting in subluxation (partial joint dislocation), ankylosis (joint fusion), and consolidation of the affected joints.

Onset of rheumatoid arthritis often occurs between the ages of 25 and 55 and is three times more prevalent in women. It is probably the most debilitating and painful form of arthritis, having significant deleterious life-style effects on women in their childbearing years, individuals during otherwise productive work years, and older adults.

Clinical Manifestations The primary signs and symptoms of rheumatoid arthritis are joint pain and swelling, warmth, and decreased ROM. Systemic manifestations that precede localized symptoms include vague muscle aches, anorexia, and fatigue. The characteristic morning stiffness in multiple joints usually lasts longer than 30 minutes and frequently involves symmetric joints. Firm, nontender nodules grow over bony prominences. Characteristic deformities include swan-neck deformity of the hands (hyperextension of the proximal interphalangeal joints), boutonniere deformity (flexion of the proximal interphalangeal joints), and ulnar drift. The small joints of the hands, wrists, and feet are most commonly affected. Systemic symptoms such as malaise, anorexia, weight loss due to chronic pain, and low-grade fever may continue as the disease progresses.

Laboratory studies reveal an elevated ESR, normochromic or hypochromic anemia, and a positive rheumatoid factor (reactive immunoglobulin M [IgM] molecule with elevated titers). Many clients also have antinuclear antibodies and elevated immunoglobulin G (IgG). Radiological studies reveal soft tissue swelling and osteoporosis in the early disease state and joint space narrowing with destruction of cartilage, deformities, ankylosis, and subluxation in later stages. Analysis of synovial fluid reveals inflammatory effusion.

Assessment Nursing assessment should include evaluation of joint pain, deformity, swelling, erythema, warmth, and limitation of movement. Systemic symptoms such as fever, malaise, and weight loss are also assessed. As with other chronic conditions, the nurse should evaluate the effects of the disease on the client's quality of life, including work, recreation, family roles, and alterations in body image. Because rheumatoid arthritis may be induced or exacerbated by stress, the nurse should assess the client's response to daily stressors and any recent, stressful life events.

Therapeutic Management and Nursing Care The goals of therapeutic management include pain management, maintenance of joint function, and minimization of joint destruction. The primary objective is to reduce inflammation before the joint is permanently damaged.

Treatment may include the use of braces or assistive devices to limit joint use. Cold therapy using cold packs or heat therapy using warm, moist compresses applied to affected joints 30 minutes prior to activity help to decrease pain and increase mobility. Whirlpool, ultrasound, and frequent position changes help prevent muscle spasms, contractures, and minimize stress on joints. The nurse should help the client find the proper balance between rest and activity unique to his or her life style and stage of disease. The use of diversional activities, imagery, and relaxation techniques allows the client active participation in his or her care and facilitates pain relief. Transcutaneous electric nerve stimulation (TENS) may be another option for pain management. ROM, isometric and isotonic exercises, and recreational activities can help maintain joint function, prevent stiffness, and strengthen surrounding muscle groups (Table 8-8). Pharmacological treatment usually begins with high doses of salicylates, 8–10 tablets per day. Nonsteroidal anti-inflammatory drugs (NSAIDs) such as ibuprofen (Motrin), indomethacin (Indocin), sulindac (Clinoril), ketoprofen (Orudis),

🔯

TABLE 8-8

Exercise for Clients with Arthritis

Educate the client to:

- Keep the body in best possible physical condition. Control weight, rest, and exercise.
- Exercise daily, even if there is pain. Do specific exercises, not just daily work.
- Apply heat before exercising to lessen pain. Do not overdo because of lessened pain.
- Prepare for exercise with gentle stretching.
- Do active exercise (self-movement) when possible. If not possible, do isometrics or have someone do passive exercise. May use continuous passive motion machine.
- Do low-impact exercises such as swimming, slow walking, or bicycling.
- Stop exercising if pain becomes severe.
- Use adaptive devices or corrective corset or brace if needed.
- Prevent contractures: turn doorknobs to radial (thumb) side when possible. Flatten hands as much as possible.

NOTE: From *Textbook of basic nursing* (6th ed., p. 1007), by C. B. Rosdahl, 1995, Philadelphia, PA: J. B. Lippincott. Reprinted with permission.

and misoprostol (Cytotec) have become the mainstays of treatment (see Table 8-7). NSAIDs are usually effective in 80% of clients and should be used at least 3–6 months before progressing to disease-modifying drugs such as corticosteroids, hydroxychloroquine, gold compounds, and cytotoxic drugs. Clients treated with these medications must be monitored for side effects. Finally, surgical management, including joint replacement, osteotomy, synovectomy, and arthrodesis, may be necessary if continued physical impairment and chronic pain are unresponsive to medical management.

Ankylosing Spondylitis

This inflammatory arthritis of the spine (sometimes referred to as rheumatoid arthritis of the spine) primarily affects the facet joints and stabilizing ligaments of the spinal column and may lead to eventual fusion. Ankylosing spondylitis affects three times as many men as women and usually manifests before the age of 50.

Clinical Manifestations Early symptoms include chronic lower back and hip pain with stiffness that usually improves with activity. As the disease progresses, there may be cervical and thoracic involvement, and the client may report neck stiffness and impaired breathing if chest expansion is impeded. If the disease progresses to a severe state, kyphosis and curvature of the chest may develop. The diagnosis is based on a clinical presentation demonstrating a reduction of motion of the lumbar spine or chest wall and/or radiographic evidence of sacroiliitis. X-ray studies usually reveal erosions of the sacroiliac joint that result in widening and eventually complete ankylosis. Ankylosing spondylitis seems to have a genetic association with the human leukocyte antigen (HLA) haplotype, HLA-B27, but testing is rarely necessary. Approximately 25–30% of clients experience an associated eye disorder known as uveitis.

Therapeutic Management and Nursing Care Therapeutic management is directed toward maintaining ROM and proper posture. Treatment and nursing care are basically the same as for other types of arthritis and include the administration of NSAIDs and physical therapy for the back.

Gout

Gout is an asymmetric arthritis (monoarticular) with associated hyperuricemia. This inflammation usually affects the peripheral joints, most commonly the metatarsophalangeal joint of the great toe, and is caused by monosodium urate crystal deposition. The etiologic factors associated with primary disease are (1) an inborn error in purine metabolism and production and (2) excessive ingestion of alcohol or a high-purine content diet. Secondary gout can be due to acquired diseases such as myeloproliferative disease, lymphoproliferative disease, hemolytic anemia, glycogen

Throughout history, **gout** has been considered a disease of kings and queens because of its association with protein-rich diets.

storage disease, psoriasis, renal insufficiency, and sarcoidosis. It also can be associated with obesity, starvation, lead intoxication, and the ingestion of certain drugs (salicylates, diuretics, pyrazinamide, ethambutol, nicotinic acid, and alcohol). The peak incidence of gout occurs between the ages of 40 and 60 and primarily affects men.

Uric acid crystals are the end product of purine metabolism and are deposited in the joints and connective tissues as a result of excessive purine intake or abnormal metabolism. Although the knees, wrists, and proximal interphalangeal joints may be affected, the deposits are most commonly found in the metatarsophalangeal joint of the great toe.

Clinical Manifestations

The characteristic manifestations of gout are inflammation and swelling of the affected joint, pain, elevated temperature, and hyperuricemia. The acute phase often begins with an attack of pain, which occurs at night, involving one joint (usually the great toe) and lasting 3–7 days. The attack may be precipitated by sustaining a trauma, taking diuretics (which cause increased tubular resorption of uric acid crystals), drinking alcohol, or eating a high-purine content diet. An intercritical period follows during which the client is asymptomatic. As the disease progresses to the chronic phase, the asymptomatic intervals shorten and more joints are affected. Morning stiffness, joint deformity, and synovial tissue thickening occur. Tophi, nodular formations of uric acid crystals, may develop on the ears, fingers, hands, and Achilles tendons. Fever, renal disease, hypertension, tachycardia, and malaise are systemic manifestations that may accompany the local symptoms.

Assessment

Nursing assessment should include evaluation of local manifestations such as pain, erythema, tenderness, swelling, and limitation of movement. The nurse also should assess for any systemic manifestations, precipitating causes, previous attacks, and family history of gout.

Diagnostic studies include elevated serum uric acid levels (greater than 7.5 mg/dL), analysis of joint fluid for monosodium urate crystals, and ESR and WBCs during an attack. Radiological studies may be ordered to rule out other conditions and may show tophi and soft tissue edema.

Therapeutic Management and Nursing Care

Therapeutic management includes a combination of joint rest, diet therapy, and pharmacotherapy. The client should be instructed to elevate the affected part, to avoid weight bearing and pressure from bed clothing, and to apply cold compresses for pain relief. Acute attacks can be managed with NSAIDs or colchicine for the client who cannot tolerate NSAIDs. Chronic gout (more than three attacks per year) is treated with urate-lowering agents such as allopurinal (Zyloprim) or probenecid (Benemid) preceded by low-dose NSAIDs or colchicine (Table 8-9). Diet therapy includes limiting high-purine content foods (e.g., organ meats, poultry, meat extracts, fish, yeast, asparagus, spinach, mushrooms) and alcohol and weight management. The nurse should encourage the client to drink 3 L of fluids each day to avoid renal calculi formation and instruct him or her to avoid salicylates.

TABLE 8-9

PHARMACOLOGY SUMMARY: URICOSURICS FOR GOUT

Drugs	Dosage	Side Effects	Nursing Considerations
Probenecid (Benemid)	0.5 g twice daily	Headache, nausea, vomiting, anorexia, urinary frequency	Encourage liberal fluid intake to minimize calculus formation Monitor serum uric acid levels Take with food or antacids Avoid concurrent use of salicylates (they decrease uricosuric effect)
Sulfinpyrazone (Anturane)	400–800 mg/day	Upper gastrointestinal disturbances (nausea, dyspepsia); reactivation of peptic ulcer disease	Administer with food, milk, or antacids Maintain adequate fluid intake
Uric acid inhibitors Allopurinol (Zyloprim)	200–600 mg/day	Skin rash, fever, chills, bone marrow depression, gastrointestinal irritation	Monitor liver and renal function in initial month Administer with food Maintain adequate fluid intake Maintain alkaline urine (avoid large doses of vitamin C)
Colchicine	0.5–1.8 mg/day (prophylaxis); 0.5–1.2 mg every 1–2 hours (acute attack)	Bone marrow depression, aplastic anemia, granulocytopenia, leukopenia, thrombocytopenia, nausea, vomiting, diarrhea, cramps, skin rashes	Monitor complete blood count for blood dyscrasias with long-term use Client should avoid alcohol when taking oral form (increases gastric toxicity and decreases drug's effectiveness) Oral form given with food Do not give more than 12 tablets in 24 hours Give at first sign of impending attack Administer intravenous dose over 2–5 minutes Do not give with dextrose 5% or bacteriostatic water (incompatible) Prevent extravasation of intravenous form into surrounding tissue (apply cold compress and give analgesic if this occurs Do not give more than 4 mg/24 hours intravenously

NOTE: From *Principles and practice of adult health nursing* (3rd ed., p. 1301), by P. G. Beare and J. L. Myers, 1998, St. Louis, MO: Mosby. Reprinted with permission.

OTHER MUSCULOSKELETAL DISEASES

Fibromyalgia Syndrome

This insidious, chronic condition consists of a constellation of musculoskeletal symptoms and primarily affects women over the age of 50. The etiology is unknown, although there may be a precipitating physical or emotional event.

Clinical Manifestations The primary manifestations are joint and muscle pain and stiffness, easy fatigability, and sleep difficulties. Clients often report a lack of energy and diffuse pain that causes significant functional impairment affecting work and recreational activities. The pain is usually described as widespread aching and stiffness that is usually worse in the morning and lasts several hours, or in some people, all day. Clients often describe their sleep as nonrestorative, leaving them tired in the morning. Other associated symptoms include paresthesis, headache, anxiety, subjective swelling, and irritable bowel syndrome. Clients may also experience associated psychological disturbances such as depression and anxiety.

This condition is often frustrating for the client, practitioner, and nurse. Characteristically, there is an absence of physical findings on assessment, with the exception of the presence of tender points or trigger points. Diagnostic studies are usually normal and of little value, except to rule out other causes (e.g., hypothyroidism, chronic infection) (Table 8-10).

◙

TABLE 8-10

AMERICAN COLLEGE OF RHEUMATOLOGY 1990 CRITERIA FOR CLASSIFICATION OF FIBROMYALGIA

For classification purposes, clients must satisfy both criteria. Widespread pain must have been experienced for at least 3 months.

1. History of widespread pain
   Definition Pain is considered widespread when all of the following are present:
   • Pain in the left and right sides of the body
   • Pain above and below the waist
   • Axial skeletal pain (cervical spine, anterior chest, thoracic spine, or low back
   In this definition, shoulder pain and buttock pain are considered as pain for each involved side. "Low back" is considered lower segment pain.
2. Pain in 11 of 18 tender point sites on digital palpation
   Definition Pain must be present in at least 11 of the following 18 tender point sites:

- Occiput: bilateral, at the suboccipital muscle insertions
- Low cervical: bilateral, at the anterior aspects of the intertransverse spaces at C5–C7
- Trapezius: bilateral, at the midpoint of the upper border
- Supraspinatus: bilateral at origins, above the scapula spine near the medial border
- Second rib: bilateral, at the second costochondral junctions, just lateral to the junctions on upper surfaces
- Lateral epicondyle: bilateral, 2 cm distal to the epicondyles
- Gluteal: bilateral, in upper quadrants of buttocks in anterior fold of muscle
- Greater trochanter: bilateral, posterior to the trochanteric prominence
- Knee: bilateral, at the medial fat pad proximal to the joint line

For a tender point to be considered "positive," the client must state that the palpation was painful.

NOTE: From "The American College of Rheumatology 1990 criteria for the classification of fibromyalgia," by F. Wolfe, 1990, *Arthritis and Rheumatism*, 33 (2), pp. 160–173. Reprinted with permission.

Therapeutic Management and Nursing Care Treatment is primarily symptomatic and focuses on long-term goals of the maintenance of functional abilities and pain management. Due to the vague, nonspecific nature of the symptoms, clients often need to have their diagnosis reconfirmed and to be reassured that the disease is not life threatening. Nursing care centers on emotional and psychological support, as the nurse recognizes and validates the client's symptoms despite the lack of significant physical findings. Physical therapy including ultrasound, heat, and massage may be helpful. The nurse should instruct the client to get adequate rest and regular sleep at night and encourage him or her to participate in gentle, low-impact exercise late in the day. Pharmacotherapy involves analgesics (acetaminophen [Tylenol] or NSAIDs), low-dose psychotropics (amitriptyline [Elavil]) at bedtime, and sleeping pills (temazepam [Restoril], triazolam [Halcion]). Some practitioners inject trigger points with local anesthetics and steroids. Referral to chronic pain centers should be considered. The nurse should be cognizant of the client's assimilation of this chronic condition into his or her life and assess for indications of depression and anxiety.

CASE STUDY: FIBROMYALGIA

Jean, a 54-year-old woman, has been experiencing musculoskeletal "achy" pain for the past 6 months. She has had sleep difficulties for nearly 1 year with frequent nocturnal awakening since the tragic death of her oldest son. Often she awakens in the morning without feeling rested. She describes her pain as "all over" and indicates her neck, thoracic spine, and lower torso. Her physician examines her and finds pain on digital palpation in 12 tender point sites throughout her body. Various diagnostic tests show a negative serum rheumatoid factor; ESR is within normal limits, and no abnormalities are found on the x-rays. CBC indicates mild anemia, and the chemistry panel is normal. Based on the criteria from the American College of Rheumatology, Jean's physician diagnoses her with fibromyalgia. She is prescribed iron supplements, naproxen sodium (Anaprox) 275 mg every 6–8 hours, physical therapy treatments, and weekly counseling sessions with a psychiatric mental health nurse practitioner. She is also referred to Good Grief, a support group for individuals who have recently lost loved ones. The nurse in the medical clinic provides her with education and literature about her newly diagnosed disease, and Jean is scheduled to follow up with her primary care practitioner in 2 months.

Osteitis Deformans (Paget's Disease)

In this disease, there is excessive bone destruction characterized by accelerated bone resorption, causing cavities in the lamellar bone and resulting in deformity and increased risk of fracture. Paget's disease is more common in men, and the rate of incidence increases with age. The etiology is unknown, although there is some supporting evidence that suggests a slow viral infection. Affected bones are soft, large, and deformed with a rate of bone turnover that is sometimes greater than 20 times normal. Dense trabecular bone replaces normal bone.

Clinical Manifestations Clinical manifestations depend on the bones affected, but many clients are asymptomatic. The bones most commonly affected are the lumbar spine, sacrum, pelvis, femur, and skull. Clients may report pain in the affected part, swelling or deformity, and disturbance of their gait due to unequal leg lengths. If skull enlargement occurs, they may experience headache, blindness, deafness, or neuralgia. Laboratory studies reveal elevated alkaline phosphatase, but usually normal serum calcium and phosphorus. Radiological studies show the underlying pathology of microfractures and a characteristic mosaic pattern within the affected bone.

Assessment The nurse should assess the client for pain, fatigue, and specific skeletal findings such as bowlegs, shortened stature, enlarged skull, and pathological fractures.

Therapeutic Management and Nursing Care Therapeutic management is based on the degree of deformity and severity of pain. Complications such as spinal cord compression, osteosarcoma, and, rarely, high cardiac output failure may develop. Pharmacotherapy involves analgesics (aspirin, NSAIDs), calcitonin (Calcimar) to reduce osteoclastic activity, and etidronate disodium (Didronel), which can promote remission of the disease (Table 8-11). Ongoing care centers on safety precautions in the home and basic first aid instruction should potential injuries or fractures occur.

TABLE 8-11

PHARMACOTHERAPY FOR OSTEITIS DEFORMANS

Drug	Dosage	Side Effects	Nursing Implications
Calcitonin	50–100 IU daily	Nausea Flushing Feeling of warmth	Monitor serum alkaline, urinary hydroxy-proline excretion; use of salmon calci-tonin hormone approved
Plicamycin	15 μ/kg daily for 10 days	Thrombocytopenia Elevated serum glutamic-oxaloacetic transaminase (SGOT), blood urea nitrogen (BUN), and creatinine Anorexia Nausea, vomiting	Contraindicated for clients with impaired bone marrow function
Etidronate sodium	5–10 mg/kg daily for 6 months maximum	Gastrointestinal irritation Diarrhea Metallic taste or loss of taste Abdominal discomfort	Cautious use with impaired renal function Large doses may result in fracture or osteomalacia Contraindicated with immobilized patients

NOTE: From *Principles and practice of adult health nursing* (2nd ed., p. 1618), by P. G. Beare and J. L. Myers, 1994, St. Louis, MO: Mosby. Reprinted with permission.

Osteomalacia

Osteomalacia is the lack of normal calcium and phosphorus deposition in the bone matrix that results in uncalcified bone. Calcium, phosphorus, and vitamin D are needed for normal bone mineralization. Vitamin D facilitates the absorption of calcium from the gastrointestinal tract, and calcium is the transport medium for phosphorus. Inadequate vitamin D prevents the calcium and phosphorus from being deposited into the bone matrix, resulting in unmineralized bone. Risk factors include dietary deficiency of calcium or vitamin D, intestinal malabsorption of vitamin D, inadequate vitamin D synthesis (limited ultraviolet exposure, increased melanin pigmentation), long-term anticonvulsant therapy, chronic renal failure, cirrhosis, and long-term parenteral nutrition. Bone consistency is soft, and bowing often occurs.

Clinical Manifestations

The primary symptoms are bone pain, tenderness on palpation, and muscle weakness. The pain usually increases with activity, most commonly affecting the lower extremities, spine, pelvis, and ribs. Laboratory studies usually reveal elevated alkaline phosphatase and other abnormalities, depending on the underlying etiology. X-rays may reveal small discontinuities in the bone cortex and fractures in advanced disease states.

Therapeutic Management and Nursing Care

Therapeutic management is based on the underlying etiology of the disease, but vitamin D supplementation is the usual treatment. Additional treatments may include calcium supplements and ultraviolet light exposure. The goals of nursing care are directed toward pain management, injury prevention, and preservation of a healthy body image. The nurse should assess the client's environment for safety and fall risks. The nurse also coordinates consultations with a nutritionist for dietary counseling and administers any exogenous vitamin D or calcium, as ordered. The client should be encouraged to participate in outdoor activities to increase exposure to ultraviolet light. Client education includes the identification of dietary sources of calcium and vitamin D, safety precautions, and the use of any needed ambulatory devices.

Osteomyelitis

This is an infection of the bone, classified as either (1) hematogenous (acute), which is bloodborne from a distant source, or (2) contiguous (chronic), which develops from adjacent soft tissue infection. The infecting organism may be bacterial, viral, or fungal.

Acute hematogenous osteomyelitis occurs primarily in children under 12 years of age and usually affects rapidly growing long bones. In chronic osteomyelitis microorganisms invade the bone tissue through blood, extension of adjacent infected soft tissue, or direct entry. *Staphylococcus* is the primary pathogen; gram-negative bacteria and anaerobes are the second most common.

In adults, hematogenous osteomyelitis usually involves the spine. Hemodialysis, urinary tract infections, and bacterial endocarditis often provide the source for bloodborne infections. Pressure sores, soft tissue trauma, necrosis associated with malignancy, and radiation therapy and burns can also extend an infectious process to the bone. Sinus and ear infections and abscessed teeth may result in osteomyelitis of the mandible or skull. Compound fractures, surgical procedures, and puncture wounds that traumatize underlying bone are common causes of *traumatic osteomyelitis*. Osteomyelitis is found most often in older adults, because many of the precipitating conditions are associated with aging.

Clinical Manifestations Clinical manifestations depend on the etiology and location of the infected bone. Pain, fever, localized tenderness, erythema, and edema may be reported. The development of these symptoms in a postoperative period or after the initial treatment for a soft tissue infection may indicate osteomyelitis. If the vertebral bodies are affected, nonspecific complaints of fever, chills, and backache may be reported. Laboratory studies may reveal an elevated WBC count and ESR; blood cultures can identify the causative organism. Radiographic studies, a bone scan, and a CT scan can confirm the diagnosis.

Assessment The nurse should assess the client for predisposing factors (such as diabetes, prosthetic joint implantation, sinus and oral infections), localized pain, erythema, swelling, and fever.

Therapeutic Management and Nursing Care The goals of therapeutic management include resolution of the infection, management of pain, and avoidance of complications of immobility. Treatment is based on the type of osteomyelitis. Long-term antibiotic therapy is the foundation of treatment and is often effective alone in acute hematogenous osteomyelitis, if administered before there is extensive bone damage. However, antibiotics alone are not effective in chronic osteomyelitis or when it is associated with a foreign body. In these cases, surgical removal of necrotic bone and tissue must be included for effective treatment. Parenteral antibiotics should be administered as ordered, often for as long as 6 weeks. The client may require prolonged bed rest; and home health nursing and coordination with community resources and social services for additional assistance may be required. Client education should include everything pertaining to home antibiotic therapy—site care, preparation and storage of medication, equipment use, and phone numbers for assistance. Prescribed analgesics and imagery and relaxation techniques may help the client control his or her discomfort. The nurse should encourage the client to perform ROM, isotonic, and isometric exercises to maintain muscle strength and joint flexibility.

Neoplasms

There are two types of bone tumors (neoplasms), primary and metastatic. Tumors that originate in the bone (primary) include benign lesions such as osteomas, chondromas, giant cell tumors, cysts, and osteoid osteomas. *Primary benign tumors* are slow growing, well circumscribed, and rarely spread. *Primary malignant tumors* are rare in adults and include osteosarcoma and multiple myelomas. Malignant tumors often metastasize to the lungs during early development. Osteosarcoma is a primary bone malignancy that is found in children and adolescents. Metastatic bone tumors usually originate in the lungs, breast, prostate, kidneys, ovaries, or thyroid. They are more common than primary bone tumors and have a poor prognosis. Carcinomas metastasize to bone more often than sarcomas.

Clinical Manifestations The most common clinical manifestations are pain, swelling, restricted movement, aching, and pathological fractures. Radiographical studies, MRI, and CT scans of the affected bone provide diagnostic information. A needle biopsy is the definitive diagnostic procedure. A chest x-ray is performed to evaluate possible metastasis.

Therapeutic Management and Nursing Care The goals of treatment are preservation of the affected part and, of course, cure if the tumor is malignant. Therapy includes surgical intervention, chemotherapy, and radiation, depending on the type of tumor and extent of the disease. Treatment of metastatic bone tumors is often palliative. Nursing care should be directed toward client comfort, pain management, safety, and prevention of pathologic fractures. The nurse should be cognizant of the emotional and psychological factors associated with a diagnosis of metastatic disease and support the client and his or her family throughout the process.

Muscular Dystrophy (MD)

MD describes a group of degenerative, inherited diseases of the skeletal muscles characterized by slowly progressive, symmetric weakness. Various dystrophies are distinguished by age at onset, pattern of weakness, associated symptoms, and heredity pattern.

Myotonic dystrophy is the most common form of the disease and affects adolescents or young adults. The characteristic symptom is myotonia, persistent muscle contraction caused by uncontrolled electrical discharges resulting in stiffness or incoordination. Muscle weakness affects the distal extremities involving the ankle dorsiflexor, plantar flexor, and the hands. Atrophy of the facial muscles occurs and results in ptosis. Clients develop "swan neck," the narrowing of the lower part of the face and forward curvature of the neck. Myotonic dystrophy is associated with cardiac arrhythmias, cataracts, and mild diabetes. Clients often live into their fifth decade, and death usually occurs as a result of cardiac complications.

Duchenne's muscular dystrophy affects males only (X-linked recessive pattern) and is usually diagnosed between the ages of 3 and 5, when parents seek advice because their child falls frequently when attempting to run. Duchenne's is the most devastating of the dystrophies, with a steady progression of weakness, causing the child to be wheelchair-bound by the age of 10. This disease is characterized by weakened pelvic muscles, wide stance with a waddling gait, lordosis, protuberant abdomen, and muscle atrophy. Despite excellent supportive care, most clients die between the ages of 18 and 25 due to complications of an underlying cardiomyopathy or respiratory problems.

Becker's muscular dystrophy is genetically similar to Duchenne's but milder and more variable and usually does not appear until the adolescent or young adult years. The clients have difficulty rising from low positions and eventual arm weakness. Some have very little skeletal muscle destruction but experience disproportionate muscular pain. The disease progression is variable. Some clients remain ambulatory for their entire life, while others are wheelchair-bound in their thirties. Becker's differs from Duchenne's as the former lacks the prominent cardiomyopathy. Some clients do not develop cardiomyopathy, while others have mild skeletal disease but severe cardiomyopathy resulting in heart failure.

Fascioscapulohumeral muscular dystrophy is a slowly progressive disease involving atrophy and weakness of the shoulder and facial muscles. The characteristic facial muscle weakness usually involves the eye muscles. There is no associated cardiomyopathy, and most clients remain ambulatory at the age of 40 and live a nearly normal life span.

Limb-girdle muscular dystrophy, once considered one of the major dystrophies, may actually represent more of a syndrome than a specific disease. Many clients previously diagnosed with this dystrophy are now diagnosed with Becker's dystrophy. Characteristics of this disease are slowly progressive atrophy and weakness of the hip and shoulder muscles. Clients often live a normal life span.

Therapeutic Management and Nursing Care Diagnosis of MD is based on clinical presentation, serum creatinine phosphokinase (CPK), electromyography, and muscle tissue biopsy. Serum CPK is related to muscle degeneration and may be extremely elevated. Electromyography determines nerve conduction and muscle innervation and is essential for evaluating clients with MD. Because MD is relatively rare, it is most accurately and economically evaluated in a neuromuscular clinic. The Muscular Dystrophy Association supports many clinics throughout the United States.

Because there is no cure for MD, therapeutic management focuses on slowing down the progression of immobility and managing symptoms. The nurse should assess the client's muscle strength, degree of mobility, contractures, and cardiovascular and respiratory status. Nursing interventions are primarily supportive as there is no known therapy that can arrest the progression of MD. The nurse should encourage clients to maintain independence and self-care abilities, which can enhance their sense of autonomy. If the client is ambulatory, an exercise regimen is important. Teach clients how to splint their arms and legs at night to help slow the development of contractures. Address safety issues such as fall precautions, the use of assistive devices (braces, canes, walkers, helmet), and environmental adaptations. If the client is bedridden or wheelchair-bound, suggest frequent turning and repositioning for comfort with the use of bolsters, pillows, alternating pressure mattress, or a water bed. It is important to perform frequent skin assessments to prevent breakdown. Dependent edema can be reduced by the use of support stockings, leg elevation, and passive exercise. Encourage the client to eat a balanced, healthy, high-fiber diet to prevent constipation and obesity. As with any progressively deteriorating condition, provide the client and his or her family with emotional support and encouragement throughout the course of the disease.

Overuse Syndromes—Bursitis and Epicondylitis

The bursae are small, fluid-filled sacs located between the muscles and joints. *Bursitis* is the inflammation of this sac, usually caused by repeated use or trauma to the joint. Inflammation is accompanied by an increase in fluid that causes distention. In time, the wall of the bursa hardens and becomes calcified. The most commonly affected joints are the shoulders and hips.

Epicondylitis, often called tennis elbow, is caused by damaged tendons of the medial or lateral radial and ulnar epicondyles that become inflamed, resulting in tissue scarring. Repeated use that requires pronation and supination of the hand, such as tennis or hammering, can lead to epicondylitis.

Clinical Manifestations Symptoms of both bursitis and epicondylitis include pain, limited ROM, swelling, and erythema. The client with epicondylitis may also have a weakened hand grip and decreased arm strength.

Therapeutic Management and Nursing Care The goals of treatment are relief of pain and swelling and restoration of normal mobility. Therapeutic management includes joint rest, cold and moist heat therapies, NSAIDs, and corticosteroid injections. The nurse should assess joint involvement by evaluating pain, swelling, erythema, and any limitation of motion. Bilateral hand grasps should also be evaluated. Modified activities to decrease joint use and trauma and to promote healing are fundamental to therapy. Activities may be restricted for as long as 4–6 weeks. If conservative measures are unsuccessful, some practitioners give corticosteroid injections into the affected site. Nursing interventions should promote self-care activities and encourage the client to continue to participate in social and work activities despite the limitations of the affected joint.

$\mathcal{S}$UMMARY

The musculoskeletal system works harmoniously to allow human beings independence and discovery. Any disorder of this system, traumatic or chronic, can potentially limit the client's ability to function independently in daily life. The nurse must be prepared to provide appropriate assessment, planning, implementation, and evaluation of a wide range of problems requiring immediate acute treatment to long-term supportive care. As clients are encouraged to participate in health promotive activities such as exercise and outdoor recreational activities, the incidence of injuries may continue to increase. Additionally, as the elderly make up an ever-growing proportion of the general population, the morbidity rate of chronic musculoskeletal diseases is likely to rise. Although alterations in this system are among the oldest known conditions, the current trends of the 1990s continue to require the nurse to have a strong foundation in the function and disorders of the musculoskeletal system.

KEY WORDS

Alignment	MRI
Cast	NSAID
Compartment syndrome	ORIF
Dislocation	Osteomyelitis
DJD	ROM
Fracture	Splint
Gait	Sprain
Immobility	Strain
Internal fixation	Tendon
Joint	Traction
Ligament	

QUESTIONS

1. RICE is
   A. a means of measurement of joint and extremity range of motion (ROM).
   B. the foundation for treatment of the muscular dystrophy diseases.
   C. the primary treatment for soft tissue injuries, such as strains and sprains.
   D. a representation of active ROM exercises.

2. Which of the following statements about rheumatoid arthritis is not true?
   A. Rheumatoid arthritis most commonly affects individuals between the ages of 25 and 55.
   B. This form of arthritis is more common in women than men.
   C. Clinical manifestations include both local joint symptoms and systemic symptoms.
   D. Characteristic physical signs include Herberden's and Bouchard's nodes.

3. An adult client recovering from a fractured femur exhibits confusion; a respiratory rate of 36 breaths/min; dyspnea; and a flat, red skin rash. Which of the following complications is the most likely cause?

   A. compartmental syndrome
   B. fat emboli syndrome
   C. osteomyelitis
   D. osteoporosis

4. Client education for the individual with gout includes:

   A. dietary instructions to limit meat, poultry, organ meats, and alcohol
   B. dietary instructions to limit complex carbohydrates such as flat bread, rice, and pasta
   C. instructions for proper cast care
   D. signs and symptoms of compartment syndrome, a major complication

5. Bursitis and epicondylitis are

   A. caused by an inherited genetic abnormality and characterized by muscle fiber degeneration.
   B. usually caused by long-term immobility and treated with increased exercise and activity.
   C. associated with trauma or overuse of a joint and treated with restriction of activities for up to 4–6 weeks.
   D. best treated with skeletal traction.

ANSWERS

1. *The answer is* C. RICE stands for rest, ice, compression, and elevation, the primary treatment for soft tissue injuries such as contusions, strains, and sprains.

2. *The answer is* D. Herberden and Bouchard's nodes are characteristic of osteoarthritis. Swan neck deformity and ulnar drift are common deformities of rheumatoid arthritis.

3. *The answer is* B. Symptoms of fat emboli syndrome are dyspnea, restlessness, agitation, confusion, tachypnea, tachycardia, fever, petechial skin rash, and diffuse rales.

4. *The answer is* A. Treatment of gout includes dietary restriction of high-purine content foods such as meats, poultry, fish, yeast, certain vegetables, and limitation of alcohol intake.

5. *The answer is* C. Overuse syndromes such as bursitis and epicondylitis involve inflammation and tissue scarring. They are treated with joint rest, cold and heat therapies, NSAIDs, and occasionally corticosteroid injections.

ANNOTATED REFERENCES

Beare, P. G., & Myers, J. L. (1994). *Principles and practice of adult health nursing* (2nd ed.). St. Louis, MO: Mosby.

This comprehensive text offers a thorough examination of nursing care of the adult individual based on a body systems approach. Nursing assessment and management of common disorders of each system are explained, taking into consideration the nursing process and changes throughout the life span.

Clark, C. C. (1996). *Wellness practitioner: Concepts, research, and strategies* (2nd ed.). New York: Springer Publishing.

This book provides a resource for the development of health care professionals as wellness practitioners. It is also useful for the lay public who may want to provide self-care measures to enhance wellness. It includes topics such as stress management, nutritional wellness, exercise and movement, self-care, and therapeutic touch.

Giger, J. N., & Davidhizar, R. E. (1995). *Transcultural nursing: Assessment and intervention.* St. Louis, MO: Mosby.

This text provides a framework for cultural assessment that focuses on the key cultural phenomena of communication, space, social organization, time, environmental control and biological variations. The authors explore how different cultural groups in the United States vary in the six phenomena and how to take these variations into account when planning care.

Kee, J. L. (1995). *Laboratory and diagnostic tests with nursing implications* (4th ed.). Norwalk, CT: Appleton & Lange.

This resource presents laboratory tests alphabetically and includes reference values, test descriptions, clinical problems, nursing implications, and client education.

Lilley, L. L., Aucker, R. S., & Albanese, J. A. (1996). *Pharmacology and the nursing process.* St. Louis, MO: Mosby.

This book presents pharmacotherapeutics in an easy-to-read and accessible format, including excellent visual graphics of tables and charts. Drugs are classified by body system and drug function. The text includes cultural, legal, and ethical implications, research and home health issues, and life-span considerations.

Selfridge-Thomas, J. (1995). *Manual of emergency nursing.* Philadelphia: W. B. Saunders.

This manual provides a quick reference to common health problems seen in the emergency department and is organized according to the nursing process. It has a chapter on musculoskeletal conditions and immediate primary treatments.

Werbach, M. R. (1996). *Nutritional influences on illness: A sourcebook of clinical research* (2nd ed.). Tarzana, CA: Third Line Press.

This is a compilation of recent research on the dietary influences on various disease states. Each chapter presents statements concerning relevant nutrients that are followed by a brief description of selected literature which may substantiate or refute the statement. Abstracts are presented for the readers to identify possible literature review to expand their knowledge about each disease state and its nutritional considerations.

INTERNET SITES FOR ADDITIONAL INFORMATION

Arthritis Foundation
  http://www.arthritis.org/

Muscular Dystrophy Association
  http://www.mdausa.org/

March of Dimes
  http://www.modimes.org/

Legacy of Health for Rheumatic Clients
  http://www.rheumatic.org/

National Fibromyalgia Research Association
  http://www.teleport.com/~nfra

Paget Foundation
  http://www.osteo.org/paget.htm/

National Institute of Arthritis and Musculoskeletal and Skin Diseases
  http://www.hih.gob/niams/

☙ THE NEUROLOGICAL SYSTEM

*I*NTRODUCTION

All of the body's systems depend upon an adequately functioning neurological system. The **nervous system** directly and indirectly controls many of our bodily processes and systems. It is the center for thought, recollection, reasoning, feeling, communication, language, movement, cognition, character, and conduct. Most nurses at some point treat clients with disorders either directly or indirectly related to the nervous system. Individuals with neurological system deficits such as an acute head injury or more chronic disorders such as Parkinson's disease may face life-threatening emergencies. Learning about the nervous system may seem like an overwhelming challenge. However, if you learn a little at a time, and apply the basic anatomy and physiology you already know as well as what is presented here, you will develop expertise in caring for neurologically impaired clients.

*A*NATOMY AND PHYSIOLOGY REVIEW

The nervous system is composed of two major parts. The central nervous system (CNS) includes the brain and spinal cord, and the peripheral nervous system includes 12 pairs of cranial nerves and 31 pairs of spinal nerves to facilitate communication with all parts of the body. The cranial

The **nervous system** includes the central nervous system (brain and spinal cord) and the peripheral nervous system (12 pairs cranial nerves, 31 pairs spinal nerves).

Three basic functions of the nervous system are to:

1. Receive stimuli from external and internal environments.
2. Interpret stimuli.
3. Transmit messages for action.

A **neuron** is the active conducting cell or basic unit of the nervous system. Neurons may be unipolar, having a single branch from the nucleus, bipolar, having a single axon and a single dendrite, or multipolar, having several processes serving as either axons or dendrites.

An **axon** is the process of a neuron that carries an impulse away from a nerve cell body and is capable of releasing a neurotransmitter such as acetylcholine.

and spinal nerves branch from the brain and spinal cord to nerve endings throughout the body. The nervous system has **three basic functions**: (1) to receive stimuli from the external and internal environments, (2) to interpret stimuli, and (3) to transmit messages for action.

The 10 billion nerve cells in the nervous system are termed **neurons**. The neuron is the active conducting cell or basic unit of the nervous system; it does the work (Fig. 9-1). The neuron is composed of three parts. The first part is a central cell body termed the *soma*, which is composed primarily of nucleic cytoplasm. The second part is the **axon**, or central cylinder, which is a nerve fiber. Each neuron has one axon that carries information away from the cell body. Some axons are surrounded by myelin sheaths. A myelin sheath is composed of white lipoprotein (a fatty substance) that speeds the transmission of impulses and protects and insulates the axon. This outer covering is termed the neurolemma. In addition to the myelin sheath, or neurolemma, nodes of Ranvier are located along the axons between the lengths of myelin sheaths. The third component of the neuron is the **dendrite**. Most neurons have many dendrites and only one axon. Dendrites are tree-like branches that carry information toward the cell body. The axon and dendrites comprise the neuron's structural components (Fig. 9-2).

Neurons are classified as sensory, motor, or internuncial. Sensory neurons, also termed afferent neurons, receive messages from the skin and other sense organs that are then carried to the brain and spinal cord. The second class of neuron is the motor neuron. These carry messages from the brain and spinal cord to muscles and glands. Motor neurons are also termed efferent neurons. The third class, internuncial neurons, connect motor neurons to sensory neurons. Internuncial neurons are located only in the CNS (i.e., the brain and spinal cord).

Impulses are conducted by neurons electrically and chemically. The electrical aspect involves conduction along nerve fibers. For example, the

FIGURE 9-1
◙
Diagram of neuron.

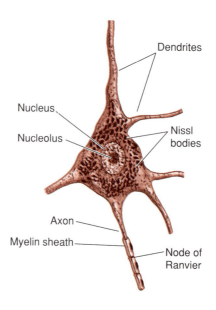

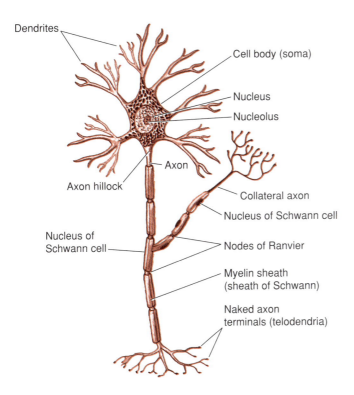

Dendrites

Cell body (soma)

Nucleus

Nucleolus

Axon

Axon hillock

Collateral axon

Nucleus of Schwann cell

Nucleus of Schwann cell

Nodes of Ranvier

Myelin sheath
(sheath of Schwann)

Naked axon
terminals (telodendria)

FIGURE 9-2

Peripheral nerve.

heart contains electrically charged nerve cells that facilitate the flow of electrolytes. When depolarization occurs, sodium (Na^+) moves into the cell, and potassium (K^+) moves out. Then, during repolarization the reverse occurs. This action takes place via the nodes of Ranvier (see Chapter 4 for more information on electrical nerve conduction). Chemical nerve conduction involves a chemical located at the end of the axon. At the end of each axon are axon gaps termed *synapses*. The axon sends impulses across the synapse to another nerve cell, muscle, or gland but does not touch the recipient of its message. A chemical mediator is required to successfully convey the message. These chemical mediators are produced in the nerve endings. The three major neurotransmitters or chemical mediators are (1) **acetylcholine**, (2) **epinephrine**, and (3) **norepinephrine.** Epinephrine is known as "Adrenaline in a bottle" and norepinephrine as "Levophed in a bottle." Chemical mediators alone are responsible for chemical conduction of nerve impulses. The neurotransmitter waits in little sacs or vesicles at the end of the axon. The vesicles merge with the membrane, and the neurotransmitter is released into the synaptic gap. The neurotransmitter travels across the gap and binds to receptor sites in the receiving membrane. This process occurs very rapidly. Chemical and electrical conduction only occurs in one direction. Axons conduct impulses away from cell bodies, and dendrites conduct impulses toward cell bodies. Some chemical mediators are inactivated, some recycled, and some destroyed after conduction occurs (Fig. 9-3).

A **dendrite** is a branching process of a neuron that has neurotransmitter receptors or specialized endings for the reception of stimuli. Dendrites conduct impulses toward the neuron cell body.

Three Classes of Neurons

1. Sensory neuron
2. Motor neuron
3. Internuncial neuron

Three Major Chemical Mediators

1. Acetylcholine
2. Epinephrine
3. Norepinephrine

Acetylcholine is an acetic acid ester of choline; in humans, it is the most widely used transmitter of impulses between nerves and across junctions of nerves and muscles.

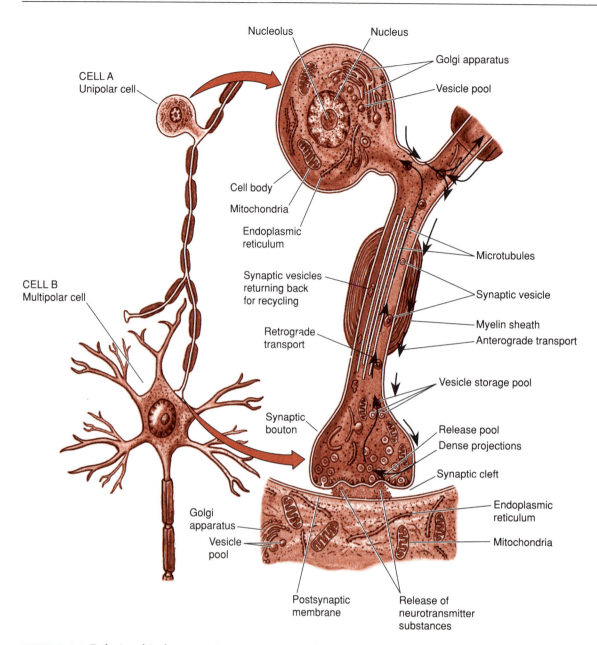

FIGURE 9-3 Relationship between 2 neurons in a pathway.

Epinephrine is the primary stimulatory hormone released by the adrenal glands located above the kidney. It is the "fight-or-flight" hormone.

Supporting cells are another type of nerve cell in the nervous system. Examples of supporting cells are **neuroglial cells** and peripheral cells. These glue-like cells are considered the "housekeepers" because they support, protect, and nourish the nervous system. Supporting cells are often affected by tumors. Examples of peripheral cells are Schwann cells and satellite cells.

Major Sections of the Brain

In embryos, the brain is primarily **gray matter**. As the fetus develops the brain grows in leaps and bounds, folding in upon itself. Each person's brain is unique. In children, the brain continues to grow until approximately 5 years of age. At this point it weighs about 3 lb. After 5 years of age the brain continues to grow until approximately age 20, but at a much slower pace. After 20 years of age, growth virtually stops; in the elderly, the brain actually begins to shrink. People can still learn after 20 years of age, but their brains will not grow any larger while they are learning!

The brain is divided into three major sections: the forebrain, midbrain, and hindbrain. The midbrain and hindbrain are often termed the brain stem. The forebrain is divided into the cerebrum, basal ganglia, thalamus, and hypothalamus.

The largest part of the forebrain is the **cerebrum**, which comprises seven-eighths of the brain's weight. The cerebrum is divided into two parts, or halves, termed the right and left hemispheres. The hemispheres are connected by several fibers collectively termed the corpus callosum. Additionally, the cerebrum comprises **six lobes:** the frontal, parietal, temporal, olfactory, occipital, and limbic lobes (see Fig. 9-4).

The *frontal lobe* is the anterior portion of the brain that extends posteriorly to the central sulcus. A **sulcus** is a shallow grove on the brain's surface that runs longitudinally (from front to back) or transversely (from side to

Norepinephrine is the neurotransmitter found in the sympathetic nerves and adrenal glands. It differs from epinephrine by the absence of the N-methyl group.

Neuroglial cells are the **supporting cells** of the central nervous system. They originate from neural ectoderm and consist of astrocytes, oligodendrocytes, or microglia.

The **gray matter** is primarily composed of nerve cells with few nerve fibers. It is located on the exterior of the brain, or cortex, and at the center of the spinal cord.

The **midbrain,** or mesencephalon, is the center of the three basic portions of the brain. It carries motor and sensory fibers between the pons and cerebrum

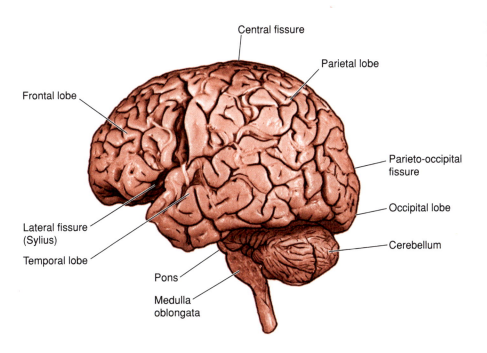

Central fissure

Parietal lobe

Frontal lobe

Parieto-occipital fissure

Occipital lobe

Lateral fissure (Sylius)

Cerebellum

Temporal lobe

Pons

Medulla oblongata

FIGURE 9-4

Lateral view of the brain.

and has two pigmented nuclei, the substantia nigra and the red nucleus, both of which are important in eliminating undesired muscle contraction.

The **cerebrum** is the largest and most anterior portion of the brain; it is the center for thought, reasoning, sensation, and motion. It is divided into two parts or halves, termed the right and left hemispheres.

Six Lobes of Cerebrum

1. frontal
2. parietal
3. temporal
4. olfactory
5. occipital
6. limbic

A **sulcus** is a shallow groove on the surface of an organ such as the interventricular sulcus of the heart or the sulci between the gyri of the brain. They may be longitudinal, going from front to back, or central, going from side to side.

The **limbic system** is a system of nerve tracts associated with the lateral and third ventricles. It includes the limbic lobe in the cerebrum, the hippocampus, the amygdaloid nucleus, thalamus, and hypothalamus and is concerned with emotion.

Three Major Brain Fibers

1. Transverse
2. Projection
3. Association

The **thalamus** is part of the diencephalon that makes up a portion of the walls of the third ventricle of the brain; it serves as a distribution center for sensory and voluntary motor tracts and is important in arousal and emotional expression.

side). The frontal lobe is responsible for "willed" or voluntary movement, emotion, behavior, intellect, memory, judgment, and personality. Individuals who undergo lobectomies experience altered behavior. Although this is an uncommon procedure today, removal of the frontal lobe of the cerebrum is still performed.

The *parietal lobe* is located just under the crown of the head. This lobe is responsible for sensation; it receives information from the skin, mucous membranes, mucosa, muscles, joints, and tendons. The parietal lobe is responsible for the sensations of pain, pressure, and temperature. However, it does not receive information from the special sense organs and thus is not responsible for the sensations of taste, hearing, and smell.

The *temporal lobe*, located under the temporal bones of the skull, is responsible for hearing and understanding speech on the dominant side. For 90% of us, the left temporal lobe or left hemisphere is the dominant side.

The *olfactory lobe* is located just under the temporal lobe. This is the location of cranial nerve I, which is responsible for our sense of smell. (Cranial nerves are discussed later.) The *occipital lobe*, located under the base of the skull, is responsible for vision and houses cranial nerve II.

The sixth part of the cerebrum is the *limbic lobe*. The limbic lobe sits deep within the cerebrum below the corpus callosum, where the frontal, parietal, and temporal lobes come together in the center of the cerebrum. The limbic lobe is responsible for primitive behavior and emotions such as love, hate, rage, and fear. This lobe also controls recent memory. There is still a lot of research being conducted to determine additional functions of the limbic lobe.

Three types of fibers pervade the cerebrum: transverse, projection, and association fibers. Transverse fibers connect the right and left hemispheres. The corpus callosum is the most important of the transverse fibers. Projection fibers connect the cerebrum to the lower part of the brain. Association fibers connect various parts of the brain within the same hemisphere.

The second part of the forebrain is the **basal ganglia**. Basal ganglia are islands of gray matter that inhibit voluntary movement. A defect in the basal ganglia may result in tremors, such as those associated with Parkinson's disease, Sydenham's chorea, and Huntington's chorea. Individuals with deteriorated basal ganglia or those who have incurred an injury to that part are unable to control their movements. The basal ganglia must be intact for control of voluntary movement.

The **thalamus** is the third part of the forebrain. This structure acts as the traffic director in the brain by sorting sensory impulses and sending them in the proper direction. Cranial nerve II travels through the thalamus.

The fourth section of the forebrain is the **hypothalamus**, which has a number of important functions and contains many nuclei (groups of cell bodies). The hypothalamus actually functions as a gland in that it makes hormones, primarily *antidiuretic hormone (ADH)*. The body's "thermostat" is located within the hypothalamus; the hypothalamus is responsible for maintaining the body's temperature at approximately 98.6°F. Our true thirst center is also located within the hypothalamus and is responsible for water balance. In addition, the satiety center is located within the hypothalamus, regulating our appetite and thus our intake of food. The hypothalamus houses the reticular activating system (RAS) that regulates our sleep cycle and conscious state (Fig. 9-5). The RAS is a series of fibers that extend up through the base of the brain and pervade the entire cortex; these fibers control wakefulness. When these fibers are depressed (such as in a head injury), the intracranial pressure (ICP) rises.

The hypothalamus regulates growth, metabolism, and reproduction through its interrelationship with the endocrine system. (The pituitary gland sits just below the hypothalamus.) In concert with the limbic lobe, the hypothalamus affects our behavior, particularly aggressive and sexual behavior. Clearly, the hypothalamus has a major influence on all of us, and its functions are very complex.

The second section of the brain is the **midbrain**, a short, narrow segment that contains the nuclei for cranial nerves III and IV. The midbrain functions as a major pathway because of an abundance of nerve fibers. A major responsibility of the midbrain is the "righting" reflex that enables us to remain upright. Our pupillary reflexes and movements also are controlled by the midbrain. The oculocephalic or doll's eye reflex indicates an intact midbrain. To test for the doll's eye phenomenon, place the client in a supine position with the head and eyes facing straight ahead and quickly rotate the head to the right or left. In a normal response or reflex, the eyes rotate to the left as the head is turned to the right, or conversely, the eyes rotate to the right as the head is turned to the left. In an abnormal or absent reflex, the eyes remain centered as the head is turned (Fig. 9-6).

The third section of the brain is termed the **hindbrain**. The hindbrain is composed of three major lobes: the *cerebellum*, *pons*, and *medulla*. The cerebellum comprises two halves connected by a band of tissue termed

The **hypothalamus** is the portion of the floor of the third ventricle of the brain that links the pituitary and the brain as well as being a center for many functions, such as the control of blood pressure, the thirst reflex, and control of reproduction.

Antidiuretic hormone, also known as ADH or vasopressin, is secreted by the posterior lobe of the pituitary. It increases the permeability of the collecting tubules of the nephrons to water, thereby increasing blood volume and decreasing urine volume.

The **cerebellum** is the part of the brain located behind the cerebrum and dorsal to the brainstem. Like the cerebrum, it is divided into two hemispheres. It is concerned with coordinating motor impulses.

FIGURE 9-5

Reticular activating system.

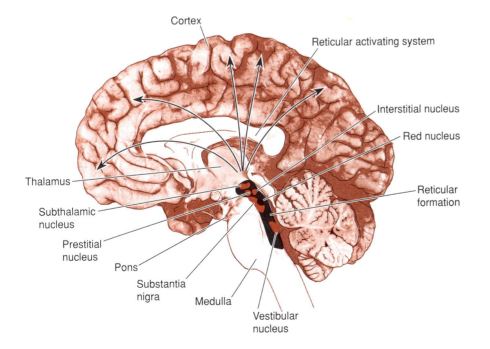

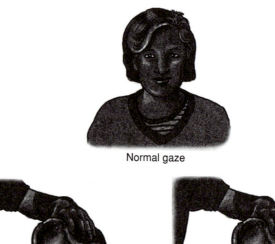

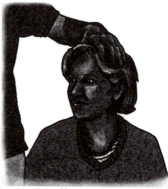

Normal gaze

Normal reflex   Absent reflex

FIGURE 9-6

☒

Doll's eye reflex.

The **pons** is the expanded part of the brainstem between the medulla and the midbrain. It carries nerve fibers into the cerebellum as well as between the medulla and midbrain. It also has nuclei for facial feeling, facial movements, and eye movements.

The **medulla** is the central portion of an organ or structure, as contrasted with the cortex or outer layer.

Sections of the Brain

1. Forebrain
   • Cerebrum
   • Basal ganglia
   • Thalamus
   • Hypothalamus
2. Midbrain
3. Hindbrain
   • Cerebellum
   • Pons
   • Medulla

the vermis. It is frequently referred to as the "little brain" because of its many important functions. The cerebellum maintains balance by influencing equilibrium, is responsible for locomotion through its influence on muscle tone and posture, and synchronizes muscle coordination. The second lobe of the hindbrain, termed the pons, contains both motor and sensory pathways. The pons connects the midbrain to the medulla; helps to control breathing through its influence on the rhythm of respiration; and contains nuclei for cranial nerves V, VI, VII, and VIII. The third lobe of the hindbrain is the **medulla oblongata,** the last part of the brain before the spinal cord. The medulla connects the spinal cord to the brain and contains the nuclei for cranial nerves IX, X, XI, and XII. Basic reflexes controlled by the medulla include coughing, swallowing, and gagging. The medulla is of utmost importance as it controls blood pressure, heart rate, and respiration.

When referring to the nervous system, many have stated that the top of the brain is "who we are" and the bottom of the brain is "where we live." Damage to the "bottom" part of the brain can dramatically affect us, as it can seriously impair our vital functions.

Circulation to the Brain

Two major sets of vessels provide circulation to the brain, the vertebral arteries and the internal carotid arteries. The vertebral arteries are located posteriorly and arise from the subclavian arteries. They join to form the basilar artery, which feeds the brain stem (composed of the midbrain and hindbrain) and branch off to the posterior cerebral artery, which feeds the posterior medial aspect of the cerebrum (i.e., the occipital lobe). The internal carotid arteries are located anteriorly and arise from the common carotid arteries. The internal carotid arteries branch into the anterior, middle, and posterior cerebral arteries. The anterior cerebral artery supplies blood to the medial aspect of the cerebrum. The middle cerebral artery feeds the lateral surface of the cerebrum (Fig. 9-7). Damage to the anterior cerebral artery can affect memory and cause a deficit in the lower extremities. Damage to the middle cerebral artery can affect the face and speech. The circle of Willis connects the anterior, middle, and posterior arteries. The meningeal arteries (branches of the external carotids) supply the dura mater (the outer covering of the brain).

The spinal cord is approximately 17 inches long and has an oval shape. It is as thick as an adult man's finger and extends from the medulla to L1 or L2. Within the spinal cord lie posterior and anterior horns. Sensory impulses enter through the posterior horns; motor impulses exit through the anterior horns. These impulses enter and exit the cord as one but travel through the cord separately. Internuncial neurons are located within the cord to connect sensory and motor neurons. The spinal cord is responsible for simple and complex reflexes. Simple reflexes involve a reflex arc. For

The **medulla oblongata** is located at the base of the brainstem. It transmits impulses between the spinal cord and the rest of the brain and contains the pyramids where most of the motor fibers of the brain pass to the opposite side of the spinal cord. The medulla oblongata is the center for regulation of heart rate, breathing, and blood vessel diameter.

The **meninges** comprise the three protective membranes covering the brain: the outer, tough dura mater; the vascular arachnoid layer; and the delicate pia mater that resides adjacent to the surface of the brain.

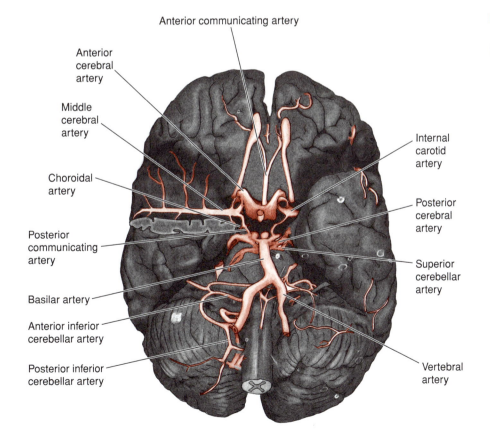

Anterior communicating artery

Anterior cerebral artery

Middle cerebral artery

Choroidal artery

Posterior communicating artery

Basilar artery

Anterior inferior cerebellar artery

Posterior inferior cerebellar artery

Internal carotid artery

Posterior cerebral artery

Superior cerebellar artery

Vertebral artery

FIGURE 9-7

Blood supply of the brain.

The **dura mater** is the outermost of the meninges. The tough dura mater protects the brain from penetration by bone fragments in the event of severe skull fracture.

The **arachnoid layer** is the middle layer of the meninges, the membrane between the dura mater and the pia mater surrounding the brain. It is associated with a web-like network of blood vessels.

The **pia mater** is the innermost layer of the three meninges covering the central nervous system. It follows the contours of the gyri and sulci of the brain.

A **ventricle** is a cavity of the brain that contains the cerebrospinal fluid.

Cerebrospinal fluid is the ionically balanced liquid that bathes the brain and spinal cord and protects them from physical

example, an impulse is first felt on the skin. The impulse travels to an afferent (sensory) neuron in the posterior root of the cord, is carried forward by an internuncial neuron to the efferent (motor) neuron in the anterior root of the cord, and then to the muscle where the response occurs. The impulse is carried very quickly (Fig. 9-8). Imagine touching a hot stove or perhaps the boiling water in a pot on the stove. The rapid response of pulling away and feeling pain is a simple reflex and may take less than 1 second. For complex reflexes involving the spinal cord, the brain is also involved. The spinal cord contains ascending fibers that carry impulses to the brain as well as descending fibers that carry impulses back down for action. Neurons that travel from the brain to the cord are termed upper motor neurons, while neurons that travel out from the cord are termed lower motor neurons.

The CNS has several protective mechanisms, including bones, meninges, cerebrospinal fluid (CSF), and the circle of Willis. The bones that protect the CNS are the skull and vertebrae. **Meninges** are membranes that cover the brain and spinal cord. The **dura mater** is the outermost layer of the meninges. It is a tough, fibrous membrane that closely adheres to the brain. The inner layer of the dura mater folds to form the falx cerebri, which further folds down to the corpus callosum of the two hemispheres of the cerebrum and the tentorium cerebelli that folds into the cerebellum and cerebrum. The middle meningeal layer is a light lacy covering termed the **arachnoid layer**. The inner layer of the meninges is termed the **pia mater**, which means "little mother." This inner layer lies on the surface of the brain and spinal cord. Blood vessels arise from the vascular, pink pia mater to form the choroid plexus. The space between the pia mater (inner layer) and the arachnoid layer (middle layer) is filled with spinal fluid and large blood vessels (Fig. 9-9).

FIGURE 9-8 Reflex arc.

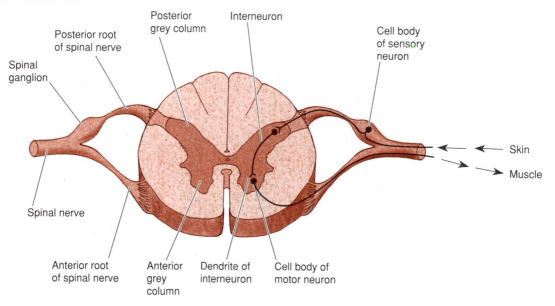

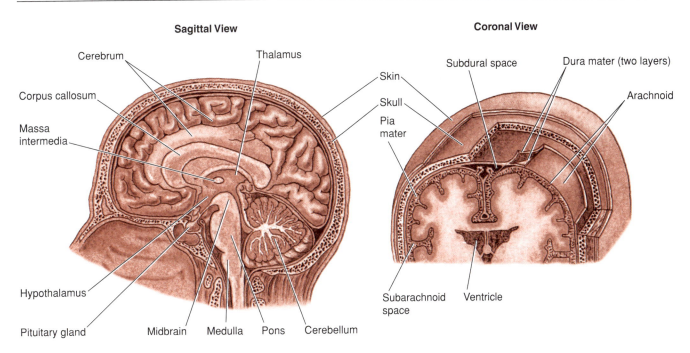

FIGURE 9-9 The meninges of the brain.

The CSF is another protective mechanism of the CNS. The choroid plexus is the principal source of CSF. The lateral **ventricles** (cavities of the brain) produce and house 95% of the CSF. A smaller amount is made in the third and fourth ventricles (Fig. 9-10). A fraction also may be produced by blood vessels of the brain and meningeal linings. As a procedure of the brain, the CSF (1) decreases the force of any impact to the brain, (2) nourishes the brain, and (3) returns tissue fluid to the brain. The CSF

shock. It is secreted by the choroid plexes in the ventricles of the brain and is absorbed by

FIGURE 9-10 Cerebral ventricles.

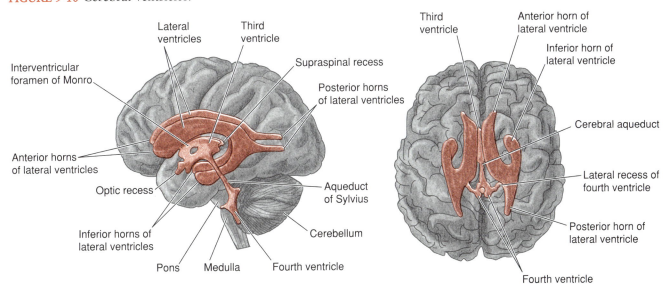

the arachnoid granulations located under the arachnoid layer of the meninges.

Functions of the Cerebrospinal Fluid

1. Decreases force of any impact to the brain
2. Nourishes the brain
3. Returns tissue fluid to the brain

circulates from the lateral ventricles of the brain through the interventricular foramen to the third ventricle, from the aqueduct of Sylvius to the fourth ventricle, and finally to the cisterns of the brain and the subarachnoid space. Normal CSF is clear, colorless, and odorless with a specific gravity of 1.003–1.009 and a pH of 7.35. The electrolyte contents of the CSF are 120–150 mEq/L of Na^+, 60% serum glucose concentration, and 40 mg/100 mL of protein.

Voluntary Nervous System

In addition to the CNS and autonomic nervous system, the voluntary nervous system includes the peripheral nervous system. The peripheral nervous system is comprised of 12 pairs of cranial nerves and 31 pairs of spinal nerves. The nurse must learn and know the cranial nerves to assess thoroughly neurologically impaired clients. Table 9-1 depicts the cranial nerves, what they control, and how to assess their various functions. Table 9-2 lists a mnemonic device to help remember the cranial nerves.

◙

TABLE 9-1

CRANIAL NERVES

Cranial Nerve	Regulates	Assessment
I—Olfactory (sensory)	Smell	With client's eyes closed, occlude one nostril on the client and ask the client to identify odors, such as coffee, cloves, alcohol, or vinegar. Repeat on the other nostril.
II—Optic (sensory)	Vision	Use a Snellen chart or newspaper to assess visual acuity. Ask client to tell you how many fingers you are holding up. Assess visual fields by having the client sit directly in front of you and stare at your nose. Move a finger slowly from the periphery toward the center of the client and have the client tell you when he or she can see your finger. Check color vision by having the client tell you the color of several items around you or use Ishihara's Test for Color-Blindness.
III—Oculomotor (sensory)	Pupillary constriction Upper eyelid elevation Most eye movement	These cranial nerves overlap in their motor functions and can be tested together. Check client's eyelids for ptosis. Assess ocular movements and note any eye deviation.
IV—Trochlear (motor)	Downward and inward eye movement	Test for accommodation and direct and consensual light reflexes.

Cranial Nerve	Regulates	Assessment
V—Trigeminal (sensory and motor)	Sensation to the corneas, nasal and oral mucosa, and facial skin Mastication	Test motor function by having client close jaws tightly. Try to separate clenched jaw. Test corneal reflex by lightly touching client's corneas with a *wisp* of cotton. Test sensory function by having the client close his or her eyes. Lightly touch forehead, cheeks, and chin.
VI—Abducens (motor)	Lateral eye movements	
VII—Facial (sensory and motor)	Facial muscles Taste perception (anterior ⅔ of tongue)	Have client puff out cheeks, close eyes against resistance, and smile widely. Put a small amount of sugar, salt, or vinegar on the front of client's tongue to identify different tastes.
VIII—Acoustic (sensory)	Hearing (cochlear) Equilibrium (vestibular)	Rub a few strands of hair between your fingers near the client's ear, and have the client identify the ear. Check ability to hear a watch ticking or a whisper. Observe client's balance. Perform Romberg test, if indicated.
IX—Glossopharyngeal (sensory and motor)	Swallowing and phonation Sensation to the pharyngeal, soft palate and tonsillar mucosa Taste perception (posterior ⅓ of tongue) Salivation	Have client identify tastes on the back of the tongue. Inspect soft palate. Check for symmetry of tongue elevation when client says "aah." Elicit palatal reflex by touching the soft palate's mucous membrane with a swab. Elicit gag reflex by touching the client's posterior pharyngeal wall with a tongue blade.
X—Vagus (sensory and motor)	Swallowing and phonation Sensation to the exterior ear's posterior wall and behind the ear Sensation to the thoracic and abdominal viscera	
XI—Spinal accessory (motor)	Uvula and soft palate movement Sternocleidomastoid muscle Upper portion of trapezius muscle (shoulder and neck movement)	Inspect and palpate the sternocleidomastoid muscle as client pushes chin against examiner's hand. Inspect and palpate the trapezius muscle by having client shrug his or her shoulders against your resistance. Have client stretch out hands to you.
XII—Hypoglossal (motor)	Tongue movement involved in swallowing and speech	Observe tongue for asymmetry, atrophy, deviation to one side, and fasciculations. Ask client to push tongue against a tongue blade. Have client move tongue rapidly in and out and side to side.

✦

TABLE 9-2
CRANIAL NERVES MNEMONIC

	Cranial Nerve	First Initial of Each	Sensory, Motor, or Both
I	Olfactory	On	Some
II	Optic	Old	Say
III	Oculomotor	Olympus	Marry
IV	Trochlear	Towering	Money
V	Trigeminal	Top	But
VI	Abducens	A	My
VII	Facial	Finn	Brother
VIII	Acoustic	And	Say
IX	Glossopharyngeal	German	Bad
X	Vagus	Viewed	Business
XI	Spinal accessory	Some	Marry
XII	Hypoglossal	Hops	Money

Involuntary Nervous System

A **ganglion** is a group of nerve cell bodies outside the nervous system (i.e., a "gang" of cells). A ganglion cyst is an example of this group of nerve cell bodies. It comprises any concentration of neurons outside the CNS that functions as a nerve distribution center.

The involuntary nervous system includes the **sympathetic nervous system (SNS)** and the **parasympathetic nervous system (PNS)**. The SNS takes over when the body is threatened or overwhelmed by too much stress, including psychological or physical injury. It is often referred to as the "fight-or-flight" system. Initiation and sustenance of the SNS requires a large amount of energy, particularly in the form of adenosine triphosphate (ATP). Nerve fibers for the SNS originate in the thoracic and lumbar areas of the spinal cord and travel to preganglionic fibers, then to **ganglions** (a group of nerve cell bodies outside the nervous system), and then to postganglionic fibers. Each type of fiber has specific chemical mediators. Acetylcholine is the chemical mediator for alpha and beta preganglionic fibers. The chemical mediator for alpha fibers is norepinephrine and for beta fibers, epinephrine. These chemical mediators are present at the nerve endings of preganglionic fibers. The nerve endings of postganglionic fibers include sympathetic adrenergic fibers and sympathetic cholinergic fibers. These fibers also have norepinephrine and epinephrine or acetylcholine chemical mediators. Sympathetic adrenergic fibers travel to either alpha or beta receptors. Alpha receptors are mediated by norepinephrine, and beta receptors are mediated by epinephrine.

Alpha receptors are found in the skin, kidneys, and gastrointestinal (GI) tract. A few fibers are found in the heart, primarily in the sinoatrial (SA) node. The transmission of norepinephrine by these fibers stimulates the SNS, which constricts vessels in the skin, kidneys, and GI tract. Beta receptors are found in the heart and lungs. Thus, when the SNS stimulates these areas in response to stress, the heart's rate and force of contraction increase, and the bronchi in the lungs dilate, increasing tidal volume. Beta receptors are stimulated by drugs such as dopamine (Inotropin) and isoproterenol (Isuprel). Some cholinergic receptors are located in skeletal muscle and blood vessels within the SNS. These receptors respond to acetylcholine. Most of the cholinergic receptors, however, are located in the PNS.

The PNS predominates in peaceful states and in sleep. It is designed to conserve energy. The PNS affects only our large internal organs. Fibers for the PNS originate from the cervical and sacral areas of the spinal cord. Acetylcholine, the only mediator for the PNS, works to calm the body down and to return it to a normal state. When the PNS is stimulated, everything slows down except for the stomach (digestion) and the intestines (elimination). Stimulation of cranial nerve X, the vagus nerve, initiates the PNS. The vagus nerve is stimulated by straining to have a bowel movement, by carotid artery massage, by suctioning, and by stimulating the gag reflex. Table 9-3 presents a summary of the SNS and PNS.

SENSES AND PERCEPTION

We receive a great deal of information through our sense organs and stimulation from the external and internal environment. The sensory organs are stimulated by sensation, perception, and response. When particular stimuli are recognized, the sensory portion of the nervous system is working effectively. Sensory receptors are responsible for our vision, hearing, taste, touch, smell, and position sense. We are constantly bombarded by stimuli. As these stimuli are received by somesthetic receptors, a great

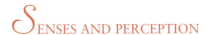

TABLE 9-3
SUMMARY OF INVOLUNTARY NERVOUS SYSTEM

Sympathetic Nervous System	Parasympathetic Nervous System
Dilates pupils	Constricts pupils
Dilates bronchioles	
Relaxes smooth muscle (GI tract)	Contracts smooth muscle of stomach, intestine, and bladder
Elevates blood pressure	
Increases heart rate	Decreases heart rate
Increases secretions from adrenal medulla	Stimulates secretions of most glands

deal of information is taken in. To use the information, we must be able to perceive it. Perception is the ability to receive, interpret, and assimilate information effectively. Our previous experiences assist in assigning meaning to the information we receive. After interpreting the sensory input, we respond to the information by taking action.

In addition to the sense organs described above, peripheral sensory receptors are found in many other areas. These receptors deliver certain messages and include (1) exteroceptors, receptors that are provoked by pain, pressure, temperature, odor, sound, and light; (2) proprioceptors, receptors that communicate a sense of position, movement, and muscle coordination; (3) interoceptors, receptors that send visceral information about pain, cramping, and fullness; and (4) chemoceptors, receptors that are activated by an assortment of chemicals. The transmission of sensation occurs when peripheral receptors recognize stimuli and send information (impulses) by either afferent (sensory) or efferent (motor) neurons.

The RAS in the hypothalamus is responsible for keeping the brain aroused and alert. It must be functioning for perception and appropriate action to take place. Adequate stimuli are required for an individual to remain aroused and alert. However, the nurse must remember that adequate stimuli for one person may be too much or too little for another. Harm can result from insufficient stimulation or overstimulation. An elderly person certainly prefers less noise than a teenager!

Altered sensation and perception can result from a change in the amount, pattern, or interpretation of incoming stimuli. Some examples of factors that can alter the senses and perceptions are presented in Table 9-4.

Sensory Alterations

Individuals respond to stimulation in different and unique ways. Sensory alteration depends on past exposure and, occasionally, adaptability. A *sensory deficit* refers to an impairment in sight, hearing, taste, touch, smell, or the position sense. The deficit is in the sense organ itself and may be the result of genetics or chance. Many people are able to adjust very well to sensory deficits. Helen Keller, for example, was born without hearing or sight but was able to compensate for her deficits. Some adjust quite well, while others may never accept the changes in their perception. A deficit that occurs gradually is generally easier to adapt to than one that occurs suddenly. *Sensory deprivation* results from faulty receptors or inefficient perception of environmental stimuli. Deprivation may be physiological (sensory deficit) or may result from an insufficient amount or variety of stimulation. The lack of appropriate stimuli can result in impaired judgment or the inability to solve simple dilemmas. Sensory deprivation may also lead to confusion, disorientation, or even delusions and hallucinations. *Sensory overload* refers to a situation in which environmental stimuli overwhelm the client. This is a major problem in the hospital setting, where clients are constantly exposed to new and strange sights and sounds.

☒

TABLE 9-4
FACTORS THAT ALTER SENSES AND PERCEPTION

Factor	Examples of Sensation/Perception
Developmental	1. Visual acuity usually decreases after age 60. 2. Hearing is most acute at age 10; after age 65, 55% of population have some hearing loss. 3. Most people over age 60 lose some sense of taste. 4. Smell declines after age 70.
Cultural	Customary stimuli may vary based upon ethnicity, religion, or income level.
Occupational	Many individuals have high levels of noise inflicted upon them because of their occupation (e.g., pilots, air traffic controllers, factory workers).
Pathologic	Clients with diabetes may suffer from visual impairment as a result of complications of their disease.
Therapeutic	1. Clients may be excessively stimulated simply from being in a high-noise or high-traffic area, such as an intensive care unit (ICU). 2. Clients in isolation may suffer sensory deficits. 3. Restriction of visitors, such as occurs in an ICU or coronary care unit (CCU), can lead to deficits.
Pharmacologic	1. Aminoglycosides can impair hearing. 2. Analgesics and sedatives can depress perception.

Alterations in Perception

Individuals with altered perception may be unable to differentiate between sensory stimuli or to categorize and apply meaning to incoming stimuli. This can result from a sensory deficit, sensory deprivation, sensory overload, or a pathological process. Examples of alterations in perception include confusion, delusional thinking, illusions, and hallucinations.

Confusion is a disruption of awareness or consciousness. The individual feels distracted and anxious. A confused client may be unable to respond appropriately to normal stimuli and may have an altered perception of person, place, time, or events. Confusion may be fleeting (lasting just a few minutes) or long-term (lasting for years). Confusion may be pathophysiological, treatment-related, or situational. Pathophysiological causes include autoimmune diseases such as systemic lupus erythematosus, degenerative diseases such as Alzheimer's disease, infections, metabolic disorders such as diabetes or electrolyte imbalances, brain tumors, seizures, trauma, and vascular deficits resulting from stroke or transient ischemic attacks (TIAs). Treatment-related confusion may result from electroshock therapy or the side effects of certain medications, such as those used to treat Parkinson's disease. Situational confusion may occur with depression, schizophrenia, or toxins such as carbon monoxide and alcohol.

To assess for confusion, ask the client open-ended questions that cannot be answered with a "yes" or "no." For example, ask the client to tell you his or her name; to identify a relative or other visitor; to tell you where he or she is; to tell you the day and year. Be sure that you are speaking the client's language; that he or she can hear and speak; and that you are asking relatively simple, easily answered questions. When documenting your assessment, be specific about your observations.

Delusional thinking is a cognitive mechanism that helps a person maintain an essence of power and authority when his or her defenses are threatened. Delusions are simply false beliefs with no basis in fact or reality. The thoughts of delusional individuals cannot be changed by presenting them with the reality. Affected individuals are guided by their delusions in interpreting events and making decisions. Delusions can be comforting or threatening; their presence indicates mental illness.

An *illusion* is a visually inaccurate judgment of physical or environmental stimuli, in other words, a disorder of perception. An individual sees something that exists but believes it is something else. There is an inaccurate connection between what is seen and how it is interpreted. For example, a person may see cracks on a ceiling or wall and think they are blood or insects. Anyone can experience illusions, but mentally ill individuals are more likely to do so. If the individual is just having an illusion, an appropriate explanation can clarify the situation. This is not true for delusional individuals.

Hallucination is a disorder of sensory perception that has no physical or environmental stimulus. All of the senses—seeing, hearing, smelling, tasting, or feeling—can be affected by hallucinations. Hallucinations are self-induced, incorrect perceptions in one of these senses. For example, an individual may see bugs on the wall when there is absolutely nothing there. Individuals who hallucinate can be taught that these are misinterpretations, but the hallucinations may still occur, even with medication.

Individuals at Risk for Sensory and Perceptual Alterations

Clients most at risk for developing sensory or perceptual alterations include elderly and hospitalized persons, individuals with occupational risks, and those who already have a sensory deficit. Normal physiological changes occur with the aging process, causing a gradual loss of acuity; for example, hearing and sight gradually decline. Thus, an 80-year-old person may be less aware of his or her environment than someone 20 years of age.

Hospitalized clients are naturally at higher risk for sensory and perceptual alterations because of the increased stimulation from the environment. Clients in isolation may experience a decrease in stimulation, while clients in a semiprivate room may experience sensory overload. Researchers have documented that clients placed in intensive care units (ICUs) experience many adverse effects. This is labeled "ICU psychosis," and clients are frequently moved out of critical care units as a result. Nurses who work in these units may suffer adverse effects from the environment as well (an example of occupational risk). Individuals who already have a sensory or perceptual deficit such as blindness may do well in a familiar environment but may become disoriented in a strange new place, such as a nursing home or hospital.

To assess a client for sensory or perceptual deficits, the nurse must observe for the presence of factors known to affect sensory perception (see Table 9-4). Question the client about factors that may have caused the alteration and factors that may have aggravated the condition. In addition, inquire how often the alterations occur, how long they last, and what measures bring relief. Symptoms of sensory or perceptual alterations include emotional lability, which may be apparent in mood swings, irritability, anxiety, apathy, or fear. Clients may be unable to differentiate their thoughts and feelings from those that occur in the real world. These altered processes may occur in the form of visual or auditory hallucinations, delusional thinking, illusions, inability to concentrate, memory deficits, or disorientation. Clients may have difficulty in communicating as a result of sensory or perceptual alterations.

In addition to obtaining an accurate, thorough history and assessing for sensory or perceptual deficits, the nurse must determine the client's response to any sensory or perceptual deficits (i.e., what characteristics describe the deficit). If a sensory or perceptual deficit has been identified, what is it related to? This is termed a nursing diagnosis and is generally used with each problem identified by the nurse and client. Nursing diagnoses are commonly used in some institutions. Nursing diagnoses were developed by a national group of nurses to individualize and separate nursing from medicine. Eventually, this may allow direct reimbursement for nursing care. However, some see it as a separatist movement that has served only to divide nursing and medicine. Whatever problem the nurse identifies in the client, there will always be causative factors and a client response to the deficit.

Planning is an important step in the assessment of clients with sensory or perceptual deficits. Planning must be specific to the medical and nursing diagnoses (if used) and the client's response to the deficit. As the nurse develops a plan, the client and his or her family or significant other should be included. The nurse must also focus on setting goals and how to attain a favorable outcome. **Nursing interventions** are the actions taken to arrive at planned outcomes. For example, if there is a sensory deficit, nursing interventions should focus on assisting the client to compensate for the deficits. If there is a sensory overload, interventions should focus on decreasing the overload and compensating for possible alterations in the nervous system. Clients with altered perceptions require interventions to help them communicate effectively.

Assessment

A detailed neurological assessment is time-consuming and requires skill. It is your task as a nursing student to acquire this skill. When beginning the assessment, start with the client's history. Determine the client's chief complaint from the client him- or herself if possible. If the client's consciousness is altered, the nurse must rely on family and others who know the client well. Gather details concerning the client's present illness, medical history, family history, and social history. Determine when the signs and symptoms first occurred, any patterns, and any activities that the disorder has limited. The nurse should ask if medical treatment has already been sought, and if so, what the treatment is. Determine whether the client is taking medication and if it has helped. To obtain a comprehensive history, the nurse must also complete a review of systems. The following guide will help to complete this part of the history.

Review of Systems

1. **Neurological.** Do you have headaches? How often? Dizziness? Any experiences of tingling, prickling, or numbness on your body? Where? Have you had seizures or tremors? Any weakness or paralysis in your arms or legs? Any trouble walking? How is your memory and ability to concentrate? Any trouble speaking? Any trouble understanding what someone says to you? Do you have trouble reading or writing?

2. **Eyes.** Do you wear glasses or contacts? Have you ever experienced blurred vision or temporary vision loss? Have you ever experienced double vision? Do you have any blind spots?

3. **Ears, Nose, and Throat.** Any trouble hearing clearly? Wear a hearing aid? Any ringing in your ears? Any hay fever, frequent earaches, sinus problems, sore throats, hoarseness, or difficulty swallowing?

4. **Respiratory.** Any difficulty breathing, shortness of breath, or wheezing? Are you a smoker? How much do you smoke? How long have you smoked? Do you sleep with more than one pillow to ease your breathing? How many? Any cough or cold for a prolonged period? Do you cough up any sputum? If so, what does it look like?

5. **Cardiovascular.** Have you ever had any chest pain? Rapid or irregular pulse? High blood pressure? Are you on any medications for hypertension? Have you ever been on medication? Have you ever had any blood clots in your legs?

6. **Gastrointestinal.** Do you have a normal appetite? Have you gained or lost weight in the past 6 months without trying? Do you have food allergies? What is your normal bowel movement routine? Do you use laxatives or antacids? Do you drink alcohol? If yes, how much?

7. **Genitourinary.** Do you have trouble urinating? Any problem controlling your bladder? Any burning sensation when you urinate? Any unusual color or odor to your urine? Do you have to get up at night to urinate? How often? Any history of kidney or bladder infections?

When the nurse obtains a neurological nursing history, he or she should confirm answers with the client's significant other if possible and be alert as to how the client interacts with family members and others. Additionally, the nurse must assess the speed and accuracy of the client's responses and his or her attention span. Observe emotional responses as well as motor function at rest. Note slow, sudden, or jerky movements; flaccid, rigid, or atrophied muscles; tremors or contractures; and abnormal gait or posture. Pay attention to signs and symptoms of degenerating motor function such as dysarthria; dysphagia; irregular or abnormal respirations; loss of muscle tone or strength; poor balance and coordination; incontinence; and changes in appetite, sleep patterns, dietary habits, and libido.

The nurse must first determine the chief complaint. Ask, for example, Why have you come to the hospital? Did something specific occur that brought you here?

Second, investigate the client's present illness. If, for example, the client is in the hospital because he or she is dizzy, ask if it feels like the room is spinning or like he or she is spinning. Is there ringing in your ears? Can you identify anything that makes it better or worse? If the client has had seizures, try to get as accurate a description as possible of precipitating factors; history of head trauma, heart disease, diabetes, hypertension; exact events that occurred during the seizure; how long the seizure lasted; and what occurred afterwards. Determine what medications the client is taking. Noncompliance with anticonvulsant drug therapy frequently causes recurrent seizures. The nurse should ask questions to elicit the client's reason for being in the hospital.

Third, the nurse should obtain information concerning the client's medical history, including all previous major illnesses, minor illnesses that recur frequently (e.g., sore throats), accidents or injuries the client has sustained, surgeries, and allergies. In addition, the nurse should ask about health and dietary habits and social habits such as smoking, drinking, or drug use (both illicit and over-the-counter [OTC] drugs). Document all positive answers carefully. If clients cannot remember, check any bottles they have with them.

Fourth, inquire about the health of the client's family to discover hereditary disorders. Ask about diabetes, heart problems, kidney problems, high blood pressure, cancer, bleeding disorders, strokes, and mental problems.

Fifth, examine the client's social history, including cultural background. Ask about religious preference and if anything particularly offends him or her. What is the client's occupation and highest level of education? Ask if he or she is employed and for how long. If the client does not live alone, who does he or she live with? Does the client have children? What are their ages and availability? What are the client's hobbies and what does he or she think about this illness?

Physical Assessment Nursing students are not expected to perform a perfect assessment the first time they examine a neurologically impaired client. The student may not perform the initial physical examination but must know its components. As a registered nurse, you will perform certain aspects of the physical examination, and you may be the first person to encounter and assess the client. An accurate baseline assessment is vital for future comparison. Refinement of nursing skills takes time, patience, and experience. It is important, however, that you become familiar with what is required to conduct a thorough neurological physical assessment. This examination includes assessment of cerebral function, cranial nerve function, and motor and cerebellar function.

1. Evaluate **cerebral function** by assessing the following:
   - **Mental Status.** Note the client's general appearance, dress, and hygiene. Is he or she alert, anxious, or apathetic? What is the speech pattern like? Is it fast or slow, slurred or clear, shrill or gruff, soft or loud, smooth or pressured? Can the client maintain his or her train of thought?
   - **Orientation.** Assess the client's orientation to person, place, and time. Ask his or her name and the date. Can the client identify the season and upcoming or past holidays? Ask the names of the attending physician, spouse, siblings, and relatives.
   - **Attention and Concentration.** Can the client answer questions without having them repeated? Does the client fidget or appear distracted? Observe the client's facial expression and body posture.
   - **General Knowledge.** Ask the client about current events such as who is the president of the United States.
   - **Memory and Retention.** Assess the client's recall of the immediate, recent, and distant past. Ask the client to repeat three objects you name in 5 minutes, as illustrated in the mini-mental status examination. Ask about things that have occurred in the past week, the past year, and even in grammar and high school.
   - **Reasoning.** Assess *judgment* by asking the client to make an imaginary decision that involves an emergency, such as a fire on a stove. Evaluate *insight* by having the client tell you why he or she is in the hospital. Test *interpretation* by having the client explain a common saying such as "People who live in glass houses should not throw stones."
   - **Mood or Affect.** Describe the client's mood and evaluate his or her emotional responses. Is the client laughing or crying, withdrawn or happy? Does the client hear or see things that are not there?
   - **Calculation.** Have the client subtract 7 from 100 five times, as described in the mini-mental status examination. Have the client add something simple or figure change from a dollar bill.
   - **Reading and Writing.** Have the client read from a book or newspaper. Have the client copy something or write his or her name and address.
   - **Object Recognition and Ability to Perform Purposeful Tasks.** Show the client an object and then have him or her use it, such as a pen, comb, or phone.
2. Evaluate **cranial nerve function** (see Table 9-1). This is usually done as part of the regular examination. Special tests are required to assess hearing or vision loss.
3. Evaluate **motor** and **cerebellar function** by assessing the following:
   - **Muscle Size.** Palpate and inspect individual muscle groups. Check and document atrophy or decreased muscle tone.
   - **Muscle Strength.** Test arm, leg, and foot strength. Check the

major muscle groups as well as flexion and extension.

- **Muscle Tone.** Do passive range of motion (ROM) exercises, and grade the muscles as spastic, rigid, or flaccid. *Spastic* muscles are hypertonic with increased tone; rigid muscles are stiff or inflexible; and *flaccid* muscles have decreased or absent tone or are hypotonic.
- **Abnormal Movements.** Look for fasciculations, tremors, tics, choreiform, and dystonic movements. *Fasciculations* occur when the muscles are at rest and are the localized, uncoordinated, involuntary twitching of a single muscle group. Fasciculations may indicate a dietary deficiency, cerebral palsy, or an adverse side effect from a medication.

  Tremors are rhythmic, purposeless, quivering movements that result from involuntary contraction and relaxation of opposing muscle groups. They can be continuous or activity-induced (intention tremor). Tremors are caused by Parkinson's disease, multiple sclerosis, hyperthyroidism, hepatic or renal failure, and pulmonary insufficiency.

  Tics are characterized by involuntary, coordinated, stereotyped movements of small muscle groups and often involve the neck or shoulder. Tics are psychogenic (of mental origin) and are aggravated by stress or anxiety.

  Choreiform movements are the hallmark of chorea. The movements are rapid, jerky, and purposeless, such as flexing and extending the fingers or grimacing.

  Dystonic movements are slow, twisting, irregular muscle spasms that usually affect the muscles of the trunk, shoulder, and pelvis.
- **Fine Motor Skills.** Assess fine motor skills by having the client rapidly touch each finger to the nose in succession. Have the client unbutton and button the shirt and open and close a safety pin.
- **Gait and Posture.** If able, have the client walk across the room, turn around, and come back. Note the posture, stride strength, balance, footing, arm swing, hip stability, and rhythm.
- **Balance and Coordination.** If able, have the client walk heel-to-toe in a straight line. Look for ataxia (uncoordination) and poor balance. Perform the Romberg test by having the client stand with the feet together and eyes open for 30 seconds, then have the client close the eyes for 30 seconds. Some swaying is normal. The shifting of feet to regain balance is a positive sign and indicates neurological impairment.

4. Evaluate **sensory function** by testing for superficial and cortical, or discriminatory, sensation.
   - **Superficial sensation** includes light touch, pain, temperature, vibration, deep pressure, and proprioception.
   - **Cortical sensation** includes two-point discrimination, stereognosis, graphesthesia, and extinction phenomenon.
5. Evaluate **reflexes** including superficial and deep tendon reflexes (DTRs) (Figs. 9-11 and 9-12). Use a dull object such as a tongue blade to test the *superficial reflexes*. Check the *abdominal reflex* by

Babinski's reflex

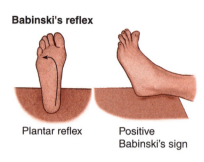

Plantar reflex   Positive
                        Babinski's sign

Brudzinski's sign

Kernig's sign

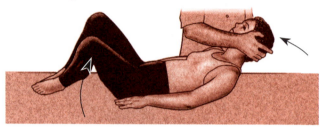

FIGURE 9-11

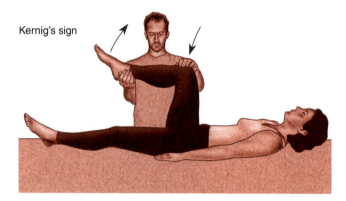

Assessment procedures for
abnormal reflexes.

stroking the abdomen from periphery to the center. The umbilicus should move toward the stimulus. For men only, test the *cremasteric reflex* by stroking the inner thigh. The sensation should cause the testicle on the side stroked to rise slightly. Test the *plantar reflex* by stroking the lateral aspect of the client's foot from the heel upward. The great toe should rise, and the remaining toes should fan out. Test the *gluteal reflex* by stroking the client's buttocks. Watch for the muscles to tense; if they do not, it is an abnormal response.

6. Assessing **pupillary** changes is a vital part of the neurological examination. The pupils are generally described as dilated, mid-sized, small, or pinpoint. However, pupil size measured in millimeters is more accurate for closely monitoring and detecting minute changes, which can be quite significant (Fig. 9-13). Both pupils usually constrict when exposed to light and dilate when the light is taken away.

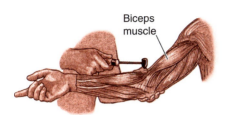

Biceps reflex
Place the client's elbow in your hand and place your thumb over the biceps tendon; then percuss your thumbnail and observe forearm flexion.

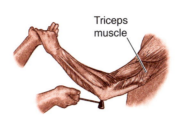

Triceps reflex
Flex the client's arm slightly, using your hand to steady the arm. Percuss the tendon above the back of the elbow. Observe elbow extension.

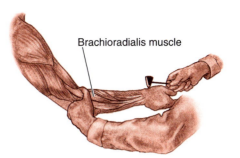

Brachioradialis reflex
Ask the client to rest his or her hand on the thigh with the palm down. Percuss the radius and observe forearm flexion.

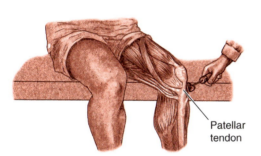

Patellar reflex
Have the patient sit on atable dangling or crossing the legs. Percuss the tendon below the patella. Observe leg extension at the knee.

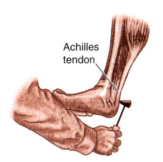

Achilles reflex
Support the client's foot in your hand. Rotate the foot and leg outward and percuss the Achilles tendon. Observe the ankle for plantar flexion.

FIGURE 9-12 Assessment of deep tendon reflexes (DTR).

One or both pupils can be abnormal and may foretell damage to cranial nerves II and III, a brain tumor, increased ICP, or brain stem damage. A thorough assessment of the pupils includes the following:

- **History**
  - Are the pupils normal and equal in size? Do they both react normally to light?
  - Is the client having any eye pain? If so, where? Is it accompanied by headache, nausea, or vomiting? Have the client describe the pain and vomiting if present and whether it is getting worse or better.
  - Has the client noticed vision disturbances such as blurred or double vision? Does he or she see halos around lights at night?
  - Has the client suffered a head injury? If so, investigate the cause and nature of the injury. Inquire about loss of consciousness and seizures. If the client has had seizures, determine when they occurred and how long they lasted.

Unilateral, dilated (4 mm), fixed,
and nonreactive

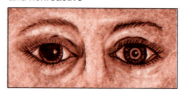

Bilateral, dilated (4 mm), fixed,
and nonreactive

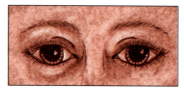

Bilateral, midsized (2 mm),
fixed, and nonreactive

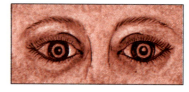

Unilateral, small (1.5 mm),
and nonreactive

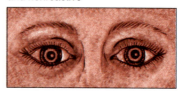

Bilateral, pinpoint (less than 1 mm),
and usually nonreactive

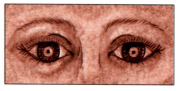

FIGURE 9-13

🔯

Pupillary assessment.

- Does the client wear an eye prosthesis? Does he or she have a neurological problem such as a tumor or a cardiovascular disorder? Is the client diabetic? Does he or she have glaucoma or increased intraocular pressure?
- What medication is the client currently taking? Does he or she use eyedrops? If yes, when? Does the client use street drugs?
- **Physical Examination of the Eyes**
    - **Inspection.** Note the size and assess the light reflex of the pupils. In a dark room, cover one eye while you assess the other. Bring the light toward the client from the side and shine it directly on the eye. This should cause a brisk constriction

termed the *direct light reflex*. Next, test the *consensual light reflex* by holding both eyes open and shining the light into one eye while watching the pupil of the opposite eye. Repeat on the other eye, checking the direct and consensual light reflex. While inspecting the eyes, be alert to bilateral or uni-lateral nonreaction or deviation. Examine the cornea and iris for abnormalities, assess the conjunctivae, check for swelling of the eyelids, and determine visual acuity. Test accommoda-tion; pupils should constrict together when the client shifts his or her gaze from a distant object to one nearby.

- **Palpation.** Place your fingers over the client's closed eyelids and the eyeball. If it is very hard to the touch, the client may have increased intraocular pressure.

7. **Evaluate the level of consciousness.** Assess the level of consciousness by determining the client's orientation to person, place, and time. This can be done during the neurological assessment when the client provides the history; his or her name, address, and current location; the name of the physician; and the date. Be alert to subtle changes between assessments and pay particular attention to complaints of headache, restlessness or unusual quietness, slurred speech, or a change in the level of orientation. The Glasgow Coma Scale (GCS) is a reliable and objective tool for assessing the level of consciousness and coma in adults (Table 9-5). Be aware that 18% of individuals

⌷

TABLE 9-5

GLASGOW COMA SCALE*

Parameter	Response	Score
Eye opening	Spontaneous	4
	To voice	3
	To pain	2
	None	1
Verbal response	Oriented	5
	Confused	4
	Inappropriate	3
	Incomprehensible sounds	2
	None	1
Motor response	Localizes pain	5
(Arouse with painful stimuli,	Withdraws to pain	4
if necessary; should not cause	Flexion response to pain	3
harm to client)	Extension response to pain	2
	None	1

*The Glasgow Coma Score is most useful in triage situations and monitoring clients post-triage. An initial score of less than 7 is indicative of a poor prognosis if trauma is the only identifiable cause. Assessment of the Glasgow Coma Score should be done frequently (i.e., with each neuro-logic check).

with a GCS score of 15 have abnormal computed tomography (CT) scans, and 5% with a GCS of 15 require neurosurgical intervention.

8. **Monitor vital signs.**

- **Temperature.** If the temperature is elevated, the client may have an infection; the hypothalamus may be injured; or a subarachnoid hemorrhage (SAH) may have occurred. If the temperature is below normal, consider a brain stem lesion, an overdose, or an insulin coma. In addition, the client may have had overexposure to cold.
- **Pulse.** If the pulse is rapid (over 100 beats/min, tachycardia), consider increased ICP. Shock, pain, and a distended bladder may also increase the pulse. If the pulse is slow (less then 60 beats/min), it may be normal or may indicate compensation for increased ICP or meningeal irritation.
- **Blood Pressure.** Does the blood pressure increase with each neurological check? If it does, the client may have increased ICP related to cerebral edema or a bleed.
- **Respiration.** Be alert for any difficulty breathing. Assess the rate and quality of the respirations.

9. **Perform the mini-mental status examination.** While assessing the client, remember that physical examination of the elderly requires special skills. Only some of the elderly require extra time, respond more slowly, have vision and hearing problems, have a short attention span, or have difficulty with cognitive questions as a result of education or physical impairments. However, the nurse should be prepared for all of these eventualities when examining older persons. If the client's responses seem appropriate, the examination may be shortened. Inappropriate behavior requires a more in-depth examination. When assessing neurological status, especially in the elderly, the mini-mental status examination should be performed (Table 9-6).

While doing the mini-mental status examination, be sure that the client is comfortable and does not feel pressured to "perform." Be nonjudgmental, and do not show disappointment should the client fail any part of the examination. Do not press for answers. A score of 20 or less indicates dementia, delirium, schizophrenia, or an affective disorder.

Diagnostic Assessment A variety of laboratory tests may be ordered by the physician. If an infection is suspected, blood should be drawn for cultures. Based on the potential diagnosis, other tests may be performed, including a complete blood count (CBC) with platelet count, erythrocyte sedimentation rate (ESR), prothrombin time (PT), partial thromboplastin time (PTT), fibrinogen, glucose level, electrolytes [Na^+, K^+, Cl^-, carbon dioxide (CO_2)], cholesterol level, and triglyceride level. Other required laboratory tests may include a blood urea nitrogen (BUN), calcium (Ca^{2+}), magnesium (Mg^{2+}), and urinalysis. A toxicity screen may be ordered as well. The physician may perform a lumbar puncture (LP) to obtain samples of CSF for analysis.

TABLE 9-6

MINI-MENTAL STATUS EXAMINATION

Points	Orientation
5	What is the (year)(season)(date)(day)(month)?
5	Where are we (state)(country)(town)(hospital)(floor)?
	Registration
3	Name three unrelated objects. Ask for all three. Repeat until the client knows all three. Record the number of trials.
	Attention and Calculation
5	Serial 7s. Stop after 5 or spell "world" backwards.
	Recall
3	Ask for three objects you had client learn earlier.
	Language
2	Naming pencil and watch
1	Repetition: "No ifs, ands, or buts."
3	3-Stage command: "Take the paper in your right hand, fold it in half, and put it on the floor."
1	Reading: "Close your eyes."
1	Writing: "Write a sentence."
1	Copying: intersecting pentagons

In the event of a spine injury, *spinal x-rays* are usually ordered to determine if there are any fractures, abnormal curvatures, bone erosion, or bone dislocation. In cerebral angiography, contrast medium is injected through a catheter into the carotid or vertebral artery. This examination helps to diagnose aneurysms, vascular malformations, and leaking or occluded blood vessels. A CT scan assesses ventricle size and shows cortical atrophy, hemorrhage, or tumor. CT is an important and useful diagnostic test. Using a computer, multiple horizontal pictures are taken at various levels in the brain and spinal cord. CT scans provide invaluable information concerning tumors, infarctions, hemorrhage, hydrocephalus, and bone malformations. Magnetic resonance imaging (MRI), one of the newer diagnostic tools used to detect neurological impairment, produces cross-sectional images of the brain and provides information about neuronal hyperactivity and structural changes. In MRI, a large magnetic field is absorbed by the body, and energy is emitted, which is converted to an image on a screen. MRI aids in the diagnosis of multiple sclerosis, meningiomas, acoustic neuromas, and arteriovenous malformations (AVMs), but is usually not available on an emergency basis. A positron emission tomography (PET) scan is a dynamic study of brain function that highlights foci of seizure activity in a resting or active state.

Probably the most frequently used diagnostic tool in determining the etiology of a neurological impairment is the lumbar puncture (LP). The physician inserts a needle into the subarachnoid space between the third and fourth or fourth and fifth lumbar vertebrae. This study is conducted to check for readings with a manometer, to obtain CSF for analysis, to check for spinal cord blockage, and to reduce ICP in certain situations. Table 9-7 lists normal CSF findings and possible conditions linked to specific findings.

An electroencephalograph (EEG) records the electrical activity of the brain. The test is performed more often on outpatients but is also done on inpatients. Electrodes (16–24) are attached to the scalp with electrode jelly according to a standard procedure. The client must remain still or engage in specific activities as instructed by the technician or physician to elicit certain responses that are then recorded. Each aspect of the test is designed to produce certain tracings that determine the following: general cerebral activity, origin of seizure activity, decreased or increased activity related to certain diagnoses, the etiology of the disease (organic or hysterical), sleep disorders, and brain death.

Nursing Care

Individuals with a temporary or permanent impairment in vision, taste, hearing, touch, smell, or position sense are often at risk for injury, self-care deficits, impaired nutrition, and sensory deprivation. In such cases, nursing interventions must focus on preventing injury, maintaining independence, improving nutrition, and providing activities for diversion.

Individuals with *visual* impairment must receive **nursing care** to prevent sensory deprivation, promote self-care, and provide a safe environment. To help prevent sensory deprivation, it is important for the nurse to speak as he or she enters the room, to use large-print or recorded books, to provide instructions in large print or record them, and to simply talk with the client. To promote self-care, the nurse should assist as needed in bathing, feeding, dressing, and toileting.

◙

TABLE 9-7

CEREBROSPINAL FLUID FINDINGS IN LUMBAR PUNCTURE

Condition	Protein (mg/dL)	Fasting Sugar (mg/dL)	White Blood Cell (per mm*)
Normal	15–45	45–80	0–10L*
Viral meningitis or encephalitis	20–200	Normal	10–500, mainly L, may be P* dominant in acute disease
Bacterial meningitis	50–1500	0–45	25–10,000; mainly P, may be L dominant if partially treated
Tuberculosis meningitis	45–500	10–45	25–1000 mainly L
Cryptococcal meningitis	<500 in 90%	Moderately decreased in 55%	<800, mainly L

*L = lymphocyte; P = polymorphonuclear leukocyte

The nurse can create a safe environment by arranging the furniture to prevent injury. Do not rearrange the furniture without informing and consulting the client. Adequate lighting and an easily accessible light switch help clients with visual impairment. To provide a safe environment for the hearing impaired, the nurse should use appropriate visual aids such as a blinking light as one enters the room, a flashing alarm clock, or flashing lights to warn of fire. To enhance hearing, clients may need to use phone amplifiers. When driving, they may require additional mirrors on their cars and should keep the windows lowered. Individuals with impaired hearing may experience social isolation. Nurses must anticipate this and promote increased social interaction. Hearing-impaired clients should be spoken to face-to-face to amplify their hearing. The nurse should speak in a normal, clear voice and use simple phrases. A lower pitch should be used with those who are partially hearing impaired. Prevent extraneous noises by turning off the radio or television when communicating. For the profoundly deaf, the nurse should communicate in writing. An interpreter may be needed.

Nurses must ensure a safe environment for persons with a decreased or absent sense of touch. A thermometer should be provided for bath water, and the client must be instructed to assess his or her body for signs of injury that may have been missed. Loss of the ability to taste or smell may affect the client's nutritional intake. Frequent mouth care and offering flavorful food help. For those who have lost their sense of smell, smoke detectors and carbon monoxide detectors are essential. Finally, discard dates should be placed on all refrigerated food.

Individuals who suffer from dizziness or vertigo experience a loss of position sense that is likely to lead to injury. The most common cause of dizziness is orthostatic hypotension: the drop in blood pressure when moving from a prone to a sitting position or from a sitting to a standing position. Cardiac dysrhythmias, dehydration, side effects of medications, staying in bed too long, and a sudden change in position can all contribute to postural hypotension. Thus, individuals who suffer from dizziness must learn to rise and change positions slowly. Using a chair, walker, or cane can help the client when getting out of bed. In addition, clients should be taught to drink adequate fluids to avoid dehydration and its sequelae.

Individuals who are ill are at increased risk for sensory overload. Factors that contribute to sensory overload include an unfamiliar routine or environment, too much light or noise, pain, and an altered pattern of sleep or rest. Dimming the lights at night or turning them off when possible facilitates sleep. In addition, nonessential equipment should be turned off, and the client's sleep should not be interrupted except when absolutely necessary. The nurse should explain unfamiliar noises to the client. If a client has become disoriented, explain everything to him or her in simple terms. The nurse can promote normal sleep and rest periods by keeping the client active and engaged during the day. Clients should be encouraged to care for themselves as much as possible. For clients who are restrained, the restraints should be released and ROM exercises should be performed every 2 hours. Finally, clients in pain should be given medication per the primary care provider's or the specialist's orders.

Evaluation

The nurse should ascertain whether outcomes or goals have been met. Most importantly, the nurse must assess whether a sensory or perceptually impaired client has improved since the deficit or alteration was sustained. As a health care professional, the nurse must evaluate both the care that has been provided to the client and its effect on the client.

$\mathcal{H}$EADACHE

Most of us experience an occasional headache. They are usually self-treated, and medical treatment is not sought unless self-treatment fails. Approximately 50 million Americans have a significant headache at least once a year. A headache occurs when pain-sensitive areas are stimulated. Pain-sensitive areas include the skin; some extracranial and intracranial vessels; the eyes, ears, nasal cavity and sinuses; the dura mater of the base of the brain; and cranial nerves I, II, III, V, IX, and X. Non–pain-sensitive areas include the skull; most of the pia, arachnoid, and dura mater; and the choroid plexus (Table 9-8).

Assessment

A detailed history is vital to make the correct diagnosis. A thorough history must include determining the nature of the headache, family history, psychosocial history, and current medications. The nurse should ask about factors that may precipitate a headache such as smoking, alcohol, medications, or certain foods like chocolate and red wine. The use of oral

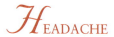

TABLE 9-8

DIFFERENTIAL FEATURES OF HEADACHES

Headache	Quality	Location	Duration	Associated Symptoms
Common migraine	Throbbing	Unilateral or bilateral	6–48 hr	Nausea, vomiting, photophobia
Classic migraine	Throbbing	Unilateral	3–12 hr	Visual prodrome, nausea, vomiting, photophobia
Cluster	Boring	Unilateral, especially the orbit	15–120 min	Ipsilateral tearing, nasal stuffiness
Tension or psychogenic	Dull	Diffuse bilateral	Unremitting	Depression

contraceptives and pregnancy can relieve or worsen headaches. The nurse must investigate analgesic overuse, which can contribute to rebound headache. The physical examination should ascertain the presence of neurological deficits; papilledema; retinal hemorrhage; cranial bruit; thickened, tender temporal arteries; trigger points for facial pain; dilated pupils; and stiff neck. The physician will order a CT scan if a lesion is suspected; LP is performed if the CT scan does not reveal a suspected infection or SAH. The client should undergo MRI if an aneurysm is suspected, and an ESR must be obtained in elderly clients with new-onset headaches. Common causes of headache include sinusitis, tooth infection, and temporomandibular joint (TMJ) syndrome.

Migraine Headache

A migraine is an acute, periodic vascular disorder that typically manifests as pain on one side of the head, although the pain may become generalized. Some clients experience migraines as often as twice a week; others may only have them once a year. Migraines usually last 4–24 hours, although some may last longer. Migraines are frequently accompanied by nausea, vomiting, blurred vision, phonophobia, photophobia, light-headedness, scalp tenderness, and cold extremities; they may be preceded by an aura. Migraines accompanied by an aura are termed *classic*; those without are termed *common*. Approximately 20–30% of clients with migraines experience an aura, or visual warning sign, such as spots, lights, or lines. Clients may also note a strange odor before the migraine attack. The appearance of an aura (i.e., classic migraine) may help the client to seek treatment more rapidly. Clients without an aura may experience another type of premonition 2–72 hours prior to the migraine, such as a feeling of well-being, depression, restlessness, hunger, energy, or fatigue. Clients usually experience the same clinical manifestations each time they have a migraine and may actually be incapacitated for several days.

In the early (prodromal) phase of a migraine, cerebral arterial vasoconstriction occurs. In the next stage, the intracranial and extracranial vessels dilate, stretch, and swell, with subsequent distention and pulsation on the affected side. In the final stage, the neck and scalp vessels may contract as the walls of the cerebral vessels become rigid and edematous, stretch, and dilate. Fluctuating estrogen levels during episodes of premenstrual tension often cause migraines.

Migraines appear to be inherited. Stress is a well-known precipitating factor, as are oral contraceptives, which can increase the frequency and severity of migraines. Migraines occur in 10% of the general population and in 15% of child-bearing women. Women experience them three times more frequently than men. Migraines usually begin in the second or third decade of life or later and continue into middle age. For some women, the onset of menopause can bring relief from migraines. Others experience them well into old age, although this is unusual.

Migraine sufferers have been described as overly neat, compulsive, rigid, and perfectionistic. They often create a climate for themselves that is impossible to maintain without some relief, which, in an odd way, is obtained by having a migraine. The origin and mechanism of action of migraines are not yet fully understood, although many new drug therapies are currently becoming available. Some established therapies for migraines or severe tension headaches are discussed below.

Treatment

Nonpharmacological Treatment The initial therapy for migraine sufferers is the reduction of triggers that contribute to the headache. For example, eliminating oversleeping, excessive tiredness, bright lights, and missed meals may prove beneficial. Reducing factors that contribute to stress, depression, fear, and anxiety is also helpful. Some authors advocate a change in diet by eliminating vasoactive substances such as tyramine that may trigger migraines. This altered diet eliminates alcohol; products that are aged, dried, fermented, smoked, or pickled; certain breads; certain beans and sauerkraut; nuts, peanuts, peanut butter, and seeds; and mince-meat pie. Clients who choose to alter their eating habits to bring their migraines under control require specific instructions concerning diet. In addition, they need instruction in stress reduction, relaxation training, and occasionally may require psychological counseling.

Acute Treatment Acute (abortive) therapy treats the headache after it has started. The following methods are used:

1. Sumatriptan succinate (Imitrex) is a serotonin-receptor agonist. It is administered subcutaneously in a 6-mg dose and may be repeated in 1 hour (up to 12 mg in 24 hours). This drug inhibits the release of 5-hydroxytryptamine, norepinephrine, acetylcholine, and substance P. Sumatriptan succinate (Imitrex) blocks inflammation and produces vasoconstriction. Currently available as a nasal spray (20 mg), sumatriptan succinate (Imitrex) is the agent of choice for abortive therapy. Many clients use the oral form or learn to inject themselves. Regardless of the method used, a 5-day hiatus should be observed between treatments. Major side effects include flushing, neck and chest discomfort, tingling, and nausea. This medication is contraindicated for clients with ischemic heart disease or Prinzmetal's angina and should not be used with medications containing ergotamine.

2. One or two tablets of an ergotamine derivative (i.e., ergotamine tartrate-caffeine [Cafergot]) are administered orally. The client can take up to five per attack or ten per week. Conversely, 2 mg of ergotamine can be taken orally or sublingually and can be repeated in 30 minutes (up to 8 mg/24 hours or 16 mg/week). Ergotamine is also available as a suppository. This α-adrenergic blocking agent affects the smooth muscles of cranial and peripheral blood vessels. Side effects include nausea, vomiting, diarrhea, cramping, dizziness, stroke, hypertension, and myocardial ischemia or infarction. It is contraindicated for clients over the age of 60 and for those with peripheral or coronary artery disease. Prochlorperazine (Compazine), 5 mg, is

A plethora of new drugs for migraine headaches are coming on the market as this text goes to press. Similar to sumatriptan (Imitrex), but improved, they included: naratriptan (Amerge), dihydroergotamine mesylate (Migranal), zolmitriptan (Zomig), and rizatriptan (Maxalt and Maxalt-MLT). Each of these new drugs has specific indications and guidelines.

administered intravenously, followed by dihydroergotamine (D.H.E. 45, 0.75 mg), a derivative of ergot. Another 0.5 mg of D.H.E. 45 may be administered in 30 minutes. D.H.E. 45 is also available as a nasal spray. The side effects are short term and include nausea, flushing, leg cramps, diarrhea, and chest or throat tightness.

3. Isometheptene (Midrin) is a combination product that constricts dilated cranial and peripheral blood vessels and contains a mild sedative and acetaminophen (Tylenol). Two capsules are administered initially, followed by one capsule every hour (up to five in 12 hours). This medication works well on mild-to-moderate migraines when taken as early as possible. Isometheptene (Midrin) has few side effects but is contraindicated for clients with hypertension, organic heart disease, and severe renal or hepatic disease and those on monoamine oxidase inhibitors (MAOIs).

4. Nonsteroidal anti-inflammatory drugs (NSAIDs) such as indomethacin (Indocin, 50 mg three times a day with food) or naproxen (Naprosyn, 550 mg two or three times a day with food) are administered to clients with mild-to-moderate migraines. NSAIDs are an excellent first choice, as they inhibit prostaglandins and may interfere with serotonin activity. The side effects are usually minor and include nausea, dyspepsia, diarrhea, and dizziness, but bleeding can result from long-term use. NSAIDs should not be administered to clients with peptic ulcer disease or renal dysfunction.

A migraine that lasts for several days or weeks and cannot be resolved by the previously mentioned treatments is termed a *status migraine*. If there are no contraindications, repetitive use of dihydroergotamine (D.H.E. 45) is the treatment of choice. Dihydroergotamine (D.H.E. 45) can be administered repeatedly with metoclopramide (Reglan), another antiemetic such as promethazine (Phenergan, 25–50 mg intramuscularly), or prochlorperazine (Compazine, 5–10 mg intramuscularly). Additional medications for intractable migraines include long-acting steroids such as dexamethasone (Decadron) with dihydroergotamine (D.H.E. 45). The treatment should be limited to less than once a month.

Prophylactic Treatment Prophylactic therapy is required for those experiencing two or more migraines a month. It is indicated for individuals whose attacks affect their quality of life and ability to function, for those in whom acute therapies do not work, or for those who cannot receive acute therapy. Each medication should be administered for a trial period of 4–6 weeks before another medication is tried.

1. Beta blockers such as propranolol (Inderal, 20–40 mg four times a day) are the medications of choice. The long-acting daily dose form, Inderal LA, is used. If this particular beta blocker fails after a 6–8-week trial, a different beta blocker should be used, such as timolol (Blocadren) or nadolol (Corgard). Common side effects include fatigue, GI disturbances, insomnia, hypotension, bradycardia, and sexual dysfunction. Beta blockers are contraindicated for clients

with asthma, heart failure, or diabetes. However, cardioselective beta blockers such as metoprolol (Lopressor) or atenolol (Tenormin) may be used.

2. Valproic acid (Depakote) should be the first choice for migraine sufferers who also have seizures, mania, or anxiety. Major side effects include nausea, GI distress, sedation, tremors, and hepatotoxicity. CBC and liver function tests should be obtained when the medication is first administered and frequently during the first 6 months. In addition, valproic acid (Depakote) blood levels should be checked every 6 months.

3. Calcium-channel blockers such as verapamil (Calan, Isoptin, 40–80 mg twice a day) inhibit arterial vasospasms and block serotonin release and aggregation. Diltiazem (Cardizem) and nifedipine (Procardia) are less effective, providing more benefit to clients with aura or cluster headaches. They should be administered for a trial period of 2 months. The most common side effects are constipation, flushing, hypotension, rash, and nausea. Calcium-channel blockers are contraindicated for clients with heart failure or heart block. The nurse should inform clients not to stop taking the medication abruptly, as chest pain or rebound angina may occur.

4. Antidepressants are often used to treat migraines.
   • Tricyclic antidepressants block serotonin reabsorption and some norepinephrine release at nerve endings. The medication takes 2–3 weeks to have a therapeutic effect. Antidepressants are helpful for some clients. Specific medications include the more sedating amitriptyline (Elavil), doxepin (Sinequan), nortriptyline (Pamelor), and imipramine (Vivactil) and the less sedating protriptyline (Tofranil) and desipramine (Norpramin). These medications may cause constipation, weight gain, dry mouth, tachycardia, hypotension, sexual dysfunction, and urinary retention.
   • Selective serotonin reuptake inhibitors (SSRIs) operate specifically at serotonin receptor sites. Fluoxetine (Prozac), sertraline (Zoloft), and paroxetine (Paxil) have proven beneficial. The common side effects include nausea, insomnia, weight loss, and sexual dysfunction. Bupropion (Welbutrin) and trazodone (Desyrel) have shown limited usefulness in migraine prophylaxis.

5. The medication methysergide (Sansert, 1–2 mg four times a day) is reserved for clients with frequent, severe migraines. Long-term use has been linked to retroperitoneal fibrosis, pleuropulmonary fibrosis, and thickening of heart valves. Methysergide (Sansert) must not be used for longer than 4–6 months without a 1–1½-month hiatus; this drug holiday is required to avoid fibrosis. The medication should not be administered to clients with peripheral or coronary artery disease.

6. NSAIDs have anti-inflammatory and analgesic properties. Because of the possible side effects, the lowest effective dose should be used (see above discussion on NSAIDs).

Approximately 60–70% of women with migraines note a relationship to their menstrual cycle. Certain agents used during the menstrual cycle help many women, including NSAIDs; methylergonovine (Methergine); methysergide (Sansert); a combination of ergotamine, phenobarbital, and bellafoline; and other previously mentioned therapies. Treatment should begin 3 days before the onset of menses and continue throughout the menstrual period. Short courses of corticosteroid therapy and transdermal estrogen patches may also be beneficial.

Symptomatic Treatment Narcotic analgesics are necessary for some clients, but those who have chronic migraines should avoid them. An injectable NSAID, such as ketorolac (Toradol, 60 mg intramuscularly), is a good choice for emergencies and the clinic setting. Butorphanol (Stadol) nasal spray is effective for some clients and often works well in clients who become nauseated with other medications. This drug should only be used every 3–4 days. For clients with nausea and vomiting, suppositories are an option for relief. Prochlorperazine (Compazine) and chlorpromazine (Thorazine) have proven helpful, but long-term use is not recommended because of the potential irreversible extrapyramidal effects.

Cluster Headache

Cluster headaches are another form of vascular headache. They manifest unilaterally, on one side, with severe pain that has been described as excruciating, boring, constant, knife-like, and nonthrobbing. The headaches typically occur on a daily basis at the same time for 1–3 months, followed by a remission for 9–12 months. A cluster headache lasts 10–45 minutes. Although these headaches do not last long, they may occur more than once a day. The site is usually consistent during a series. Some clients experience chronic cluster headaches for a full year before the period of remission begins. Signs and symptoms include tearing of one eye, rhinorrhea or congestion, ptosis, facial flushing or pallor, and sweating. Clients may also experience bradycardia, elevated intraocular pressure, and elevated skin temperature. The temporal artery may be prominent, and clients may pace the floor or sit and rock. Onset is associated with relaxation, napping, and rapid eye movement (REM) sleep. The etiology is unknown. There is no familial, dietary, or personality link. Cluster headaches occur more commonly in younger men, as much as seven times more often than in women.

Treatment
Abortive Treatment These headaches are acute but painful and incapacitating. Therefore, treatment must be quick and effective. Low-dose ergotamine (Ergomar), methysergide (Sansert), prednisone (Deltasone, 60 mg/day for 1 week with a rapid taper), verapamil (80–160 mg three times a day), and lithium carbonate (300 mg twice or three times a day) are used. Sumatriptan succinate (Imitrex) has also been approved for treatment of cluster headaches. If possible, oxygen (delivered via a nonrebreathing mask at 7 L/min for 10–15 min) may be helpful along with the previously mentioned treatment.

Prophylactic Treatment Prophylactic therapy is preferred for decreasing the frequency of attacks and to resolve the series. Because cluster headaches have a short duration, the agent of choice is methysergide (Sansert, 2 mg three times a day). Corticosteroids may be added to the usual treatment regimen for cluster headaches. Since these headaches are self-limiting, the short-term use of corticosteroids may be beneficial. Methylprednisolone (Depo-Medrol, in a tapering dosepak), prednisone (Deltasone, 30 mg daily and then tapering), and triamcinolone (Aristocort, 4 mg four times a day) are all acceptable alternatives. Verapamil (Calan) may be helpful if used concomitantly with steroids in divided doses (240–480 mg/day). Finally, lithium carbonate (Eskalith, Lithobid, 90 mg/day in a divided dose) has been shown to have some usefulness through its effect on ADH and REM sleep. Lithium levels should be checked monthly and should not exceed 2.0 mEq/L. Side effects are usually mild; however, if severe side effects such as persistent nausea and vomiting, blurred vision, or fasciculations occur, the drug should be stopped.

Histamine Desensitization Histamine desensitization should be considered for refractory cluster headaches. This procedure is usually done on an inpatient basis by a qualified physician. In one study, histamine desensitization resulted in at least a 50% improvement in as many as 64% of clients. Thus, this therapy effectively decreased the frequency and duration of headaches 4 weeks after treatment.

Tension Headache

Tension headaches are chronic headaches that occur episodically. They are usually described as a steady, nonpulsatile ache. Pain manifests as tightness bilaterally or at the base of the head, either as a band-like sensation around the head or as a vise-like pressure. Tension headaches are often accompanied by neck pain and tightness and are typically linked to some type of emotional disorder or fatigue. Most clients do not seek medical advice or treatment. These clients report daily, continuous headaches with multiple other complaints. They usually appear after the third decade, are more frequent in women, and are often associated with depression. A complaint of early or frequent awakening is the classic sign of tension headache.

Treatment *Prophylactic Treatment* Narcotics, barbiturates, and tranquilizers should be avoided, as tension headaches are continuous and chronic, and these medications are habit forming. Tricyclic antidepressants are very helpful for the client with tension headaches. Amitriptyline (Elavil) and doxepin (Sinequan) are recommended in large doses at bedtime for those with sleep disorders. Other choices include nortriptyline (Pamelor, 25 mg at bedtime), protriptyline (Vivactil, 5–10 mg three times a day), imipramine (Tofranil, 75–150 mg/day in divided doses), or trimipramine (Surmontil, 75–200 mg/day in divided doses). The SSRIs (fluoxetine [Prozac], sertraline [Zoloft], and paroxetine [Paxil]) have also proven beneficial. In some studies, newer medications such as trazodone (Desyrel) and venlafaxine (Effexor) have shown some efficacy in the treatment of tension headache.

Abortive Treatment OTC medications designed to relieve headache pain are usually effective. Those containing caffeine should be avoided because of the tendency to overuse them. If the client is having headaches from overuse of medication (i.e., rebound headaches), it is necessary for him or her to gradually taper off the medication.

Seizures

Seizures involve aberrant, abrupt, intense discharges of electrical activity within the brain. They result from brain or CNS irritation that can cause neurological dysfunction, such as disturbances in consciousness, motor function, sensation, or behavior. Seizures may indicate an underlying CNS dysfunction such as a tumor or meningitis. The term *epilepsy* comes from the Greek word "epilepsia," which means a condition of being overcome or seized. Epilepsy refers to a chronic disorder of recurrent seizures that are typified by abnormal electrical activity in the cerebral cortical neurons. This disorder affects approximately 2% of the population, with 100,000 new cases diagnosed annually. Children under the age of 18 comprise 30% of seizure cases. The underlying etiology of a seizure is unknown in approximately 70% of all cases. What is known about seizures is that a triggering mechanism exists that produces an abrupt, aberrant discharge of electrical activity, disrupting normal nerve conduction. When the disturbance is widespread, a general seizure can occur; when limited or localized, a partial seizure may occur.

The most common known causes of seizures include head trauma, anoxia at birth, brain tumor, cerebral scar tissue, and infections of the brain. Seizures are also caused by metabolic disorders, alcohol withdrawal, and electrolyte imbalances. Precipitating factors (i.e., those elements contributing to the onset of a seizure) are physical stress, chemical imbalance, metabolic and endocrinological disorders, and drug and alcohol abuse. There is no identifiable cause for primary (idiopathic, essential, genetic) seizures. They are often inherited and age-related. Secondary (symptomatic, organic, acquired) seizures occur secondary to an identifiable cause such as head trauma, vascular disease, tumor, aneurysm, or an infection. A *convulsion* is a seizure in which motor signs predominate. Seizures are classified as *partial* or *generalized*.

There are two types of partial seizures, simple and complex. *Partial seizures* (focal, local) begin focally (i.e., on one side of the brain) and may become secondary generalized seizures. *Simple partial seizures* do not involve a loss of consciousness. *Complex partial seizures* present with impaired consciousness and, typically, automatic behaviors such as walking and driving. A simple partial seizure may be motor, sensory, or autonomic. Focal motor seizures usually begin in the face or hands but may spread and affect other areas. The client may experience a certain smell, thought, or prickling and tingling sensation during this seizure. Complex partial seizures have bilateral brain involvement and impaired consciousness. A temporal lobe seizure can alter behavior and cause automatisms such as lip smacking, chewing, grimacing, and patting or picking hand movements. Clients experiencing such seizures may have rare outbursts of rage or violence followed by amnesia. In addition, a variety of sensory experiences may occur, such as olfactory, visual, and auditory hallucinations. Temporal lobe seizures usually last only about 30 seconds to a few minutes, followed by confusion. Partial seizures also include automatic signs and symptoms. For example, flushing, dilated pupils, or abdominal cramping may be a partial seizure. Simple seizures can become complex, and complex seizures may develop into generalized seizures.

Generalized seizures (convulsive or nonconvulsive) are usually idiopathic, bilateral, and symmetrical without a focal onset. A generalized seizure may first present as a loss of consciousness. There may or may not be an aura (i.e., a sensory warning such as a smell, flash of light, or metallic taste) preceding the seizure. Electrical and motor signs occur bilaterally, and clients experience widespread neuronal hyperactivity. There are several types of generalized seizures: tonic–clonic, absence, myoclonic, and atonic. Tonic–clonic and absence seizures are the most common forms. Tonic–clonic seizures, once called grand mal seizures, affect all age groups. In the tonic phase, there is a sudden loss of consciousness with muscle spasms. If the throat and diaphragm muscles contract, the client emits a cry or scream. Apnea and cyanosis usually occur. In the clonic phase, hyperventilation and rapid, synchronous muscle jerks occur. Clients may bite their tongues; lose bladder and bowel control; become hypertensive, tachycardic, and diaphoretic; salivate heavily (foaming at the mouth); and have dilated pupils. These types of seizures last 2–5 minutes and are followed by fatigue, confusion, headache, memory loss, muscle weakness, and irritability. It may be several hours before the client recovers fully. Complications of seizures include hypoxia, aspiration pneumonia, and injuries.

Absence seizures, formerly called petit mal seizures, are characterized by a brief, 15–30-second loss of consciousness. No aura precedes these seizures. Clients stare and may occasionally blink their eyes or smack their lips during the seizure. After the seizure, normal activities are usually resumed. This type of seizure typically affects children, although adults can also be affected. Absence seizures can occur as often as 100 times a day, which can affect the individual's concentration and attention span. This type of seizure usually diminishes during adolescence and disappears by the age of 20, although some clients develop generalized tonic–clonic seizures.

A major complication of seizure, **status epilepticus**, occurs when a seizure lasts over 4 minutes or a series of seizures occurs in rapid succession. Status epilepticus can occur with any seizure. Causes of status epilepticus include sudden withdrawal of anticonvulsant medication, infection, acute alcohol withdrawal, head trauma, cerebral edema, and metabolic disorders. Clients may have focal signs or symptoms and a prolonged

Status epilepticus is an emergency condition. It is defined as a seizure that lasts more than 15 minutes or as repetitive seizures with incomplete recovery to baseline neurologic function. This prolonged seizure can increase the risk of anoxia, cardiac dysrhythmias, and systemic lactic acidosis. Prompt treatment and management is absolutely essential!

postictal state (longer than usual recovery time after a seizure). Clients with status epilepticus may also have a fever. A history of seizures is common. During an emergency, and after stabilization, the nurse should look for causes of the prolonged seizure, including metabolic, toxic, hypoxic, and infectious causes; intracranial lesions; and poor compliance. In the client who has a history of seizures and who is on prescribed medication, the level of the drug's concentration in the body should be determined to assess compliance. Phenytoin (Dilantin, 50 mg/min administered intravenously) is the drug of choice for seizure clients in status epilepticus. Since prolonged seizures can cause hypoxia, it is important to be alert for an impaired airway (the most important consideration in *all* clients). Any identifiable, underlying metabolic cause should be corrected.

Diagnosis

Diagnosis is made predominantly by history. This necessitates the need for a very thorough and accurate interview with the client (Table 9-9). An EEG is absolutely necessary but does not reliably diagnose or exclude the diagnosis of epilepsy because abnormal EEGs are not necessarily indicative of epilepsy. Required laboratory tests include a CBC, BUN, glucose level, electrolytes (Na^+, K^+, chloride [Cl^-], CO_2), Ca^{++}, Mg^{++}, and urinalysis. A drug screen may also be ordered. The physician may also perform a LP, and skull x-rays may be obtained to demonstrate calcified areas of the brain. CT scan, MRI, and PET scan may be ordered as well.

Assessment

The nurse should obtain a complete history of seizure activity to help identify the cause and plan the client's care. Determine the frequency of seizure activity, obtain a description of each seizure, and determine if more than one type of seizure has occurred. Additionally, record the sequence of

TABLE 9-9

SEIZURE ETIOLOGY BY AGE

Age of Onset	Probable Cause
Adolescence	Idiopathic, trauma
Early adulthood	Idiopathic, trauma, tumor, alcohol, or hypnotic drug withdrawal
Middle age	Trauma, tumor, vascular disease, alcohol, or drug withdrawal
Late life	Vascular disease, tumor, degenerative disease

seizure progression, the length of time they last, when the last seizure occurred, if the seizures are accompanied by an aura, if the client is conscious of having had the seizures, what occurs after the seizure, how long it takes the client to resume normal activity after the seizure, or whether bladder and stool incontinence occurs. It is important to ascertain if the client is currently taking anticonvulsant medication, and, if so, what it is, the dose and frequency of administration, when it was last taken, and whether the client is actually taking the medication. If the nurse witnesses a seizure, it is vital to record an accurate description.

Treatment

Most seizures can now be controlled with anticonvulsant medications which prevent and reduce the frequency of seizures. One or more medications may be prescribed by the primary care provider or neurologist. Some drugs work well in combination while others do not. Blood levels should be monitored closely to ensure the efficacy and safety of each of these drugs and the client's compliance. The primary health care provider and nurse must be alert for signs of drug interactions, toxicity, and other adverse effects. If at all possible, clients should not be given multiple anticonvulsants. Carbamazepine (Tegretol) and phenytoin (Dilantin) are the drugs of choice for first-line treatment of partial seizures. Valproic acid (Depakote), phenytoin (Dilantin), and phenobarbital (Luminal) are the medications of choice for generalized seizures. Ethosuximide (Zarontin) and valproic acid (Depakote) are used for absence seizures (Table 9-10).

▨

TABLE 9-10
ANTI-SEIZURE DRUGS

Generic (Trade Name)	Daily Dose (mg)	Major Indications	Serum Half-Life (hrs)	Treatment Level (mg/L)
Phenobarbital (Luminal)	60–200	Generalized, absence, simple and complex partial	24 ± 12	10–40
Phenytoin (Dilantin)	300–400	Generalized, simple, and complex partial	24 ± 12	10–20
Carbamazepine (Tegretol)	600–1200	Generalized, complex partial	12 ± 3	4–10
Valproic acid (Depakote)	1000–3000	Absence, generalized, complex partial	8 ± 12	50–100
Primidone (Mysoline)	750–1500	Generalized, simple, and complex partial	12 ± 6	5–15
Ethosuximide (Zarontin)	750–2000	Absence	40 ± 6	50–100
Clonazepam (Klonopin)	1.5–20	Absence, myoclonic	18–50	0.01–0.07

It is important, when administering anticonvulsant medications, that the nurse be keenly aware of their serious side effects. These drugs can alter or impair liver function, cause teeth and gum problems, and depress the production of bone marrow in long-term therapy. They can also cause serious adverse effects if used in conjunction with many other medications. Thus, it is important that clients understand the expected effects and potential side effects of the medications they are taking. The nurse should warn the client of the importance of not stopping any anticonvulsant medication suddenly, as this can precipitate status epilepticus. Sudden withdrawal can also cause subsequent seizures to be longer and more severe. Some clients require lifelong drug therapy; others may be weaned gradually after 1–2 years. Clients must be warned to avoid alcohol while taking these medications. The nurse must also stress the importance of good nutrition. Clients with intractable seizures may require surgery.

Major side effects of anticonvulsant medications include drowsiness, sedation, mental dullness, fatigue, dizziness, irritability, GI upset, and ataxia. Seizure thresholds can be lowered with the addition of phenothiazines or tricyclic antidepressants. There can be adverse drug reactions to phenytoin (Dilantin) when it is combined with any of the following: alcohol, chloramphenicol (Chloromycetin), isoniazid (Nydrazid), trimethoprim, cimetidine (Tagamet), disulfam (Antabuse), folic acid (Folvite), oxyphenbutazone, valproic acid (Depakote), or levodopa (Dopar). Phenobarbital (Luminal) and valproic acid (Depakote) can potentiate phenobarbital toxicity. Carbamazepine (Tegretol) can be more toxic when combined with phenobarbital, erythromycin, or propoxyphene (Darvon).

Nursing Care

A client having a seizure should be placed on his or her side to prevent aspiration. Gum, food, and dentures should be removed, if possible. However, never place your fingers inside the mouth of a client who is actively having a seizure! If available, provide nasal oxygen. Protect the client's head from injury with pillows. Protect the client from other injury by guiding the arms and legs without forcibly restraining seizure movements. The nurse should provide privacy, if possible, and not leave the client during a seizure. Administer anticonvulsants intravenously as ordered, if an access is available. When the seizure has ended, the nurse should provide appropriate care for any injuries and assist in stabilizing the client. As the client regains consciousness, reorient him or her and encourage rest. When it is safe to leave the client, document the details of the seizure while they are still fresh in your mind. Documentation should include the time the seizure started, the parts of the body affected, the seizure's progression, the type and character of movements, the client's condition throughout the seizure, and the postictal status. The nurse should describe the duration of each component of the seizure, changes in consciousness, pupillary changes, eye deviations, and automatisms (if they occurred).

Clients who have seizures should be instructed to never smoke in bed and to never take baths or swim alone. In addition, they may not be

When **documenting seizures**, the nurse must note the following:

- Size and reactivity of pupils
- Eye direction
- Head turning
- Motor activity and progression
- Level of awareness
- Vocalizations
- Incontinence
- Skin color changes
- Confusion after seizure
- Paralysis of any extremity
- Reports of subjective feelings or sensations

allowed to drive, operate machinery, or work in high places. The nurse must remind the client that alcohol interferes with the effectiveness of anticonvulsant drugs. The client and family should be taught about the disorder, and emotional support should be provided.

Evaluation

To evaluate your nursing care, first determine whether the client is free of injury. Next, assess the client's knowledge and understanding of the medications and whether he or she is taking them as prescribed. Third, determine if the client understands and utilizes the appropriate precautions to prevent injury when a seizure occurs. Finally, determine whether the client is working to decrease the risk for seizures by employing stress management techniques, relaxation therapy, and getting adequate rest.

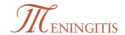

$\mathcal{M}$ENINGITIS

Bacterial meningitis is an infection of the pia mater, arachnoid membrane, and CSF-filled subarachnoid space. It may result from a bacterial infection in the bloodstream or from bacteria entering the brain through a cranial structure (nose, ears, sinuses). Any disruption in the blood–brain barrier, such as a skull fracture, may provide a port of entry for bacteria. Most bacterial meningitis is caused by *Haemophilus influenzae, Streptococcus pneumoniae, Staphylococcus aureus,* and *Neisseria meningitidis. H. influenzae* has decreased dramatically during the past 10 years, with a 0.2% incidence per 100,000 population, primarily as a result of the vaccine now available. There also has been a decline in the incidence of meningitis from *N. meningitidis.* However, there has not been a decrease in the number of cases caused by *S. pneumoniae*; the incidence rate has remained stable at 1.1% per 100,000 population over the last 10 years.

Bacterial meningitis is most often transmitted by direct contact, including droplet spread. Factors that predispose individuals to acquiring meningitis include sinusitis, otitis media, and mastoiditis. Other individuals at risk are those who are immunosuppressed (e.g., persons with acquired immunodeficiency syndrome [AIDS]) and those with otorrhea (ear discharge) or rhinorrhea (nasal discharge) that may occur secondary to a basilar skull fracture.

Bacteria multiply after they enter the subarachnoid space and spread to the ventricles of the brain, which results in inflammation. Blood vessels that have enlarged from the high volume may rupture or thrombose. Furthermore, bacteria can cause a great deal of irritation to the brain, leading to increased subarachnoid exudate, vascular congestion, and increased capillary permeability. Purulent material may extend into the cranial or spinal nerves or block the flow of CSF, causing hydrocephalus. If the surface of the brain adjacent to the meninges becomes affected, secondary encephalitis and neuron degeneration may result. Fever and focal neurological signs should raise the possibility of a brain abscess. In such cases, the nurse should look for the source or cause. A lung abscess is an example of a source. Opportunistic organisms such as *Cryptococcus meningitis* and *Tuberculosis meningitis* must be ruled out whenever suspected.

Viral meningitis occurs frequently and is generally benign. It frequently results from a viral illness such as measles, mumps, herpes simplex, and herpes zoster. Inflammation occurs over the meninges, **cerebral cortex**, and **white matter.** Depending on the virus, cell dysfunction occurs, and there can be neurological deficits.

The very young and the very old are most susceptible to developing meningitis. Others at risk include those who are malnourished, immunosuppressed, chronically ill (cancer, tuberculosis), or have sustained CNS trauma. Despite newer antibiotics, the morbidity and mortality rate for bacterial meningitis is still quite high. In one study, 25% of afflicted adults died.

The characteristic signs of meningitis are fever, severe and unrelenting headache, nausea, vomiting, papilledema, a stiff neck (nuchal rigidity), altered level of consciousness (LOC), behavior or personality changes, and altered motor or sensory abilities. Other signs include an impaired ability to communicate, ocular palsies, photophobia, **nystagmus, ptosis,** cranial nerve palsies, vision and hearing changes, positive **Brudzinski's** and **Kernig's signs,** seizures, vomiting, tachycardia and dysrhythmias, and respiratory distress. Mental status changes or seizures may indicate encephalitis.

Diagnosis

In the absence of focal neurological signs and papilledema, an LP should be performed immediately by a qualified physician for CSF analysis. In the event of increased or suspected increased ICP, an LP is usually not done. If an LP cannot be done, antibiotics should be administered immediately. Once a successful LP is performed, the first tube of CSF is marked for protein and glucose, the second tube for Gram stain and culture and sensitivity, and the third tube for CBC and differential. A more sophisticated test called a counterimmunoelectrophoresis (CIE) may be used to examine the CSF and is most helpful if antibiotics have already been started. CIE can identify viruses or protozoa in the CSF. Additional diagnostic laboratory studies include a CBC, which includes a white blood cell (WBC) count that may point to an infection if elevated; a serum glucose to compare to that of the CSF; a urinalysis, which may reveal the red blood cell (RBC) count and WBC count, as well as albumin; and nasopharyngeal, skin lesion, and blood cultures to identify a causative organism.

Skull and spine x-rays may be ordered to help diagnose sinusitis, mastoid infection, fractures, or osteomyelitis. Chest x-rays may reveal pneumonia, lung abscess, tuberculosis lesions, or granulomas secondary to fungal infection. In the client whose consciousness is markedly changed, a head CT or MRI is recommended.

The **cerebral cortex** is the layer of gray matter on the surface of the cerebral hemispheres that integrates high mental functions and is, therefore, the center for thought.

The **white matter** is comprised of nerve fibers covered with myelin; it has few, if any, nerve cell bodies. White matter is located in the interior of the brain and the perimeter of the spinal cord.

Nystagmus is a tremor of the eyeball. It may be horizontal, vertical, rotating, or mixed.

Ptosis is a drooping of the upper eyelid, usually caused by lack of nervous innervation.

Kernig's Sign. To assess Kernig's sign flex the client's leg at the hip, place the knee and lower leg at a 90-degree angle, and attempt to extend the knee. Pain and spasm of the hamstring muscle will occur in the presence of bacterial meningitis, indicating a positive Kernig's sign.

Brudzinski's Sign. To assess Brudzinski's sign, gently flex the client's head and neck toward the chest. If the hips and knees flex, the test is positive.

Assessment

The nurse needs to perform a thorough neurological assessment to detect subtle changes that may occur during the course of the illness. He or she should begin by assessing the client's LOC; orientation to person, place, and time; pupillary reactions and eye movements; and motor response. The nurse must look for the following signs of early disease: mild lethargy, memory changes, short attention span, bewilderment, and personality and behavioral changes. These will deteriorate as the disease progresses. Determine the presence of meningeal irritation by checking for nuchal rigidity and assessing for Kernig's and Brudzinski's signs, which are positive in the presence of bacterial meningitis. Nuchal rigidity is a stiff, sore neck when the neck is flexed. To elicit Kernig's sign, flex the client's leg at the hip, place the knee at a 90° angle, and then attempt to extend the knee. Pain and spasm of the hamstring muscle (a positive Kernig's sign) will occur in the presence of bacterial meningitis. To assess for Brudzinski's sign, flex the client's head and neck gently toward the chest. If the hips and knees flex, the test is positive (see Fig. 9-11).

Additional assessment requires that the nurse determine the presence of increased intracranial pressure (ICP), which can occur in the presence of bacterial meningitis. Increased ICP can cause cerebral edema, hydrocephalus, eventually brain herniation, and death. Seizure activity can also ensue as a result of increased ICP.

In the neurologically impaired client, a neurological assessment and vital signs check must be obtained every 2–4 hours or more often if warranted or ordered. In addition, assessment of the cranial nerves is a routine part of the neurological assessment. Damage to cranial nerve VI may indicate hydrocephalus. The development of hydrocephalus is also indicated by the presence of urinary incontinence as the LOC decreases. A complete neurological assessment includes a vascular assessment, with particular attention paid to pulses, color, capillary refill time, and temperature. Normal capillary refill time is less than 3 seconds. The nurse should take seizure precautions as the client with meningitis may have one or more seizures. Furthermore, a client with meningitis may have severe headaches and will require careful pain control. Elevating the head of the bed 30 degrees, avoiding neck flexion, eliminating restrictive linens and clothing, using an ice cap, providing a dark and quiet environment, and even restricting visitors can ease the pain of a headache. The only pain medication that may be prescribed is acetaminophen (Tylenol). It is important that the client's LOC is not compromised by medication.

Treatment and Nursing Care

Treatment of the client with meningitis is aimed at eliminating the causative organism, preventing the spread of infection, maintaining optimal neurological function, and preventing complications. Fluids should be limited to 1000 mL/day, and 5% dextrose in water (D5W) should not

TABLE 9-11
ANTIBIOTIC THERAPY FOR BACTERIAL MENINGITIS

Bacterial Pathogens	Standard Drug Therapy	Alternative Drug Therapy
Streptococcus pneumoniae	Penicillin G or ampicillin	Cefotaxime or ceftriaxone; chloramphenicol; vancomycin
Neisseria meningitidis	Penicillin G or ampicillin	Cefotaxime or ceftriaxone; chloramphenicol; fluoroquinolone
Haemophilus influenzae		
β-Lactamase-negative	Ampicillin	Cefotaxime or ceftriaxone; chloramphenicol; aztreonam
β-Lactamase-positive	Cefotaxime or ceftriaxone	Chloramphenicol, aztreonam, fluoroquinolone
Pseudomonas aeruginosa	Ceftazidime	Aztreonam, fluoroquinolone
Listeria monocytogenes	Ampicillin or penicillin G	Trimethoprim-sulfamethoxazole
Streptococcus agalactiae	Ampicillin or penicillin G	Cefotaxime or ceftriaxone; vancomycin
Staphylococcus aureus		
Methicillin sensitive	Nafcillin or oxacillin	Vancomycin
Methicillin resistant	Vancomycin	
Staphylococcus epidermidis	Vancomycin	

be used if cerebral edema is suspected. Narcotics also should be avoided as they impede an accurate assessment of consciousness, and they may hamper breathing and worsen cerebral edema. Oxygen may be ordered to prevent **hypoxia**.

The drug of choice for the client with bacterial meningitis who is not immunocompromised or allergic is penicillin G (2 million units intravenously every 4 hours) or ampicillin (3 g intravenously every 6 hours for 10–14 days). In elderly or alcoholic clients and clients who do not demonstrate any organisms on Gram stain, it is suggested that a third-generation cephalosporin be added, such as cefotaxime (Claforan, 2 g intravenously every 4 hours) or ceftriaxone (Rocephin, 2 g every 12 hours). Remember that these combinations are not effective against *S. aureus*, Pseudomonas, or anaerobes; however, those organisms are very rare in uncomplicated adult meningitis. The specific course of antibiotic therapy varies according to the individual primary care provider and the length of treatment (7–21 days).

In addition to antibiotic therapy, clients may require antipyretics to control temperature, antiemetics to control vomiting, anticonvulsants to prevent seizures, and sedatives or tranquilizers to promote rest. In the event of cerebral edema, osmotic diuretics such as mannitol may be ordered to decrease the edema. Some physicians use corticosteroids to control or decrease cerebral inflammation. It is important for the nurse to become very familiar with the drugs that he or she administers to the client with meningitis, as many of them can have serious side effects.

Hypoxia is characterized by inadequate oxygen levels in the lungs or bloodstream.

In the event of viral meningitis, clients are usually hospitalized and antibiotics are begun as described above, if the exact diagnosis is uncertain. Otherwise, clients are treated at home with hydration, antiemetics, and analgesics for headache. If signs of encephalitis such as mental changes should occur, hospital admission is warranted.

Clients with herpes encephalitis are treated with acyclovir (Zovirax) (10 mg/kg intravenously every 8 hours) for 10 days. This treatment should be initiated immediately in clients who experience an abrupt onset of fever, changes in behavior, or altered consciousness with or without focal neurological changes, especially when CSF abnormalities are moderate, which suggests a viral CNS infection. A neurologist should be consulted, as characteristic but subtle changes that indicate temporal lobe abnormalities may be demonstrated by MRI.

CASE STUDY: WOMAN WITH MENINGITIS

A 28-year-old woman is seen in a physician's office complaining of a stiff neck and feeling feverish. She states that she has some trouble turning her head, but it hurts most when she tries to touch her chin to her chest. She has just recovered from the flu. While she had the flu, she had a fever of up to 101°F with body aches and a dry cough. This lasted for about 72 hours, and then she felt much better; however, she does not feel well now. In addition to her complaint of a stiff neck, she has a low-grade fever of 99.8°F, a headache, and nausea. On examination, the client has positive Brudzinski's and Kernig's signs, a heart rate of 120 beats/min, and a respiratory rate of 28 breaths/min (see Fig. 9-11). The woman is alert and oriented to person, place, and time; her pupils are equal and accommodate and react to light; however, she is a little lethargic and her attention span does not seem up to par.

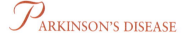

PARKINSON'S DISEASE

Parkinson's disease is a slowly progressive disease associated with degenerative changes in the substantia nigra of the brain. This disease produces a resting tremor in the early stages and progresses to paralysis.

Parkinson's disease is a slowly progressive chronic movement disorder of unknown cause that mainly affects the pigmented, dopamine-containing neurons of the pars compacta in the **substantia nigra** of the brain. The supply of **dopamine** in the brain becomes more and more depleted, causing the characteristic symptoms. Dopamine normally *inhibits* the function of acetylcholine-producing neurons that usually transmit *excitatory* messages throughout the basal ganglia, thus allowing for fine coordination. In Parkinson's disease, there is slow, widespread degeneration of the feedback mechanism that assists in the control of movement, coordination, and posture as the amount of dopamine is depleted; however, the amount of acetylcholine is not depleted, thus creating an imbalance between inhibitory and excitatory nervous activity. Most of the signs and symptoms are related to the loss of dopamine-containing neurons. The clinical signs and symptoms of Parkinson's disease do not occur until 70% of the affected neurons are destroyed. Parkinson's disease is characterized by muscle rigidity, bradykinesia, slow movement, and tremor. It usually presents in late adult life (around age 60) but may appear as early as the fourth decade. There is usually no family history, although more than 10% of sufferers do have a family history. It afflicts 1 in every 100 persons and affects men and women equally. Syndromes can occur that are similar to the disease as a result of drugs or from postencephalitic, neurosyphilitic, or arteriosclerotic origins.

Diagnosis

A clinical diagnosis is made based on six major symptoms: (1) resting tremor ("pill-rolling"), (2) akinesia or bradykinesia (slowed voluntary movements), (3) muscle rigidity, (4) loss of postural reflexes, (5) stooped posture, and (6) freezing phenomenon. At least two of these features must be present for a positive diagnosis. Other features include a masked face, decreased blinking, and a festinating gait (rapid propulsion forward with an inability to stop). Depression and dementia also may occur. Most clients eventually have difficulty in performing the activities of daily living (ADLs). A positive response to the administration of L-deoxyphenylalanine (L-dopa, Sinemet) strongly suggests Parkinson's disease (Table 9-12).

The **substantia nigra** is a pigmented body located in the mesencephalon (midbrain) that functions to filter out unwanted impulses from motor pathways. Degeneration of the substantia nigra produces Parkinson's disease.

Dopamine is a neurotransmitter produced by the substantia nigra in the brain. Deficiency in this compound produces the condition known as Parkinson's disease.

L-**Dopa** (levodopa) is the synthetic compound L-deoxyphenylalanine. It is closely related to dopamine, a neurotransmitter, and is used in the treatment of Parkinson's disease.

TABLE 9-12

STAGES OF PARKINSON'S DISEASE

Stage	Description	Signs and Symptoms
1	Initial	Unilateral limb involvement Minimal weakness Hand and arm trembling
2	Mild	Bilateral limb involvement Mask-like facies Slow, shuffling gait
3	Moderate disease	Gait disturbance increase
4	Severe disability	Akinesia Rigidity
5	Complete dependence	

Assessment

Obviously, obtaining an accurate history is vital. The nurse must determine when the symptoms of the disease first occurred and how the symptoms have progressed. Very early symptoms such as fatigue, tremor, and problems with manual dexterity may have been ignored by the elderly client. The client should be asked about gait problems and bradykinesia. The nurse must determine if the client has difficulty performing two activities at the same time such as walking and talking. Tremors occur in approximately half of Parkinson's disease clients. Observe the client for tremors, which can occur at rest, during times of stress, while sleeping, or during voluntary activities. The nurse must also assess for problems with speech, swallowing, and bladder and bowel control. Handwriting may become very small, difficult to accomplish, and slow.

During the physical examination, the nurse must determine if there is muscle rigidity by checking for resistance to passive movement. Rigidity is classified as follows: (1) *cogwheel*, exhibited by a rhythmic interruption of the muscle movements; (2) *plastic*, manifested by restrictive movement; or (3) *lead pipe*, confirmed as total resistance to movement. The client should also be assessed for changes in posture and gait. Clients with Parkinson's disease usually have a stooped posture and truncal rigidity. Rolling over and moving from lying to sitting to standing is not an easy task. The client may have a propulsive gait that is difficult to start, but once started it is difficult to stop. The severely impaired client may not be able to move at all. The client's respiratory movement should be assessed, as respiratory compromise is not uncommon. There may be chest wall restriction, labored respirations, and decreased breath sounds. The nurse should be alert for speech impairments such as a low-pitched, soft voice; repetitiveness; and echolalia.

Some Parkinson's clients suffer from orthostatic hypotension, so the nurse should check the blood pressure while the client is lying, sitting, and standing. A decrease of 20 mm Hg signifies orthostatic hypotension. The nurse must observe for excessive sweating, flushing, and changes in skin texture. The client should be asked about constipation, and this should be addressed in the plan of care.

Many clients with Parkinson's disease are emotionally labile and suffer from depression. They also may be paranoid. Furthermore, some clients become easily upset and have mood swings. The client should be assessed for cognitive impairment, which may be either a sign of the disease or a side effect of medication.

Treatment and Nursing Care

The primary aim of therapy is to control symptoms. The disease is always progressive, which, to date, cannot be prevented. Major principles of treatment include keeping the client as active, mobile, and independent as possible for as long as possible; individualizing treatment; establishing drug therapy that can slow the progression of the disease; and instituting the appropriate medication regimen as soon as possible.

Common complications with Parkinson's disease include aspiration of food due to impaired voluntary movements, altered bowel and bladder function, and skin breakdown in the client with severely impaired mobility. Medical and nursing care goals should be aimed at preventing complications for as long as possible and ensuring an acceptable quality of life for the client.

Treatment of the bradykinesia associated with Parkinson's includes selegiline (Eldepryl), a monoamine oxidase B (MAOB) inhibitor, 5 mg in the morning and again at noon, or tranylcypromine (Parnate), an MAOB and MAOI inhibitor, 10 mg three times a day. One of these medications should be given to all clients as soon as the diagnosis of Parkinson's disease is confirmed because it seems to slow the progression of the disease. If tranylcypromine (Parnate) is used, the client will need to be placed on an MAOI diet that contains both MAOB and MAO enzyme inhibitors. Tranylcypromine (Parnate) does have some rather unpleasant side effects such as insomnia and male impotence that may require adjustments in the dosage if they occur, but it does have the beneficial side effect of lifting depression. With both of these drugs, meperidine (Demerol) and SSRIs should be avoided because of the potential for fatal psychiatric and autonomic reactions (i.e., severe hypertension).

The tremor may be decreased with anticholinergics such as trihexyphenidyl (Artane, 5–10 mg a day) or benztropine (Cogentin, 0.5–4 mg twice a day). Side effects of these drugs include blurred vision, constipation, and urinary retention. In elderly clients, there also may be mental status changes, which limit the use of these drugs in the geriatric population. Amantadine (Symmetrel, 100 mg 1–3 times a day) also is used for tremor, but its side effects include congestive heart failure (CHF), pedal edema, and confusion.

Dopamine agonists have also proven to be helpful for some clients. Bromocriptine (Parlodel, 1.25 mg twice a day) or pergolide (Permax, 0.05–0.25 mg at bedtime) are the dopamine agonists of choice. Bromocriptine (Parlodel) can be increased by 2.5 mg/week up to a maximum of 100 mg/day, and pergolide can be increased by 0.25 mg/day, each week, to a maximum of 5 mg/day. Side effects of these drugs include orthostatic hypotension and confusion with visual hallucinations. These drugs are indicated for younger clients and may delay the need for L-dopa, but they may require several months before they become fully effective.

For moderate-to-severe bradykinesia, selegiline (Eldepryl) should be continued. **Carbidopa**, 25 mg, and L-dopa, 100 mg (Sinemet, 25/100 1:4 ratio, three times a day) is started with meals to minimize nausea. This medication is slowly increased by one tablet every 3–4 days to reach the minimal effective dose while not exceeding more than 1 g/day of L-dopa. Only 25–50% of clients maintain their initial improvement after 5–6 years of therapy. The major side effect of carbidopa and levodopa is a peak-dose dyskinesia similar to tardive dyskinesia. This occurs 20–90 minutes after a dose and requires the dose to be gradually decreased. Also, a wearing off phenomenon can be seen when it is almost time for the next dose. In these cases, the L-dopa may need to be given more frequently in smaller doses. Sinemet CR, which is given every 6 hours, requires a 25% higher daily

Carbidopa is the synthetic compound used to reduce the formation of dopamine outside the brain, thus reducing the side effects of treatment of Parkinson's disease with L-dopa.

Two new drugs for Parkinson's disease have come on the market as this text goes to press. These include tolcapone (Tasmar) and pramipexole (Mirapex). Mirapex, indicated for idiopathic Parkinson's disease, is a dopamine agonist. Tasmar is a COMT inhibitor and is used as an adjunct to carbidopa/levodopa in idiopathic Parkinson's disease.

dose to be effective. The onset of this medication is delayed for 5–6 hours. The literature recommends that regular Sinemet be used in the morning to prevent morning symptoms. If this drug should cause nausea and vomiting, trimethobenzamide (Tigan, 250 mg three times a day) is helpful or a higher dose of carbidopa can be added. The efficacy of the Sinemet can be decreased by vitamin B_6 and high-protein diets.

In addition to drug therapy, nursing care includes monitoring for side effects of ordered medications, facilitating mobility through planning and collaborating with occupational and physical therapists, providing time for the client to complete activities by him- or herself, and preventing complications (constipation, decubiti, contractures). The nurse must teach the client to speak slowly and clearly, assess the client's ability to chew and swallow, and stress a positive body image by focusing on the client's strengths. After discharge from an acute care facility, clients may need home care follow-up, psychosocial support, and referrals to appropriate health care resources.

Controversial Treatment of Parkinson's Disease

Parkinson's disease is typically treated with drug therapy. However, the effectiveness of medications tends to dissipate as the disease progresses. Experimental surgeries have been conducted in Sweden, Mexico, China, and the United States. These include adrenal transplants and fetal tissue transplants. In the adrenal transplant procedure, tissue from the client's own adrenal glands is transplanted into the caudate nucleus to enhance dopamine production. According to researchers in Mexico, the procedure has been successful in a few clients. Researchers in Mexico have also reported success with fetal substantia nigra and adrenal tissue transplantation into the brains of individuals with Parkinson's disease. Repeat experimentation in the United States has not yielded the same results obtained by Mexican and Swedish surgeons. At least 80 clients have undergone adrenal transplants in the United States thus far, with only marginal success. Fetal tissue transplants have reportedly been more successful, but immunosuppressive therapy is required indefinitely after surgery. The procedure is fraught with ethical concerns regarding informed consent and pregnancies for the purpose of selling aborted fetuses.

Evaluation

As always, the nurse must evaluate the **nursing care** that has been provided to the individual client. The person with Parkinson's disease should be evaluated based on ability to care for himself or herself, mobility, lack of contracture development, participation in structured exercise, utilization of strategies to assist in communicating, adequate intake of fluids and solid foods, and projection of a positive self-image. Each of these items is essential for an overall positive outcome for the client with Parkinson's disease.

ALZHEIMER'S DISEASE

Alzheimer's disease, also called **senile dementia Alzheimer's type (SDAT)**, is a chronic and progressive degenerative disorder. It is responsible for 60% of the dementias that occur in clients over the age of 65. However, it is not restricted to the elderly. Alzheimer's disease that affects people in their fifth and sixth decades is called *presenile dementia*. Clients with Alzheimer's have loss of memory of recent events, persons, and places. Eventually, cognitive impairment worsens, followed by physical deterioration and, finally, death. The exact cause is not yet known.

Approximately 10–15% of clients with dementia have partially reversible conditions. Some of these clients suffer from dementia that is caused by side effects of certain medications, infections, dehydration, depression, schizophrenia, Wernicke-Korsakoff syndrome, uremia, liver failure, hypothyroidism, hyponatremia, hypercalcemia, hypoglycemia, vitamin B_{12} deficiency, subdural hematoma, stroke and neoplastic disease. Alzheimer's-type dementia, Parkinson's-related dementia, multi-infarct dementia, and dementia associated with Huntington's chorea are incurable causes of dementia.

Diagnosis

As we age, our brain shrinks in size and takes up less space in the cranium. Other changes that occur with aging include cerebral sulci widening, gyri narrowing, and ventricular enlargement. In clients with Alzheimer's disease, these changes occur much more rapidly. Specific areas of the brain that are affected by Alzheimer's disease include the precentral gyrus of the frontal lobe, the superior gyrus of the temporal lobe, the **hippocampus,** and the substantia nigra. Furthermore, there are chemical changes in the brain, particularly abnormalities in the transmission of acetylcholine, norepinephrine, dopamine, and serotonin. Acetylcholine may be reduced by 75%, interfering with cholinergic innervation in the cerebral cortex. Thus, the client may have impaired cognition, loss of recent memory, and the inability to acquire new memories.

If dementia is suspected in a client, an accurate diagnosis is vital. This requires a thorough physical examination, including a neurological examination. A positive Babinski's sign and asymmetry of reflexes suggest multi-infarct dementia or focal CNS deformity rather than an Alzheimer's-type dementia.

Additionally, diagnosing dementia requires appropriate laboratory tests: a CBC, electrolytes, Ca^{++}, BUN, and thyroid-stimulating hormone (TSH). Further tests may be ordered as indicated by the history and physical examination. These could include vitamin B_{12}, Venereal Disease Research Laboratories test (VDRL), liver panel, ESR, heavy metal screen via blood and urine, electrocardiography (ECG), chest x-ray, head CT, oxygen saturation, and LP.

Alzheimer's disease is a rapidly progressive dementia beginning before age 80. It is characterized by atrophy, with formation of neurofibrillary tangles, especially in the hippocampus of the brain. A similar condition after age 80 is now called **senile dementia of the Alzheimer's type (SDAT).**

Pathology of Deterioration in Alzheimer's Disease

- Neurofibrillary changes
- Neuritic plaques
- Decreased oxygen metabolism and cerebral blood flow
- Thickening of capillary walls in blood–brain barrier
- Absence of the perivascular neural plexus in the cortex
- Loss of cortical, hippocampal, and hypothalamic cells, as well as acetylcholine

The **hippocampus** is the curved structure in the floor of a portion of the lateral ventricles of the cerebrum. It plays a part in learning, memory, and rage and is an important part of the limbic system.

Laboratory tests are generally not helpful in diagnosing Alzheimer's disease, but they may be ordered to rule out other disorders. The physician may order the following studies: folate levels, thyroid function tests, liver function tests, serology for syphilis, and a drug screen. A CT scan may be ordered as well, which will reveal cerebral atrophy and ventricular enlargement if the disease is in the second or third stage. MRI may be ordered to rule out other causes of dementia, and an EEG may be required, which will demonstrate slow-wave delta activity in clients with Alzheimer's disease.

Assessment

Clients may initially present with confusion. A thorough history obtained from the client and significant others is needed to determine whether the cause of the confusion is Alzheimer's disease. The nurse must ascertain the onset, duration, and course of the client's symptoms. The client must be asked about memory changes; changes in driving ability, employment, and ability to perform routine household responsibilities; and changes in language and communication skills.

There are typically three stages in the progression of Alzheimer's disease, although they are by no means well delineated. One stage may be bypassed, or the client may have signs and symptoms from more than one stage simultaneously. A summary of the three stages is presented in Table 9-13.

During the assessment, the nurse should focus on determining the client's cognitive abilities (language, personality, behavior). Seizures,

◙

TABLE 9-13
STAGES OF ALZHEIMER'S DISEASE

Stage	Signs and Symptoms
1 (lasts 1–3 years)	Forgetfulness Mild memory loss Short attention span Decreased interest in personal affairs Subtle changes in personality and behavior Minimal visual spatial impairment
II (lasts 2–10 years)	Confusion, problems with judgment Profound memory loss Significant cognitive impairment Severe loss of judgment
III (lasts 8–12 years)	Severe impairment of all cognitive functions Complete disorientation to time, place, and event Physical impairment Total loss of ability to perform self-care

tremors, and ataxia may occur late in the disease's progression. To quantify the client's loss of cognition, use the mini-mental status examination (see Table 9-6). A client with Alzheimer's disease can be expected to score very low on this examination, perhaps as low as 5.

Nursing Care

Hospital admission is very traumatic for the client with dementia. The client with Alzheimer's disease may become abusive or even combative. Nursing interventions for working with the client with altered thought processes include orientation to person, place, and time and decreasing or eliminating episodes of agitation. The nurse should provide a structured, consistent environment without overstimulation for the client and assess for manifestations of Alzheimer's that can be addressed in **nursing care.** The nurse must avoid arguing with the confused client but work to reorient the person to reality without increasing his or her agitation. Encourage as much independence and self-care as the client can handle. Schedule specific times for going to the bathroom to avoid incontinence, which may become inevitable. The client may need a great deal of assistance in recognizing himself or herself, family, and significant others. Clients may also talk to themselves in the mirror, which is not harmful and requires no intervention. Help the client in promoting communication. The nurse can prevent injury by properly positioning the bedrails and commode and placing the client in a room near the nurse's station. If restlessness or wandering is a problem, encourage exercise and redirection of the client's energy. Clients should not be restrained unless absolutely necessary, as this usually worsens their agitation and confusion.

Alzheimer's clients and their families require a great deal of assistance to cope with the disease. They should be encouraged to seek legal counsel, when indicated; be referred to a support group; be helped in maintaining their social activities; have their questions answered; and be allowed to verbalize their feelings and frustrations. Clients and their families may need assistance through the provision of home health care, health instruction, and psychosocial preparation for what lies ahead. Individuals who care for a family member or friend with Alzheimer's need guidance and assistance in reducing their own stress. The nurse can teach the caregiver to be realistic, take one day at a time, use humor, think positively, set aside time for themselves if possible, seek respite care, use available resources, explore optional care settings, and establish advanced directives for the client.

Evaluation

The nurse can evaluate the care provided by assessing if the client (1) remains at home for as long as possible, (2) maintains as much independence as possible in self-care activities, and (3) stays free from injury (i.e., falls, seizures, environmental hazards).

Drug therapy may include ergoloid mesylate (Hydergine) to improve cognitive abilities in the early stages. Other approved medications include tacrine (Cognex) and donepezil (Aricept) for use in the early to middle stages of Alzheimer's. Both drugs can cause insomnia, GI problems, and liver damage, but if tolerated they have been shown to slow the progression of the disease for 6–12 months. In some clients, antidepressant, antianxiety, or antiagitation therapy may also be required.

𝓜ULTIPLE SCLEROSIS

Multiple sclerosis is a disease characterized by the progressive destruction of the myelin sheaths of nerves in the CNS. The sheaths deteriorate to sclerosis or plaques in multiple regions. Remissions occur, but each new attack results in loss of additional function.

Multiple sclerosis (MS) affects young adults and is characterized by multiple areas of demyelination (plaques) and sclerosis in the CNS. MS is a chronic, progressive, and degenerative disease of the white matter, sparing the peripheral nerves. Sporadic areas of demyelination develop in the myelin sheath, causing disintegration of the myelin, which slows or stops impulse conduction (see Fig. 9-14). Plaques can form anywhere in the CNS but usually develop in the spinal cord, brain stem, and optic nerves. The exact cause of MS is not yet known. It has been theorized that it is a slow viral infection or an autoimmune disease. Familial incidence has typically been low, but this is changing. Caucasians are more susceptible than African Americans and Asians. However, in recent studies, it has been found that children of adults with MS have a 30–50% greater risk of developing the disease than the general population, which is 0.1%. Daughters of mothers with MS have approximately a 5% risk. If both parents have MS, the child has a risk of 10–15%. A specific gene associated

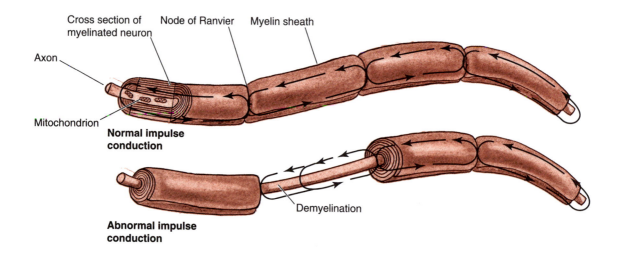

FIGURE 9-14 Cross section of myelinated and demyelinated neuron.

with MS has not been discovered. MS rarely occurs in children. It occurs most commonly in women 18–35 years of age who live in northern climates and urban areas and who are from higher socioeconomic groups. The average age at onset is 33 years. Pregnancy decreases the risk of exacerbations, but the exacerbations increase as soon as the pregnancy is over. It is estimated that 500,000 individuals in the United States have MS. The life expectancy is approximately 35 years after the onset of the disease.

There are four types of MS: (1) benign, (2) exacerbation–remission, (3) chronic relapsing/progressive, and (4) chronic progressive (combined). Twenty percent of those with MS have the benign type, characterized by mild, infrequent attacks. Twenty-five percent have the exacerbation–remission type, which is characterized by increasingly frequent attacks. Progressive or chronic relapsing MS is the most common type. It has few or no periods of remission. Combined or chronic progressive MS is similar to relapsing MS; however, its initial presentation is more covert. The combined type eventually progresses to MS without remissions.

Diagnosis

Clinical Manifestations The onset of MS is acute. Symptoms generally last for several weeks or longer, but they also may persist for only a few minutes or hours. A history of fluctuation in the clinical course and signs of neurological deficits consistent with multiple lesions in the white matter of the CNS are classic indicators for MS. Initially, symptoms usually include weakness or numbness of a limb, monocular visual loss, diplopia, vertigo, facial weakness or numbness, ataxia, and nystagmus. Sometimes clients state that their symptoms are aggravated by a hot bath, another classic symptom. The hallmark of MS is unpredictable periods of exacerbation and remission, and the progression of MS is unpredictable. Because of this, complications can vary and may include any or all of the following: immobility, bowel and bladder alterations, emotional lability, visual disturbances, and muscle spasms. The 25-year mortality rate was found to be 26% in one study, compared with 14% in the general population. Furthermore, after 25 years, two-thirds of those with MS were still ambulatory. Clients with MS may experience temporary episodes of immobility following an exacerbation; aggressive therapy and treatment may restore mobility. Generally, 75% of clients with MS experience prolonged remissions and remain mobile.

Laboratory Findings Typically, 90% of clients have abnormal findings in the CSF, such as a mild mononuclear pleocytosis, increased total protein, increased γ-globulin fraction, a high immunoglobulin G (IgG) index, the presence of oligoclonal bands, and increased myelin basic protein. An MRI is as sensitive as CSF analysis and is now the neuroimaging test of choice for diagnosing MS. During the MRI procedure, gladolinium enhancement differentiates new lesions from old ones.

Assessment

A thorough history is required, as MS may be mistaken for other diseases. The nurse should question the client about visual, motor, and sensory changes. Symptoms are typically vague, but the client probably will report some ambiguous manifestations that were ignored years earlier because they seemed unimportant. The nurse should focus on the progression of symptoms and determine whether they are intermittent and worsening. Try to ascertain the month and year the symptoms were first noticed. The client should be questioned about activities that seem to exacerbate symptoms such as fatigue, stress, overexertion, temperature extremes, or a hot shower or bath. Interrogate the family or significant others about changes in behavior or personality as well as a possible family history of MS.

The nurse needs to perform a thorough neurological assessment, perhaps beginning with the client's motor status. Ask the client about fatigue and spasms, especially of the extremities. Deep tendon reflexes may be increased, there may be a positive Babinski's sign, abdominal reflexes may be absent, and the client's gait may be unsteady. In addition, the client may have an intention tremor and be unable to direct or limit movement. Clumsiness and other signs of poor coordination may be apparent as well. When the nurse assesses the cranial nerves, the client may divulge that he or she has tinnitus, vertigo, and hearing loss. There also may be facial weakness, dysphagia, and speech problems. Visual acuity may be impaired with blurred vision, diplopia, decreased acuity, scotomas (changes in peripheral vision), and nystagmus. Regarding sensory function, the client may report numbness, tingling, burning, or crawling sensations. In the event that demyelination has occurred, there may be bladder or bowel dysfunction and changes in sexuality. Finally, the nurse should assess cognitive function, which generally does not change dramatically until the later stages of the disease. Expect changes in the client's psychosocial status possibly exhibited as apathy, emotional lability, or depression. There may be some evidence of drug side effects.

Treatment

Researchers are currently working on treatments for victims of MS. To date, no current therapy completely halts the progression of the disease. The major goals of therapy are to provide psychological support, slow the course of the disease as much as possible, and provide relief from symptoms.

Corticosteroids are frequently used to shorten acute exacerbations, but their worth has not been proven in research studies. Typically, clients receive 60 mg of prednisone (Deltasone) for 10 days, then taper the dose over a 3-week period. Some clients improve rapidly with high-dose intravenous methylprednisolone (Solu-Medrol, 250–1000 mg/day for 2–7 days), followed by a short course of oral prednisone. Major side effects of corticosteroids include hypo- or hypernatremia, hypokalemia, fluid retention and pedal edema, heart failure and hypertension, gastric ulcer, hyperglycemia, increased chance of infection, and changes in personality. Interferon beta-1a (Avonex) and interferon beta-1b (Betaseron) have been used to treat MS. A newer drug, glateraner (Copaxone), has also proven effective in reducing the effect of exacerbations. These medications are used to treat the relapsing form of MS. Clients are generally taught to give themselves these drugs, after the first supervised dose. Major side effects include injection site and postinjection reactions, chest pain, infection, pain, nausea, and arthralgia. Antidepressant and antipsychotic drugs may be given to clients with MS, as well as drugs to control spasticity, such as diazepam (Valium), dantrolene (Dantrium), or baclofen (Loresal). Severely affected clients may need medication for paresthesias, such as carbamazepine (Tegretol), and drugs for fatigue, such as amantadine hydrochloride (Symmetrel).

Nursing Care

The nursing plan of care should revolve around goals of maintaining maximum mobility for the client, decreasing the sequelae of immobility, teaching the client appropriate strategies for adaptation to changes in self-care activities that may be necessary for episodes of impaired mobility and visual and sensory losses, assisting the client to adjust to changes in body image, and encouraging the client to participate in planning care. Interventions focus on an appropriate exercise program and administering and teaching the client about ordered medications (purpose, dosages, side effects). If the client is on steroid therapy, the nurse must monitor fluid and electrolyte balance, test the blood for glucose and K^+, provide K^+ if indicated, observe for signs or symptoms of GI bleeding, document personality changes, and monitor the client's exposure to others who may transmit an infection. Assist the client in developing compensatory strategies if visual or sensory loss has occurred. Alternating eye patches from one eye to the other every few hours usually relieves diplopia. To accommodate for peripheral vision changes, the client should move his or her head from side to side. Protect the client from injury and avoid overexposure to heat, cold, or pressure. The nurse should encourage maintenance of independence and usual activities as the client's condition permits. Finally, the nurse can provide useful information for the client and significant others and assist in setting short- and long-term goals.

Evaluation

Of course, the nurse needs to evaluate the care provided to the client with MS. Determine if the client has few or no complications from immobility, if appropriate, and assess whether the client has maintained maximum activity and mobility for his or her level of disability. Finally, ascertain whether the client knows about and understands the medications and is able to state the names of the drugs, the dosages and times of administration, their actions, and the major side effects of each medication.

CASE STUDY: WOMAN WITH MULTIPLE SCLEROSIS AND COMPLICATIONS

A 33-year-old Caucasian woman comes into the clinic with complaints of visual difficulties and numbness and weakness in her legs. She reports that she has been having some progressive numbness in her lower extremities that has now reached the middle of her thighs. She also has noticed a loss of sensation in her bladder, although she has not experienced incontinence. She feels extremely tired. Her family history is noncontributory. She is not taking medications and does not drink or smoke. A review of her systems reveals no prior medical illnesses; she has always been well. Her vital signs are blood pressure, 124/76 mm Hg; temperature, 98.9°F; pulse, 88 beats/min; and respirations, 24 breaths/min. The woman weighs 138 lbs. The client is well developed, well nourished and in no acute distress, but anxious. She is alert and oriented to person, place, and time. Physical examination reveals dry oral mucous membranes; a supple neck with good ROM; clear lungs; regular heart beat; a soft, nontender abdomen with good bowel sounds; and deep tendon reflexes that are hyper-reflexic in both arms (radial and brachial).

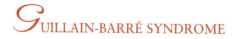

GUILLAIN-BARRÉ SYNDROME

Guillain-Barré syndrome (GBS) is an acute inflammatory process that involves loss of the myelin sheath around the axons, which causes slowed nerve impulse transmission between the nodes of Ranvier. This syndrome (also referred to as infectious polyneuritis) develops rapidly but is reversible. It is characterized by varying degrees of motor impairment and paralysis. There is no specific known cause, but GBS is frequently associated with upper respiratory or GI viral infections. This disease most often affects young people between the ages of 16 and 25 and more men than women. It can affect older people, and when it does their recovery period is much longer. Guillain-Barré typically affects its victims in an ascending manner, from the lower extremities to the head, and resolves in a descending fashion. It can cause respiratory arrest, and clients may require mechanical ventilation before it reaches that stage.

Symptoms of GBS include hypertension, bradycardia, respiratory failure, and cardiovascular failure in the acute phase. As the client recovers, it is important that the nurse be alert to complications of rehabilitation, which may include nosocomial infections, decubiti, and pulmonary emboli.

Diagnosis

Clients usually have a history of an acute illness with fever 1–4 weeks prior to the onset of the disorder (i.e., before neurological signs and symptoms occur). Analysis of CSF helps confirm the diagnosis of GBS. Protein levels in the CSF increase as GBS progresses, and the CSF pressure increases in both mild and severe cases. There may be a mild leukocytosis revealed in the CBC, but this usually returns to normal quickly.

Assessment

The nurse needs to complete a thorough medical and surgical history. Determine if there was an acute febrile illness a few weeks prior to the onset of symptoms. Ask the client to chronologically describe the symptoms if possible. Most clients report an abrupt onset. The most common complaints include numbness or tingling, charley horse–like pain, facial weakness, difficulty walking, motor weakness, and sometimes problems with bladder control. There may be a labile blood pressure, cardiac dysrhythmias, or tachycardia secondary to autonomic dysfunction. DTR may be decreased or absent. Cranial nerve involvement may be indicated by dysphagia, diplopia, or facial weakness. Cranial nerve VII, the facial nerve, is most often affected. A common complication is respiratory difficulty or failure. The nurse should be alert for evidence of dyspnea, decreased breath sounds, and decreased tidal volume and vital capacity (revealed by pulmonary function tests). Typically, weakness begins in the lower extremities and ascends. There may be mild to total quadriplegia, with respiratory compromise occurring in 50% of affected individuals. GBS can also begin in the face and descend, but this is rare.

The nurse should determine the client's usual role and responsibilities and his or her occupation. It is also important to assess the client's support system and ability to cope with a potentially devastating illness, which is so often accompanied by fear and anxiety. This may occur initially, followed by anger and depression; this is a long illness with a prolonged recovery time.

Treatment

Effective treatment of this disorder relies on ventilator assistance when required and extremely supportive **nursing care.** The client's very survival depends on the nurse's expertise. Although controversial, drug therapy generally consists of corticosteroids that suppress the inflammatory response during the acute stage. Adrenocorticotropin (Corticotropin, 25–40 units subcutaneously three times a day) is usually ordered, or prednisone (Deltasone, 45–60 mg/day in two to four doses) is given by mouth. Azathioprine (Imuran, 3–5 mg/kg/day initially, then 1–2 mg/kg/day) may be given by mouth. Cyclophosphamide (Cytoxan, 2–4 mg/kg/day for the first 10 days, then 1.5–3 mg/kg/day) is another option.

Plasmapheresis may be performed to separate whole blood from plasma, removing the abnormalities from the plasma or exchanging the plasma and reinfusing the solution. It has been found that this procedure reduces the duration of severe weakness or paralysis and thus decreases (1) the length of hospitalization, (2) the ventilator dependency period, and (3) the time needed for the client to begin walking again. This procedure needs to be done fairly early in the course of the syndrome to be effective. Plasmapheresis is generally performed daily for 5 consecutive days, with approximately 75% of the circulating plasma proteins removed each day.

Nursing Care

The client's very survival may well depend on intensive, excellent, and expert nursing care. The nurse must maintain an adequate airway, suction frequently as indicated, provide mechanical ventilation, prevent respiratory aspiration and subsequent infection, treat pneumonia if it occurs, provide adequate hydration, and maintain electrolyte balance. These factors are key to the client's successful recovery from GBS. Thus it is vital that these interventions, as laid out in the plan of care, be well thought out and specific.

There are several major areas on which the nurse needs to focus on when planning the care of a client with GBS. Clients with this disorder need frequent neurological assessments at least every 4 hours. In addition, nurses must pay particular attention to the client's breathing pattern and prevent complications from an impaired respiratory pattern, such as ineffective gas exchange secondary to weakness or paralysis of the respiratory muscles. Maintaining physical mobility is a priority, as these clients have weakness and possibly paralysis. Clients also receive passive ROM exercises, but this must be done cautiously because too much activity can worsen this disorder. Braces, splints, and related devices may be used to assist in gaining independence. If the client's ability to communicate is impaired, the nurse must find other ways to communicate. Clients with GBS often feel powerless and frightened and have high levels of anxiety related to their feelings of powerlessness, the uncertain prognosis, and the fear of the unknown. There may be active grieving as the disease progresses and remits. These clients may also experience pain secondary to paresthesias. Finally, the nurse needs to plan for self-care deficits, which can range from minimal to total dependence.

The need for very supportive **nursing care** for clients with GBS cannot be overemphasized. Kindness, reassurance, thorough explanations, and a caring attitude are essential for a successful outcome in the client with this disorder.

Evaluation

The nurse must evaluate nursing care by determining if the client demonstrates an effective breathing pattern with adequate gas exchange and is ventilator support free. The client should be effectively participating in efforts to increase and strengthen mobility. The client must be able to verbalize his or her feelings about the illness and effectively use available resources, such as his or her family and the nurse. Assess the client's development of effective coping strategies. Finally, the nurse must evaluate the client's ability to perform ADLs and other self-care activities as motor function returns and improves.

CASE STUDY: MAN WITH GUILLAIN-BARRÉ SYNDROME

On July 3, an 88-year-old retired businessman woke up and could not walk. He had been feeling quite well except for a stomach virus 2 days prior, which had not slowed him down at all. Mr. E. had always been very active. He and his wife travel within the United States quite a bit. He often helps his only son and daughter-in-law with some of their household repairs and gardening. He has always been healthy and has never been hospitalized before. On this particular day, he called his son, who came to his home, got him into the car, and took him to his doctor. At first the doctor thought that Mr. E. had had a stroke, but there were no objective signs to support this diagnosis. During the next 2 days, Mr. E. began to get worse, with a noticeable inability to swallow normally and weakness in his hands and arms. A lumbar puncture was performed and a diagnosis of GBS was made. Eventually, Mr. E. was placed on a ventilator and subsequently underwent a tracheostomy for long-term ventilator support.

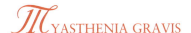

ℳYASTHENIA GRAVIS

Myasthenia gravis (MG) is a chronic autoimmune disease in which affected individuals have altered neuromuscular transmissions that weaken muscles, leading to muscle fatigue on exertion. The term means "grave muscle weakness." This disease affects 2–10 people per 100,000 population. Women aged 18–25 are most often afflicted. It is not a hereditary disorder, but its specific nature and origin are unknown. The most widely accepted theory postulates that an autoimmune malfunction blocks, deactivates, or destroys postsynaptic acetylcholine receptor sites. Thus, nerve impulses are not transmitted to muscles. This defect is apparently caused by acetylcholine deficiency. Circulating antibodies to acetylcholine receptors (AChR) have been documented in 60–90% of individuals with MG. Muscles usually appear normal with no apparent atrophy. In this disease, the thymus gland is often abnormal; this is called thymoma and occurs in 15% of clients with MG. Eighty percent of the remaining individuals have hyperplasia of the thymus gland. Because of

Myasthenia gravis is an autoimmune condition of progressive weakness of the muscles, especially of the face or throat, as a result of loss of acetylcholine receptor sites. Difficulty in swallowing often results. The disease sometimes progresses to death by respiratory failure.

limited development of compound action potentials and inhibition of muscle contraction, clients with MG have increased weakness with increased activity. This disease has a variable and unpredictable course and is characterized by exacerbations and remissions.

Clinical manifestations of MG include any or all of the following: double vision and ptosis (drooping of one or both eyelids, usually a first sign); weak, nasal-sounding speech; weak facial movements; tendency for the head to fall forward or for the client to hold the jaw closed with a hand; increased weakness on exertion; some improvement with rest; upper and lower extremity involvement; compromise of respiratory muscles (diaphragm) with dyspnea or arrest. Complications may include respiratory distress, pneumonia, and chewing and swallowing problems that can lead to choking and aspiration of food.

Clients with MG may have a crisis characterized by severe weakness in breathing and swallowing. This may happen subsequent to an infection, surgery, or an exacerbation that occurs if corticosteroids are tapered too quickly. In the event that a crisis does occur, the client will require immediate hospitalization and artificial respiratory assistance on a mechanical ventilator. A vital capacity below 25% of normal or less than 1L indicates a need for mechanical ventilation in an ICU. Weaning a client from mechanical ventilation may be a lengthy and arduous process.

Diagnosis

A panel of four tests can assist the accuracy of diagnosing MG. All of the components of this panel can be assessed with one blood sample. Baseline serum levels of certain antibodies are measured. The AChR-binding antibody test detects antibodies directed at several sites on solubilized AChR protein. The AChR-modulating antibody test detects antibodies that bind to AChR sites on the surface of intact muscle membranes and cause weakness. The third test, the AChR-blocking antibody test, assesses for antibodies that bind near the AChR neurotransmitter-binding site. More than 50% of MG clients have positive AChR-blocking antibodies. Finally, the fourth test in the panel, the striational antibody test, detects antibodies that bind to the contractile elements of skeletal muscle. In 80% of clients with MG-related thymoma, this test is positive for these antibodies.

Intravenous anticholinesterase is a reliable test for MG. An anticholinesterase such as edrophonium chloride (Tensilon) is administered, and the client's response is subsequently evaluated. If 1–2 mg of the drug improves muscle function in 1 minute, the client may have the disorder. Electron microscopic studies of biopsied muscle tissue may reveal postsynaptic membrane changes with a reduction of AChR receptor sites, which is also indicative of MG.

Thymoma commonly occurs in clients with MG. The thymus is an H-shaped gland located beneath the sternum in the anterior mediastinum. This is the one organ where AChR antibodies are found. Thymomas are neoplasms that originate from thymic tissue and are typically benign and

Differentiation of Myasthenia Gravis and Guillain-Barré. To differentiate myasthenia gravis from Guillain-Barré syndrome, it may be necessary to perform electromyography and nerve conduction studies. A decreasing impulse conduction *amplitude* with repeated nerve stimulation suggests myasthenia gravis; a reduced impulse *speed* indicates Guillain-Barré syndrome.

encapsulated. Thymoma can sometimes be seen on a routine chest x-ray, but clients usually undergo a CT scan to detect the neoplasm.

Electromyography (EMG) may be performed, as it detects muscle contraction, which may be decreased in the client with myasthenia gravis. An overall decrease of 10% in muscular response between the first and fifth responses may be indicative of the disorder. Several muscles are usually tested after exercise or after exposure of the muscle to curare or ischemia.

Assessment

The history and physical examination are of utmost importance in assessing the client with m MG. As the nurse obtains the usual biographical data and history, the client should be assessed for rapidly occurring fatigue. Clients typically complain of muscle weakness that worsens as the day progresses and improves with rest. The client should describe the symptoms, and the nurse should question him or her about specific muscle groups that tire and any functional impairment. The nurse must inquire about ptosis, diplopia, chewing and swallowing difficulty, respiratory difficulty, choking sensation, and weakness of the voice. Assess for problems with holding up the head, brushing teeth, combing hair, or shaving, and ask about paresthesias, muscle aches, and any known history of problems with the thymus gland. Determine if the client has recently had an infection, received anesthesia, been pregnant, or been upset emotionally. Some clients may have an increase in weakness after receiving a vaccination, after menstruation, or after being exposed to extremes in climate.

The nurse should perform a physical and neurological assessment based on the client's history. The client must be assessed for ocular palsies, ptosis, diplopia, and weak or incomplete eye closures. These symptoms of lavatory palpebrae or extraocular involvement occur in 90% of clients with MG. The muscles for facial expression, chewing, and speech are affected. Assess the client's smile, tendency to prop up the jaw, and chewing and swallowing difficulty. Ask about weight loss that is related to eating difficulties. Some clients may have tongue fissures.

Limb weakness is usually proximal, so the muscles of the neck and shoulders may not have as much involvement. Thus, clients may have the most difficulty climbing stairs, raising their arms, walking, or maintaining a sitting position. In advanced cases, all muscles are weak, including those that help control bowel and bladder function and respiratory function. Atrophy is uncommon, DTRs are not usually affected, and pain is not usually a problem for these clients; however, the nurse should assess for these. Paresthesias, which are uncommon, are not usually associated with loss of sensation.

A psychosocial assessment is performed by obtaining information about the client's occupation, usual roles and responsibilities, coping methods, motivation, acceptance of the condition, and support systems. MG can be devastating for the client, his or her family, and significant others because the disease's progression is uncertain.

Treatment

Anticholinesterase drugs such as neostigmine (Prostigmin) and pyridostigmine (Mestinon) may be ordered. These medications inhibit ACh destruction and permit the accumulation of ACh at the synapses, thereby increasing stimulation of the existing receptor sites. This effect, in turn, promotes nerve impulse transmission and improves muscle strength. These medications are given with meals. Another drug that may be used with these medications is kaolin to treat GI side effects such as cramping and diarrhea that often occur with anticholinesterases. Corticosteroids may also be administered to clients as an adjunct to the aforementioned therapy, but should be given with antacids to reduce their GI side effects. Other medications that are often used for clients with MG are immunosuppressants, such as azathioprine (Imuran) and cyclophosphamide (Cytoxan).

Plasmapheresis is routinely used for the client with MG. This procedure removes circulating antibodies, including ACh antibodies, which are suspected of compromising the AChR. Thymectomy may also be performed on these clients. This procedure involves excision of the thymus gland, which often improves symptoms of this disorder, although remission may not occur for several years postprocedure. It is theorized that removal of the thymus, the source of antigens, shuts off the immune response.

Nursing Care

The primary focus of nursing care is maintenance of an effective respiratory pattern and adequate gas exchange. The nurse is responsible for performing an ongoing assessment of the client's respiratory status and maintenance of respiratory function. Undermedication as well as overmedication can bring on a crisis that affects the diaphragm and intercostal muscles. Dysphagia may lead to the aspiration of food, which can also compromise breathing. The nurse needs to monitor and assess the client for dyspnea, complaints about respiratory difficulty, air hunger, labored respirations, and confusion and restlessness that may result from hypoxia. The rate, rhythm, and depth of respirations and other vital signs must be assessed on a regular basis. The client should be encouraged to turn, cough, and breathe deeply every 2 hours. Auscultate the lungs at least once every 8-hour shift. The nurse should obtain arterial blood gases (ABGs) as ordered or indicated by protocol if available. Oxygen, suction equipment, and an Ambu bag must always be available at the client's bedside with a crash cart and emergency resuscitation equipment nearby in the event of respiratory failure or arrest.

The major problem in MG is muscle weakness, so the nurse must plan for maintaining or increasing the client's mobility without causing excessive fatigue or other complications. The client's motor strength must be assessed before and after exercise. The nurse can assist the client in ADLs and other activities (ambulation, transfers, position changes) as needed to ward off fatigue. Teach the client to participate in desired or essential activities early in the day or after taking medication that enhances energy levels. Active or passive ROM exercise should be performed every 2–4 hours. Use heel and elbow protectors, egg crate mattress (or a special bed), and other devices to prevent decubiti. If the client is severely impaired and unable to perform ADLs, help the client maintain his or her self-esteem and cope effectively with the deficits. These clients are at high risk for sensory and perceptual impairment, so plan to assist them in ways that prevent further damage. For example, artificial tears may be required to prevent corneal abrasions and alternating eye patches to assist with diplopia. Encourage the client to verbalize feelings and ask for assistance whenever it is needed.

When damage to the brain stem paralyzes a client's face and limbs and leaves only the eyes capable of movement, the client is experiencing **locked-in syndrome**. The client is alert but can only respond to stimuli with the eyes. The condition results from an injury that damages the descending motor tracts to the face and limbs but not the RAS, thus sparing the innervation of the eyes. Thus, the client can respond to questions that require a yes or no answer by blinking his or her eyes A locked-in client requires skilled **nursing care** to prevent respiratory failure and complications from immobility, and time and patience for effective communication. Signals may need to be developed, such as blinking, paper and pencil, magic slates, and picture and word cards. Maintaining adequate nutrition can also be problematic and needs to be addressed. The nurse must assess the client's gag reflex frequently, provide oral hygiene often, and ensure delivery of food that the client prefers. Encourage the client to eat slowly, observe for choking and aspiration, and be prepared to assist as needed. If warranted, consult with a speech or occupational therapist.

The nurse needs to monitor and assess the client's response to ordered medications. Whatever medications may be ordered, it is vitally important for the client with MG to receive them *on time* for full therapeutic effect; therapeutic blood levels are essential for the best effect. Administration of medications is usually time-specific to enhance the client's well-being at certain times of the day. For example, anticholinesterase should be given 30–60 minutes before meals to maximize the client's muscle strength and to prevent aspiration.

Locked-in Syndrome. When damage to the brainstem paralyzes a client's face and limbs and leaves only his eyes capable of movement, it is called locked-in syndrome. The client is alert, but cannot respond to stimuli, other than with the eyes. The condition results from an injury that damages descending motor tracts to the face and limbs but not to the RAS, thus sparing the innervation of the eyes. The client can respond with the eyes to questions that require a "yes" or "no" answer by blinking. A locked-in patient requires skilled nursing care to prevent respiratory failure, complications of immobility, and time and patience for effective communication.

Evaluation

Nursing care is evaluated by ascertaining that the client has an effective breathing pattern, is as mobile and ambulatory as possible, and can perform self-care activities independently or with appropriate assistance. The nurse should ensure that the client is oriented to person, place, and time and is free from injury. If appropriate goals have been set and met, the client should be able to communicate effectively and verbalize his or her feelings. Furthermore, the nurse should determine whether the client has maintained a body weight within 10% of his or her weight when admitted.

CEREBRAL VASCULAR ACCIDENT

Risk Factors for CVA

- Age
- Atherosclerosis
- Cardiac disease
- Diabetes mellitus
- Family history
- Hypertension
- Nonprescription diet pills containing phenyl-propanolamine
- Oral contraceptives

Signs and Symptoms of a Vertebrobasilar TIA

- Dizziness
- Double vision, dark or blurred vision, visual field defects, or ptosis
- Dysarthria (impairment of tongue or other muscles needed for speech)
- Dysphagia
- Unilateral or bilateral weakness and numbness in the fingers, arms, legs, or all three
- Staggering or veering to one side

Signs and Symptoms of a Carotid TIA

- Transient blindness in one eye
- Altered level of consciousness
- Numbness of the tongue
- Unilateral or bilateral weakness and numbness in the fingers, arms, legs, or all three
- Seizures

Cerebral vascular accident (CVA), or stroke, is listed as the third leading cause of death in the United States. It is generally associated with atherosclerosis and results from an interruption of cerebral blood supply caused by an occlusion or rupture of a cerebral artery. A clot or a plaque can occlude a vessel, causing ischemia or a cerebral infarction; the vessel can rupture, which can produce increased ICP or even brain herniation. A CVA can occur in anyone, but it most often affects the elderly. Individuals who are intravenous drug users or those with congenital disorders such as sickle cell anemia can have a CVA at an earlier age. Men typically have more strokes than women, and African Americans have more strokes than do European Americans.

Cerebrovascular disease may be classified as an *infarction* or a *hemorrhage*. Infarctions may be classified as vertebrobasilar or carotid. TIAs are diagnosed when there are neurological symptoms or deficits that clear in less than 24 hours. TIAs usually last 5–20 minutes, and all signs and symptoms dissipate within 24 hours. Causes of TIAs include vascular disorders, such as extensive extracranial atherosclerosis; blood disorders, such as hypercoagulability, polycythemia, and embolism; and cerebrovascular insufficiency from decreased cardiac output, carotid artery stenosis, or subclavian steal syndrome. TIAs may be classified as vertebrobasilar, resulting from inadequate blood flow through the vertebral or subclavian arteries; or carotid, resulting from occlusion along the common, internal, or external carotid arteries. Reversible ischemic neurological deficits (RIND) are diagnosed when signs of **ischemia** last more than 24 hours but less than 7 days.

There are two types of intracranial hemorrhage: *intracerebral hemorrhage (ICH)* and *subarachnoid hemorrhage (SAH)*. Hypertension is the usual culprit in ICH. An ICH involves a local area of bleeding in the brain from a ruptured intracranial artery. Bleeding occurs in the subarachnoid space with an SAH. A ruptured aneurysm or ruptured AVM in a major cerebral artery or one of its branches is the usual cause of SAH. In either case, the occlusion or hemorrhage distorts the perfusion pressure in the cerebral circulation and leads to ischemia and dilatation of collateral vessels. Electrical activity ceases, and CSF pressure increases.

A person with a progressing stroke, or a *stroke in evolution,* demonstrates unstable, progressing neurological deficits. A person with a completed stroke is stable with nonprogressing neurological deficits. A lacunar infarction is a stroke that is caused by hyaline thickening of the small penetrating arteries of the subcortical brain and is commonly associated with hypertension. This type of infarction is frequently asymptomatic but often results in pure motor strokes, pure sensory strokes, clumsy hand-n-dysarthria syndrome, or ataxic hemiparesis. A CT scan may show small subcortical infarcts; MRI is a more sensitive diagnostic test.

Diagnosis

A detailed history and physical examination are required to diagnose cerebrovascular disease. A rapid or sudden onset of signs and symptoms suggests infarction, but brain abscess, tumor, granuloma, and subdural hematoma must be ruled out. A differential diagnosis includes epilepsy, MS, and hysteria. The physician looks for embolic causes of the disease, such as atrial fibrillation, valvular disease (mitral stenosis, mitral prolapse), recent myocardial infarction (MI), ventricular aneurysm, carotid stenosis, and a history of intravenous drug abuse. The workup should also include an echocardiogram and carotid Doppler examination. Transesophageal echocardiography may reveal an abnormality that was missed by transthoracic echocardiography.

There are several possible predictors of CVA. German researchers have found that individuals with high-normal WBC counts have four times the risk for a MI and possibly a CVA. A high WBC count may also predict the risk of a second MI or stroke. In addition, researchers from the Framingham Heart Study have discovered that low levels of TSH, or thyrotropin, may be a warning sign for a CVA. Low TSH levels indicate an overactive thyroid gland, which means there is a greater risk of developing atrial fibrillation. Today, experts believe that all women age 50 and older and men age 60 and older should have their TSH levels routinely checked. A fairly large number of individuals with atrial fibrillation (35%) eventually incur a CVA.

No particular laboratory studies confirm the diagnosis of a stroke. However, laboratory tests should include a CBC with platelet count, ESR, PT, PTT, fibrinogen, glucose, electrolytes, cholesterol and triglyceride levels, ECG, and chest x-ray. These laboratory studies are conducted for a variety of reasons. Electrolyte studies reveal fluid and electrolyte balance, providing guidance for restoring fluids and electrolytes and preventing increased ICP. A CBC provides information regarding the oxygen-carrying capacity of the blood as well as the blood's viscosity and assists in determining who may be predisposed to developing thromboses, which can lead to cerebral infarction. Clients who have atherosclerosis may have elevated cholesterol and triglyceride levels. Finally, the clotting profile, including PT, PTT, platelet count, and fibrinogen values, assists in ruling out clotting abnormalities, especially with ischemic stroke. The PT and PTT also give information for guiding anticoagulation therapy.

A noncontrast CT is usually done; however, the area of infarct may not be visible for 36 hours, and this test misses about 10% of subarachnoid bleeds. A contrast CT should be obtained if an abscess, tumor, or granuloma is suspected. The CT scan provides the physician with informationto identify pathological changes in the brain such as hemorrhage or aneurysm, ischemia, and a baseline for future examinations. MRI is more sensitive for detecting infarction, particularly if there is a lesion in the brain stem or posterior fossa, but it is difficult to obtain on an emergency basis.

If an SAH is suspected, LP is usually done. The physician looks for bloody fluid initially, which should taper off, and yellow fluid (yellow supernatant) if the hemorrhage occurred more than 6 hours previously.

Ischemia is an inadequate blood supply to a tissue or organ. It can produce pain, itching, or death of tissue.

Suspected Causes of Cerebral Hemorrhage

- Hypertension
- Ruptured aneurysm
- Ruptured arteriovenous malformation
- Septic embolism
- Vascular inflammatory disease
- Trauma
- Complications of anticoagulation therapy
- Smoking

Possible Predictors of CVA

German researchers have found that individuals with high-normal WBC counts have four times the risk of having an MI and possibly a stroke as well. A high WBC may also predict the risk of a second MI or stroke. In addition, researchers with the Framingham Heart Study have discovered that low levels of TSH, or thyrotropin, may indicate a warning sign for CVA. Low levels mean an overactive thyroid gland and can indicate a greater risk of developing atrial fibrillation. A fairly large number of individuals with atrial fibrillation (35%) eventually have a CVA. Experts today believe that all women age 50 and older and men age 60 and older should have their TSH levels routinely checked.

Although it may not be especially helpful, an ECG is ordered. An inverted T wave, ST depression, and QT elevation and prolongation are unusual findings in the presence of neurological disease. An ECG is obtained if a cardiac embolism is suspected (i.e., which might occur with atrial fibrillation). A Doppler examination of the carotid arteries is indicated to determine stenosis of the arteries. If the client is young, relatively healthy, or poses a diagnostic dilemma, angiography may be indicated as well.

Assessment

An accurate history is essential in the diagnosis of a CVA. The information the nurse obtains can be vital in identifying the area of a stroke. The nurse should ask what the client was doing when the stroke began. Ischemic strokes tend to happen during sleep, whereas hemorrhagic strokes happen during activity. Ask how the symptoms progressed, how severe they were, when they were worse, and when they began to improve. Observe the client's LOC during the interview and assess for intellectual defects, impairment in memory, and speech and hearing impairments. Question the client and family about his or her medical history, paying special attention to any mention of head trauma, diabetes, hypertension, heart disease, obesity, anemia, and headaches. Find out what prescribed and OTC medications the client has been taking.

The nurse must perform a thorough neurological assessment, focusing on evidence of hemiparesis; sensory defects such as impaired vision, hearing, and touch; spatial and perceptual deficits; an altered LOC; **aphasia,** amnesia, agraphia, **ataxia,** and **dysphasia;** choreoathetoid movements; headache; bruit; grasp and sucking reflex; confusion; and coma. The client may have dysfunction in a few or several areas, which provides clues about the type of stroke. Expect the client to exhibit a variety of cognitive problems and an altered LOC. For example, the right hemisphere is more involved with spatial and visual awareness and proprioception. Thus, the client with a right hemispheric stroke may not be aware of any problems and may be quite confused. The left hemisphere, which is dominant in 80%–90% of us, is the center for language and thought. A stroke in this area causes aphasia, alexia, and agraphia; that is, the inability to use or comprehend language, problems with reading, and problems with writing, respectively.

If paralysis occurs on the right side, the left side of the brain is affected; if paralysis occurs on the left side, the right side of the brain is affected. Motor changes can be determined by assessing motor strength; muscle tone, including hypertonia (spastic paralysis); and ROM. Sensory changes are assessed by determining the client's response to touch and painful stimuli as well as his or her ability to differentiate two tactile stimuli presented at the same time. Clients with unilateral neglect syndrome are unaware that one side is paralyzed. In some cases, the client may only wash or dress one side. The nurse must perform a visual assessment as part of the sensory assessment. There may be pupillary abnormalities, visual field problems, and ptosis. *Amaurosis fugax* is the brief occurrence of blindness in one eye; hemananopsia is blindness in half of the visual field. Most often, blindness

Types of Aphasia

- **Broca's aphasia**—motor or expressive; affects ability to speak or write.
- **Wernicke's aphasia**—sensory or receptive; affects ability to understand written or oral communication.
- **Global aphasia**—affects ability to understand *and* communicate.
- **Anomic-amnesic aphasia**—affects ability to name objects.

Ataxia is the inability to coordinate muscles enough to move effectively.

Dysphasia is a failure to coordinate words or put them in proper order, often resulting from a CVA.

occurs on the same side of both eyes, requiring head turning to scan the total range of vision. Some clients may, for example, eat only half of their meal because that is all they see. The nurse must assess cranial nerve function with particular attention to cranial nerves V, VII, IX, and XII. Damage to these nerves may cause problems with chewing, facial paralysis or paresis, dysphagia, loss of gag reflex, or impaired tongue movement.

After conducting the neurological examination, examine the cardiovascular system to detect possible heart murmurs, dysrhythmias, and hypertension. Blood pressure on admission may be very high. Assess the client's reaction to his or her illness (i.e., how he or she is coping with it), identify any problems related to the disorder, and look for personality changes. Ascertain emotional lability, which may be demonstrated by inappropriate laughter or crying spells.

The nurse must focus on several problems while developing a plan of care for the client who has had a stroke. Altered cerebral tissue perfusion, impaired physical mobility and self-care deficits, altered senses and perception, unilateral neglect, impaired verbal communication, impaired swallowing, and urinary and bowel incontinence all must be considered in the nursing care plan.

Treatment

In general, after a CVA or SAH, the blood pressure should not be lowered too rapidly during the first 10 days after the injury unless the diastolic pressure is greater than 120 mm Hg in a client with a CVA or is persistently elevated in a client with an SAH. A 10-mg capsule of sublingual nifedipine (Procardia) is often used because it begins acting in 30 minutes. This capsule can be pierced or chewed in an emergency situation. When the blood pressure is lowered quickly, vomiting frequently occurs; therefore, the nurse should be prepared with an emesis basin and suction equipment. Clients experiencing neurological deficits such as a CVA or SAH should not receive large amounts of fluid, particularly intravenously, as this can worsen cerebral edema. D5W should not be the intravenous fluid of choice.

In the event of a cardiogenic embolus, systemic anticoagulation is indicated to prevent the development of more emboli. The timing of systemic anticoagulation remains controversial, as hemorrhage into an infarcted area can develop 1–7 days after injury and can be fatal. If there is a large embolic infarct, anticoagulation is usually withheld for 1–7 days, unless a thrombus is discovered in the heart. Otherwise, anticoagulation is initiated and titrated to prolong the aPTT (activated partial thromboplastin time) to 1.5–2.5 times longer than normal. Anticoagulation is begun with a 5000–10,000 unit bolus of heparin, and then 1000–2000 units per hour intravenously. This rate is adjusted periodically based on the aPTT, which may be obtained as often as every 4 hours. On the second day, oral anticoagulation is started with warfarin (Coumadin), usually 10 mg/day for 3 days, and then adjusted based upon the PT, which is also kept at 1.5–2.5 times longer than control. INR is a standard international method of determining anticoagulation. A level of 2–3 is optimal. Once warfarin

Common Complaints of Clients with Neurologic Disorders

- Headaches
- Motor disturbances (i.e., weakness, paresis, paralysis)
- Seizures
- Sensory deviations
- Altered level of consciousness

Acute Complications of Open Head Injury

- CSF leakage
- Hematomas
- Subarachnoid hemorrhage
- Increased ICP
- Hydrocephalus
- Seizures

Suspected Causes of Cerebral Embolism

- Dysrhythmias, especially atrial fibrillation
- Myocardial infarction
- Cardiac valve disease
- Valve prosthesis
- Congenital septal defect
- Cardiac surgery complications

(Coumadin) is started and a steady PT is obtained, heparin is stopped. The PT is then checked every 2 weeks.

One-third of the clients who have had a TIA or RIND will have a cerebral infarction within 5 years. The time of greatest risk is immediately after a cardiac event. These individuals should be placed on 325 mg/day of aspirin. Ticlopidine (Ticlid, 250 mg twice a day) is also used but is usually reserved for clients who have failed aspirin therapy. Carotid endarterectomy is also an option but is generally reserved for those with high-grade stenosis (70–99%) and only if the client is symptomatic.

In the event of a progressing stroke, intravenous heparin should be used, although studies regarding the efficacy of heparin have not shown any real benefits to date. A noncontrast CT scan should be obtained to rule out hemorrhagic infarction. Thrombosis (atherosclerosis) and lacunar infarctions are treated with aspirin or ticlopidine as outlined above. Risk factors, particularly hypertension, should be treated. The diagnosis of ICH requires a neurosurgical consult for possible evacuation for clients with cerebellar hematomas and large superficial cerebral hematomas. Immediate neurosurgical consultation is imperative for those with SAH.

Other drugs that may be administered include anticonvulsants such as phenytoin (Dilantin) to prevent seizures; epsilon-aminocaproic acid (Amicar) to stabilize a cerebral clot; and a calcium-channel blocker such as nimodipine (Nimotop) to treat cerebral vessel spasms. Some clients may also require sedation.

Nursing Care

The major goals of nursing interventions include maintenance or improvement of the LOC and prevention of additional neurological problems resulting from the stroke. Nursing care should be planned around the medical management, which usually focuses on drug therapy and aggressive rehabilitation. For clients with altered cerebral tissue perfusion, the nurse must monitor for increased ICP and perform a complete neurological examination at least once every 8 hours. Use the GCS and other tools available for assessing the client once per shift or more often as indicated. Keep the head of the bed elevated to enhance venous cerebral drainage and avoid activities that increase the ICP. Stagger the procedures to conserve the client's energy. Do not suction unless needed, as this procedure increases ICP. Monitor and assess the vital signs at least once every 4 hours, paying special attention to the client's blood pressure. Blood pressure higher than 150/100 mm Hg should be reported to the physician.

The nurse must set goals for clients with impaired physical mobility and self-care deficits, such as increasing tolerance and endurance for therapy, reducing or eliminating the complications of immobility, and achieving maximal independence while performing ADLs. Passive ROM exercises should begin within 24–48 hours after the stroke has occurred. The nurse should change these to active ROM exercises as soon as possible. Clients should be positioned carefully to maintain proper body alignment. The hand or lower extremity on the affected side may need to be splinted.

Furthermore, seek to avoid the complications of immobility such as deep vein thrombosis by using antiembolism stockings, frequently changing the client's position, and mobilizing the client as soon as possible.

Clients who have suffered a stroke have alterations in senses and perception. The nurse's plan of care must address ways to assist the client in adapting to impairments and preventing injury. It is necessary for the nurse to assist the client in adapting to certain inabilities in performing ADLs. One way to accomplish this is to break large tasks down into smaller, more manageable ones. The client should be approached from the unaffected side and placed in bed so the unaffected side faces the door. The nurse must teach the client to turn the head to gain visual depth and to scan with the eyes. Provide a safe environment by removing clutter from the room. Reorient the client as often as needed to the year, month, date, and day of the week. The nurse should establish a structured, consistent schedule and use a step-by-step approach with the client for the most effective attainment of goals.

Clients with unilateral neglect syndrome should be taught how to use compensation techniques. This syndrome occurs most often in clients who have had a right cerebral stroke. Unilateral neglect increases the client's risk for injury. Teach the client to use the sense of touch and to use both sides of the body. The nurse can also encourage the client to wash both sides of the body and to dress the affected side first. The client should be taught to scan by turning the head from side to side.

Clients with impaired verbal communication require assistance in developing alternative ways to communicate. Aphasia results from cerebral hemisphere damage; dysarthria is a consequence of motor function loss in the tongue or speech muscle, resulting in slurred speech. Nursing interventions for this problem should be planned in collaboration with a speech therapist. Clients with impaired communication need to have directions repeated to them to finish a task, need to be faced when spoken to, talked to slowly, and allowed adequate time to respond. Names of objects must be repeated. Providing pictures of the object and the activities associated with it is helpful.

Clients who have had a stroke may have impaired swallowing, which can lead to many problems. The goals are for the client to eat and drink without aspirating fluid or food and to maintain an ideal or usual body weight. Always assess the client's ability to swallow before giving food and be alert to facial drooping; drooling; and a weak, hoarse voice. To assess the client's ability to swallow, place your thumb and forefinger on either side of the client's Adam's apple and ask him or her to swallow. Check the cough and gag reflex as well. Position the client to enhance swallowing, that is, preferably sitting in a chair or sitting straight up if in bed. Soft or semisoft foods are generally better tolerated than liquids. Work with the dietitian and the speech therapist to ensure that the client does not choke or aspirate while eating. Broths and sweet, sour, and salty foods tend to stimulate saliva production, which makes swallowing easier.

An important goal for all stroke clients is gaining bowel and bladder control. This may be a major problem initially because of an altered LOC, cognitive deficits, and muscle weakness. The client may be unable to communicate his or her need to urinate or defecate. Most clients can relearn these important functions, but the nurse must have time and patience to plan and implement a bowel and bladder retraining program. Unless contraindicated, encourage a fluid intake of 2000 mL/day. Establish and follow a regular schedule for urination and perform intermittent catheterizations as indicated to assess for residual urine. Ascertain the client's normal bowel habits before starting a retraining program and establish the client's normal routine if possible. Work with the dietitian to provide a high-bulk and high-fiber diet. Encourage the client to drink apple or prune juice to establish a regular bowel pattern.

Discharge planning needs to focus on preparing the home for the client, teaching the client about his or her health, psychosocial preparation, and contacting appropriate and available health care resources. The nurse must work with the social worker to plan for discharge adequately. The American Heart Association offers information on strokes, and families can be referred to the National Stroke Foundation.

Evaluation

Nursing care is evaluated by assessing whether there is adequate cerebral tissue perfusion and whether the client's LOC has improved. Has the client adapted to changes in perception and senses? The nurse determines the client's endurance and appropriate use of assistive or adaptive devices. The nurse assesses the client's bowel and bladder control. Does the client communicate in an understandable way with gestures, speech, or phrases? Finally, the nurse evaluates the client's ability to eat without choking or aspirating.

HEAD AND SPINAL CORD INJURIES

Diagnosis

Head Injury Head injury involves a traumatic injury to the brain from an external force that may be followed by a decreased or changed LOC in the affected individual. Head injuries can lead to cognitive or physical disorders and emotional or psychological disturbances. Neurological disorders resulting from a head injury may be temporary or permanent. Head injury is the leading cause of death in the United States among those aged 18–34 years. The total cost from head injuries is approximately 50 billion dollars annually, including hospitalizations, rehabilitation, and lost wages and productivity.

Head trauma is frequently associated with other severe traumas. Critical attention to the airway, breathing, and circulation (ABCs) is vital to save the client. Head injuries are often classified as low risk, moderate risk, or high risk. *Low-risk injuries* include scalp wounds and those with no signs of intracranial injury or LOC. *Moderate-risk injuries* are those with symptoms consistent with intracranial injury, including (1) vomiting, transient LOC, post-traumatic seizures, amnesia, evidence of basilar fracture (CSF, rhinorrhea, Battle's sign, raccoon eyes, hematotympanum); and (2) nonfocal neurological examination without localizing signs. Treatment of moderate-risk injuries includes observation and frequent neurological checks. Based on clinical judgment, a CT scan may be done. The client should be admitted for observation and monitoring.

The criteria for *high-risk injuries* include those clients with LOC, focal neurological signs, a penetrating injury of the skull, or a palpable depressed skull fracture. These clients require an immediate CT scan and a neurosurgical consultation. Emergency supportive measures while awaiting definitive neurosurgical consult include intubation and hyperventilation to maintain adequate oxygenation; maintenance of normal cardiac output with hypertonic saline (3% or 7% normal saline solution); and administration of an appropriate beta blocker if the client is hypertensive. Emergency treatment of increased ICP involves hyperventilation; mannitol (Osmitrol, 1 g/kg body weight over 20 minutes) for osmotic diuresis, furosemide (Lasix, 20 mg intravenously), and elevation of the head of the bed 30 degrees. If hypotension is present, the nurse should look for possible causes other than head trauma.

Head injuries may result from skull fractures, concussions, or contusions. Skull fractures are classified as *simple*, or *linear*, with a simple crack; *comminuted*, more than one broken bone; depressed, the fracture has penetrated the meninges of brain; compound, involving a break in the scalp with the fracture; or *basilar*, a fracture or crack from the frontal bone to the roof of the orbit of the eye, resulting in raccoon eyes and possible CSF discharge from the ears. Approximately 80% of skull fractures are linear (i.e., a simple, clean break). Penetrating skull injuries usually result from a knife or gunshot wound. Clients may have a simple fracture or a combination of fractures.

A concussion involves a jarring of the brain. If a client goes into a coma following a concussion, it is usually transient, lasting less than 24 hours. In contrast, a contusion involves trauma that leads to alterations in the brain. The severity of the contusion depends on the location and extent of injury. When a contusion is accompanied by unconsciousness, the coma usually lasts more than 24 hours, and there may or may not be a fracture involved.

Head injuries can also cause various types of bleeding under the skull or in the brain. A SAH is the rupture of a blood vessel or vessels in the subarachnoid space. The bleed remains in the subarachnoid space, and signs and symptoms may vary. The most common symptom is a severe headache. A subdural hematoma is an accumulation of blood in the subdural space that occurs when a vein ruptures. With this type of bleed, ICP increases. A subdural hematoma can be acute, occurring within 48 hours of injury; subacute, occurring 48 hours to 10 days after the injury; or chronic, occurring 10 days to 1 month after the injury. Chronic subdural hematomas occur more commonly in the elderly and alcoholics due to brain atrophy. An epidural bleed occurs when there is an arterial rupture in the epidural space, the area that separates the dura mater from the skull. An epidural bleed is most common with fractures of the temporal bone. With this type of trauma, there is usually a lucid interval after the trauma, and the client's condition suddenly and rapidly deteriorates. The client has signs and symptoms of increased ICP.

An ICH can result from trauma, rupture of an arteriosclerotic vessel, or a blood dyscrasia. The chief signs and symptoms of this type of hemorrhage are LOC and paralysis. Injury can also occur to the brain stem as a result of a contusion or increased ICP. Abnormal respiratory patterns and decerebrate posturing (hyperextension of the arms and legs in response to a painful stimulus) are common when there is a bleed into the brainstem.

Spinal Cord Injury Spinal cord injuries should be suspected in clients who are unconscious from a head injury and those who are wounded in the face, head, or shoulders. Approximately 10,000 persons incur spinal cord injuries annually. Most individuals survive these injuries today because of trauma centers located throughout the United States and the widespread use of mechanical ventilators and antibiotics. Spinal cord injuries may result from a concussion or cord penetration and transection. The injury may be temporary or permanent with fragments actually penetrating the cord. The most common *open injuries* occur from knives, ice picks, and bullet wounds. The most common *closed injuries* result from motor vehicle accidents and falls.

Assessment of Head Injury The nurse must obtain as thorough a history as possible. As the client may be unconscious, it may be necessary to talk with the client's family and friends to find out what happened. Ask when, where, and how the trauma occurred. Did the client lose consciousness? If yes, for how long? Has there been any change in consciousness since the trauma? Ascertain as much information as possible about events after the injury. Some clients may be immediately unresponsive and stay that way, while others may be quite alert but deteriorate later. Question the client about seizure activity, and obtain a description. In some cases, it may be necessary to determine if the client fell or had a stroke. Ask about allergies, such as to contrast media. Inquire about alcohol and drug use, and check the client's breath. The nurse must obtain information about the client's prior medical status. The major goal is to obtain baseline data for comparison and evaluation throughout the client's hospital stay. The early detection of changes in the baseline data is very important in the care and treatment of clients with head injuries. Clients with head injuries often have cervical neck involvement and are treated for both injuries unless the physician determines that there is no neck injury.

The nurse's first priority is to assess and maintain adequate oxygenation. Clients with head injuries must undergo a thorough neurological assessment to ensure a positive outcome. The major aspects of a neurological checklist include evaluating vital signs, assessing the LOC, checking motor and sensory responses, determining pupillary response, observing and evaluating signs and symptoms of increased ICP, and assessing posturings.

Vital Signs Vital signs are very important in the neurological assessment. The nurse must assess blood pressure, temperature, pulse, and respirations. An elevated temperature may indicate damage to the hypothalamus; this may increase cellular metabolism, increasing demand for oxygen and dilatation of the blood vessels. When this occurs, the resulting increased blood flow can subsequently increase ICP, which must be avoided. Increased ICP eventually leads to a rise in blood pressure, but this is a late finding. Assessment of the quality of respirations is an essential component of the neurological assessment. Respirations can be quite irregular; there may even be a pattern to the irregularity. *Cheyne-Stokes respirations* involve deep inspirations and long pauses between inspirations and expirations. This can be normal in elderly men. *Central neurogenic hyperventilation* can occur when there is a disorder in the pons. With this type of respiratory disorder, the rate and depth of respirations are increased. *Apneustic breathing* also indicates a disorder in the pons. This is a breathing pattern in which inspiration is held much longer than expiration. *Biot's breathing* is a totally erratic pattern of respiration. *Cluster breathing* is clusters of erratic breathing, sometimes in inspirations and sometimes in expirations. This respiratory pattern indicates a problem in the medulla (Fig. 9-15). Changes in blood pressure are often the last vital sign to reflect a noticeable change in the client.

Signs and Symptoms of Increased Intracranial Pressure

- Decreased level of consciousness
- Headache
- Motor changes
- Irregular or slowed respirations
- Papilledema
- Vomiting without nausea
- Widened pulse pressure
- Bradycardia

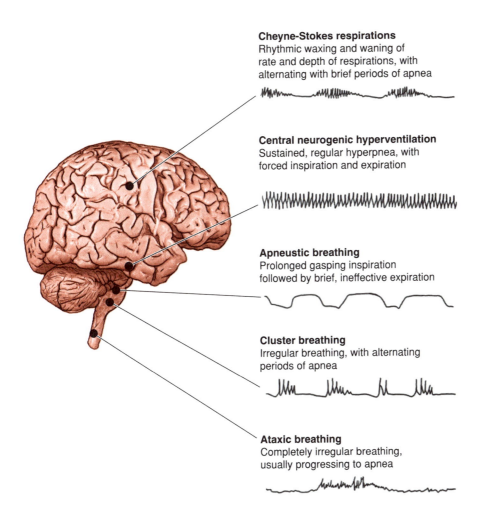

Cheyne-Stokes respirations
Rhythmic waxing and waning of rate and depth of respirations, with alternating with brief periods of apnea

Central neurogenic hyperventilation
Sustained, regular hyperpnea, with forced inspiration and expiration

Apneustic breathing
Prolonged gasping inspiration followed by brief, ineffective expiration

Cluster breathing
Irregular breathing, with alternating periods of apnea

Ataxic breathing
Completely irregular breathing, usually progressing to apnea

FIGURE 9-15

Abnormal respiratory patterns.

Key Signs and Symptoms of Increased Intracranial Pressure

1. Increased restlessness, confusion, disorientation, or a subtle decrease in level of consciousness
2. Sluggish pupillary reactions; unequal or fixed and dilated pupils (may be one-sided)
3. A combination of vital sign changes, known as Cushing's triad:
   - Decreased blood pressure with widening pulse pressure (the difference between the systolic and diastolic blood pressures becomes greater than normal, with the primary reason being an increased systolic blood pressure)
   - Bradycardia in the 30–50 beats/min range
   - Respirations that are irregular or arrhythmical

Monro-Kellie Hypothesis. There is 1800–1900 mL of fluid in the cranial vault. Of this, 80% is brain tissue, 10% is blood, and 10% is CSF. Normal ICP is 3–11 mm Hg; 15–40 mm Hg is a moderate increase; 40+ mm Hg is a severe increase. The Monro-Kellie hypothesis states that the volume of the brain plus the volume of CSF, plus the volume of blood equals the volume of the intracranium. Nothing can take up space within the cranium without subtracting space from another part of the intracranium.

Level of Consciousness Is the client alert and awake? Is the client oriented to person, place, and time? Is the client lethargic or restless? How does the client respond to verbal commands? How does the client respond to painful stimuli such as a sternal rub or gentle pinch? Does the client withdraw purposefully (i.e., have purposeful movement), or does the client grimace with irrelevant or nonpurposeful movement? Is there no response to stimuli at all? How much stimulation is needed to obtain a response? (Note that nurses should never cause severe pain or injury to a client to assess LOC. Bruising and hard pinches are unethical.)

Mobility and Sensation To assess sensory response, the nurse should use a light touch and ask clients to say where the cotton ball is touching. Use a safety pin to assess for sharp and dull sensations. Check for *stereognosis* by placing an object in the client's hand and have the client tell you what it is. Check for *graphesthesia* by writing a letter or number on the client's palm and have him or her tell you what you wrote. Assess the client's ability to move her arms and legs by asking her to move, raise her arms, squeeze your hands, wiggle her toes, and touch an ear. Check the client's facial muscles by having her smile and show her teeth, having her shut her eyes tightly while you try to open them, and having her wrinkle her forehead. Check for unusual movements such as grasping or spontaneous rigidity. Check Babinski's sign by running a rough, firm object up the outside bottom of the foot. The great toes should rise and the remaining toes should fan out. Any other response is abnormal in those older than 18 months.

Pupil Response Check the pupils for their shape, size, and equality. Test pupillary reactions to direct and consensual light and determine how much they dilate. The nurse should look for unusual eye movements and ensure that both eyes move together. Finally, assess the corneal reflex.

Increased Intracranial Pressure ICP is the most common cause of death in neurologically impaired clients. There is 1800–1900 mL of fluid in the cranial vault. Of this, 80% is in brain tissue, 10% is blood, and 10% is CSF. Normal ICP is 3–11 mm Hg; 15–40 mm Hg is a moderate increase; and 40 mm Hg is a severe increase. The *Monro-Kellie hypothesis* states that the volume of the brain plus the volume of the CSF plus the volume of blood equals the volume of the intracranium. Nothing can take up space within the cranium without subtracting space from another part of the intracranium; there is only room for what nature provides. Therefore, in the event of increased ICP, there must be compensation in one of the other components. Thus, CSF is shunted to the spinal cord, arterial blood is shunted to the veins, and brain tissue may be compressed.

Factors that influence cerebral blood flow include ABGs, mean arterial pressure (MAP), and autoregulation. Concerning ABGs, an elevated P_{CO_2} causes vasodilatation; a decreased P_{CO_2} causes vasoconstriction; and a decreased P_{CO_2} (< 50 mm Hg) also causes vasodilatation. The mean arterial pressure minus the ICP equals the cerebral perfusion pressure (CPP). This is an advanced concept and requires ICP monitoring, which is not discussed in this textbook. However, you should remember that normal cerebral perfusion pressure needs to be 70–80 mm Hg, and that a pressure less than 45 mm Hg is incompatible with adequate brain function. MAPs less than 50 mm Hg can result in vascular collapse and cellular death. Furthermore, MAPs greater than 170 mm Hg can cause cerebral edema and intracranial bleeding. Failure of the brain's autoregulatory function can result from hypotension, hypoxia, brain trauma, and CVA. ICP is caused by increased brain volume, increased blood volume, increased CSF pressure, lesions, tumors, or abscesses.

Increased blood volume can result from hemorrhage (including trauma and hematomas), seizures, vasodilatation, and hydrocephalus. Seizures contribute to increased blood volume by increasing oxygen demand, causing vasodilatation. This increases ICP, which increases lactic acid production, causing further dilatation. In hydrocephalus, the production of CSF exceeds its absorption. This can be hereditary or result from tumor, hemorrhage, or meningitis.

Cerebral edema can occur as a result of increased ICP hours or days after a head injury. An increase in brain volume can be the result of edema from a closed head injury. Furthermore, fluid overload and alcohol or drug intoxication can lead to cerebral edema. When cerebral edema occurs, local hypoxia in the brain may result. Excessive or prolonged cerebral edema can result in cellular ischemia and possibly death of brain cells. The *key signs and symptoms* of increased ICP include: increased restlessness, confusion, disorientation, or a subtle decrease in the LOC; sluggish pupillary reactions and unequal or fixed and dilated pupils (may be unilateral); widened pulse pressure (the difference between the systolic and diastolic blood pressures is greater than normal because of increased systolic blood pressure); a combination of vital sign changes, known as Cushing's triad: (1) decreased blood pressure with widening pulse pressure, (2) bradycardia in the 30–50 beats/min range, and (3) respirations that are slowed irregular, or arrhythmical; headache; motor changes; papilledema; and vomiting without nausea.

Treatment of increased ICP involves

1. elevating the head of the bed at least 30 degrees;
2. oxygenating with 90–100% oxygen;
3. hyperventilating to keep P_{CO_2} below 24–30 mm Hg;
4. using osmotic diuretics, such as mannitol (Osmitrol), to decrease the pressure;
5. giving steroids intravenously to decrease edema; and
6. administering barbiturates or anticonvulsant medication.

The health care provider must be alert for signs of CSF leakage. This may be apparent when the "halo" effect is seen (i.e., when CSF drainage leaves a blood-tinged spot with a lighter halo on the sheets or pillow). The nurse can check for CSF leaks by testing for the presence of sugar with a Dextrostix. Head injuries should be dressed but not packed too tightly and examined periodically.

Posturings The final part of a thorough neurological assessment is checking for posturings (Fig. 9-16). *Decorticate posturing* is the flexion of the arms and extension of the legs. *Decerebrate posturing* is the extension of all extremities and indicates damage to the brainstem. *Opisthotonos*, the extreme extension of all extremities, is often accompanied by seizures, tachycardia, tachypnea, clenched teeth, and diaphoresis.

Assessment of Spinal Cord Injury

To determine whether a client has incurred a spinal cord injury, it is important to assess for sensory and motor deficits as well as the location of the injury. Injury levels can be determined by the following:

1. C_2 or C_3: Complete respiratory paralysis, complete flaccidity, and absence of reflexes; death occurs without mechanical ventilation
2. C_5 or C_6: Paralysis of intercostal muscles, diaphragmatic respirations, complete loss of motor power in trunk and lower extremities resulting in quadriplegia, anesthesia below the clavicles, and bladder and bowel retention
3. T_1–T_{12}: Paraplegia, anesthesia below the affected level, and bowel and bladder retention
4. L_1–L_5: Partial flaccid paraplegia; anesthesia of the perineum, sacral area, and lower extremities; temporary bowel and bladder retention. Some sensation may be retained.

FIGURE 9-16

◼

Abnormal posturing.

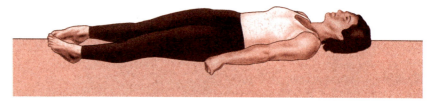

Extensor (decerebrate) posturing
The patient stiffly extends one or both
arms and legs.

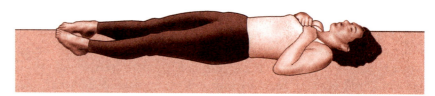

Flexor (decorticate) posturing
The patient flexes one or both arms on
the chest and stiffly extends the legs.

Nursing Care of Head and Spinal Cord Injuries

While planning the care of the client with a head or spinal cord injury or both, a major goal is to ensure adequate cerebral tissue perfusion by maintaining normal ICP and appropriate vital signs, as well as improving the client's LOC if possible. Most clients with head injuries are admitted for at least 24 hours of observation. Some require neurosurgical intervention. The nurse initially assesses the vital signs and performs a neurological assessment every 1–2 hours. This varies depending on the injury and the client's response. Clients with suspected or confirmed increased ICP are placed on a mechanical ventilator and hyperventilated to keep their carbon dioxide (CO_2) levels below normal; this helps to prevent vasodilatation, which can worsen cerebral edema. Some physicians may actually place these clients in a "barbiturate coma" with pentobarbital sodium (Nembutal, Novopentobarb) to decrease the metabolic demands on the body. Other drugs ordered may include corticosteroids and osmotic diuretics. As in any client, it is important for the nurse to maintain the client's fluid and electrolyte balance.

The second goal is to develop strategies to assist head-injured clients in adapting to perceptual or sensory alterations. Such changes may result from a decreased LOC, parietal lobe injury, or damage to the olfactory lobe. Thus, the client's sense of smell, ability to taste and swallow, ability to feel pain and temperature, and vision may be altered. This may place the client at risk for nutritional deficits, falling, and burns. The nurse should plan interventions that decrease these risks. For example, meals should be attractive, flavorful, and presented in a pleasant environment that is hazard free; explanations need to be clear and related to pictures, if possible; and the nurse should never assume that the client can remember things from one minute to the next.

Gas exchange may be impaired as a result of pooling of secretions, poor cough reflex, and an altered respiratory pattern. Nurses should ensure that the client does not develop a respiratory infection and that measures are taken to ensure normal or ordered blood gases. The client may require chest physiotherapy (i.e., frequent turning and suctioning). Suctioning must be done very carefully, according to established protocol, to ensure that the ICP is not inadvertently increased. The client should be suctioned for only 5 seconds at a time, with rest allowed between suctioning episodes. Be sure to turn the client every 2 hours as well.

Clients with head injuries are at high risk for further injury. They may be agitated, restless, confused, and seizure-prone. The bed should be kept in a low position with the side rails raised. Hand restraints or mittens may be required, but should only be used as a last resort because restraints often make the client worse and increase metabolic demands on the body. A physician's order is required for restraints; they must be removed at least every 2 hours with the affected body part massaged. Closely monitor the client's response to the external environment, including television and visitors. Clients often require reorientation.

Impaired physical mobility resulting in a self-care deficit may occur in these clients, depending on the extent of trauma. The nurse must ensure that the client does not incur complications from immobility while working towards the primary goal of ambulation and independent performance of ADLs by the time of discharge. It is very important that respiratory complications be prevented as they can worsen the client's neurological status. Turn the client every 2 hours, provide or oversee the administration of chest physiotherapy, and apply antiembolism stockings to prevent pulmonary embolus or deep vein thrombosis. Passive ROM exercises should be performed at least every 8 hours. Some clients may require splints or supportive shoes. This intervention should be employed with physician's orders and after consultation with an occupational therapist.

Head-injured clients may have difficulty chewing and swallowing because of an injury to a specific lobe of the brain or cognitive impairment. They are therefore at risk for malnourishment. Nursing goals include maintaining adequate hydration and the client's body weight at no less than 90% of the ideal or usual body weight. Intravenous fluid administration or tube feedings via a nasogastric or gastrostomy tube may be required. Weigh the client daily, and check serum albumin levels frequently to assess for adequate protein intake. Also, assess the client for signs of dehydration such as dry mucous membranes and poor skin turgor.

The client may have some difficulties with his or her body image as a result of a head or spinal cord injury. Nurses can create ways for clients to develop confidence in their abilities and to begin adapting to changes in appearance and abilities. Helping clients adjust to overwhelming changes in their appearance and abilities requires developing trust, being nonjudgmental, encouraging open communication, answering questions honestly, and facilitating their involvement in making decisions about treatment.

Evaluation

The nurse can evaluate nursing care provided to the head-injured client by answering some pertinent questions. Was adequate cerebral tissue perfusion maintained? Did the client's LOC improve or at least not worsen? Were seizures prevented? If they occurred, was injury prevented? Did the client remain free from injury? Has the client begun to develop strategies to adapt to sensory or perceptual changes? Has the client's mobility level improved noticeably, with minimal spasticity? Was a patent airway maintained? Finally, was adequate and appropriate nutrition and hydration maintained?

Coma

A coma, also called *unarousable unresponsiveness*, may be a complication of a variety of neurological problems, such as brain herniation, SAH, or head trauma. Coma may be the result of a failure of the brain stem's RAS, or it may be a bihemispheral failure. Emergency treatment includes implementation of the ABCs of resuscitation with cervical spine immobilization.

Causes of coma may be *metabolic*: hypoglycemia, uremia, nonketotic hyperosmolar coma, Addison's disease, diabetic ketoacidosis, hypothyroidism, hepatic coma; *respiratory*: hypoxia or hypercapnia; *intoxication*: barbiturates, alcohol, opiates, carbon monoxide poisoning, benzodiazepines; *infection*: sepsis, pneumonia, typhoid fever; *shock*: hypovolemic, cardiogenic, septic, anaphylactic; *epilepsy*; *hypertensive encephalopathy*; *hyperthermia* (heat stroke); and *hypothermia*. A coma with meningeal irritation and no localizing signs may be caused by meningitis, a SAH from a ruptured aneurysm, or an AVM. If focal brain stem or lateralizing signs are present, a coma can be caused by a pontine hemorrhage, CVA, brain abscess, or subdural or epidural hemorrhage. If the client appears to be awake but is not responsive, it may be due to one of the following: (1) *abulic state*: a depression of frontal lobe function in which the client may take several minutes to respond; (2) *locked-in syndrome*: a destruction of the pontine motor tracts, only allowing the client to look up; and (3) *psychogenic unresponsiveness*.

Two brain lesions can cause a coma, bilateral cortical disease and RAS compromise. To differentiate between a cortical and a brain stem lesion, the physician may use the caloric test in which ice water is injected into each ear. If both eyes deviate toward the injected side and have nystagmus, the client is not comatose. If both eyes deviate toward the injected side without fast return, the brain stem is intact and the coma is due to a cortical problem. If there is no eye movement, it indicates that there is no brainstem function. This may or may not be permanent and can be related to severe hypothermia or a drug overdose. Movement of only one eye on the ipsilateral (same) side after injection of ice water reveals brainstem damage and requires rapid evaluation to determine whether there is a correctable lesion.

Pupillary examination and testing also differentiates between a cortical and a brain stem lesion. The pupils are generally resistant to metabolic insults. It is important to remember that a dilated eye may result from topical or systemic medications. If the client is alert and has a dilated eye, there is probably no increased ICP and herniation. However, a dilated pupil in an unconscious person may be a warning of imminent uncal herniation. If the pupils are small and reactive, a metabolic or diencephalic lesion is usually the cause. A unilateral, dilated, and fixed pupil indicates a third nerve lesion or uncal lesion. Bilateral pinpoint pupils are indicative of a pontine lesion. If pupils are fixed in mid-position, a midbrain lesion is suspected. Large and fixed pupils indicate a tectal lesion. Propoxyphene (Darvon) and other drugs can cause a coma with pinpoint pupils. Eyes deviate toward the side of a physiologically inactive lesion, such as a CVA, and away from an active lesion, such as a seizure. It is also important to remember that 5% of the general population have anisocoria, or unequal pupils.

Diagnosis

In the event of a coma, the following studies should be obtained: CBC, electrolytes, BUN, creatinine, glucose, Ca^{2+}, Mg^{2+}, ABGs, toxicity screen,

Recovery from Coma

A typical "wake-up" pattern may occur (agitation may take place during any phase of waking up) and includes the following:

- Spontaneous eye-opening without recognition of the environment
- Visual tracking about the room
- Response to sounds
- Response to simple commands

To Assist in Coma Recovery:

1. Provide a structured environment, with a regular schedule, periodic care, naps, therapy, and visitors. Write out the schedule, and post it where the client can see it.
2. Personalize the client's room with things like pictures from home, music, or a clock.
3. Control stimulation. Close the door and draw the blinds during normal sleeping hours.
4. Talk slowly and provide instructions one at a time. Provide time for processing of information.

Prognosis of Recovery from Coma

- Extent of lesion
- Personality before injury
- Environment

carboxyhemoglobin, and liver enzymes. A CT scan and LP should be done if meningitis is suspected. Antibiotics should not be withheld while waiting for a LP or CT scan if meningitis is suspected.

Assessment

Examination and treatment of the comatose client requires expert assessment and nursing skill. Initially inspect the head for evidence of trauma such as an overt head injury. Check for raccoon eyes (bruising around the orbits and the bridge of the nose) and Battle's sign (bruising on the mastoid process behind the ear). Palpate the skull for bogginess or depression. Check the skin for needle tracks, myxedematous changes, uremic frost (rare), jaundice, a sallow or cherry red complexion, skin lesions or rashes, and poor skin turgor. The nurse should also check the client's breath for alcohol or acetone odors, assess the vital signs, and check for hypothermia and hyperthermia.

Assessing the cranial nerves can be done fairly quickly (see Table 9-1) after gaining experience. The nurse must assess cranial nerves II and III with direct light. Cranial nerves III, VI, and VIII should be checked for doll's eyes reflex and cold caloric reflex (oculocephalic and oculovestibular reflexes). Cranial nerves V and VII should be checked for the corneal reflex, and cranial nerves IX and X, for the gag reflex. The nurse must be alert to the client's breathing pattern (see Fig. 9-15 to determine the breathing pattern and location of the corresponding lesion).

$\mathcal{S}$UMMARY

While planning the nursing care of the neurologically impaired client, it is vital to prioritize rapidly. Begin with assessing and maintaining ABCs (airway, breathing, circulation). Clients with neurological deficits who have come through the emergency room should be somewhat stable, although this certainly may not be the case in the critical care setting. In the medical-surgical setting, these clients should be fairly stable, but the nurse must always ensure that ABCs are maintained. Neurologically impaired clients are at increased risk for developing complications as a result of an impaired airway, inadequate breathing, or compromised circulation. Once the client is stabilized and diagnosed, the nurse can proceed with planning his or her care.

Pay particular attention to maintaining an effective airway, because the client may have an altered LOC and be unable to cough. Always keep oral airway and suction equipment available and ready. The client must be protected from injury, especially if he or she is having seizures. If the client is unable to communicate verbally as a result of a speech impairment or coma, the nurse must use another method of communication. Furthermore, in light of the neurological deficits, the nurse needs to be attentive to the client's nutritional needs, mobility, tissue perfusion, and general health. The client and family often have a poor understanding of the deficit. This can create anxiety and fear. Finally, the client will most likely have a deficit in self-care, and the ADLs that most of us take for granted must be relearned and assisted.

Always provide explanations regardless of whether the client seems to understand. Include the family in your teaching and use language that they can easily understand. Describe what you are doing and why and the expected changes that occur with the client's diagnosis. Teach the client and the family the purposes and names of medications, the dosages, and the possible side effects that should be reported to the physician. Stress the importance of adequate nutrition and exercise.

If indicated, the following general nursing diagnoses should be included for neurologically impaired clients: inadequate oxygenation; impaired physical mobility; high risk for injury; high risk for impaired skin integrity; altered nutrition and altered bowel elimination (constipation); altered urinary elimination (incontinence); knowledge deficit; bathing or hygiene self-care deficit; impaired verbal communication; ineffective individual coping; and powerlessness. You will become more familiar with these diagnoses as you gain experience. A nursing diagnosis is developed by identifying the client's problems or potential problems and then relating the identified problem to a possible cause. The nurse may reference a specific nursing diagnosis textbook and a medical-surgical textbook when working with neurologically impaired clients.

In some cases, a problem-focused approach to planning care rather than a nursing diagnosis is used. Nursing diagnoses can easily be "converted" into problems. For example, constipation is a nursing diagnosis, a problem, and a medical diagnosis. The use of nursing diagnosis or problems as the central focus on which the plan of care is based depends on the nursing school. There are a multitude of appropriate resources to assist with forming nursing diagnoses.

Nursing interventions for neurologically impaired clients may include providing emotional support, proper nutritional support, adequate rest and exercise, and being attentive to signs and symptoms of infection. In addition, arranging for occupational and physical therapy may need to be included in the plan of care. Administering ordered medications and teaching the client about the medications are also important parts of the plan.

The following are some general nursing measures to include in the plan of care.

1. **Respiratory Care.** Unless contraindicated, turn the client frequently, and encourage him or her to cough and breathe deeply if able. If increased ICP is present or a risk, this will probably not be done.
2. **Cardiovascular Care.** Assess cardiac status and check vital signs, including apical and radial pulses; monitor for hypertension and signs of CHF, such as crackles, restlessness, and tachycardia.
3. **Skin Care.** Use antiembolic hose to decrease the risk of deep vein thrombosis and position the client to prevent pressure on the calves. Perform ROM exercises. If the client is in a coma, be especially alert

for skin breakdown. Pad bony prominences and change the client's position at least every 2 hours unless contraindicated. Be aware that the thin, immobile, febrile, and hypotensive client is also at risk for skin breakdown and development of decubiti.

4. **Client Positioning.** Maintain good body alignment and work to prevent contractures, abnormal limb rotations, and deformities. Use a footboard, pillows, hand rolls, and a trochanter roll as indicated. Be alert to preferences for abnormal positioning, particularly in the hemiplegic client, such as elbow and wrist flexion, external hip rotation, and arm adduction.

5. **Exercise and Mobility Care.** Perform ROM exercises 4–5 times a day. When they are able, clients should do these exercises by themselves. Provide support as needed, especially for CVA clients, and encourage ambulation as soon as possible. Clients at risk, such as those with a ruptured aneurysm, should be treated cautiously when moved (i.e., turn the client only to prevent venous stasis, pressure sores, and respiratory problems).

6. **Bladder and Bowel Care.** Neurologically impaired individuals may not have full control of the bladder and bowel. Clients may initially have a Foley catheter in place and be incontinent of stool. If there is paralysis, constipation may also be a problem. Bladder and bowel retraining may be required. Intermittent catheterization (every 6 hours) may be done to begin bladder retraining until the client can void spontaneously. Once that occurs, the client is catheterized after voiding to assess for urinary retention. If more than 200 mL is obtained from the postvoid catheterization, the client should be catheterized every 8 hours until postvoiding catheterization results in 150 mL or less of urine. Wait several days before checking again. Encourage the client to drink plenty of water. Clients with cerebral injuries should avoid constipation and straining during bowel movements. Use stool softeners, mild laxatives, enemas, or glycerine suppositories as ordered to facilitate normal bowel movements. Bowel control can be re-established by adhering to a regular schedule, a high-fiber diet, and increased fluid intake. Constipating foods should be avoided as well.

7. **Speech Care.** The CVA client may have a weak tongue and facial muscles or damaged speech and language centers. Clients with sensory or receptive aphasia (Wernicke's encephalopathy) cannot understand oral or written communication. Clients with motor or expressive aphasia (Broca's) can comprehend speech but cannot speak or write. Global aphasia affects both reception and expression. A consult with a speech therapist is often needed to re-establish communication with the neurologically impaired client. Speech may return spontaneously, it may require many months of speech therapy, or it may never return. Clients with speech impairments require a great deal of patience. The nurse should face the client when speaking; speak clearly; be patient; use nonverbal communication; encourage the client to talk and use different ways of communicating; simplify as much as possible; and assist the family.

8. **Emotional Care.** Neurologically impaired clients may become irrational, express anger in unusual ways, swear, or cry. They require patience and understanding from everyone. Families, in particular, may need a great deal of emotional support and assistance to understand that this is not unusual behavior for these clients. Clients who have seizures may suffer from poor self-esteem, especially because of the social myths and fears about seizures.

The nurse needs to establish some expected outcomes to guide the evaluation of the client's progress as goals are reached. For example, the nurse, client, and his or her family may establish the following as expected outcomes: The client is able to state the name, dosage, purpose, and potential side effects of prescribed medications. The client is able to identify the effects of the disorder. The client will actively participate in his or her care. Others might include the client's ability to maintain adequate cell oxygenation, remain free of infection, remain seizure-free, or maintain normal body weight. These are just a few examples of goals or outcomes to include in the plan of care and to evaluate at appropriate times. Furthermore, the nurse should pay particular attention to communication and the client's progress in this area. To determine if goals have been met, ask the client how he or she feels about the disorder. Assess the client's reaction to therapy and interaction with family members and significant others. To evaluate goals or outcomes, the nurse must answer questions that pertain to the client's status and the effectiveness of nursing and medical care. Assist the client in contacting an appropriate support group.

Working with neurologically impaired clients is one of the most challenging fields in professional nursing. The professional nurse needs to be familiar with the basic anatomy and physiology of the nervous system to assess, diagnose, plan, intervene, and evaluate nursing care accurately. These clients have many needs whether they are acutely ill and require hospitalization or are ambulatory and care for themselves independently. It is vital to remain alert to prevent potential complications and sequelae.

KEY WORDS

Alzheimer's disease
Autonomic nervous system
Brain
Cerebrovascular disease
Central nervous system
Cluster headache
Coma
Concussion
Confusion
Contusion
Convulsion
Cranial nerves

Delusion
Epidural hemorrhage
Generalized seizure
Glasgow Coma Scale
Guillain-Barré syndrome
Hallucination
Head trauma
Illusion
Intracerebral hemorrhage
Intracranial pressure
Involuntary nervous system
Migraine headache

KEY WORDS *(cont'd.)*

Multiple sclerosis
Myasthenia gravis
Parasympathetic nervous system
Parkinson's disease
Partial seizure
Peripheral nervous system
Sensory deficit
Sensory deprivation
Sensory overload

Skull fractures
Spinal cord
Status epilepticus
Subarachnoid hemorrhage
Subdural hematoma
Sympathetic nervous system
Tension headache
Voluntary nervous system

QUESTIONS

1. Fasciculations are best described as
    A. rhythmic, purposeless, quivering movements.
    B. involuntary, coordinated, stereotyped movements.
    C. slow, twisting, irregular spasms.
    D. focal, uncoordinated, involuntary twitching.

2. If your client has a fever, which one of the following would you suspect is the source?
    A. Brain injury
    B. Infection
    C. Insulin coma
    D. Drug overdose

3. When a client responds to a crisis situation or an acute injury, the sympathetic nervous system will respond in which of the following ways?
    A. It will increase blood flow to the abdominal organs
    B. It will decrease blood flow to the vital organs
    C. It will stimulate the adrenals to release epinephrine

4. During the clonic phase of a generalized seizure, you may expect to see
    A. pupil dilatation, tachycardia, and muscle spasms.
    B. bladder incontinence, elevated blood pressure, and diaphoresis.
    C. loss of consciousness, cessation of breathing, and cyanosis.
    D. contracted throat muscles, hyperventilation, and salivation.

5. Which of the following signs may be exhibited by the client with meningitis?
    A. Fever and seizures
    B. Normal temperature and nuchal rigidity
    C. Cranial nerve palsies and cerebellar ataxia
    D. Steppage gait and ptosis

6. Prognosis for the client recovering from a coma depends on all of the following EXCEPT the
    A. clients' pre-coma personality
    B. coma's duration
    C. lesion's extent
    D. client's environment during recovery

ANSWERS

1. *The answer is D.* Fasciculations occur when muscles are rested. They are localized, uncoordinated, and involuntary twitching of a single muscle group.

2. *The answer is B.* A fever does not always accompany a brain injury, insulin coma, or a drug overdose. The most common cause of a fever is an infection of some kind. Fever *may* occur with a brain injury.

3. *The answer is C.* The sympathetic nervous system prepares the body for emergency responses (fight-or-flight), increasing heart rate and contractility, stimulating the adrenal medulla to release epinephrine and norepinephrine, increasing respiratory rate, increasing blood flow to the cardiorespiratory systems, decreasing blood flow to non-priority organs, releasing red blood cells to increase oxygen-carrying capacity of the blood, and stimulating the liver to release glucose to provide more energy for the body in crisis.

4. *The answer is B.* In the clonic phase of a seizure, hyperventilation and rapid synchronous muscle jerks occur. The client may bite his or her tongue, have bowel and bladder incontinence, have dilated pupils, tachycardia, diaphoresis, and salivate heavily. Hypertension may also be present.

5. *The answer is A.* An infection is a reaction to an invading organism. Meningitis is an infection and is typically accompanied by fever. Seizures may occur because of irritation to the brain's underlying structures. Nuchal rigidity may also occur in the presence of meningitis, but not a normal temperature.

6. *The answer is B.* Research has shown that clients have a better chance of recovery from a coma based on their pre-coma personality, the extent of the lesion, and the climate during recovery. Furthermore, young adults and children typically have the greatest potential for recovery.

ANNOTATED REFERENCES

Christiansen, J. L., & Grzybowski, J. M. (1993). *Biology of aging.* St. Louis: Mosby.

This text presents a comprehensive focus on the older adult, with attention, by chapter, to each body system. There are excellent chapters on the nervous system and the sense organs, as well as an excellent glossary.

Hogstel, M. O. (1994). *Nursing care of the older adult.* Albany N.Y.: Delmar.

This is a helpful, basic text on caring for the older client. It includes a chapter on mental disorders, with a brief discussion of the client with organic mental disorder (e.g., dementia) in basic, easily understandable language.

Hudak, C. M. & Gallo, B. M. (1994). *Handbook of critical care nursing.* Philadelphia: J. B. Lippincott.

This is a quick reference on assessment, diagnosis, and care of the client with acute illness. It contains many figures, tables, and screening tools for neurologically impaired clients, with a specific focus on the critically ill client.

Ignatavicius, D. D., Workman, M. L., & Mishler, M. A. (1995). *Medical-surgical nursing: A nursing process approach.* Philadelphia: W. B. Saunders.

This is a 77-chapter, two-volume advanced medical-surgical nursing textbook, which is very detailed and comprehensive. It is an excellent resource for the student who wishes to know a great deal about a particular nursing topic.

Rakel, R. E. (Ed.) (1998). *Conn's current therapy.* Philadelphia: W. B. Saunders.

This is an excellent comprehensive medical textbook, which provides the latest information for practice. It is a good resource for nurses who are interested in the most recent research and treatment for almost any disorder.

Karch, A. M. (1996). *Lippincott's nursing drug guide.* Philadelphia: J. B. Lippincott.

This text alphabetically lists drug monographs and provides clinically useful drug information, with drug-specific client teaching points.

Lubkin, I. L. (1995). *Chronic illness impact and interventions.* Boston: Jones & Bartlett.

This text focuses on factors and issues that affect clients and their families as they deal with chronic conditions. Geared toward upper-level students, it provides information on ways to assist clients in developing self-management skills in the chronically ill individual.

Lutz, C. A. & Przytulski, K. R. (1997). *Nutrition and diet therapy.* Philadelphia: F. A. Davis.

This text covers a wide variety of topics related to nutrition, with specific focus on the role of nutrients in the body, family and community nutrition, and clinical nutrition. Of major interest is the chapter on food, nutrient, and drug interactions. The book contains detailed discussion and presentation of many drugs, including those that the neurologically impaired client may be expected to have prescribed.

Pagana, K. & Pagana, T. (1995). *Diagnostic and laboratory test reference.* St. Louis: Mosby.

Tests are presented in an alphabetical fashion for quick reference. The text includes normal and abnormal drug levels, with patient education content for specific studies.

INTERNET SITES FOR ADDITIONAL INFORMATION

Transient Ischemic Attacks
   http://www.strokewatch.org/tia.htm

Strokes
   American Heart Association
      http://www.amhrt.org

Parkinson's Disease
   http://james.parkinsons.org.uk/parkinsons.htm
   http://www.parkinsoninfo.com

National Institute of Neurological Disorders and Stroke
   http://www.ninds.nih.gov/

Parkinson's Disease Menu
   http://dem0nmac.mgh.harvard.edu/neurowebforum/
      ParkinsonsDiseaseMenu.html

Stroke Prevention
   http://www-cme.erep.uab.edu/courses/stroke/stroke.htm

Multiple Sclerosis
   http://www.coin-neuro.com/multscler.html
   http://www.ifmss.org.uk

Alzheimer's Disease
   http://www.alzheimers.org
   http://med-www.bu.edu/alzheimer/home.html

Meningitis
   http://www.thehealthconnection.com/DiseaseCenter/diseases/
      meningitis.asp
   http://www.merck.com

Guillain-Barré Syndrome
   http://www.mayohealth.org/mayo/9708/htm/guillain.htm
   http://www.idiom.com/~drjohn/gts.htm/

Myasthenia Gravis
   http://pages.prodigy.com/myasthenia
   http://www.merck.com

Miscellaneous
   http://www.nursingworld.org/nindex.htm

Men's and Women's Health

Sexually Transmitted Diseases

Environmental factors and life-style choices have an enormous impact on public health. This is particulary true for sexually transmitted diseases (STDs) and other diseases influenced by life-style choices, such as diet, smoking, alcohol consumption, and the amount and type of exercise. Although the organisms, transmission routes, and complications of STDs are known, health care professionals have been unable to control their spread. The incidence of STDs has increased over the last few decades. They are the most common reason women seek outpatient, community-based treatment (Ladewig, London, & Olds, 1998). The dramatic spread of STDs demonstrates that health care workers must address the social determinants of these diseases. Nurses must know about the social dimensions of STDs and be able to teach and offer guidance to clients of all ages.

STDs are caused by a variety of organisms. More than 100 disorders and syndromes are currently recognized as sexually transmitted. Although some STDs affect only one anatomical area, such as the urethra in men or the labia or cervix in women, other organisms ascend the reproductive tracts of both sexes, where further invasion may occur. In women, organisms can ascend from the vagina, through the cervical canal, into the uterus, where further colonization into the fallopian tubes, ovaries, and entire pelvis may occur (Fig. 10-1). In men, an infection that spreads to the testicles, termed orchitis, can be caused by gonococci (Fig. 10-2). Infections such as *Chlamydia*, gonorrhea, syphilis, herpes, and acquired immune deficiency syndrome (AIDS) can seriously threaten future

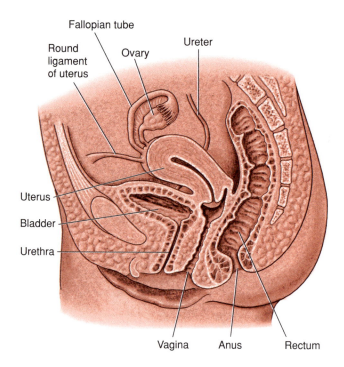

FIGURE 10-1

Cross section of the female reproductive system.

reproductive ability as well as life itself. Each organism requires a unique diagnostic strategy and treatment, as symptoms and treatment options vary. A general guide for major STDs in the United States is provided in this chapter. The information is not comprehensive; other textbooks and resources should be consulted for more detail. The Centers for Disease Control and Prevention (CDC) remains the authority on treatment protocols for STDs.

FIGURE 10-2

Cross section of the male reproductive system.

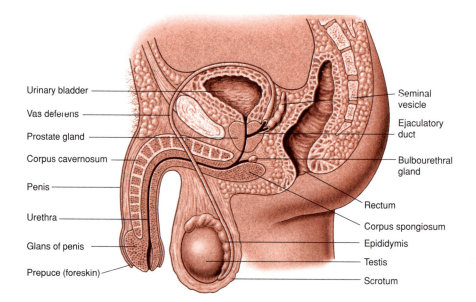

Social Dimensions of STDs

STDs are thought to be "biologically sexist," because women experience STDs and their complications (sterility, perinatal infections, genital tract neoplasm, and death) disproportionately to men. Although STDs in women are often asymptomatic, the silent process is both infectious and damaging. Vertical transmission of the disease in the perinatal period places the fetus at risk for illness, congenital anomalies, mental retardation, and death.

For both men and women, considerable stigma accompanies a diagnosis of a STD, regardless of the organism. Many still equate STDs with immorality, promiscuity, and low social status. The nurse should display a nonjudgmental attitude that conveys to the client that he or she is still an acceptable person who happens to have an infection.

Cultural and emotional dimensions complicate efforts to provide public health education. Prevention and treatment programs for STDs cross all racial, ethnic, and economic strata, but the social dimensions of sexual choices differ greatly among individuals. Sexual behavior is not always logical and rational. For example, prostitutes may wear condoms with their clients but not with their boyfriends. Teenage girls may believe condoms are unnecessary because a boyfriend has declared his love.

Strategies are required to convey factual information and to address the social context of the client and partner. Young teenagers must be taught the correct use of condoms. Some communities are successful in providing school and community clinic programs on sexuality and its social dimensions. However, many communities still struggle with conflicts over what is considered appropriate information for school-age students and teens. Furthermore, lack of funding makes STD services and sex education for homosexuals and heterosexuals unavailable in some neighborhoods.

Commonly Acquired STDs

The most frequently seen STDs are *Chlamydia*, gonorrhea, syphilis, genital herpes, condyloma, human immunodeficiency virus (HIV), and AIDS. Nurses are encouraged to use more detailed resources from the CDC when treating these diseases.

Chlamydia *Chlamydia trachomatis* is the most common bacterial STD in the United States (CDC, 1994; Allen & Phillips, 1997). Although many women are asymptomatic, any one of the following symptoms may appear 1–3 weeks after contact: frequent, uncomfortable urination; cervicitis with scant cervical discharge, lower abdominal pain, and pelvic inflammatory disease (PID). *Chlamydia* is a major cause of nongonococcal urethritis (NGU) in men (Ladewig, London, & Olds, 1998).

Men are usually diagnosed with NGU first, and women are diagnosed with NGU after the male partner has been treated. Symptomatic women who test negative for gonorrhea are often diagnosed with NGU, as are asymptomatic women who are screened routinely in pregnancy. Laboratory tests are now more sophisticated, and specific monoclonal antibodies for *C. trachomatis* can be detected from a smear.

Antibiotic treatment includes the administration of a 1-g dose of azithromycin (Zithromax) or a course of doxycycline (Vibramycin) (CDC, 1994).

Gonorrhea Gonorrhea, caused by the bacteria *Neisseria gonorrhoeae*, was once the most prevalent STD in the United States. The decline in the incidence of gonorrhea is one of the relatively few successes in the fight against STDs. Men with gonorrhea experience extreme burning on urination, and a penile discharge is often present. Women also experience burning on urination, often with increased vaginal discharge. Many women are asymptomatic early in the disease. This STD is transmitted vaginally, orally, or anally (by sexual activity), or from the mother to the newborn during delivery. Gonorrhea is diagnosed in men with a culture of a discharge sample and in women with a culture of the cervical area. Untreated gonorrhea, in both men and women, may spread throughout the urogenital system. Since strains of gonorrhea exist that are resistant to penicillin, the drug of choice is usually a single injection of ceftriaxone (Rocephin).

Syphilis Syphilis is a bacterial STD caused by the spirochete *Treponema pallidum*. Although syphilis is not as widespread as gonorrhea, it is more serious because of the harmful effects the untreated bacterium has on the heart, eyes, central nervous system (CNS), and fetus. Syphilis, like gonorrhea, is transmitted vaginally, orally, or anally (through sexual activity), and from the pregnant woman to the fetus. In the first stage of syphilis, a painless ulcer-like lesion termed a chancre appears at the site of infection. The chancre disappears within a few weeks, but if left untreated, the bacteria continue to proliferate within the body. Thus, untreated syphilis may progress through secondary, latent, tertiary, and fatal stages. Diagnosis is established by blood tests (rapid plasma reagin [RPR] or Venereal Disease Research Lab [VDRL]), which determine the presence of antibodies in the blood. Treatment includes antibiotics such as penicillin, doxycycline, tetracycline, and erythromycin. Clients not allergic to penicillin are usually given 2.4 million units of benzathine penicillin G intramuscularly as a single dose.

Genital Herpes Genital herpes is caused by the herpes simplex virus type 2 (HSV-2). Like agents for other STDs, HSV-2 may be transmitted vaginally, orally, or anally (through sexual activity), and to the newborn during delivery. Herpes is most contagious during active outbreaks of the disease when lesions are present, but cells may be shed at other times. Latex condoms are effective barriers to HSV-2. Genital lesions or sores typically appear 6–8 days after infection. These papules develop into blisters and may become extremely painful ulcers. Although these outbreaks may disappear, the virus remains in the body permanently. Recurring outbreaks may be related to stress, hormonal changes, or fatigue. Diagnosis of HSV-2 is made by clinical inspection and culture of the sores. Herpes does not have a cure, but antiviral drugs such as acyclovir (Zovirax) and famcyclovir (Famvir) can help relieve pain, speed healing, and possibly decrease the incidence of outbreaks.

Human Papillomavirus (HPV) HPV causes condyloma (genital warts). It is the most common viral STD and highly prevalent among young sexually active teenagers. Women are more susceptible to HPV infection because cervical cells divide swiftly, facilitating the spread of the virus. The genital warts appear as bumps or cauliflower-like shapes along the genital tracts of both sexes. Diagnosis is made by inspection, biopsy, or Papanicolaou (Pap) smear. HPV is prevented by practicing safer sex. Individuals should limit the number of partners, use latex condoms, and have annual Pap smears. HPV is treated by electrocautery, laser, or surgical removal. Currently, the carbon dioxide laser used under local anesthetic is the most effective method to destroy the condyloma (CDC, 1994). Public health officials are particularly concerned because of the dramatic increase (50–85%) in cases of cervical cancer in women with HPV (Bobak, Lowdermilk, & Jensen, 1995; Ladewig et al., 1998).

HIV and AIDS HIV is the virus that causes AIDS, a STD that is pandemic wordwide. Safer sex practices to prevent HIV include limiting the number of partners, avoiding anal intercourse, always using latex condoms (with nonoxynol-9), and avoiding contact with the blood, semen, and vaginal secretions of others. The current level of HIV transmission among heterosexual couples and the increased incidence in women are alarming. A detailed description of HIV and AIDS and nursing care for the disease can be found in Chapter 13.

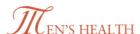

MEN'S HEALTH

As men age, prostate problems develop that threaten sexual and urinary function (see Fig. 10-2). Other common disorders of the male genitourinary system also may pose a risk to fertility and can even be life-threatening. The nurse must be aware that these disorders can significantly affect the man's ability to function and his self-esteem.

Prostate Cancer

Prostate cancer rarely occurs before 50 years of age. The incidence increases with advancing age, with 80% of all cases occurring in men older than 65 years of age. The exact cause has not been determined; however, scientists know it is androgen dependent in the early stages. Prostate cancer progresses slowly, thus early detection improves the survival rate. According to the American Cancer Society (ACS), if prostate cancer is detected early, the survival rate is 85% (1994, 1995, 1996). African

Americans are more likely to develop prostate cancer. Almost all primary prostate cancers are adenocarcinomas that can metastasize to the pelvic lymph nodes and skeletal sites of the vertebral column. Clinical manifestations include urinary symptoms of nocturia, dysuria, frequency of urination, and hematuria. If the cancer has metastasized, low back pain, bone pain, muscle spasms, weight loss, and fatigue may be present. When the cancer is confined to the prostate gland, clients may be asymptomatic.

Primary prostate cancer cannot be prevented. Therefore, men older than 40 years of age should be screened regularly for early detection and treatment. Diagnostic screening and tests include the following:

- **Annual digital rectal examination.** Men over 40 years of age should undergo this procedure in which the clinician inserts a finger into the rectum and feels for abnormalities in the prostate gland.
- **Annual Prostate Specific Antigen (PSA).** Men over 50 years of age should have PSA levels measured. If the PSA test is positive (i.e., PSA is high), transrectal ultrasonography and tissue biopsy offer a more definitive diagnosis.
- **Bone scan and pelvic computed tomography (CT).** These tests help to stage the tumor and detect metastasis. The grade and stage of the cancer aid the practitioner in deciding what treatment to use. The tumor is staged to determine if it is localized to or extends beyond the gland.

Treatment   Treatment decisions are based on diagnostic test results and the tumor stage. Prostate cancer is occasionally treated surgically or with radiation. Surgery may involve both the testicles and the prostate. Orchiectomy, an excision of the testicles, is performed to decrease androgen production. Prostatectomies are simple or radical. A radical resection of the prostate gland includes removal of the entire prostate gland, including the capsule and adjacent tissue (Phipps, Cassmeyer, Sands, & Lehman, 1995). Transurethral resection of the prostate (TURP) may relieve urinary obstruction of the urethra. Approximately 6–8% of men experience impotence following prostate surgery, although the exact cause for failure to have an erection is unknown. Hormone therapy, an alternative to orchiectomy, is used for metastatic cancer, and as a palliative treatment of advanced prostate cancer (Wilson, Shannon, & Stang, 1998). Estrogen compounds such as diethylstilbesterol (DES), leuprolide (Lupron), or megestrolacetate (Megace) are effective palliative treatments. Irradiation is another form of palliative treatment.

Nursing Care   Nursing care for clients undergoing prostate surgery includes explaining the procedures and expected outcomes to the family and client preoperatively. The client should be prepared for postoperative tubes such as a urinary catheter for continuous bladder drainage. The client usually undergoes a bowel preparation prior to surgery. Postoperative nursing care includes taking strict measurements of intake and output, monitoring vital signs every two hours, monitoring the urine color in the urinary catheter, and monitoring the continuous bladder irrigation (CBI), if present. Depending on the amount of bleeding expected after TURP or prostate surgery, CBI is used to maintain the patency of the urinary catheter, facilitate removal of clots, and cleanse the surgical area to prevent hemorrhage. During CBI, saline solution runs through a three-way Foley catheter for approximately 24 hours postoperatively. The rate of flow should be adjusted to keep the urine pink. Bladder spasms may be present, and the surgeon should be notified if these occur. The client should be given a stool softener and instructed to avoid straining during bowel movements. The client also should drink 2–3 L of fluids per day.

When the client is to be discharged, the nurse must explain that urinary incontinence may be expected. Depending on the surgical procedure, stress incontinence as a result of abdominal pressure may be present. Urge incontinence, in which the urge to void is followed by the involuntary passing of urine, is also common. Nocturnal incontinence, involuntarily passing urine while in bed, may be especially troublesome. Nursing care should focus on the type of incontinence the client is experiencing and strategies to help him cope with the accompanying anxiety. The nurse should teach and encourage the client to use Kegel exercises to strengthen the pelvic floor muscles. The client also should be reminded to increase his water intake. Sexual dysfunction is another common postoperative complication. Erectile and ejaculatory functions may be affected, depending on the treatment used. Clients should abstain from sexual intercourse for 6 weeks after prostatic surgery. The nurse should assess the quality, location, radiation, and rating of any pain and offer the client the analgesia ordered by the surgeon. The client should avoid strenuous activity and lifting for 6–8 weeks postsurgery.

Benign Prostatic Hypertrophy (BPH)

BPH is an enlargement of the prostate gland. The prostate typically becomes enlarged in all men over 50 years of age. The enlarged prostate constricts the urethra, causing urinary symptoms such as frequency, urgency, nocturnal frequency, and difficulty in starting the flow of urine. Although the exact cause is unknown, BPH may be be linked to endocrine control. Men who undergo an orchiectomy before puberty never develop BPH. Other clinical manifestations include diminished urinary stream, urinary retention, hematuria, dysuria, incomplete emptying, and urge incontinence.

Diagnostic tests include a urinalysis to exclude urinary tract infections, serum creatinine and blood urea nitrogen (BUN) concentrations to exclude renal disease, acid phosphatase and PSA tests to exclude prostate cancer, urodynamic tests to evaluate the degree of urinary obstruction, and cystoscopy.

Treatment BPH is treated pharmacologically or surgically. Finasteride (Proscar) is a commonly prescribed medication. It specifically inhibits an enzyme that converts testosterone to dihydroxytesterone (DHT), a potent androgen that mediates prostate growth (Wilson, Shannon, & Stang, 1998). BPH is treated surgically by transurethral resection of the prostate (TURP). In TURP, some of the prostate tissue is excised surgically by cystoscope. This resection is generally successful for a period of time, but the gland may regrow. Transurethral incision of the prostate (TUIP) is a procedure in which small incisions are made in the prostate to enlarge the prostatic urethra, and relieve obstruction. Regular postoperative management and nursing care are performed. In addition, for men with TURP and BPH, problems of urinary incontinence, sexual dysfunction, and body image disturbance should be discussed. The client should be advised to drink at least 2–3 L of fluids per day to decrease the chance of dysuria and urinary tract infection (UTI). The client should be instructed to restrict fluids at night to facilitate uninterrupted sleep.

In caring for the TURP client postoperatively, the nurse should monitor the client for fluid volume excess by documenting accurate intake and output, daily weight, and assessing lung sounds frequently. CBI is usually ordered by the surgeon to keep the catheter patent. Serum electrolytes should be monitored frequently, as fluid and electrolyte imbalances may occur. Restriction of fluids will cause sodium to be retained, and this may be desirable in some clients since dilutional hyponatremia may occur during surgery. It is possible that during TURP a patient may absorb as much as 1000 mL of fluids due to the prostate venous sinuses being open.

CASE STUDY: POSTOPERATIVE CARE FOR A CLIENT WHO HAS UNDERGONE A TURP

Mr. J. has just returned from the postanesthesia care unit (PACU) area after undergoing TURP for obstructive BPH. An intravenous line infuses intravenous (IV) fluid into a heplock in his right forearm, and the nurse makes sure that the site is clear and the IV line is patent. A three-way Foley catheter has been inserted to gravity drainage, and two bags of CBI saline irrigation hang on an intravenous pole. One bag is full, and the other is open at full constant drip. The urine in the catheter tubing is bright red with small dark red clots. The nurse assesses Mr. J.'s bladder, which is nondistended. Mr. J. does not complain of bladder spasms, thus the nurse decides correctly not to irrigate the catheter by syringe.

The following nursing actions should be taken: The nurse should determine how many milliliters are left to infuse into the bladder and how many milliliters have been infused since the CBI was started. The Foley catheter drainage bag should be emptied and the output, less the CBI intake, should be recorded. Every hour, the nurse should observe the CBI, examine the color of the drainage in the catheter tubing, check for the presence of clots, and look for bladder distension. The CBI infusion rate should be adjusted so that the urine is yellowish pink. An accurate intake and output must be kept until the catheter is removed and the client is voiding normally. One CBI saline bag should always be kept full and clamped and only opened when the previous bag is empty. Extra bags must be kept in the room at all times until CBI is stopped. The CBI is recorded as intake and subtracted from the output; none of the CBI is absorbed into the bladder. Output should be approximately 1mL/kg/hr. Vital signs should be taken frequently in the postoperative period to monitor for possible bleeding. The nurse must always be aware of the estimated blood loss (EBL) during surgery. The EBL should be documented on the progress notes, anesthesia record, or PACU record. If ordered by the physician, oral fluid intake should be encouraged. The nurse should encourage early ambulation (when ordered by the physician) to facilitate peripheral circulation and prevent thrombosis, especially deep vein thrombosis in the legs.

If bladder spasms occur, the bladder should be checked for distension. If it is distended, under physician's orders stop the CBI and syringe irrigate the catheter. The primary care nurse's main concern is to keep the catheter free-flowing. When urinary catheter drainage is once again clear yellow without CBI infusion, the catheter is usually removed upon the physician's order. The nurse must provide the client and family with extensive discharge instructions and emphasize the need to call the physician if fever, inability to void, or bright red hematuria occurs.

Prostatitis

Prostatitis results from infectious agents that inflame the prostate. An acute bacterial, chronic bacterial, or nonbacterial inflammation of the prostate can occur; nonbacterial inflammation is the most common. The chief symptoms are an ache or pain between the scrotum and anal opening and painful ejaculation. The presence of bacteria in cultures of urine and prostate secretions confirms the diagnosis. Prostatitis is usually treated with antibiotics. Nonsteroidal anti-inflammatory drugs (NSAIDs) such as ibuprofen (Motrin) are administered for pain. Although aspirin and ibuprofen may relieve the pain, persons with these symptoms should consult a physician. Anticholinergic medications may reduce the urge to void. In severe cases, surgeons perform TURP to excise infected prostatic calculi. Clients should be instructed to increase fluid intake to 3 L per day, to void frequently, and to avoid straining during bowel movements. Sitz baths may help to relieve pain and irritation.

Testicular Cancer

Testicular cancer remains relatively rare, accounting for approximately 1% of newly diagnosed cancers in men (ACS, 1994–1996). However, it is the most common cancer in men between 15 and 35 years of age. If it is caught at an early stage, 90–100% of clients are cured. The etiology is unknown; however, a relationship exists between undescended testicles at birth (cryptorchidism) and testicular cancer. Those with cryyptorchidism are 40% more likely to develop testicular cancer. Therefore, infants with cryptorchidism should undergo an orchiopexy between one and two years of age.

The first signs and symptoms of testicular cancer are the painless swelling of one testicle or the formation of a nodule. Diagnostic tests include serum studies for tumor markers, liver function tests, and CT or magnetic resonance imaging (MRI) to determine if the cancer has metastasized. Treatment includes surgical removal of the diseased testis, radiation, and chemotherapy. A radical orchiectomy is performed to remove the cancerous testis. Retroperitoneal lymph node dissection is done to look for metastasis to the lymph nodes. Cyclic chemotherapeutic protocols (lasting from ten months to two years) of cisplatin, bleomycin, or vinblastine or a combination of VP-16, bleomycin, and cisplatin effectively treat testicular cancer. Irradiation of the retroperitoneal nodes and other lymph nodes may be necessary.

Treatment Postoperative nursing care for clients who have undergone an orchiectomy includes applying scrotal support and an ice bag to the scrotum. If one testicle remains, the client should be taught and encouraged to perform monthly self-examinations. An orchiectomy does not cause impotence or infertility if the remaining testis is normal. The nurse should encourage the client to openly discuss sexual function postoperatively.

Nurses have the vital task of teaching the public to perform testicular self-examinations. Men are advised to examine themselves once per month after reaching puberty. Unfortunately, only 50% of testicular cancers are discovered in the early stages. This is the leading cause of death from cancer in males aged 15–35 years (ACS, 1994–1996).

Testicular Torsion

Testicular torsion, a twisting of the testes and spermatic cord, is a potential surgical emergency. Torsion can occur between birth and 20 years of age. Signs and symptoms include the sudden onset of scrotal pain that may be related to trauma and, often, nausea and vomiting. Men with testicular torsion have a history of scrotal pain. Surgical intervention is required to untwist the testicle and affix it to the scrotum.

Infections of the Male Genitourinary Tract

Epididymitis Epididymitis is an infection or inflammation of the epididymis. Trauma or the spread of a UTI or urethral infection to the vas deferens causes epididymitis. Signs and symptoms are pain, edema, and erythema of the scrotum. Treatment includes the application of cool packs to the scrotum, scrotal support, and antibiotics. Occasionally, hospitalization with intravenous antibiotic therapy is necessary.

Orchitis Orchitis is an infection or inflammation of the testicle. It is the most common complication of epididymitis. Trauma, vasectomy, and untreated gonorrhea may also cause this condition. Acute orchitis can occur in a variety of infectious diseases, including syphilis, pneumonia, or mumps. Orchitis is detected by performing a urine culture and sensitivity, and the treatment is the same as that for epididymitis.

Priapism

Priapism is a sustained, painful erection lasting 4 hours or more that is not associated with sexual arousal. The erection may be the result of trauma to the perineal area that has torn the cavernous artery; of certain diseases such as leukemia, sickle cell disease, metastatic cancer, or spinal cord trauma; or of drugs such as marijuana, alcohol, or some psychotrophic agents. Treatment includes applying ice to the perineal area or penis and administering vasoconstrictive medications. Enemas with warm water or ice water or vigorous prostatic massage may be effective, and surgery may be required. Nursing care includes carefully monitoring intake and output and administering anxiety-relieving medication.

Phimosis

In phimosis, the foreskin constricts so it cannot retract over the glans penis. This condition may be genetically inherited. Phimosis is treated with antibiotics and warm water soaks and circumcision may be required.

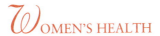

WOMEN'S HEALTH

In the last few years a "knowledge explosion" has occurred in gynecological and reproductive sexual health. Nurses must constantly update their knowledge of the changing roles of women in culture, society, and politics. Nurses should not characterize health as the absence of illness or disability. The emotional, spiritual, and social aspects must be considered as well. Women's health no longer focuses solely on reproductive health. The Association of Women's Health, Obstetric, and Neonatal Nursing (AWHONN) defines women's health as "the health care of nonpregnant women across the life span from adolescence to senescence with a focus on health issues distinctive to women" (AWHONN, 1998).

Demographic changes in the United States include both a lower birth rate and an aging population. Approximately 50% of women will be older than 50 years of age by the year 2000. The number of women over 85 years of age will grow most rapidly. American women outlive their male counterparts by approximately seven years (Allen & Phillips, 1997). Racial and ethnic diversity are also expected to increase in women over the next several decades.

The nurse must share responsibility and decisions with the client. Excellent communication and interviewing skills must be developed to foster a partnership with female clients. The basis of the contemporary philosophy of women's health care is that women have the right and responsibility to control their bodies and make their own health decisions. Health education must be provided so that women can make informed choices. Women receive support from other women, family, nurses, communities, church groups, and other support systems.

This section is divided into four topics: gynecological health and gynecological cancers; menstruation through menopause; breast health and breast cancer; and cardiac health, osteoporosis, nutrition, and exercise. Many of the health problems that plague women can be alleviated by public health education. For example, studies have shown that as many as 90% of the women who died from cervical cancer never had a screening Pap smear. More health education and comprehensive prevention programs are needed to provide quality health care for all women.

Gynecological Health and Gynecological Cancer

Infections of the Reproductive Tract Genital tract infections are common. Symptoms of dysuria and vaginal discharge frequently induce women to seek care (Phipps et al., 1995). Conditions of the genital tract can cause embarrassment and misunderstanding or threaten a woman's sexuality; thus, clients may be reluctant to discuss these problems. Women should have all the necessary information to take care of themselves. Perineal hygiene and yeast infections specifically should be emphasized because of their prevalence and the reluctance of women to seek information.

Perineal Hygiene to Prevent Infection The nursing care goal is to prevent organisms such as *Escherichia coli* from causing infections like vaginitis and urethritis. Women should be instructed to wash their hands before and after genital contact and after using the restroom. Women should always wipe the perineum from front to back and discard the tissue. This front-to-back motion is used after urination, bowel movements, sex, and menses. Women should avoid products that may disturb the normal flora of the vagina or cause irritation and an allergic reaction in the genital area. Women prone to vaginitis should use only white, unscented tissue. No feminine hygiene sprays or other sprays should be used near the perineum. Deodorized tampons and pads should be avoided. When using tampons, do not let the string slip back to the rectal area. If it does, the tampon should be changed immediately. Women never need to douche unless told to do so by a physician or nurse practitioner. Distilled white vinegar (two tablespoons per quart of water) costs less and is better than commercial douches. Perfumed douches should never be used.

The warm, moist environment of the vagina encourages microbial growth. The risk of genital infection or vaginitis is decreased by wearing cotton underpants with a cotton crotch, especially while wearing panty hose, girdles, and exercise suits. Cotton pants should always be worn during exercise activities such as aerobics, jogging, or biking. Women should avoid nonabsorbent clothes. Showers are preferable to tub baths and women prone to vaginitis and urine infections must avoid bubble bath and other perfumed bath products. If a lubricant is necessary during sexual intercourse, K-Y jelly or Replens, not petroleum jelly (Vaseline), can be used. Lubrication may not be necessary if one allows adequate time for sexual stimulation. However, vaginal dryness may be unavoidable during perimenopause.

Changes in vaginal physiology such as a rise in the pH leave the woman susceptible to vaginal infections. Known risk factors include pregnancy, high-estrogen oral contraceptives, antibiotic therapy, and uncontrolled diabetes. Women with these conditions should follow the suggested techniques in addition to the protocol their specific condition requires. If a woman is taking antibiotics, eating yogurt or sour cream may help to prevent vaginal infections. Some women require prophylactic antifungal therapy in conjunction with antibiotic therapy. Vaginal itching, irritation, burning, sores, or odor should be examined to determine the exact cause. Many different types of vaginal infections exist and each has a different treatment.

Transmission of organisms between sexual partners should be avoided. While undergoing treatment for a vaginal infection, women should refrain from sexual contact or use a condom. Frequent vaginal irritations indicate that the partner's soap or other personal products may be the cause.

Yeast Infections Vaginitis is caused by a variety of organisms. A bacterial or yeast infection often causes vaginitis. These organisms can cause symptoms such as burning, itching, and vaginal discharge. Asymptomatic colonization can occur as well.

The incidence of yeast infections appears to be increasing, partly because of widespread antimicrobial therapy (Bobak, Lowdermilk, & Jensen, 1995). Vulvovaginal candidiasis is caused most often by the fungus *Candida albicans*. More healthy, asymptomatic women now harbor *C. albicans*. A change in the vaginal environment and pH causes the candidal organisms to grow, resulting in irritation. The risk of yeast infections increases when the client takes an antibiotic for an infection in another part of the body that inadvertently destroys the normal flora of the vagina. Since these bacteria normally control the growth of candidal fungi, their destruction may result in the development of a yeast infection.

Hormonal changes during pregnancy or from high-dose estrogen oral contraceptives can change the environment of the vagina and induce yeast cell growth. For example, during pregnancy vaginal secretions become less acidic as the pH changes from approximately 4 to 5–5.5 to 6.5 (Bobak et al., 1995). HIV infection or immunosuppressive medication can cause yeast infections. An impaired immune system allows yeast to grow unchecked. Diabetes can foster the growth of *C. albicans* because high blood sugar reduces the body's natural ability to resist infection. It also increases glucose levels in the body's tissues, making yeast growth more likely.

The primary symptom is vulvar or vaginal burning and itching. Candidiasis typically produces an odorless, thick, curd-like white discharge resembling cottage cheese. Symptoms tend to worsen just before menstrual periods. Men may be asymptomatic or experience a rash or excoriation of the skin of the penis (Ladewig et al., 1998). The CDC (1993) does not recommend treatment of the partner unless candidal inflammation of the penis is present or infections recur frequently.

Treatment Many over-the-counter (OTC) antifungal medications are available. Yeast infections are treated for 3–7 days with topical antifungal agents in suppository or cream form. OTC medications include clotrimazole (Gyne-Lotrimin) and miconazole (Monistat 7). If the vulva is also infected, another cream can be applied topically. These medications are convenient and inexpensive for women who know the etiology and symptoms of fungal infections. Candidiasis does not pose a serious health risk, but if OTC treatment does not eradicate the infection, the woman must see a physician or nurse practitioner to treat the symptoms and exclude other serious problems such as diabetes and HIV. Infections that do not respond to treatment are serious and may require prescription medications such as metronidazole (Flagyl) taken orally or fluconazole (Diflucan) given as a one-time dose in a 150-mg pill. Chronic yeast infections may indicate reinfection from the partner.

To confirm candidiasis, a vaginal smear is examined by wet-mount preparation. On physical examination, the woman's labia and perineum may appear cherry red, swollen, and excoriated if the fungus and pruritus are severe.

Cervical Cancer

Risk Factors Most risk factors for cervical cancer are related to sexual history. Cervical cell changes may be the result of an "insult" from viruses or multiple partners. Women with cervical cancer often report a history of cervical infections. The infections most frequently linked to cervical cancer include HSV-2; HPV types 16, 18, and 31; HIV; and perhaps cytomegalovirus (Alexander & LaRosa, 1994). These viruses alter the deoxyribonucleic acid (DNA) in the nuclei of immature cervical cells (Bobak et al., 1995). Sperm from many different partners also may promote dysplasia (Table 10-1).

Most of the predisposing factors relate to sexual activity; embarrassment may prevent early detection and treatment. The nurse must convey with sensitivity that sexual health is part of the client's total health and that the woman should not feel ashamed of a normal physiological function. Marrying later, divorcing, and remarrying, and having more than one sexual partner are now considered aspects of the norm. Nurses should

⊠

TABLE 10-1

RISK FACTORS ASSOCIATED WITH CERVICAL CANCER

Multiple sexual partners
Early age at first incidence of sexual intercourse (before 18 years)
History of sexually transmitted diseases
Human papillomavirus
Lack of access to or use of health care
A nonmonogamous male partner
Diethylstilbestrol (DES) exposure
Cigarette smoking
Belonging to a lower socioeconomic group

encourage sexually active women to seek regular gynecological checkups and Pap smears and practice safer sex.

Papanicolaou (Pap) Test The Pap test, or smear, safely and inexpensively detects cervical cancer at an early stage. Dr. George Papanicolaou, a Greek physician, developed the Pap test in the 1940s, and it began to be used regularly in gynecological examinations during the 1950s. Since then, the incidence of invasive cervical cancer and the mortality rate from cervical cancer have declined, but the number of women with cervical intraepithelial neoplasia (CIN) has increased at an alarming rate (Allen & Phillips, 1997). See also Table 10-2. When cervical cancer is diagnosed at an early stage, the cure rate is almost 100%. However, approximately 5000 women die from it annually (ACS, 1996). In the United States, only approximately 30% of women have regular gynecological checkups and Pap smears.

To obtain a cell sample for a Pap smear, the physician or nurse practitioner scrapes the cervix and endocervix with a swab, brush, or spatula

⊠

TABLE 10-2

CLASSIFICATION SYSTEM FOR PAP SMEAR

Previous Terminology	Bethesda System Terminology
Class I	Normal
Class II	Inflammation
Class III	Cervical intraepithelia neoplasia
Mild dysplasia	CIN I
Moderate dysplasia	CIN II
Severe dysplasia	CIN III
Carcinoma in situ	CIN III
	Invasive carcinoma

(Fig. 10-3). Computerized analysis of Pap smears such as "Papnet" are now available. This technique may result in fewer false-positive and false-negative reports. Most women barely feel the cervix being scraped. However, women often do not undergo gynecological checkups and Pap smears because of fear, denial, lack of information, cultural beliefs, social status, embarrassment, absence of symptoms, lack of access to health care, and the expense.

The ACS, the National Cancer Institute, and American Medical Association (AMA) recommend, as reported in the United States Preventive Services Task Force, that women should have their first Pap smear at 18 years of age or when they first have intercourse. Women 18–64 years of age should have Pap smears yearly or every three years after three normal, consecutive, annual Pap smears. After 65 years of age, women should have Pap smears yearly, or every three years after two normal, consecutive, annual Pap smears.

The American College of Obstetricians and Gynecologists (ACOG) currently recommends annual Pap tests for all sexually active women. Controversy exists regarding the screening schedule. For example, women who take birth control pills are often required to undergo an annual Pap smear before their prescriptions are refilled. Even women who do not require Pap smears benefit from regular pelvic and breast examinations, as these checkups may detect potential problems. There is concern that women who do not need a Pap smear may find it easy to delay a checkup. Women should consult their physicians or nurse practitioners to determine how often they should have a Pap smear. Women at high risk, such as those with multiple sex partners, a history of a STD (especially HPV), a nonmonogamous male partner, those of African-American heritage, elderly women who have not been screened, those with a family history of cervical cancer, and women whose mothers used DES during pregnancy should undergo more frequent screenings. In addition, nurses must make efforts to test those who have not been screened.

Cervical cells often go through a series of changes. The older classification system, dysplasia and carcinoma in situ, described two separate entities. The newer classification system, the Bethesda System, is preferred

FIGURE 10-3

◙

Pelvic examination with Pap smear.

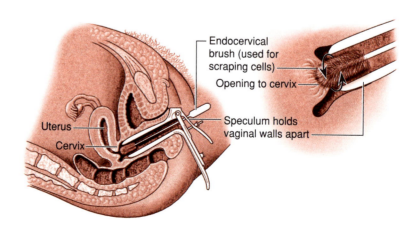

because it represents a neoplastic continuum and is more descriptive of the changes that occur at the cellular level. CIN I, II and III are now used to describe these epithelial abnormalities (Bobak et al., 1995).

Nurses must inform women that the new system improves the identification and treatment of cervical cell changes. Additionally, researchers are only beginning to understand the pattern of changes cervical cells undergo over months to years. If the Pap test shows an abnormality, the physician or nurse practitioner then performs more tests to determine the cause. Since a vaginal infection may cause an abnormal Pap test, the practitioner should treat the infection and repeat the test in three months. If there is no infection, the practitioner may perform a colposcopy and biopsy. The nurse should discuss psychosexual factors and the risk of cervical cancer with compassion.

Treatment The goal is to eradicate the central cervical disease and prevent lymph node spread. Following an abnormal Pap smear, treatment depends on the results of a cervical biopsy. Most women with an abnormal Pap smear have an easily treated precancerous condition termed mild dysplasia or CIN I. Treatment for dysplasia, depending on its severity, consists of cryosurgery, colposcopy, laser therapy, or a loop electrodiathermy excision procedure (LEEP). CIN I, or mild dysplasia, may not require treatment but should be checked regularly for changes. CIN II, or moderate dysplasia, is usually treated by colposcopy, cryotherapy, or laser therapy. Colposcopy is both a diagnostic and treatment procedure for mild-to-moderate dysplasia, because the magnified view of the cervix allows the practitioner to locate and define the size and distribution of the CIN. Colposcopy is an office procedure in which a microscope permits close examination of the cervix and vagina as well as biopsy and removal of the abnormal tissue. Cryotherapy destroys tissue by a freezing process, produces little or no discomfort, and presents a low risk for complications such as bleeding, further infection, or infertility. Recently, laser therapy has been used to treat dysplasia: a powerful beam of light destroys abnormal cells but leaves the normal cells underneath unharmed.

Treatment for CIN III (severe dysplasia and carcinoma in situ) and invasive cervical cancer depends on the extent of the disease. A total hysterectomy (removal of the cervix and uterus) or a radical hysterectomy (removal of the cervix, uterus, upper third of the vagina, supporting ligaments, parametrium, and pelvic and iliac lymph nodes) may be performed. Invasive cervical cancer is usually treated by surgery, radiation, or both.

Radiation, both external and internal, is commonly used to treat cervical cancer, as it can be used during any stage of the disease. Radiation destroys the cell's ability to grow and divide. Both normal and diseased cells are affected, but most normal cells are able to recover rapidly. Radiation treats cancer that has spread to the pelvis, lower part of the vagina, or ureters. External beam radiation to the pelvis treats regional nodes and disease, while intracavitary radiation implants target the central cancer.

Radiation therapy causes minimal complications. Morbidity may result from the tumor, not the actual therapy. Women undergoing treatment must understand that radiation therapy delivers the highest curative dose

Hysterectomy. A hysterectomy is the surgical removal of the uterus. Although it is commonly performed in the United States, controversy remains over its necessity. Women are encouraged to seek a second opinion and discuss all treatment options. Indications for hysterectomy include fibroid tumors, cervical and uterine malignancies, premalignancy, endometriosis, severe prolapse, and debilitating bleeding.

- **Vaginal Hysterectomy.** Vaginal hysterectomy is the removal of the uterus via the vagina. Clients recover more rapidly because no abdominal incision is made.
- **Abdominal Hysterectomy.** The uterus is removed through the abdominal wall in an abdominal hysterectomy.
- **Total Hysterectomy.** In a total hysterectomy, the uterus and cervix are completely excised.

of radiation to the cervix and pelvic lymph nodes while limiting normal tissue damage. Possible complications during or shortly after therapy include irritation of the small bowel and rectum that causes diarrhea, irritation of the bladder that causes cystitis, reactions in the skin folds, radiation-induced menopause, and mild bone marrow depression that manifests as fatigue. In addition, the implant phase of treatment produces some degree of vaginal stenosis and loss of vaginal lubrication.

Women undergoing radiation therapy or implant treatment must be taught vaginal dilation techniques to minimize the effect of vaginal stenosis. The woman's sex life is part of her health, and normal sexual activity can be resumed after cancer treatment. Some women may not feel comfortable discussing sex. Nurses should be sensitive to their feelings and advocate sexual rehabilitation to help them. The nurse should expect and discuss the grief premenopausal women will experience from the loss of childbearing ability. More younger women are being diagnosed with cervical cancer. The nurse should emphasize the necessity of follow-up examinations and reporting any vaginal bleeding.

CASE STUDY: WOMAN WITH HPV AND CERVICAL DYSPLASIA

Mandy, a 21-year-old student, goes to the health clinic at her college for an annual examination and to renew her prescription for birth control pills. Mandy has been involved in a serious relationship with a fellow student for one year. Following the results of her examination and Pap smear, she is diagnosed with HPV and cervical epithelial abnormalities. Mandy is upset and embarrassed, and angry at both herself and her boyfriend. Upon confronting her boyfriend, he admits that he has been sexually involved for a short time with another woman on campus while they had briefly been separated and that this was the most likely source of the virus. Mandy's mother had been treated for breast cancer three years previously.

The nurse explores Mandy's and her boyfriend's preconceived notions of sexuality and cancer. Mandy establishes good communication with her partner, and both attend pretreatment counseling. Factual information is given concerning the recommended cryosurgery. Mandy's concerns about future problems with sexual intercourse and fertility are alleviated. The nurse discusses HPV as a risk factor for cervical epithelial changes. The couple is able to explore their relationship as well. Both partners express a desire to maintain a monogamous relationship and to get married after graduation.

Uterine Cancer The most common type of gynelogical cancer is cancer of the uterus (Fig. 10-4). The two layers that comprise the uterus are the inner layer (the endometrium) and the muscular layer (the myometrium). Cancer develops more frequently in the endometrium. Endometrial cancer

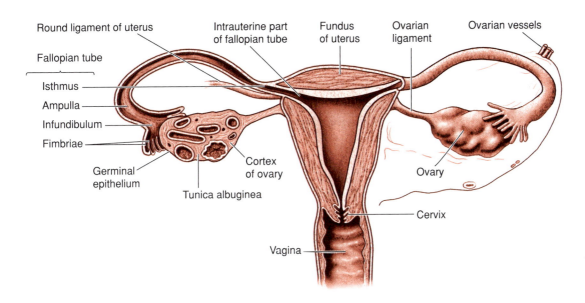

Round ligament of uterus
Fallopian tube
Isthmus
Ampulla
Infundibulum
Fimbriae
Germinal epithelium
Tunica albuginea
Cortex of ovary
Intrauterine part of fallopian tube
Fundus of uterus
Ovarian ligament
Ovarian vessels
Ovary
Cervix
Vagina

FIGURE 10-4 Frontal view of the female reproductive system.

occurs most often in older women; 75% of endometrial cancers are seen in women over 50 years of age (Allen & Phillips, 1997). Previously, unopposed estrogen therapy was the principal factor predisposing women to endometrial cancer (see Hormone Replacement Therapy). Endometrial cancer is familial, although no genetic marker is known. Women who have had breast or ovarian cancer are more likely to develop endometrial cancer.

The only sign of endometrial cancer, especially in postmenopausal women, is abnormal vaginal bleeding. Women should be instructed to seek treatment whenever this occurs. A pelvic examination with endometrial biopsy is performed. If the result of the biopsy is positive, a total abdominal hysterectomy and bilateral salpingo-oophorectomy are performed. Radiation and chemotherapy may be used, depending on the stage. Since these tumors tend to be well differentiated and localized, if detected and treated early, women with endometrial cancer have a high survival rate.

Ovarian Cancer Ovarian cancer is the most deadly cancer because it is difficult to detect and diagnose in an early stage (ACS, 1996). Frequently, by the time it is diagnosed it has already spread throughout the pelvis (Figure 10-4). Current research focuses on improving screening methods.

Ovarian cancer occurs most frequently between 40 and 70 years of age. The cause may be linked to endocrine function. The number of times a woman ovulates appears to correlate with the incidence of ovarian cancer. Women who conceive before age 25, experience early menopause, or use oral contraceptives appear to be relatively protected. Ovarian cancer is genetic; if a mother or a sister had ovarian cancer, the woman is as much as 50% more likely to develop it. Environmental risk factors include talc and asbestos exposure and a high-fat diet.

Ovarian cancer has few symptoms. The most common sign is an enlargement of the abdomen (ACS, 1996). Women may complain of an inability to fasten their pants and skirts and may experience vague abdominal fullness or discomfort, pelvic pain, and ascites. Treatment options include surgery, radiation, and chemotherapy. Paclitaxel (Taxol), a newer anticancer medication, has successfully treated progressive ovarian cancer. Because of the high mortality rate associated with ovarian cancer, an extensive case management team is required, comprising surgeons, oncologists, oncology nurse specialists, social workers, and pastoral care. Nurses must provide current information for women to make informed decisions.

To prevent ovarian cancer, women may consider removing both ovaries if they are undergoing a hysterectomy for other medical reasons. For women with a family history of the disease, prophylactic bilateral oophorectomy performed by laparoscopy is recommended at 40 years of age. This laparoscopic procedure decreases the cost, risks, and recovery time compared to abdominal surgery.

Salpingo-oophorectomy. A salpingo-oophorectomy involves the excision of the fallopian tube and ovary and may be unilateral or bilateral. This procedure may be performed by laparoscopy.

Nursing Care for Clients With Gynecologic Cancer Gynecological cancer is an invisible disease. Consequently, the cancer's full impact is occasionally minimized or hidden by the clients, their families, and health care professionals. The nurse must understand the extent of the adjustments the women and their caretakers make. Concerns about treatment, sex, and childbearing are common. The diagnosis of a gynecological condition such as cervical, uterine, or ovarian cancer is often accompanied by guilt, embarrassment, shame, and disturbances in body image. Women may resent the lack of privacy and feel defensive and angry that such a private part of themselves must be treated. Some women may associate this form of cancer with punishment for real or imagined sexual expression. This shame and guilt can be lessened if nurses adopt an accepting, nonjudgmental approach.

The nurse must assess the disease's impact on the woman's self-image and how the disease or treatment may interfere with normal sexual function. For example, it is common to experience a watery vaginal discharge for approximately two weeks after cryosurgery; thus, women should avoid intercourse and using tampons during this time. Normal sexual relations can be resumed once the discharge ceases.

The above-mentioned feelings of guilt, anger, and shame may prevent women from asking questions or discussing sexual activity. The nurse must do the following:

- Establish a rapport with the woman by thoroughly assessing her preconceived notions of cancer and the treatment's effects.
- Alleviate fears and misconceptions by providing accurate facts and answering questions.
- Provide as much privacy and comfort as possible.
- Encourage the client to discuss possible "causes" of the cancer. The nurse must emphasize that gynecological cancer has multiple risk factors, and the exact cause is unknown. The woman must **not** blame herself.

- Openly and sensitively discuss issues of fertility, sexual expression, body image, and the results of treatment.
- Encourage the woman to follow the entire treatment plan, get regular Pap smears, and use safer sexual practices in the future.
- Offer the assistance of cancer support groups.
- Be nonjudgmental.

Two out of every five women do not undergo routine Pap smears, and unscreened women account for over 50% of cervical cancers. This is far from optimal (Bobak et al., 1995). The Pap smear can prevent deaths from cervical cancer. Therefore, nurses must make health education and screening programs more readily available, especially to poorer women and minorities who experience a disproportionate amount of cervical cancer. The mortality rate is more than twice as high among African Americans as compared to Caucasians (ACS, 1996).

Menarche to Menopause

Menstruation First menstruation, or menarche, marks the onset of puberty in adolescents girls. Girls typically begin menstruating at between 10 and 16 years of age. Menarche now begins at an earlier age in adolescents in Western nations, most likely because of improved nutrition and health care. Another theory holds that reaching critical body weight and body fat triggers menarche, and children today meet these growth parameters more rapidly. Menarche occurs later in those, like athletes, who have a lower percentage of body fat. The nurse must provide facts about menstruation and clarify any myths or misconceptions that adolescents have.

Premenstrual Syndrome (PMS) PMS is a cluster of symptoms that occurs 2–3 days before the onset of menstruation and then disappears during the first few days of the menstrual period. The symptoms vary greatly among women but follow a consistent pattern. Clinicians recommend keeping a log for three months, which allows the individual's PMS patterns to be diagnosed with greater accuracy. Nursing care includes recognizing PMS as a valid syndrome and encouraging women to keep a log. Nonpharmacological treatments include decreasing sodium and sugar intake, restricting caffeine intake, and regular exercise. Supplemental vitamin therapy including B complex vitamins, especially B6, helps some individuals. Other pharmacological treatments include prostaglandin inhibitors and diuretics. Sleep and rest are important, as fatigue worsens the symptoms. Women with severe PMS should be referred to specialists and support groups.

Dysmenorrhea Painful menstruation, or dysmenorrhea, usually occurs at or one day prior to the onset of menstruation and decreases during the menstrual cycle.

Primary Dysmenorrhea Primary dysmenorrhea is painful menstruation with no detectable organic disease. Prostaglandins, produced by the uterus in high concentrations during menses, are the primary cause of the cramping pain. Prostaglandins increase uterine contractility and decrease uterine arterial flow, causing ischemia (Ladewig et al., 1998). Frequent complaints include cramps, abdominal pain, headache, malaise, and fatigue, as well as an aching back and thighs and gastrointestinal (GI) symptoms. The etiology of primary dysmenorrhea has not been determined. Drug therapy includes prostaglandin inhibitors such as ibuprofen (Motrin) and naproxen (Anaprox, Naprosyn) and oral contraceptives. Nonpharmacological treatments include moderate exercise, rest, avoidance of constipation, applying moderate heat to the abdomen, improving nutrition, and biofeedback.

Secondary Dysmenorrhea Secondary dysmenorrhea is associated with some pelvic pathology. Conditions that frequently contribute to secondary dysmenorrhea include endometriosis, PID, uterine prolapse, or the presence of an intra-uterine device (IUD). Since primary and secondary dysmenorrhea may coexist, an accurate differential diagnosis is important.

Toxic Shock Syndrome (TSS) TSS is an infectious disease that occurs during menses. The syndrome may be caused by a toxin secreted by a strain of *Staphylococcus aureus*. The use of super absorbent tampons has increased the incidence of TSS (Ladewig et al., 1998). Common signs and symptoms include high fever, a sunburn-like rash with desquamating skin on the palms and soles, hypotension, nausea, vomiting, diarrhea, alterations in consciousness, and if left untreated, death.

Clients with TSS are hospitalized and given supportive therapy for shock, IV therapy to maintain blood pressure, and antibiotic therapy. Any respiratory and renal complications are managed as well. Renal dialysis, intubation and mechanical ventilation, and vasopressor administration may be required. Early detection and treatment are vital.

Nurses are directly involved in TSS prevention. Public health education for menstruating women includes the following key points:

- TSS may be eliminated by not using tampons (CDC), but this is not a practical solution.
- Tampons, when used, should be changed every 3–4 hours.
- Super absorbent tampons should be avoided.
- Tampons should not be used at night.
- Women with a history of TSS should never use tampons.
- Contraceptive diaphragms or cervical caps should not be used during menstruation or left in for prolonged periods.
- Postpartum women should avoid using tampons for 6–8 weeks after childbirth.

Endometriosis In endometriosis, endometrial cells travel through the fallopian tubes and implant on other structures such as the bladder, rectum, ovaries, outside surface of the uterus, vulva, and vagina. The exact incidence is unknown but as many as 50% of clients seen for pelvic pain, infertility, or a pelvic mass are later diagnosed with endometriosis. The symptoms are caused by changes in the endometrial patches related to the hormonal cycle. The endometrial patches thicken and bleed during the menstrual cycle just like normally functioning endometrial tissues. The symptoms increase in severity over the years as the endometrial patches grow. Clients may complain of pain, sometimes radiating to the thighs, pelvic heaviness, and hypermenorrhea. Scar tissue, infertility, and distortion or blockage of the affected structures may result (Bobak et al., 1995).

The diagnosis is confirmed by laparoscopic identification of the patches. Treatment depends on the severity of the condition and the woman's childbearing choices. Since endometriosis may cause infertility, the decision to bear children should not be delayed. Oral contraceptives are helpful, as is treatment with danazol (Danocrine). Mild endometriosis is treated by surgically removing the endometrial patches. Women with severe endometriosis who do not wish to bear more children may consider hysterectomy. During perimenopause, the endometrial tissue atrophies; endometriosis is no longer a concern. However, hormone replacement therapy (HRT) can reactivate the disorder (Bobak et al., 1995).

Perimenopause and Menopause The negative stereotypes surrounding the "change of life" began years ago when a woman's life expectancy was short and she was valued primarily for her reproductive capacity. Generations ago, so few women reached menopause that they were considered old if they survived into their forties, and elderly if they lived beyond 50 years of age. Menopause was thus associated with the undesirable attributes of extreme old age.

In Western culture, the strong emphasis on female youth and beauty has made menopause a difficult period of adjustment for some women. Attitudes have changed, and the perimenopausal years are now considered just as important and meaningful.

Although menopause means the cessation of menses, it is a process rather than a discrete, single occurrence. Menopause is now considered a sequence of biological and cultural events over a period of months to years. Perimenopause refers to the stages of regression of ovarian function. This period can last as long as 7–10 years. It culminates in the last menstrual cycle and encompasses at least one year after menopause. Menstrual periods stop when the ovaries no longer produce progesterone and estrogen. The major source of estrogen prior to menopause is the ovarian follicle, which accounts for more than 90% of the body's total production (Figure 10-5). The estrogen deficiency can cause hot flashes, vaginal dryness, emotional changes, and weight gain, although some women are asymptomatic. Menopause is a gradual process, and occurs suddenly only by surgery or if it is medically induced by chemotherapy or radiation.

Many misconceptions surround menopause. To avoid further confusion when counseling clients, nurses should explain the change of life as a process in terms women can understand. Women may attempt to define it themselves. For example, women who have not had a period for 6 months or more are often certain they have reached menopause. Conversely, women may simply wonder when it will happen. Nurses must describe the entire

Age and Menopause. Women reach menopause in the United States between 45 and 52 years of age. The mechanisms that initiate its onset are unknown, but menstruation stops when estrogen levels fall too low.

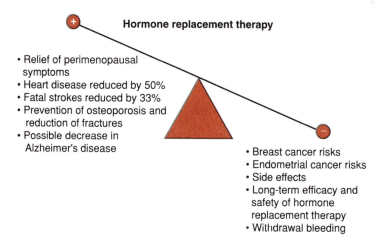

Hormone replacement therapy

- Relief of perimenopausal symptoms
- Heart disease reduced by 50%
- Fatal strokes reduced by 33%
- Prevention of osteoporosis and reduction of fractures
- Possible decrease in Alzheimer's disease

- Breast cancer risks
- Endometrial cancer risks
- Side effects
- Long-term efficacy and safety of hormone replacement therapy
- Withdrawal bleeding

FIGURE 10-5 ⊠

Risks and benefits of hormone replacement therapy (HRT).

process as a continuum leading to the cessation of menses. Contraceptive use should be discussed. Women older than 50 years of age should continue to use contraceptives for one year after their last period, as ovulation may occur sporadically during the perimenopausal period.

An average life expectancy of 78 years means that women now live one-third of their life after menopause. As the rights and roles of women in society have changed, the negative stereotypes attached to menopause have been altered; women now face middle age with good health and peace of mind. A woman's adjustment to menopause is influenced by her understanding and expectations, marital or relationship stability, financial resources, family views, physical health, and social and cultural expectations.

Cultural messages influence the perimenopausal transition. Some women view giving birth as their major role; thus, the inability to bear children is considered a great loss. Western culture values youth and physical beauty, leading some women to fear loss of attractiveness, status, energy, and value. In cultures where postmenopausal women gain status, such as in India, the Far East, and the South Pacific Islands, researchers have observed little or no depression or negative emotions. Western women, however, have little to replace what they view as their "lost youth" and are more likely to suffer from depression and low self-esteem (Bobak et al., 1995).

Many women actually welcome menopause, as it frees them from periods, pregnancy, and contraceptives. Women experiencing menopause have fewer child-care responsibilities and increased opportunities to pursue other goals. This combination of events often energizes women to improve their careers and relationships. The transition often provides more leisure time, as well as increased opportunities for self-expression and community involvement. Despite a strong cultural message that youth is valued above age, women who maintain a positive image and value themselves highly adapt well. Research has not demonstrated an increase in depression or psychosis in menopausal women.

The nursing profession views menopause as a natural event. Nurses should assess the feelings, symptoms, risk factors, and family and social support systems of a perimenopausal woman individually, and then work together with her on a realistic, acceptable, and economically feasible plan of care.

Nursing Care for Perimenopausal Women Women entering perimenopause should be informed of the normal changes they can anticipate as well as important health and life-style changes that need to be instituted. Preventive behaviors, including exercise, diet, health screening, and HRT decrease the incidence of chronic or fatal illnesses such as diabetes, osteoporosis, and heart disease.

Perimenopausal women should perform aerobic, weight-bearing exercise for 20 minutes, 3–4 times a week. This will reduce bone loss, prevent weight gain, and improve well-being.

The American Heart Association recommends eating a balanced diet that consists of 65% complex carbohydrates, 20% fat, and 15% protein. Consuming adequate amounts of vitamin D (400 to 800 IU) and calcium (1500 mg) also helps to prevent osteoporosis.

Although not without risk, HRT is considered a safe and reliable treatment both for the physical and emotional effects of menopause and for the reduction of age-related risk factors. The Women's Health Initiative (WHI) study at the National Institutes of Health (NIH) is currently studying 164,500 women in 40 clinical centers across the United States. The WHI study focuses on diet, HRT, and the incidence of chronic illnesses among middle-aged women.

Perimenopausal women should be screened routinely for early detection and treatment of health problems. A pelvic examination with a Pap smear, mammogram, cholesterol test, clinical breast examination, digital rectal examination with a fecal occult blood test, and blood pressure checks are recommended annually (or more frequently in high-risk clients).

Assessment for depression, domestic violence, and drug or alcohol dependency should also be conducted. Midlife adjustments are a time to develop future goals and pursue new interests.

Oral Contraceptives. Oral contraceptives are now commonly prescribed for perimenopausal women who do not smoke or have other contraindications for them. Oral contraceptives provide supplemental hormone therapy and contraceptive benefits until menopause. Once the woman reaches postmenopause, other medications can be used for hormone replacement.

Hormone Replacement Therapy Currently, dozens of medications are available for the treatment of menopause. HRT may help some women but is not appropriate for everyone. Understanding the physiological changes that occur during perimenopause and the implications of HRT can help women make informed choices. As natural estrogen decreases from the cessation of ovarian follicle secretion, many bodily changes occur (Fig. 10-6). While many of these changes occur in the reproductive system, other organs and systems are affected as well. These endocrinological changes appear to cause such symptoms of menopause as hot flashes, headaches, weight gain, irritability, and anxiety. Some women are asymptomatic; their transition consists solely of the cessation of menses. Hot flashes are reported by 50%–85% of women, but only 10%–20% seek treatment.

The sense of well-being is more difficult to measure than cholesterol or bone density but is just as important. Some women take hormone supplements to help relieve their physical symptoms. The resultant decrease in bothersome symptoms improves their overall quality of life and sense of well-being.

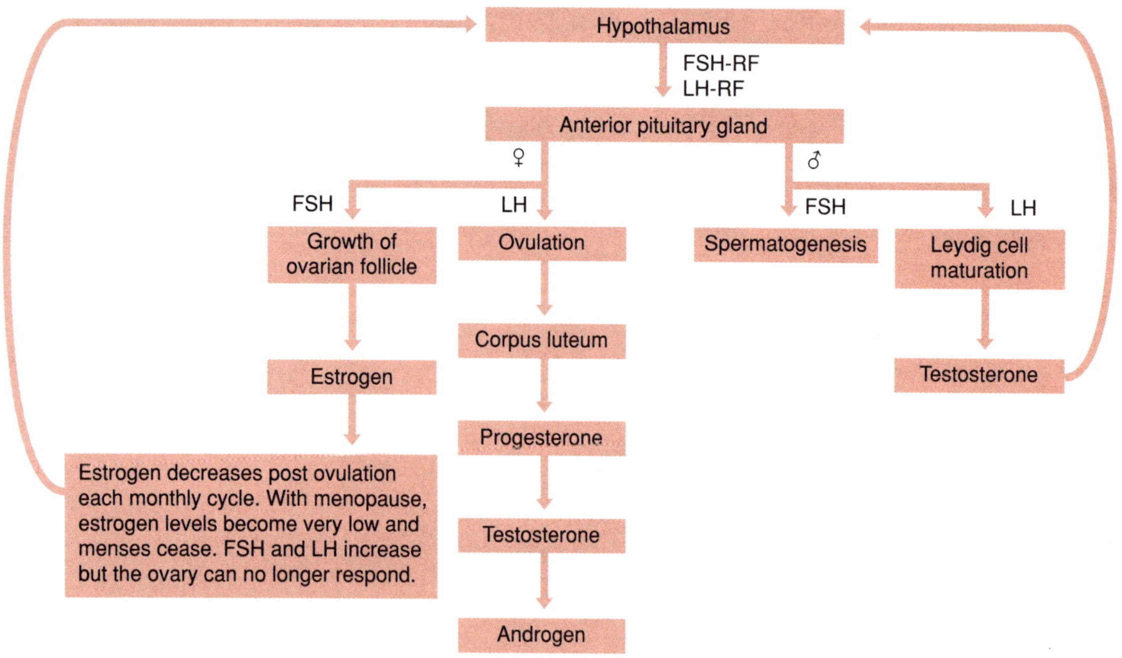

FIGURE 10-6 Feedback mechanism involving hormone secretion. FSH = follicle-stimulating hormone; LH = luteinizing hormone; RF = releasing factor.

CASE STUDY: WOMAN EXPERIENCING MENOPAUSE

A 52-year-old runner training for a marathon is experiencing no menopausal symptoms other than increased stress incontinence and "dribbling" during her training. When she seeks help, the nurse informs her that when estrogen levels decrease, the urethral epithelium becomes thin and easily inflamed. The nurse instructs the client to perform Kegel's exercises and informs her about HRT. After examining the benefits and drawbacks of HRT, the athlete chooses to take the hormones. She states: "My running serves both as my hobby and as the exercise I need to decrease other risk factors. I do not want my runs and my life style to be inconvenienced with this dribbling."

HRT and Cardiovascular Disease Cardiovascular disease is the leading cause of death in women. The incidence increases markedly after menopause. Research has shown that natural and surgically induced menopause are associated with changes in serum lipid profiles, a decline in high-density lipoproteins (HDLs), and an increase in low density lipoproteins (LDLs). These cholesterol changes may increase the risk of developing postmenopausal heart disease.

Recent research has found compelling evidence of the cardioprotective effect of HRT. Researchers from the 10-year Nurses' Health Study of almost 50,000 women reported that postmenopausal estrogen users had approximately half the risk of coronary artery disease and one-third the risk of a fatal stroke as compared with women who had never used estrogen (PhRMA, 1998). The evidence from several studies strongly suggests that postmenopausal estrogen exerts an independent, protective effect against cardiovascular disease. However, the problem with these and other studies is that estrogen was researched alone, not in combination with other hormones. For example, because of the risk of endometrial cancer, a combination of estrogen and progesterone is prescribed for any woman with an intact uterus. Until more data are available from the WHI study, the long-term effects of combination hormone therapy on cardiovascular disease cannot be determined (Stampfer et al., 1991).

HRT and Osteoporosis Osteoporosis is an important long-term concern during and after menopause. The loss of bone mass causes bones to become brittle and more likely to break. Hip fractures among elderly women are costly and debilitating, and these women often die from subsequent complications within a year.

Women reach peak bone mass in their thirties, and by approximately 40 years of age, bone resorption exceeds bone formation. In the 5–10 years following menopause, this process of bone loss markedly increases unless positive measures are taken. Methods that help to prevent bone loss include increasing calcium intake to 1500 mg/day postmenopause; taking vitamin D supplements (400–800 IU/day); stopping smoking; taking HRT; limiting the intake of alcohol, coffee, and soft drinks; and performing at least 1–3 hours of weight-bearing exercise each week.

Studies have shown that long-term estrogen use protects women from postmenopausal bone loss and osteoporosis. Estrogen therapy slows the demineralization process but cannot restore bone already lost. In addition, once estrogen replacement stops, bone loss resumes. The risk factor of osteoporosis is often enough for clinicians to advocate long-term or lifelong estrogen therapy for women without an intact uterus, and long-term combined estrogen and progesterone therapy for women with an intact uterus (Rickert, 1992).

HRT and Cancer Although HRT is widely used to prevent cardiac disease and osteoporosis, it is not an option for every woman. During the 1970s, unopposed estrogen therapy was given to all menopausal women with an intact uterus. This resulted in an increased risk of endometrial hyperplasia and cancer. Adding progesterone to estrogen decreased the risk of endometrial cancer. HRT advocates argue that the risks of endometrial cancer are low compared with the associated cardiovascular and osseous benefits. Baseline endometrial biopsy (a procedure done in an office) and annual biopsy detect early cancer development. With the advent of combined hormonal therapy, most clinicians feel even these biopsies are unnecessary unless irregular bleeding occurs. Women on HRT who experience irregular bleeding should always undergo a biopsy procedure.

The link between breast cancer and HRT remains controversial. Some studies suggest that lower doses of estrogen do not increase the risk while others suggest the opposite. Comparing existing studies is difficult because of selection biases and other methodological differences. Two major research studies by the NIH, the Nurses Health Study and the WHI, should answer some of these questions. However, the NIH studies will not be completed until approximately 2005. Therefore, until more definitive information concerning the effects of estrogen therapy and cancer becomes available, HRT is contraindicated for women with a family

Unopposed Estrogen Therapy. The administration of estrogen alone is unopposed therapy. It should be used only in women who do not have an intact uterus. If the woman has an intact uterus, unopposed estrogen therapy causes endometrial hyperplasia that can lead to endometrial cancer.

Hormone Replacement Therapy: Combined Estrogen and Progesterone. Combined estrogen and progesterone is always administered to women with an intact uterus. Estrogen (0.625 mg) and medroxyprogesterone (2.5 mg) [Prempro] and estrogen (0.625 mg) and medroxyprogesterone (5 mg) [Premphase] are examples of combined hormone medications available in one tablet. These medications may be more convenient than alternating estrogen and progesterone tablets for various weeks of a monthly cycle.

history of breast cancer. HRT is absolutely contraindicated for women who have a history of breast cancer or any other estrogen-dependent neoplasia, and for women who have a history of estrogen-related thromboembolic disease (such as those who experienced deep vein thrombosis while on oral contraceptives) (Wilson et al., 1998; Burnhart, 1998).

The decision to use HRT must be made by the individual (see Fig. 10-5). For example, if a woman's father died of a heart attack but her mother had breast cancer, is she a good candidate for HRT? Women who experience major menopausal symptoms, those at high risk for heart disease, and those who have thin bones (as measured by bone densitometry) are strong candidates for HRT. Women with a history of blood clots or breast cancer are not. Nurses must primarily educate women about estrogen, take a thorough personal and family history, and help the woman to evaluate objectively the benefits and drawbacks of HRT. Nurses and women will shortly have access to more research information to help them make these important decisions. The woman's perceptions of her experiences, her history of cancer, any uncontrolled hypertension or thrombophlebitis, and concerns about her sexuality should be assessed. Women on HRT should be warned of the possible, though inconclusive, link between estrogen replacement and breast cancer. For the duration of their HRT, they must be instructed to undergo regular mammograms and clinical breast examinations (AWHONN, 1998; Moore & Noonan, 1996; Rickert, 1992).

Pharmaceutical companies are currently developing "designer estrogens" and "selective estrogen receptor modulators" (SERMs). These medications exert estrogen-like effects that target organs like the heart and bone but block negative effects on the breast and uterus. One SERM, termed raloxifene (Evista), recently received Food and Drug Administration (FDA) approval (PhRMA, 1998) for the prevention of osteoporosis. Further clinical studies are needed to determine whether these SERMs are a better alternative to HRT.

Alternative Treatments Alternative treatments are available for women who are not good candidates for, or who chose not to take HRT. In addition, alternative treatments can be used as adjuvant therapy for women taking HRT. Greer has emphasized that holistic medicine is effective for the symptoms of menopause: "Matters are not made easier for the woman if her gynecologist treats her as a pair of dead ovaries, her rheumatologist as a collection of joints, her gerontologist as a nuisance" (1992, p. 160).

Those not using HRT may want to try herbal teas and natural remedies. Some report their hot flashes are relieved by ginseng, black cohosh, and red sage (AHWONN, 1998). Primrose oil often provides a calming effect. Consumers need to be advised that these products are not regulated by the FDA, and therefore safety and side-effect information has not been researched.

Breast Health and Breast Cancer

Men and Breast Cancer. Breast cancer also occurs in men, although rarely. Men with breast cancer account for approximately 1% of all breast cancers.

More than half of all women who menstruate regularly go through the frightening experience of finding a lump in their breast. Less than 10% of these lumps are malignant or require treatment (Alexander & LaRosa, 1994). Despite this, few conditions cause as much concern as breast cancer. Nurses should understand breast health, screening protocols, and treatment options, as early detection and treatment remain the best hopes for improving both the quality of life and survival rate. The nurse must both educate and advocate for women concerning all aspects of breast health and breast cancer.

Screening and Early Detection The breast cancer screening information is from the ACS and the National Cancer Institute (NCI).

Breast Self-Examination (BSE) During the BSE, women manually check their own breast tissue for changes and lumps. The woman should perform the BSE in two positions, while lying down and while observing herself in a mirror for physical changes in the breast. The ACS recommends that all women older than 20 years of age perform BSE; other sources suggest beginning at an earlier age if the woman seeks birth control. The early detection of potential malignancies remains the most important factor in successfully treating breast cancer. Since professional breast examinations are only performed annually, BSE should be done every month. The best time to examine the breasts is a few days after the menstrual period ends. Women detect lumps more accurately after the menstrual period, because the breasts are least affected by swelling and fibrocystic changes (Fig. 10-7). The examination is also more comfortable

FIGURE 10-7 Anatomy of the female breast.

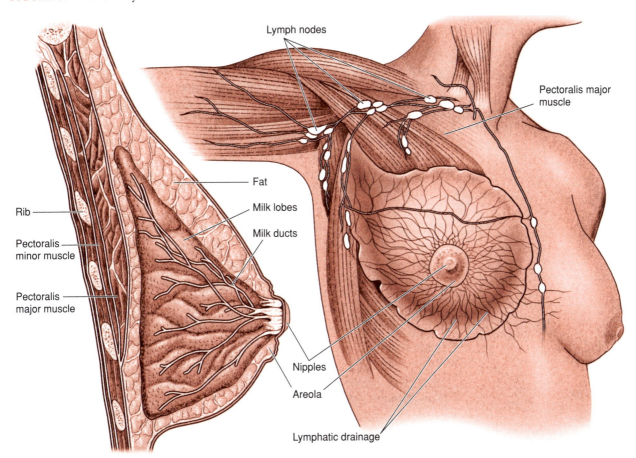

after the menstrual period because the breasts are less tender. If the woman is experiencing menopause or does not have regular periods, the BSE should be done on the same day every month, such as the first day of the month. Monthly BSE helps the woman to become familiar with the usual feel and appearance of her breasts, making it easier and more likely for her to notice any changes.

BSE, performed correctly and consistently, enables women to detect palpable masses that may not be visualized by mammography. Approximately 10%–15% of carcinomas are not detected by mammography. If the woman finds a change in her breast, she should not try to diagnose it herself; she should see a physician for further evaluation and diagnostic tests (Table 10-3).

Few women regularly perform BSE. Women often lack confidence in the technique or do not remember or take the time to do it. Shower cards illustrating the BSE technique have been helpful. All nurses must encourage and educate women to perform BSE.

Clinical Breast Examination The clinical examination is an important part of the ACS and NCI breast cancer detection guidelines. The clinical examination has a dual purpose. First, the experienced professional may find a change that the woman has missed. Second, the clinical examination is an excellent opportunity to demonstrate and explain a thorough breast examination. Modeling the correct technique reinforces the pattern women should follow at home every month.

Screening Recommendations Most breast lesions are present for several years before they can be palpated, thus mammography can detect lumps much earlier than BSE. Mammography can detect breast cancer at its earliest stage of development. When in situ breast cancer is detected this early, the survival rate is 99%. Mammography is recommended in conjunction with BSE and clinical breast examination. The NCI guidelines released in 1993 responded to the controversy surrounding mammogram schedules

✦

TABLE 10-3

SIGNS AND SYMPTOMS OF POSSIBLE BREAST CANCER
THAT REQUIRE FOLLOW-UP

Lump
Pain (breast cancer may or may not be painful)
Discharge
Skin changes
Lymphadenopathy with or without symptoms
Any unusual change in the breast

by stating that routine screening every 1–2 years with mammography and clinical breast examination may reduce breast cancer mortality by approximately one-third for women 50 years of age and older. The NCI acknowledged that experts disagree on the recommended screenings for those aged 40–49 years. A general screening schedule is provided as a guideline, but each woman must make an informed choice with her physician or nurse practitioner.

Regular mammograms should be performed annually after 50 years of age. Risk factors and informed choices determine the schedule for those younger than 50 years of age. Women at high risk should begin routine mammograms and breast examinations at 35 years of age. Because many women with breast cancer do not have any of the known risk factors, screenings are of the utmost importance (Table 10-4).

Detection and Treatment Breast cancer is the most common carcinoma in women but one of the most treatable if detected early. One in eight American women will develop breast cancer at some point in their lives (ACS, 1996). Since risk increases with age, if a woman lives to be 85 years old, her risk is one in eight. Nodal involvement is the best prognostic indicator for long-term survival. The ACS (1995) reported a 5-year survival rate of 99% for no invasion, 90% for local invasion, and 68% for regional spread. These survival rates underscore the importance of rigorous, consistent screening.

The etiology of breast cancer remains unknown, although some risk factors have been identified. These risk factors are age, gender, and personal and family history of breast cancer. The recent identification of the gene for familial breast cancer is a remarkable step forward in identifying risk factors for the prevention of breast cancer (ACS, 1995). However, BRCA1 and BRCA2 only account for approximately 5% of breast cancer cases in the United States.

Breast Ultrasound. Breast ultrasound is a painless and noninvasive method of assessing the size and consistency of a lump or tumor. Ultrasound can determine if the lump has a fluid consistency (such as a cyst) or a solid mass.

"Genetic" Breast Cancer. Genetic breast cancer is not common. More than 90% of women who develop breast cancer have no particular genetic risk for it. Their daughters and other relatives have no increased risk.

- **BRCA1.** Genes are the functional unit of heredity within the cell nucleus. Breast cancer gene 1 is a gene which is defective in about 2% of women with breast cancer.
- **BRCA2.** Breast cancer gene 2 is the other gene implicated in familial breast cancer. With the presence of BRCA1 or BRCA2, an inherited disposition to breast cancer exists. In these families, breast cancer can affect two or more close relatives, especially in premenopausal women.

TABLE 10-4

GENERAL SCREENING GUIDELINES FOR BREAST CANCER

Screening Procedure	Schedule
Breast self-examination	Monthly for those aged 20 years and older
Clinical breast examinations	Every 3 years for those aged 20–40 years
	Annually after 35 years of age if at risk
	Annually after 40 years of age
Mammography	At 35 years of age if at risk
	Every 1–2 years for those aged 40–50 years
	Annually after 50 years of age

Breast Reconstruction. Various methods of breast reconstruction involve the formation of a breast shape, and often a nipple, after a mastectomy. Breast implant surgeries have caused apparent autoimmune complications in some women, contributing to the current trend for transverse rectus abdominis myocutaneous flap (TRAM) reconstruction. TRAM reconstruction uses skin and fat from the abdomen carried on the rectus abdominis muscle that runs down the middle of the abdomen. Breast reconstruction surgeries are performed by plastic surgeons. Breast reconstruction may be performed at the time of mastectomy or at a later date. Reconstruction can be done months or even years later.

Tamoxifen (Nolvadex). Tamoxifen, a hormonal therapy, blocks estrogen's effects on the cells. Tamoxifen is more effective on estrogen-receptor positive tumors. However, it still works, although to a lesser degree, in women with estrogen-receptor-negative tumors.

Treatment Choices A diagnosis of breast cancer threatens a woman's life, but it also alters her self-image and changes her support systems and family relationships. The treatment options often contribute to the confusion that the diagnosis has caused. The choice of treatment depends on the type of breast cancer, age, menopausal status, extent of the cancer, lymph node involvement, the size of the tumor, hormonal receptors, desire to participate in a clinical trial, and general health status.

Women should discuss the treatment plan with their physicians, families, and support system. Many women prefer to get a second opinion. The nurse should emphasize that a short delay while seeking a second opinion does not compromise the success of treatment.

Advances have been made in determining the biology of cancer. Treatment is now based on the theory that breast cancer is a systemic disease, and micrometastases may be present with or without nodal involvement. Therefore, treatment may involve not only the surgical procedure, but adjuvant therapy as well. Adjuvant treatments such as chemotherapy, hormone therapy, and radiation therapy enhance survival and complement surgical effectiveness.

Only a few years ago, a diagnosis of breast cancer was usually followed by a radical mastectomy. Currently, surgery remains a primary component of treatment, but more breast tissue is conserved, and it is combined with other adjuvant therapies. A modified mastectomy or lumpectomy is performed for carcinoma in situ (noninvasive breast cancer). These surgeries remove the breast tissue and axillary lymph nodes but leave the pectoralis muscle intact. Women with small tumors (less than 4 cm), and in an early stage of cancer (Stage I or II), are often good candidates for lumpectomy. For those who are candidates, the lumpectomy with radiation has demonstrated the same survival rate as other surgical techniques, while preserving breast tissue.

For many women, breast cancer is a hormonally influenced malignancy. Cancer cells are tested following surgical removal, and hormonal therapy is used when the cancer is sensitive to estrogen (i.e., the cells are estrogen-receptor positive). Tamoxifen (Nolvadex), a synthetic anti-estrogen, effectively treats breast cancer metastases at a dose of 10–20 mg once or twice per day (Wilson et al., 1998). Research has demonstrated an increased survival rate for women with early stage disease who take tamoxifen (Nolvadex).

The National Cancer Institute study on tamoxifen in healthy women at high risk for breast cancer found a 45 percent reduction in breast cancer in the women taking tamoxifen. Further studies are being conducted. The common side effects are similar to those of menopause, including hot flashes, vaginal dryness, and weight gain.

To summarize treatment choices, local treatment includes surgery (radical, modified radical, or simple mastectomy), lumpectomy, and radiation therapy. Systemic treatment includes chemotherapy, hormone therapy, combination chemotherapy and hormone therapy, and bone marrow transplant.

The case studies below illustrate the wide range of treatment choices available and the need for nurses to have a broad knowledge base to provide information and support.

CASE STUDY: POSTMENOPAUSAL WOMAN WITH BREAST CANCER

The client describes her experiences as follows: "My mother had breast cancer when she was 60, so I was more aware of screening. When I was 50, I went in for a routine checkup to the gynecologist and went through everything. I actually said to the physician, 'By the way, don't you think I should have a mammogram?' So I did, and they discovered it. I cannot sing the praises of a mammogram any higher. The cancer could not be felt, and it was discovered as a result of the mammogram. The cancer had not spread to the lymph nodes, so I had a lumpectomy. After the surgery, the doctor just said, 'Go home, everything's great' and that I'd be fine. However, I think that fear, once you hear you have any cancer, is awful. Once I found out that it hadn't gone into the lymph nodes, I did feel a whole lot better."

This woman's experience demonstrates that women need to advocate for themselves if physicians do not perform screenings. Also, this is a good example of how breast cancer was discovered by a mammogram in its earliest stages, long before the mass was large enough to be palpated. Finally, nurses should take into account the woman's feelings about being diagnosed with cancer. Although in this particular case the woman was fortunate enough to be diagnosed early and was a good candidate for a breast-conserving treatment such as lumpectomy, she still must make serious emotional adjustments.

CASE STUDY: PREMENOPAUSAL WOMAN WITH BREAST CANCER

Another client describes her experiences in treatment decisions as follows:

"You know, I started backwards because the lump was under my arm first. It took the surgeon about 15 minutes to find the spot in my breast. We discussed my options, and I chose to have a lumpectomy. I opted for this because being 42 I was pretty young, and I could probably get by with just a lumpectomy. Unfortunately, that didn't work because when the report came back they said the tissue around the lump was not healthy. So, they left the option to me regarding further surgery, and I had 10 weeks to think about it. During that 10 weeks, I had my chemotherapy. That was a real hard 10 weeks. My husband said it didn't matter to him whether I lost a breast, and he would rather I was overtreated, but it was a hard decision. I kept thinking, How am I going to look? How am I going to feel? Am I still going to be a woman? It took me a long time, and I finally decided it didn't matter, that I was going to live. It didn't matter what I had to do in order to do it. So, I said okay and I elected to have the mastectomy done."

The younger woman in the second case study persistently sought care for the lump under her arm. Nurses must remember that breast cancer may not always present in the breast. In addition, unexpected or borderline test results make treatment decisions unclear. Nurses need to provide support and information and present a caring attitude to these women who are making emotionally difficult decisions.

Nursing Care　Most women with breast cancer undergo a full course of surgery, chemotherapy, and radiation within several months after diagnosis. At the time of diagnosis, many women worry that the cancer and its treatment may affect all aspects of their life, including their children, relationships, finances, employment, physical limitations, and body image. Women are profoundly affected by the uncertainty and vulnerabilities that accompany a diagnosis of breast cancer. Currently, many women who undergo lumpectomies or modified mastectomies are treated as outpatients or are only hospitalized for a few days. Much of the recovery process occurs after treatment is completed and the client is discharged from the hospital. The nurse must assess the adequacy of the woman's support system, her family environment, and her ability to live with breast cancer. Nurses should then offer the woman and her family community resources, cancer support groups, and ACS programs such as "Reach for Recovery" for continued emotional support.

Women with breast cancer can, throughout both their acute treatment phase and their recovery, benefit from nurses who are sensitive to their health needs and concerns. Informative and compassionate nursing care fosters the woman's personal growth, as well as that of her family and friends. Eighteen women diagnosed with breast cancer were interviewed to explore their experiences of inner strength (Roux, 1993; Roux & Keyser, 1994). The women in the study expressed the following needs: When confronted with the diagnosis, women need time and space to adjust. The nurse should provide only the necessary or requested information so as not to overwhelm the women, who are often preoccupied with thoughts, fears, and uncertainties at this time. After allowing time to adjust, the nurse should encourage the client to share her thoughts and feelings. The nurse should provide clear, factual information about treatment options, clarifying any misconceptions or unrealistic fears. She should encourage the client to work with other women in similar situations and offer the assistance of a breast cancer support group. The woman must use her basic strengths, such as keeping a journal, listening to music, imagery, humor, and quiet time, to keep a positive attitude and promote healing. The nurse should encourage positive, fun activities to release energy and encourage the woman to plan for the future. Study participants also reported that maintaining connections with family, friends, and God was crucial to their recovery. The nurse should encourage women to ask for help and to accept support and caring from others. Spouses or partners may be unable to fulfill a woman's needs, as they are also dealing with their own feelings of loss. Poetry and meditation may help her feel connected, as well as church activities and prayer.

Cardiac Health

Heart disease has traditionally been considered a "man's disease," possibly because cardiovascular disease patterns reveal interesting gender differences.

Age Women tend to show signs of cardiovascular disease later in life. Between 25 and 35 years of age, men have three times the incidence of coronary artery disease (CAD). Although menopause decreases a woman's protection from CAD, this biological advantage persists until 65–70 years of age. After 65 years of age, however, heart disease is the leading cause of death among women (American Heart Association [AHA], 1996). Older women who have heart attacks are twice as likely to die within a few weeks as men (AHA, 1996). Therefore, only slightly more men die from CAD because of the dramatic rise in the mortality of older women with the disease (AHA, 1996).

Signs and Symptoms: Gender Differences CAD signs and symptoms differ significantly between women and men. Angina pectoralis is typically the first symptom women experience; men initially have a myocardial infarction. Women rarely experience myocardial infarction initially (Allen & Phillips, 1997). Women may experience unspecified, misleading pain. Nurses must look for evidence of a heart attack in women and men equally. The nurse should ask the woman how the symptoms change in response to exercise, temperature extremes, and heavy meals. In the past, women were excluded from most CAD research studies. This has greatly compromised the discovery of facts concerning the early identification and treatment of heart disease in women, and is only now being rectified.

Morbidity and Mortality Of women who have heart attacks, 44% die within 1 year compared to 27% of men (AHA, 1996). Women 65 years of age and older experience greater mortality from myocardial infarction than men (Studies have found mortality as an outcome to be up to 50% more likely in women than men.) (AHA, 1996). Once infarction occurs, the relative immunity women enjoy in earlier years is lost; indeed, they survive less often than men. Within 6 years after the initial heart attack, 23% of men and 31% of women develop a second infarction (AHA, 1996). The survival rate 10 years after an infarction is 50% for men. For women, it is 30% because of higher early mortality. Strokes occur more often in men, but women die from strokes more often. It is the second leading cause of death in 45–64-year-old American women and much more deadly than breast cancer (National Stroke Association, 1996).

Social Factors Although CAD affects women all ages and socioeconomic classes, it is concentrated among the elderly, poor, and less educated. Many women with CAD are older than 65 years of age, widowed, living alone on less than $25,000/year, not well educated, and have other health problems such as diabetes, high cholesterol, and hypertension. For example, diabetes is more prevalent in women and is a major risk factor for cardiovascular disease. Nurses must emphasize that heart disease is not an inevitable consequence of aging; rather, it is a disease process that can be greatly influenced by behavior modification. Factors such as diet, exercise, not smoking, maintaining weight, monitoring blood pressure and cholesterol, and taking HRT are all helpful. The nurse, the aging woman, and the community must recognize that the postmenopausal years bring a higher risk for CAD.

Risk Factors and Preventive Health Behaviors Risk factors are actions, behaviors, or characteristics that place an individual at high risk of developing a condition. Women may have combinations of negative social, psychological, cultural, physical, and addictive behaviors that increase their risk. The major modifiable risk factors are cigarette smoking, high blood cholesterol levels, high blood pressure, diabetes, physical inactivity, excessive alcohol consumption, stress, and excessive weight. Women who smoke and have high blood pressure and high blood cholesterol levels are eight times more likely to develop heart disease than those who do not. Women who have diabetes are four to six times more likely to die from CAD than women without diabetes (Allen & Phillips, 1997).

Women can reduce the risk of cardiovascular disease by taking responsibility at a younger age and developing behaviors that will decrease their cardiovascular risk later in life. Childhood is the best time to develop healthy habits, but it is never too late to begin.

It remains unclear what factors are present after menopause that lead to heart attacks. Because women present with heart disease at different ages and with different signs and symptoms, their conditions have not been taken as seriously as those of men. Women are diagnosed with heart disease when they are older, more likely to be on other medications, and have other conditions such as diabetes, hypertension, and osteoporosis. Until recently, most major research studies of cardiovascular disease have excluded women. Upon completion in 2003, WHI should reveal whether HRT provides continued protection against CAD in postmenopausal women. The study is investigating the effects of diet, smoking, and hormonal therapy on a woman's risk of developing heart disease and stroke. Nurses must take an active role in teaching the facts of heart disease to their peers and clients.

Osteoporosis

In osteoporosis, the most common skeletal disorder, the bone thins, or decreases in density, as a result of the aging process. Osteoporotic bone is more porous (has more openings) and is weaker than normal bone; thus, it fractures more easily. This condition is the leading cause of bone fractures in postmenopausal women, leading to long-term disability, frailty, and enormous expense. A woman loses 2%–5% percent of bone tissue per year

Bone Densitometry. Bone strength depends primarily on bone mineral density, which is measured by a variety of noninvasive techniques termed bone densitometry. Bone densitometry quantitatively measures bone mass by calculating the mean value with a standard deviation. This diagnostic test allows the clinician to estimate the client's risk of fractures and helps to determine if more treatment is required to prevent further osteoporosis and risk of fractures.

immediately before and approximately eight years after the onset of menopause (Lutz & Prytulski, 1997). Common fracture sites are the spine, wrists, forearms, and hips. After arthritis, osteoporosis is the leading cause of musculoskeletal disturbances in the elderly.

Osteoporosis is known as the silent epidemic because no symptoms are seen during the early stages. Preventive measures are the primary defense against this debilitating disease. Improved preventive care promotes early recognition of osteoporosis before fractures have occurred. Osteoporosis is now considered a pediatric problem as well, as some children and adolescents have poor calcium intake. An early prediction of which individuals are at risk for developing osteoporosis is helpful, but elderly women are primarily at risk.

Risk Factors Women are much more likely to develop osteoporosis than men because of differences in bone mass and density. For example, almost 80% of all hip fractures occur in women. The nurse must educate and motivate women to undergo preventive screening and practice positive life-style behaviors. Women must be informed of the risk of osteoporosis as they reach menopause and as they make informed choices regarding HRT.

Many and various risk factors exist for osteoporosis. The primary factor is a family history of osteoporosis. The client's health history reveals if any female relatives have had a broken wrist or hip or development of a dowager's hump.

Hysterectomy or surgical removal of the ovaries before 50 years of age is another risk factor. Secondary osteoporosis is a reduction in bone mass that is not the result of the aging process. Young women who have had their ovaries removed surgically are at equal risk of developing osteoporosis as postmenopausal women.

Poor health behaviors include smoking and alcohol consumption. Women who smoke are more likely to develop osteoporosis. Excessive alcohol consumption causes a greater calcium loss that can result in osteoporosis. Women who drink wine, beer, or other alcoholic beverages daily increase their risk of osteoporosis.

Another risk factor is having a small, thin body frame. European and Asian women with small, slender frames develop osteoporosis more often than African-American women because of differences in peak bone mass and density. Drinking soft drinks or more than two cups of coffee per day causes calcium loss, increasing the chances of developing osteoporosis.

Inactivity is another risk factor. Women should participate in weight-bearing exercises such as walking, jogging, or low-impact aerobics.

Strenuous exercise, however, can lead to amenorrhea. Exercise that results in irregular periods or no periods at all is as harmful as inactivity. A balanced exercise and diet program promotes healthy habits that prevent osteoporosis.

A major risk factor is a low calcium intake. Women's dietary calcium intake varies widely. The nurse should determine during the health history if the client has milk allergies or lactose intolerance or has eating disorders such as bulimia or anorexia nervosa. The nurse should also determine if the client continually goes on diets that often exclude dairy products. Most women do not consume enough calcium in their young adult years to achieve peak bone mass.

Preventive Health Measures Since most postmenopausal women have osteoporosis, nurses must develop teaching methods to prevent further bone loss. The best preventive measures are early education and health-promoting behaviors before the disorder develops. Nurses should teach clients to: increase calcium intake; take vitamin D supplements; avoid excessive caffeine, soft drinks, and alcohol; avoid smoking; increase physical activity; take HRT if appropriate; and perform weight-bearing exercises to improve bone density. Since vitamin D is needed for proper calcium absorption, elderly women should increase their daily intake from 200 IU to 400–800 IU.

The nurse should take a thorough health and diet history that covers typical eating patterns. Nutritional concerns such as weight control, lowering cholesterol, and food preferences should be discussed.

Calcium Dairy products provide approximately 75% of the average American's dietary calcium. Currently, women consume only about half the recommended amount. Women who are allergic to milk products should be directed to other food sources of calcium and to calcium supplements. Cholesterol can be controlled and calcium levels increased by consuming low-fat yogurt, skim milk, pudding made with skim milk, and low-fat cheese. For example, only three 10-oz glasses of milk supply 1000 mg of calcium. The client should record her calcium intake for two weeks. The nurse can then evaluate her diet and suggest alternatives. A dietitian may need to be consulted (Table 10-5).

Dietary Calcium. Dairy products are the most common source of calcium in the American diet. One cup of skim milk has 302 mg of calcium, 8 ounces of lowfat yogurt has 415 mg calcium; and 1½ oz of cheddar cheese has 306 mg of calcium.

TABLE 10-5

NATIONAL INSTITUTES OF HEALTH
RECOMMENDATIONS FOR CALCIUM INTAKE

Age	Daily Requirement
11–25 years of age	1200–1500 mg
Pregnant, lactating	1200–1500 mg
Perimenopausal	1000–1200 mg
Postmenopausal on HRT	1200 mg
Postmenopausal not on HRT	1500 mg
Males over 50 years of age	1200 mg

The daily calcium intake, including supplements should not exceed 2000 mg. Most commercial calcium supplements are available in 200–500-mg pills. Three 500-mg pills of calcium carbonate (Os-Cal) can be taken in divided doses during the day or in a single bedtime dose; calcium seems to be absorbed more readily during sleep. GI upset is the most common side effect; constipation, flatulence, gastric distention, and nausea may be experienced as well.

The essential vitamins and minerals are adequately provided by a balanced, nutritious diet. However, women do not always have the time, education, or finances to consume balanced meals. Thus, nurses must be familiar with the common mineral deficiencies.

Iron Menstruation and a greater iron requirement during pregnancy place women at high risk for iron deficiency anemia. Nurses should be alert to situations where even a balanced diet may not supply enough iron. Heavy menstruation, diets of less than 1500 calories/day, pregnancy, and vegetarianism (not eating red meat) place women at risk for iron deficiency anemia.

Iron absorption is a complex process that varies with the amount and combination of foods consumed. Foods that are high in vitamin C facilitate the absorption of iron. Therefore, fruits, fruit juices, and vegetables should be eaten with the selected iron food source. Moderate amounts of lean meat help to maintain the correct amount of iron in the body but are not essential. Vegetarians must consume legumes and nuts for iron and protein. Iron-enriched breads, cereals, and pasta also supply adequate amounts of iron for women.

To meet general nutritional needs, the food pyramid should be used to guide choices and proportions. Vegetables, fruits, whole grain foods, legumes, fish, poultry, and lean meats should be used predominantly, and saturated fats and cooking methods that add fats and oils should be avoided. Special consideration must be given to each woman's history. For example, menopausal women must balance cholesterol levels and calcium requirements, while women who experience heavy menstrual periods are at risk for iron deficiency anemia. Nurses can adapt the dietary guidelines to meet each woman's specific needs.

Exercise Regular exercise offers many benefits, such as weight control. The relationship between diet and exercise and its effects on the metabolic rate should therefore be emphasized in the nurse's teaching plan.

The metabolic rate measures energy production or how rapidly the body burns calories. Many factors affect the metabolic rate, including gender, age, heredity, food intake, body composition, activity level, and frequent cycles of weight loss. Frequent weight loss from severe caloric restriction followed by increased caloric intake and weight gain seems to slow the metabolic rate. In what is commonly termed "starvation metabolism" or "yo-yo dieting," the body seems to fear starvation and reacts by conserving and storing energy more efficiently. This weight-loss cycling is harmful to the woman's health. It is also very discouraging and increases the woman's risk of hypertension, heart disease, and diabetes.

CDC Iron Recommendation. The CDC urges that adolescent girls and women of childbearing age consume 15 mg of iron daily. Pregnant women should take low-dose iron supplements to meet the U.S.R.D.A of 30 mg daily of iron.

The set-point theory states that certain areas of the brain may control body composition. According to this theory, severe dietary restrictions force the body to maintain the set point by decreasing energy expenditure and increasing appetite. The set point may help to control the metabolic rate through various hormonal and nervous system connections. The set point actually changes in response to caloric intake, diet components, and exercise. Aerobic exercise burns calories, lowers the set point, and promotes good health. However, too much exercise should be avoided; overexercising can send the body the same starvation message as restrictive dieting.

Summary

Nurses provide holistic health care. The client, family, and community must all be involved. Nurses must offer clients and their families information, support, economical treatment options, and community resources, whether they are confronted with the psychological and physiological stresses of breast or prostate cancer, life-altering events such as menopause, or the daily challenge of exercising and eating a balanced diet. Health care has evolved into separate specialties that focus on gender-specific care, shared responsibility, and informed treatment options. Nurses can now take leadership roles in promoting primary care, primary prevention, and healthy life styles for men and women across the lifespan.

KEY WORDS

Acquired immunodeficiency
    syndrome
Angina
Benign prostatic hypertrophy
Bone densitometry
Breast cancer
Breast reconstruction
Breast ultrasound
Cervical cancer
Chlamydia
Dietary calcium
Endometrial cancer
Endometriosis
Epididymitis
Genital herpes
Gonorrhea
Hormone replacement therapy
Human papillomavirus

Iron deficiency anemia
Lumpectomy
Mammogram
Mastectomy
Menarche
Menopause
Menstruation
Orchitis
Osteoporosis
Ovarian cancer
Pap smear
Perimenopause
Phimosis
Premenstrual syndrome
Priapism
Primary dysmenorrhea
Prostate cancer
Prostatitis

Radiation
Secondary dysmenorrhea
Selective estrogen receptor
    modulators
Set point
Sexuality
Sexually transmitted diseases
Supplemental calcium

Syphilis
Testicular cancer
Testicular torsion
Toxic shock syndrome
Unopposed estrogen therapy
Uterine cancer
Vulvovaginal candidiasis
Women's Health Initiative

MEN'S HEALTH QUESTIONS

1. Mr. T. has to urinate at least six times every night and is not getting enough sleep. Which of the following conditions will *not* cause these symptoms?

   A. Phimosis
   B. Benign prostatic hypertrophy
   C. Prostatitis
   D. Prostate cancer

2. Mr. L. underwent a transurethral resection of the prostate (TURP) one week ago. He complains that he is dribbling urine at times. How should the nurse respond?

   A. The dribbling will probably occur for the rest of his life, and he should wear an absorbent pad every day.
   B. During the TURP all of the prostate gland and sphincter were removed; thus, the dribbling will occur for the rest of his life.
   C. The dribbling will probably decrease in amount and frequency as sphincter control returns.
   D. The nurse should ask the physician to insert a Foley catheter until the dribbling stops.

3. A client returns from surgery after undergoing a TURP for obstructive benign prostatic hypertrophy. The urine varies from clear yellow to a pink-tinged color in the catheter. What should the nurse do?

   A. Note intake and output at every shift, or according to orders or protocol.
   B. Calculate intake and output every hour because of the pink-tinged output.
   C. Call the physician immediately, since the pink-tinged urine indicates an abnormal finding.
   D. Arrange for a unit of blood, since the physician will probably order an infusion.

4. Dr. G. orders ice for the scrotum of a client diagnosed with epididymitis. The nurse correctly assumes that

A. ice slows circulation and decreases peripheral edema.

B. ice should be applied in intervals, not continuously.

C. ice is placed on the scrotum continuously until the physician orders otherwise.

D. ice will not stop the pain, and it has a placebo effect.

WOMEN'S HEALTH QUESTIONS

5. All of the following situations are risk factors for yeast infection *except*

A. uncontrolled diabetes.

B. pregnancy.

C. antibiotic therapy.

D. hypertension.

6. All of the following symptoms can occur with a yeast infection *except*

A. vulvar or vaginal burning and itching.

B. thick, white vaginal discharge.

C. symptoms that lessen before menstruation.

D. no accompanying odor.

7. The first Pap smear should be performed either when the woman begins to have intercourse or at

A. 14 years of age.

B. 18 years of age.

C. 20 years of age.

D. 22 years of age.

8. All of the following infections are frequently linked to cervical carcinoma *except*

A. herpes simplex virus 2.

B. gonorrhea.

C. Human papillomavirus types 16, 18, and 31.

D. cytomegalovirus.

9. A combination of estrogen and progestin is prescribed for women with an intact uterus to

A. potentiate the action of estrogen.

B. prevent breakthrough bleeding.

C. decrease the risk of endometrial cancer.

D. increase cardiovascular protection.

10. Women reach peak bone mass in their

A. adolescence.

B. third decade.

C. fourth decade.

D. fifth decade.

11. A woman on hormone replacement therapy should undergo an endometrial biopsy if she experiences

    A. hot flashes.
    B. irregular vaginal bleeding.
    C. vaginal pH changes.
    D. urinary tract infection.

12. A good candidate for hormone replacement therapy (HRT)

    A. has a family history of breast cancer.
    B. has had breast cancer.
    C. has a family history of heart disease.
    D. has had an estrogen-dependent neoplasia.

13. The best time for menstruating women to perform a breast self-examination is

    A. right before the menstrual period.
    B. during the menstrual period.
    C. a few days after the menstrual period.
    D. 14 days after the menstrual period.

14. American women have a lifetime risk of developing breast cancer of

    A. one in twelve.
    B. one in ten.
    C. one in eight.
    D. one in six.

15. The drug tamoxifen (Nolvadex) is classified as

    A. an estrogen.
    B. a progestin.
    C. a synthetic antiestrogen.
    D. an androgen.

16. All of the following conditions place women at risk for iron deficiency anemia *except*

    A. menopause.
    B. heavy menstruation.
    C. pregnancy.
    D. adolescence.

ANSWERS

 1. *The answer is A.* BPH, prostatis, and prostate cancer frequently cause nocturia and frequency.

 2. *The answer is C.* Men require several weeks to regain urine control following a TURP procedure.

 3. *The answer is A.* Accurately noting intake and output is an important aspect of this client's care. Pink-tinged urine is a normal finding.

4. *The answer is B.* Ice therapy needs to be removed from the scrotum every 15–20 minutes.

5. *The answer is D.* Uncontrolled diabetes, prergnancy, and antibiotic therapy are risk factors for vulvocandidiasis.

6. *The answer is C.* For unknown reasons, yeast infection symptoms often increase before menstruation.

7. *The answer is B.* Guidelines specify that screening Pap smears should begin when the woman becomes sexually active or by 18 years of age.

8. *The answer is B.* Viral cervical infections seem to increase the risk of developing cervical cancer.

9. *The answer is C.* Unopposed estrogen therapy causes endometrial hyperplasia, a condition that can lead to cancer.

10. *The answer is C.* Women reach their peak bone mass between 30–35 years of age. Calcium intake in adolescence and early adulthood is crucial for women to establish peak bone mass in their thirties.

11. *The answer is B.* The only sign of possible endometrial cancer is irregular vaginal bleeding.

12. *The answer is C.* HRT may decrease the incidence of heart disease by half and the incidence of fatal stroke by one-third. A family or personal history of breast cancer or a history of estrogen-dependent neoplasia are absolute contraindications for HRT.

13. *The answer is C.* A few days after the menstrual period, the breasts have the least amount of fluid and are less tender. This may improve the accuracy and comfort of a self-examination.

14. *The answer is B.* As a woman ages, her risk of breast cancer increases. As she approaches the end of her life, the woman's risk rises to one in eight.

15. *The answer is C.* Tamoxifen is an antiestrogen hormonal drug, not a chemotherapy drug.

16. *The answer is A.* Menopausal women are not at risk for iron deficiency anemia. Menstruation, pregnancy, and adolescence place women at risk.

ANNOTATED REFERENCES

Alexander, L., & LaRosa, J. (1994). *New dimensions in women's health.* Boston: Jones and Bartlett.

This text is a very progressive and thorough resource on all aspects of women's health.

Allen, K. M., & Phillips, J. M. (1997). *Women's health across the lifespan.* Philadelphia: J. B. Lippincott.

This text is a very progressive and well-researched resource on women's health.

American Cancer Society (1994, 1995, 1996). *Cancer facts & figures.* Atlanta, GA: Author.

These booklets provide a wealth of demographical and epidemiological data on cancer.

American Heart Association (1994, 1995, 1996). *Heart and stroke facts.* Dallas, TX: Author.

These booklets provide a wealth of demographical and epidemiological data on heart disease.

AWHONN (1998). *Standards and Guidelines.* Washington, D.C.: Author.

Bobak, I. Lowdermilk, D., & Jensen, M. (1995). *Maternity care* (4th ed.). St. Louis: C .V. Mosby.

Burnhart, W. (Ed.) (1998). Physician's Desk Reference. Oradell, N.J.: Medical Economics.

This text provides information on common reproductive and gynecological health problems.

Centers for Disease Control and Prevention (1994*). Sexually transmitted disease surveillance and treatment guidelines.* Atlanta, GA: CDC.

Greer, G. (1992). *The change: Women, aging and the menopause.* New York: Alfred A. Knopf.

This classic text on menopause was written by the well-known feminist, Germaine Greer.

Ladewig, P., London, M., & Olds, S. (1998*). Maternal-newborn nursing care.* Menlo Park, CA: Addison-Wesley Longman.

This text provides information on common reproductive and gynecological health problems.

Lutz, C., & Przytulski, K. R. (1997). *Nutrition and diet therapy.* Philadelphia: F.A. Davis.

This comprehensive text covers nutrition for the mature adult and diets for persons with osteoporosis, cancer, and cardiovascular disease.

Moore, A., & Noonan, M. (1996). A nurses's guide to hormone replacement therapy. *JOGNN. 25*(2), 24–31.

This is an excellent guide to drug regimens, risks, benefits, and client education.

Phipps, W., Cassmeyer, V., Sands, J., & Lehman, M. K. (1995). *Medical-surgical nursing concepts and clinical practice.* St. Louis: C. V. Mosby.

This text discusses the alterations in the body systems and nursing care for common problems among ill adults. One section discusses altered sexual function and reproductive problems.

PhRMA (October 1997). *New medicines in development for women.* Washington, D.C.: Authors.

This newsletter, presented by American pharmaceutical research companies, provides updates on medications in development and highlights the results of clinical drug trials.

Rickert, B. (1992). Estrogen replacement: Making informed choices. *Registered Nurse 9*, 26–33.

This article discusses the advantages and disadvantages of HRT. It is a good resource for client education.

Roux, G. (1993). *Phenomenologic study: Inner strength in women with breast cancer.* Doctoral dissertation, Texas Woman's University, Denton, TX.

This research study investigated the strengths women developed as they recovered from breast cancer. The participants were 18 women who had been diagnosed with breast cancer in the preceding 6 months to 20 years.

Roux, G. & Keyser, P. (1994). Inner strength in women with breast cancer. *Illness, Crisis, and Loss, 4* (2), 1–12.

This research report details methods health professionals can use to assist women with breast cancer to develop inner strength and enjoy improved quality of life.

Stampfer, M., Colditz, G. A., Willett, W. C., Manson, J. E., et al. Postmenopausal estrogen therapy and cardiovascular disease: Ten-year followup from the Nurses' Health Study. *New England Journal of Medicine. 1991: 325;* 756–762.

This article discusses research findings from the NIH study.

Wilson, B., Shannon, M., & Stang, C. (1998). *Nurses' drug guide.* Stanford, CT: Appleton & Lange.

This comprehensive resource guides the nurse on the safe and accurate administration of drugs.

INTERNET SITES FOR ADDITIONAL INFORMATION

American Heart Association
  http://www.amhrt.org

AWHONN
  http://www.awhonn.org

CDC
  http://www.cdc.gov/cdc.html

Australian Breastnet
  http://www.bci.org.au

Avon's Breast Cancer Awareness
  http://www.pmedia.com/Avon/avon.html

Breast Cancer Clearinghouse
  http://nysernet.org/bcic

Breast Cancer Net
  http://www.breastcancer.net

CancerNet
  http://cancernet.nci.nih.gov

Cancer of the Cervix
  http://www.cancerbacup.org.uk/info/cervix/cervix-1.htm

National Alliance of Breast Cancer Organizations (NABCO)
  http://www.nabco.org

The New York Times Women's Health
  http://www.nytimes.com/women

Oncolink
  http://cancer.med.upenn.edu

Oncolink-Cervix
  http://oncolink.upenn.edu/specialty/gyn_onc/cervical/

ONS online
  http://www.ons.org

Prostate
  listserv@sjuvm.stjohns.edu

PSA: Prostate Cancer Screening
  http://kptl.tricon.net/Personal/wesley/prostate

Prostate Cancer Infolink
  http://www.comed.com/Prostate/index.html

Safer Sex Pages
  http://www.safersex.org/

Women's Health Initiative
  http://www.healthtouch.com

CLIENTS WITH DIABETES MELLITUS

INTRODUCTION

Diabetes mellitus (DM) is a chronic systemic syndrome characterized by hyperglycemia that is caused by a decrease in the secretion or activity of insulin resulting in the inability to metabolize carbohydrates, protein, and fats properly. Eventually, if diabetic clients do not follow their management plan or are unable to maintain a normal blood sugar concentration, complications will affect the heart, vascular system, kidneys, nervous system, and eyes.

Insulin is a hormone produced by the beta cells in the islets of Langerhans of the pancreas. It is continuously released into the bloodstream in small amounts and increases when food is ingested. Generally, 40–50 units of insulin are secreted daily in an average adult. This insulin regulates metabolism to maintain a fasting blood sugar level at the normal limit of 70–120 mg/dL.

Insulin is involved in the digestion of all foods. After eating, insulin levels rise, promoting the passage of carbohydrates into cells to be metabolized for energy and stimulating the liver and muscle to store glucose as glycogen. Insulin supports fat metabolism by promoting storage in the adipose tissue, and stimulates the entry of amino acids into cells, thus enhancing protein synthesis. Though secretion is greatest after eating, insulin is continuously released throughout the day. During sleep, small amounts of insulin act to release glycogen from the liver, protein from muscle, and fat from adipose tissue.

The counterregulatory hormones, that is, those that work in opposition to insulin, are glucagon, epinephrine, growth hormone, cortisol, and somatostatin. These hormones stimulate glycogen release from the liver, increase blood sugar levels, and regulate the amount of insulin in the body. For example, when a client goes into shock, epinephrine is released to stimulate glycogen release. In clients without DM, insulin and its counter-regulatory hormones maintain the body in homeostasis. Some researchers believe that diabetic clients produce abnormal amounts of one or all of these hormones. Many interconnected variables are responsible for DM; there is no single cause.

ℰTIOLOGY AND CLASSIC SYMPTOMS

There are often several factors that may predispose clients to DM, including age (over 40 years), obesity, stress, and a family history of diabetes. In some clients, a specific event such as a viral infection may be the precipitating factor. Genetic, autoimmune, viral, and environmental factors have all been linked to diabetes.

DM sometimes has familial components, but the exact genetic pattern of inheritance is currently unknown. The patterns of transmission are unpredictable and seem to depend on economic, social, emotional, or biological factors. Future DNA research may provide more answers.

The classic symptoms of DM are known as the "three Ps": *polyuria* (increased urination), *polydipsia* (increased thirst), and *polyphagia* (increased hunger). In a client with DM, glucose cannot pass through the cell membrane into the intracellular space to be metabolized, resulting in polyphagia. As the blood glucose level rises, the glucose-saturated blood circulates through the kidneys. Once the renal threshold is reached, usually at a concentration of 160–180 mg/dL, glucose enters the urine as a result of osmosis, causing glycosuria. With glycosuria, water excretion increases as a result of the osmotic effect, resulting in polyuria. The large amount of water lost by the kidneys causes excessive thirst, or polydipsia.

Diabetes was first described by the ancient Greeks as early as the first century A.D. Diabetes is derived from the Greek word for "passing through," and originates from the description of polyuria, or the excessive urine "passed through."

CASE STUDY: CLASSIC SYMPTOMS OF DIABETES MELLITUS

A young college student with undiagnosed type I DM drank eight glasses of water at one meal and had three helpings of food at dinner. Her roommate was astonished by her friend's appetite, particularly because she had just remarked that she had recently lost 15 lbs. At the roommate's urging, the student visited the student health center for an evaluation, which revealed suspected type I DM.

This young woman's body was literally starved for energy because carbohydrates were unable to enter the cells. These starved cells alert the brain, and the client experiences increased appetite (polyphagia). Despite the excessive hunger and thirst, the client most often loses weight. Other common presenting signs and symptoms of DM are blurred vision, fatigue, and recurrent vaginitis or bladder infections.

In June 1997, the American Diabetes Association (ADA) Expert Committee on the Diagnosis and Classification of Diabetes Mellitus released new criteria for the classification and diagnosis of DM, particularly as it relates to the fasting blood sugar (FBS) levels. DM is unique in that it is actually defined and diagnosed by laboratory values; however, a diagnosis cannot be made based on one abnormal laboratory value. When an abnormal value is found, the client should be tested again on the following day. The ADA criteria for the diagnosis of DM that must be present on two occasions are:

1. Symptoms of DM plus a random blood sugar level greater than or equal to 200 mg/dL.
2. FBS level greater than or equal to 126 mg/dL (fasting at least 8 hours).
3. Glucose tolerance test (GTT) result greater than or equal to 200 mg/dL 2 hours postglucose load (ADA, 1997).

It is important for practitioners and nurses to understand that, as a result of research, the FBS level as an indicator for DM was lowered from 140 mg/dL to 126 mg/dL, which is equivalent to a 2-hour GTT greater than or equal to 200 mg/dL. Also, FBS levels between 110 and 126 mg/dL are now considered a new diagnostic category, impaired fasting glucose (IFG). The ADA Expert Committee recommends screening asymptomatic individuals with the FBS rather than the GTT because it is easier, faster, more economical, convenient, and more acceptable to the client. To facilitate early detection of DM, screening is recommended for all adults 45 years and older, and if results are normal, the FBS should be checked at 3-year intervals. Screening guidelines should always be adapted to the individual client, and testing at a younger age or more frequent testing should be considered for clients with obesity, first-degree relatives with DM, delivery of a baby weighing more than 9 lbs, or a previous FBS identifying impaired fasting glucose (Zinman, 1997). Quite often, a client has been diabetic for a long period before seeking health care. The situation is often brought to the attention of the client by pure coincidence. Because the symptoms are so frequently overlooked, screening blood sugar levels according to the ADA guidelines are recommended for the early detection and treatment of DM.

CASE STUDY: COINCIDENTAL DIAGNOSIS OF DIABETES MELLITUS

A 9-year-old child was treated in an emergency room for various accidents over a 3-month period. During the fifth emergency room visit, the client required sutures for a laceration on his foot that he received when he fell. When the child had to interrupt the suturing four times to urinate, a nurse had the sound clinical judgment to check his blood sugar. The child's blood sugar was over 600 mg/dL. Extreme hyperglycemia had likely caused blurred vision and an altered sensorium, contributing to the child's previous falls and accidents.

CLASSIFICATION

There are two types of DM, type I and type II (Table 11-1). An earlier classification of DM, based primarily on the clinical presentation and type of treatment, was found by the ADA Expert Committee to have significant shortcomings. The terms insulin-dependent diabetes mellitus (IDDM) and non–insulin dependent diabetes mellitus (NIDDM) created confusion regarding the requirement for insulin because approximately 40% of clients with NIDDM require insulin therapy for disease management (Zinman, 1997). The new classification is based on disease etiology and pathology. Type I DM occurs with beta-cell destruction, usually leading to absolute insulin deficiency. Type II DM may range from predominantly insulin resistance with relative insulin deficiency to a predominantly secretory defect with insulin resistance (ADA, 1997). The classification for gestational DM remains the same. Most importantly, many clients with any form of DM may require insulin treatment at some stage of their disease. Therefore, classification as type I or type II is more accurate. Use of insulin does not by itself classify the client. This new classification highlights the underlying pathology as opposed to the clinical presentation of DM.

☒

TABLE 11-1

COMPARISON OF TYPE I AND TYPE II DIABETES MELLITUS

	Type I	Type II[ab]
Classification	Absolute insulin deficiency	See below.
Incidence	5–10% of diabetics	90–95% of diabetics
Age at onset	During childhood, under 20 years of age	Adult, over 40 years of age
Weight	Often underweight	Often overweight
Medications	Insulin required daily or insulin with oral hypoglycemic agents	Oral hypoglycemic agents Diet and exercise alone Insulin as needed
Self-monitoring blood glucose	4–8 times daily	1–2 times a day or 3 times a week
Acute complications	Prone to diabetic ketoacidosis	Prone to HHNC,[c] especially the elderly
Diet therapy	Integrate diet, exercise, and insulin Regular meals timed with insulin	Weight loss desirable

[a] Insulin resistance with deficiency.
[b] Secretory defect with insulin resistance.
[c] HHNC–hyperglycemic hyperosmolar nonketotic coma

Type I DM

In this type of DM, insulin production is reduced or absent, and insulin must be replaced. The onset of hyperglycemic symptoms is more abrupt and their progression more rapid. The client cannot survive without daily insulin injections. Type I DM was previously termed juvenile diabetes; since clients of all ages can require treatment with insulin, this term is no longer used. The onset of type I DM does, however, occur most commonly during childhood. Of the clients with Type I DM, 5–10% are insulin-dependent (Lutz & Przytulski, 1997).

After a client is diagnosed with type I DM and treated with insulin, the DM often goes into remission; this is the so-called *honeymoon phase*. Some researchers believe that this remission is the result of a final effort of the failing pancreas to produce insulin. Little or no exogenous insulin is required during this phase. The honeymoon phase can last up to 1 year, after which an increase in the amount of administered insulin is required. It is crucial for the nurse to explain this physiologic process to clients and their families, to prevent false expectations regarding their disease and the need for insulin.

Type II DM

Type II DM is the more common form of DM of which there are two sub-types, *obese* and *nonobese*. A strong genetic factor for type II DM exists, and it usually occurs in clients over 40 years of age, especially if they are overweight. When a client is overweight, the number of insulin receptors is decreased. Peripheral insulin resistance is a pathophysiologic factor linked to type II DM. This occurs when the pancreas secretes insulin, but the body cannot use it effectively. In some clients, there is reduced production of insulin. In other clients, there may be insulin overproduction but a decreased insulin response and abnormal hepatic glucose regulation.

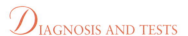

DIAGNOSIS AND TESTS

Few chronic conditions are diagnosed, defined, and managed by laboratory values to the extent that DM is. Therefore, the nurse must be knowledgeable about laboratory tests, related physiology, and the client education needed for each test. The laboratory tests required for clients with DM are summarized below.

Fasting Blood Sugar (FBS)

Blood glucose values differ depending upon the source of the sample, the site where it was obtained, the timing in relation to meals, and the time of day. Arterial and capillary plasma are higher in glucose than whole or

Prevention of Type II DM. Most clients with Type II DM are overweight and lead sedentary lives. The foods that many Americans eat are directly involved in heart disease, DM, and cancer. Performing physical activity for 30 minutes three to four times a week, decreasing the amount of fat consumed, maintaining an ideal body weight, and eating a balanced diet can prevent Type II DM.

Gestational DM. DM during pregnancy is diagnosed by a glucose tolerance test at approximately 24 weeks gestation. Individuals with gestational DM have a 25% risk of developing DM later in life. Preventive lifestyle behaviors are essential to decrease the incidence of DM as clients age.

venous blood. Glucose values are higher in the postprandial period (after meals) and in the late afternoon. For each decade after 50 years of age, add 10 mg/dL to the normal level of 70–120 mg/dL glucose. Because accuracy is essential, several tests of a client's blood sugar concentration are necessary before establishing the diagnosis of DM. Glucose values defining a diagnosis of DM are discussed under Etiology and Classic Symptoms.

Home Glucose Monitoring

Clients should use a glucose-monitoring device to follow their blood sugar pattern. Clients use a lancet to prick their finger and place a drop of blood on the monitor strip. Within 1 minute, the value of the capillary blood glucose is known. For certain clients, the physician or nurse practitioner will order regular administration of insulin if the blood glucose value reaches a certain level. Other clients with type I DM become expert enough in their own management to adjust their insulin dose themselves according to their glucose concentration, diet, and activity.

Urine Test for Glucose and Acetone

Whether this test is performed depends on age, severity of the DM, and renal function. In general, if the blood glucose is 160–180 mg/dL, the renal threshold has been reached, and glucose appears in the urine at a level of 1+ or above. Measuring glucose levels in urine is not as reliable as measuring blood glucose levels; therefore, urine testing for glucose no longer has a major role in the laboratory analysis for diabetes. Under conditions of ketoacidosis, acetone testing is useful to monitor ketones in the urine (ketonuria). Ketonuria occurs when excess ketones enter the urine as a result of diabetic hyperglycemia, which is characterized by a marked increase in serum ketones from the increased metabolism of fat to meet energy demands, rather than carbohydrates. Ketonuria is a hallmark of diabetic ketoacidosis.

Cholesterol and Triglycerides

When insulin is not functioning, blood levels of lipid, cholesterol and triglyceride are elevated. This is associated with vascular complications of DM. Nurses should frequently monitor levels of total cholesterol, high-density lipoproteins (HDLs), and low-density lipoproteins (LDLs). Exercise and dietary changes can help prevent atherosclerosis. Cholesterol-lowering medications may also be required.

Glycosylated Hemoglobin (HbA$_{1c}$)

Measurement of the HbA$_{1c}$ level is an indicator of the glucose level over the past 3 months; it reflects trends in client compliance and management of glucose levels. Normally, the HbA$_{1c}$ is 5–7% glucose. If the blood glucose level is elevated over time or fluctuates widely, the amount of glucose attached to the hemoglobin molecule increases. Glucose remains attached to the red blood cell (RBC) for the life of the cell (120 days). Therefore, HbA$_{1c}$ shows the glucose control for the past 90 days. Levels of 4–8% are considered normal for adults (Pagana & Pagana, 1995). The goal is to maintain HbA$_{1c}$ levels of 6–7% in the diabetic client. A HbA$_{1c}$ level of 6% is equivalent to an average blood sugar of 110 mg/dL. A HbA$_{1c}$ of 10% is equivalent to 250 mg/dL.

The HbA$_{1c}$ level has many advantages. The blood sample can be drawn at any time; it is the best way to evaluate the success of treatment or response to changes in treatment. The HbA$_{1c}$ level gives clients one number as a goal and it provides a reward for self-management. It gives clients a feeling of control over their DM. It is useful in determining the severity of hyperglycemia before the DM was diagnosed.

Proteinuria

Proteinuria is a sign of early nephropathy. A microalbuminuria analysis is now recommended for the early detection of nephropathy, followed by a 24-hour urine test for creatinine clearance and serum creatinine.

Doppler Studies

Doppler studies are performed to diagnose peripheral vascular disease. These studies use amplified sound to demonstrate blood flow velocity. Vascular changes result in decreased lumen size, compromised blood flow, and consequent tissue ischemia (Phipps et al., 1995).

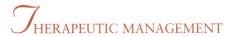

THERAPEUTIC MANAGEMENT

The goal of treatment of clients with both type I and type II DM is to keep the client as euglycemic as possible. *Euglycemia* is literally "good" sugar, or a serum glucose at the normal level of 70–120 mg/dL. Like hypertension, DM is a condition that is managed, not cured. The management of clients with DM is most effective when an individualized educational program for the client and family is supported by the entire health team. The physician, nurse practitioner, dietitian, social worker, diabetic nurse educator, ophthalmologist, and podiatrist are valuable members of the diabetic care team. The four major components of care that must be addressed by the diabetic team are diet, education of the client and family regarding self-management skills, exercise, and medications. The overall goals of therapy are (1) to correct metabolic abnormalities of DM and (2) to prevent long-term microvascular and macrovascular complications (Zinman, 1997, p. 20).

Diet

Because clients with DM are unable to metabolize food properly, it is natural that nutrition is an important component of treatment. General nutritional guidelines for diabetics are essentially the same as for anyone who follows a healthy diet and life style. The *food pyramid guide* (USDA, 1992) is a useful tool for nutrition counseling. Approximately 55–60% of calories in a diet should be from carbohydrates. Most of these are complex carbohydrates, which are easily broken down for energy. About 20% of calories should be from protein and less than 30% from fat. The diet should contain 10–15 g of fiber. The diet should be balanced and contain fruits, vegetables, oats, whole grains, and legumes. The American Diabetic Association (ADA) diet is composed of exchange lists of six categories: milk, meat, vegetables, fats, breads, and fruits.

The nurse should weigh the client and take a thorough history, as dietary needs are calculated according to ideal body weight (IBW), occupation, age, and activities. A dietary consultation is done when the client is newly diagnosed, and the nurse reinforces the information the client has received. Dietary consultations should be included periodically in the long-term treatment plan to aid clients in self-management. Home health nurses, diabetic nurse educators, and nurses working in ambulatory care need to work closely with the client, family, and health care team members to tailor the treatment to the client's daily behaviors. The daily schedule of meals, sleep patterns, and favorite activities needs to be incorporated into the diabetic individual's dietary, exercise, and life-style plans. This is an important way of individualizing and enhancing the treatment plan (Lubkin, 1997).

Education for the Client and Family Regarding Self-Management Skills

Education of the client and family regarding self-management skills is very important. Learning to live with DM is a lifelong process. The major principles that nurses should teach to clients and their families are given below.

Diet The client should be instructed never to skip meals and to eat at regular intervals. Foods should be chosen from the food pyramid guide and divided into three meals and two snacks a day. The prescribed diet should limit salt, sugar, fat, and alcohol. Alcohol consumption may cause hypoglycemia, but if the diabetic does imbibe, a dry light wine is best. Special diet foods are expensive and unnecessary. The client should avoid foods with sugar, mannitol, or sorbitol listed as the first two ingredients. Artificial sweeteners can be used, and the client should carry a sugar source at all times for emergency use.

Identification The nurse should encourage the use of a Medic Alert bracelet or other identification tag which, in case of an emergency, identifies the client as a diabetic.

Foot Care The client should inspect the feet and legs daily for sores, redness, infection, or drainage and report suspicious lesions to the physician, nurse practitioner or podiatrist. The feet should be kept clean and dry, and sturdy, comfortable shoes should be worn.

Glucose Monitoring Self-monitoring has revolutionized the ability of clients to maintain euglycemia. Clients need to be taught how to monitor themselves and how to check the quality control of the monitor to ensure continued accuracy of the machine. Clients with type I DM may need to monitor themselves four to eight times daily.

Follow-up Care The ADA recommends that clients with type I DM undergo measurement of HbA_{1c} levels every 3 months. Therefore, it is generally accepted that these clients should be evaluated every 3 months by a physician or nurse practitioner. An annual examination with a board-certified ophthalmologist is also recommended.

Exercise

Exercise should be nonstressful and performed regularly. Research studies have indicated that clients are more apt to exercise consistently if they like the activity and if they exercise with someone else. Exercise assists in weight loss, reduces triglycerides and total cholesterol, increases muscle tone, improves circulation, and contributes to an overall sense of well-being. Exercise also promotes the passage of insulin into the cells to metabolize carbohydrates for energy. Blood sugars should be checked before and after exercise. Lower doses of insulin are used when the client is exercising. Exercise should be performed 1.5 hours after meals when the glucose level is highest. For every 1 hour of strenuous exercise, the diabetic should eat a 10–15 g carbohydrate snack.

Medications

Insulin, sliding scale insulin, and oral hypoglycemic agents (OHAs) are the most commonly used medications for the treatment of DM. A more in-depth review of these medications, as found in pharmacology textbooks, is recommended.

Insulin Insulin is a protein. Usually 2–4 insulin injections daily are required for clients with type I DM. The exogenous insulin may be used temporarily in clients with type II DM during surgery, stress, or when diet, exercise, or OHAs fail.

Once opened, a vial of insulin can be stored at room temperature in a cool, dry place for 4 weeks. Many clients use a vial of insulin within 1 month. If the insulin has not been finished after 4 weeks, it should be refrigerated. Insulin should never be frozen.

Diabetics Seeking Care from Primary Practitioners. In 1996, DM was the second most common reason for seeking care with a primary practitioner, the most common being hypertension (*Levin's 1996 Year in Review*).

When a nurse administers insulin to a client in the hospital setting, policy requires that it be double-checked by another nurse. The insulin containers, the syringe containing the insulin, and the original order should be checked to ensure accuracy. If a diabetic client is going to have surgery, the nurse must ask the surgeon or anesthesiologist prior to the client's surgery if the morning insulin should be given and if the sliding scale should be used. Frequently, the diabetic client about to undergo surgery receives a decreased dose of insulin.

Various syringes are available, but the U 100 (100 units/1 mL) is most commonly used. Insulin is administered subcutaneously. The fastest and most effective absorption occurs in the abdomen, deltoid, thigh, and buttock. To protect tissues over time and prevent lipodystrophy, the site of injection is changed every few weeks. For example, the client should use different sites in the abdomen for 3 weeks and then rotate to the deltoid region. If the client engages in an activity or exercise that focuses on one area of the body, it is best to avoid using that site because of the possibility of inconsistent absorption of insulin. For example, clients who jog prefer the abdomen to the legs, because the movement of the legs in jogging results in inconsistent absorption.

Insulin pumps provide a continuous insulin infusion subcutaneously. A bolus can be injected prior to meals. The needles are changed every 48–72 hours. The advantage of the continuous infusion pump is that it closely mimics the body's normal insulin secretion. Clients using insulin pumps must be very committed to strict self-management programs.

Humulin Insulin Humulin insulin is produced by genetically altering common bacteria by recombinant DNA technology. It exhibits chemical and biological properties identical to the insulin produced by the human body. Because it has a more predictable insulin action and reduced allergic response, humulin insulin is now used for most newly diagnosed type I DM clients. Humulin insulin is available in regular, lente (insulin zinc suspension), NPH (Neutral Protamine Hagedorn, modified insulin composed of insulin, protamine, and zinc), ultralente (extended suspension), and Humalog. The newer Humalog insulin begins to act within 10–15 minutes and lasts approximately 4 hours. A major advantage of Humalog is that the client can begin eating almost immediately after the insulin is administered. Two combinations of humulin insulin are 70/30 (70% NPH and 30% regular) and 50/50 (50% NPH and 50% regular) (see Table 11-2). In general, the 70/30 combination is useful for elderly clients, clients with visual difficulties, or clients who have difficulty following a sliding scale plan. Other clients usually benefit from a more specific combination of insulin based on their individual needs, with daily adjustments according to their blood glucose levels, diet, exercise, and the presence of infections or other stressors.

Iletin Insulin Iletin insulin is commonly obtained from the pancreas of pigs and cows. Pork (pig) insulin is very similar to human insulin. Purified pork (pig) insulin has had almost all extraneous pancreatic proteins removed. These types of insulin differ in origin, purity, onset, peak, and duration of action.

TABLE 11-2
Time Cycles of Various Types of Insulin

Type of Insulin[a]	Onset	Peak	Duration	Appearance
SHORT-ACTING				
Lilly				
Regular Iletin (B/P)	½–1 hour	2–4 hours	6–8 hours	Clear
Regular Iletin II (P)	"	"	"	"
(R)Regular Humulin (H)	"	"	"	"
Novo Nordisk				
Regular (P)	"	"	"	"
Velosulin (H)	"	"	"	"
(R)Regular Novolin (H)	"	"	"	"
(R)Regular Pen-fill	"	"	"	"
INTERMEDIATE-ACTING				
Lilly				
(R)NPH Humulin (H)	1–2 hours	4–12 hours	10–14+ hours	Cloudy
NPH Iletin I (BP)	"	"	"	"
NPH Iletin II (P)	"	"	"	"
(R)Lente Humulin (H)	2 hours	8–12 hours	12–16+ hours	"
Lente Iletin I (BP)	"	"	"	"
Lente Iletin II (P)	"	"	"	"
Novo Nordisk				
(R)NPH Novolin (H)	1–2 hours	4–12 hours	10–14+ hours	Cloudy
(R)NPH Pen-fill (H)	"	"	"	"
NPH Purified (P)	"	"	"	"
NPH Standard (B)	"	"	"	"
(R)Lente Novolin (H)	2 hours	8–12 hours	12–16+ hours	"
Lente Purified (P)	"	"	"	"
MIXTURE OF NPH/REGULAR				
Lilly				
(R)70/30 Humulin (H)	Short and	Short and	Short and	Cloudy
(R)50/50 Humulin (H)	intermediate	intermediate	intermediate	"
Novo Nordisk				
(R)70/30 Novolin (H)	"	"		Cloudy
(R)70/30 Novolin Pen-fill (H)	"	"	"	"
70/30 Mixtard (P)	"	"	"	"
LONG-ACTING				
Lilly				
(R)Ultralente Humulin (H)	8 hours	18 hours	24–36 hours	Cloudy

[a]Onset and duration differ across time range according to different brands. They can also differ from person to person.
Source: From *Medical-Surgical Nursing Concepts and Clinical Practice* (p. 1296), by W. Phipps, V. Cassmeyer, J. Sands, & M. K. Lehman, 1995, St. Louis: C. V. Mosby. Reprinted with permission.
NOTE: P = pork; B/P = beef and pork; B = beef; H = human (both Eli Lilly [human] and Novo Nordisk [human] are of recombinant DNA origin); R = recombinant DNA.

Regular Insulin Regular insulin is fast acting and is the only insulin that can be given intravenously. All types of insulin begin with regular insulin as a base. Zinc is added to make lente insulin, and zinc and protamine are added to make NPH and PZI (protamine zinc insulin). These additives prolong the action of insulin. Clients are instructed to take insulin 20–30 minutes prior to meals to ensure that the onset of action coincides with meal absorption. After the administration of regular insulin, the onset of activity occurs in 0.5–1 hour, peaks in 2–3 hours, and lasts 4–6 hours. Since the half-life of intravenous insulin is 4 minutes, it is usually given in a continuous infusion.

Sliding Scale Insulin Sliding scale insulin is given in response to the glucose value that is obtained from monitoring glucose before meals and at bedtime. It is important to remember that the parameters always vary among practitioners. An example of a sliding scale order is shown in Table 11-3.

Adverse Effects All medications have side effects and adverse effects. While most clients with type I DM take insulin for years without untoward effects, nurses and clients need to be aware of its complications. Insulin has five major adverse effects.

Allergic reactions are of three major types:

- **Local reaction.** This consists of itching and erythema at the injection site that usually resolves within a few days. Another source of insulin (new species) may be used.
- **Systemic response.** This is an anaphylactic reaction and may be life-threatening. The client should seek emergency care immediately.
- **Resistance response.** This is the result of antibodies binding to insulin molecules and rendering them inactive. This response is seen with clients who require over 100 units a day.

Lipodystrophy is an atrophy or hypertrophy of the subcutaneous tissue at the injection site. It is rarely seen in conjunction with Humulin insulin. The nurse and client can avoid this problem by rotating the injection sites.

⬕

TABLE 11-3

GLUCOSE MONITORING WITH SLIDING SCALE INSULIN
AT 0730 (7:30 A.M.), 1130 (11:30 A.M.), 1630 (4:30 P.M.), AND
2100 (9:00 P.M.)

Blood Glucose	Regular Insulin[a]
0–150 mg/dL	No insulin administered
151–200 mg/dL	Administer 5 units
201–250 mg/dL	Administer 10 units
251–300 mg/dL	Administer 15 units
> 300 mg/dL	Call the physician for orders

[a]The nurse or the client administers regular insulin if the blood glucose reaches the levels above at the stated times.

The *Somogyi effect* consists of alternating periods of hyper- and hypoglycemia in early morning and after meals. Counterregulatory hormones are released that produce rebound hyperglycemia and ketosis. Clients often make adjustments by increasing the dose of insulin when they should actually be treated with less. Clients may experience night sweats, nightmares, or headaches.

In the *dawn phenomenon* fasting blood sugar is increased in the morning, and ketonuria may be present. This is attributable to the morning release of cortisol or growth hormone, counterregulatory hormones that raise blood sugar. This phenomenon may require an increase in the dose of insulin and is very common.

A *hypoglycemic reaction* can be precipitated by too much insulin, skipping meals, or other metabolic changes. Initially, clients experience feelings of hunger, nausea, diaphoresis, and bradycardia. The counterregulatory hormone epinephrine is released, causing clients to experience lethargy, diaphoresis, nervousness, tremors, palpitations, irritability, and mood changes. Clients may appear intoxicated. If not treated promptly, death can occur as a result of damage done to the brain as glucose is the only nutrient that crosses the blood–brain barrier and provides energy to the brain. Untreated hypoglycemia eventually causes double vision, convulsions, coma, and sometimes death as a result of the insult to the brain cells (Fig. 11-1).

Hypoglycemia is treated by giving client 4 oz of orange juice or apple juice immediately, if they are awake and able to swallow. Drinking a glass of milk after the orange juice is an effective way to stabilize carbohydrate metabolism by preventing the "roller coaster" secondary hypoglycemic effects. Milk is also effective instead of orange juice if the hypoglycemic reaction is at an early stage. If the client is unresponsive, 0.5–1 mg glucagon should be administered intramuscularly, subcutaneously or intravenously. In the hospital setting, a frequently used treatment is to administer 50 mL of 50% dextrose intravenous push into a large vein in hypoglycemic emergencies when the client is unresponsive. Response to the treatment can take 5–10 minutes. After the client is awake, appropriate food is ordered immediately to prevent secondary hypoglycemia. The physician may order the subcutaneous administration of 0.5–1 mL of epinephrine (1:1000) as this stimulates the conversion of glycogen to glucose.

Diabetic education programs always include specific plans for clients to follow when they recognize the onset of a hypoglycemic reaction. Diabetics should always carry foods rich in carbohydrates that are quickly available for emergencies. The nurse should instruct clients to monitor their glucose. When the level is less than 60 mg/dL or at the first signs of hypoglycemia, the client should drink 4 oz of juice or a glass of milk. The glucose should be rechecked in 15 minutes. The clients' families and significant others should also be educated about hypoglycemia and its treatment.

CASE HISTORY: INSULIN-DEPENDENT DIABETES MELLITUS

Mr. J., age 22, has had type I DM for the past 10 years. Recently, he was hospitalized for an infected ulceration on his right foot. Prior to admission he took 20 units of Humulin N at 8 A.M. and 7 units at

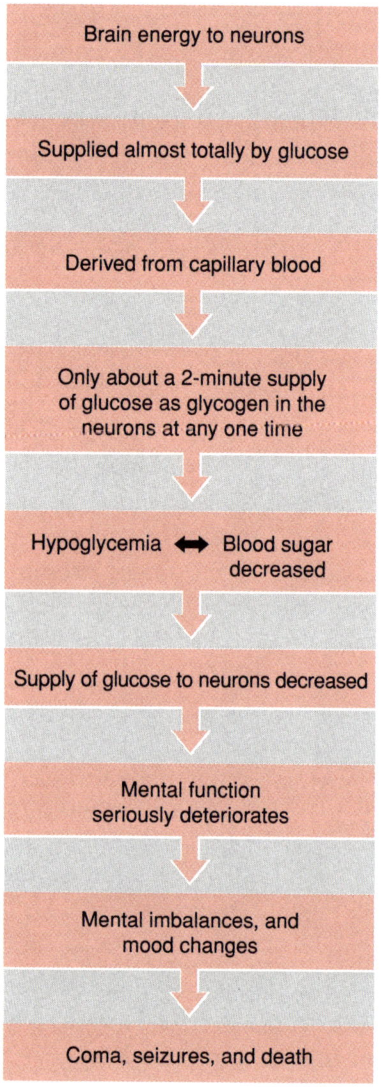

FIGURE 11-1 Effects of hypoglycemia on the brain

7:30 P.M. He checked his blood sugar four times a day, at 7:30 A.M.,
11:30 A.M., 4:30 P.M., and 9:00 P.M. and used the following sliding
scale according to his physician's order:

Blood Glucose	Humulin R (regular insulin)
0–150 mg/dL	No coverage
151–200 mg/dL	5 units
201–250 mg/dL	7 units
251–300 mg/dL	10 units
> 300 mg/dL	Call the physician

While in the hospital, at 7:30 A.M., his FBS was 148 mg/dL. The nurse injected 20 units of Humulin N U100 insulin into the client's abdomen subcutaneously. He manages himself on a 2000 calorie ADA diet and follows it exactly. He is a gardener by trade and is very active every day. When he checked his blood sugar at 4:30 P.M., it was 74 mg/dL. At 7:30 P.M., the nurse gave the client 7 units of Humulin N insulin and injected it subcutaneously into his abdomen. He continued with his diet according to proper exchanges and then watched television. At 9:00 P.M., he said that he felt nervous, nauseated, and hypoglycemic. The nurse realized that the blood sugar should be checked immediately, and if it was at 60 mg/dL or below, (it was 62 mg/dL) provides 4 oz of orange juice or some hard candy, or glipizide (Glucotrol) is ordered IM or SC by the physician. After the client had eaten a snack, the nurse rechecked the blood sugar. If the symptoms disappeared and the blood sugar approached normal limits, no further action would be necessary. If after 10 minutes the symptoms persisted and if the client's blood sugar was still low, the 4 oz of orange juice should be given again and the process repeated until the blood sugar was within normal limits (it was 72 mg/dL).

The next morning, the FBS was 68 mg/dL, and the client was asymptomatic. The nurse correctly advised the client to inject his morning insulin and to eat his breakfast since the NPH insulin does not peak until early afternoon. He then felt dizzy at 1 P.M., at which point his blood sugar was 290 mg/dL. The nurse contacted the physician, who ordered 10 units of regular insulin as a one-time order immediately. At 4:30 P.M. the client checked his blood sugar, and it was 249 mg/dL. The nurse correctly advised the client to inject 7 units of Humulin R subcutaneously.

Oral Hypoglycemic Agents These drugs are not oral insulin. Insulin is administered subcutaneously; otherwise it would be inactivated by enzymes in the stomach and gastrointestinal tract before it could be absorbed. OHAs (sulfonylureas) stimulate the pancreas to produce insulin and increase insulin sensitivity to receptors on insulin-sensitive tissues. First-generation OHAs include tolbutamide (Orinase), acetohexamide (Dymelor), chlorpropamide (Diabinese), and tolazamide (Tolinase). Second-generation OHAs include glipizide (Glucotrol) and glyburide (Micronase) (Table 11-4). Second-generation OHAs require lower doses and have fewer side effects. Clients who are 20% over their ideal body weight may not respond to oral hypoglycemic agents. The ideal client for OHAs has type II DM, is nonobese, is over 40 years of age, and has had diabetes for less than 5 years.

OHAs taken with alcohol may produce an antabuse-type reaction resulting in nausea, vomiting, respiratory distress, flushing, and chest pain. OHAs are metabolized in the liver. Sulfonylureas are metabolized by the liver and excreted by the kidneys. Hypoglycemia is the most serious side effect of sulfonylureas. Side effects may include nausea, vomiting, diarrhea, skin allergies, and hematological disorders. Clients should be instructed never to double the dose of pills or skip meals.

TABLE 11-4

FIRST- AND SECOND-GENERATION ORAL HYPOGLYCEMIC AGENTS

Brand Name	Generic Name	When It Starts to Work	When It Works the Hardest	How Long It Works	Dose Range	Dose/ Day	Excretion
First Generation							
Orinase	Tolbutamide	1 hour	4–6 hours	6–12 hours	500–3000 mg	2–3	Kidney
Tolinase	Tolazamide	1 hour	4–8 hours	Approximately 24 hours	100–1000 mg	1	Kidney
Dymelor	Acetohexamide	1–2 hours	8–12 hours	Approximately 18 hours	250–1.5 g	1–2	Kidney
Diabinase	Chlorpropamide	1 hour	3–6 hours, up to 36 hours	Up to 60 hours	100–500 mg	1	Kidney
Second Generation							
Micronase	Glyburide (nonmicronized)	1 hour	4–8 hours	12–24 hours	1.25–20 mg	1–2	50% kidney 50% bile
Diabeta	Glyburide (nonmicronized)	1 hour	4–8 hours	12–24 hours	1.25–20 mg	1–2	50% kidney 50% bile
Glynase	Glyburide (micronized)	1 hour	2–6 hours	12–24 hours	1.5–12 mg	1–2	50% kidney 50% bile
Glucotrol[a]	Glipizide	10–30 minutes	1–3 hours	12–24 hours	2.5–40 mg	1–2	80% kidney 20% bile
Glucotrolyl	Glipizide extended release		Up to 24 hours	24 hours	5–20 mg	Once a day	Feces

[a] For best results take 30 minutes before eating. All other oral agents may be taken before eating. For all medications listed, action may vary from person to person.
Source: From *Medical-Surgical Nursing Concepts and Clinical Practice* (p. 1299), by W. Phipps, V. Cassmeyer, J. Sands, & M. K. Lehman, 1995, St. Louis: C. V. Mosby. Reprinted with permission.

Anticoagulants, salicylates, alcohol, and beta-blockers enhance the action of OHAs. Thyroid drugs, corticosteroids, and thiazide diuretics block OHA action. Thiazide diuretics potentiate hyperglycemia by increasing potassium loss.

Metformin (Glucophage), a newer agent, recently has been used to treat diabetics. Within the past 2 years, the simultaneous administration of insulin and oral agents such as metformin (Glucophage) has been successful in the treatment of clients with type I DM. Nurses need to remind clients with type I DM that this dual therapy does not eliminate the need for insulin. Combined drug therapy may decrease the insulin dosage required and increase the likelihood of improved management of blood sugars. Further research needs to be conducted on dual medication regimens that use both insulin and OHAs for type I DM.

COMPLICATIONS OF DIABETES

The ultimate goal of treatment for clients with type I DM or type II DM is to maintain steady blood glucose levels, to promote well-being, and prevent complications. However, even clients who are experts in self-management may undergo surgery, experience an unexpected accident, or contract an infection that can trigger complications. Complications of DM are classified as acute and chronic. Acute complications require immediate emergency treatment. Chronic complications involve insidious damage to the heart, vascular system, kidneys, eyes, and nervous system. The chronic complications that diabetics experience contribute to a diminished quality of life and increased morbidity and mortality. Strategies to promote compliance with treatment plans and to prevent complications remain a challenge to clients, researchers, practitioners, diabetic nurse educators, and social science theorists studying behavioral changes.

DM-related death rates are unchanged for the Caucasian population but have increased among African Americans, Native Americans, and Hispanics.

Acute Complications

Four acute complications are commonly seen in clients with DM: hyperglycemia, ketoacidosis, hyperglycemic hyperosmolar nonketotic coma (HHNC), and hypoglycemia.

Hyperglycemia During hyperglycemia, metabolic dysfunction occurs, which generates damaging by-products from glucose breakdown. Glucose abnormally binds to protein structures and affects the nerves and blood vessels. Hyperglycemia deprives the body of energy from carbohydrate sources. The body compensates by breaking down fat and protein for energy. Thus, hyperglycemia often occurs synergistically with another complication, ketoacidosis. Blood sugar values of 300–1000 mg/dL are seen in clients with both hyperglycemia and ketoacidosis.

Diabetic Ketoacidosis (DKA) DKA is an acute metabolic complication of DM. It may occur rapidly or take days or weeks. DKA is seen mostly in clients with type I DM. Fat and protein are broken down and used for energy when glucose is not available. Ketones are a by-product of fat metabolism, and the presence of excess ketones causes acidosis. An increase in the loss of water, potassium and other electrolytes (e.g. bicarbonate) further complicates the metabolic condition of clients with acidosis and hypokalemia. Clients with severe ketoacidosis can lose up to 7 L of fluid and 400–500 mEq of sodium, potassium, and chloride in 1 day (Lutz & Przytulski, 1997). Severe dehydration, hypovolemia, and hypokalemia may occur. The skin is dry and loose, the eyeballs are sunken in the orbits, and urine output is decreased. The client experiences hypotension with a rapid, weak pulse. Nausea and vomiting are common. With increasing serum ketones and acidosis, Kussmaul's respirations (rapid deep breathing with dyspnea) occur. This is a compensatory mechanism that removes carbonic acid by exhaling carbon dioxide. Acetone is noted on the client's breath as a sweet, fruity odor. Renal failure occurs from hypovolemic shock. Coma and death may follow if diabetic ketoacidosis is not treated.

Treatment of diabetic ketoacidosis involves astute emergency care. The severity of the hyperglycemia and ketonemia (high levels of ketones in the blood) determines the treatment plan. The nurse must maintain the airway. Intubation with mechanical ventilation may be required. The nurse should establish fluid and electrolyte balance and reestablish carbohydrate metabolism. Continuous intravenous infusion of insulin in saline solution is initiated. The nurse must be aware that 20%–50% of the insulin infusion will be lost because the tubing absorbs it. Fluids and electrolytes are replaced. Insulin is infused intravenously until the glucose level reaches 250 mg/dL. Once the blood sugar has decreased, food is given, and 5% dextrose in normal saline is administered to prevent secondary hypoglycemia and cerebral edema, which may accompany a rapid insulin-induced fall in blood sugar. The nurse then administers subcutaneous insulin on a sliding scale to maintain the glucose level. Electrolytes are monitored and replaced as necessary. Sodium bicarbonate is given only if the pH is less than 7.0 because acidosis may reverse too rapidly, which can result in hypokalemia with fatal dysrhythmias. Nursing care requires frequent monitoring of hydration, vital signs, urine output, electrocardiogram (ECG), blood glucose, ketone levels, lung sounds, and mental status.

Hyperglycemic Hyperosmolar Nonketotic Coma (HHNC) HHNC is typically seen in elderly clients with type II DM. It can occur in persons with undiagnosed or poorly managed type II DM and is usually precipitated by an event such as an illness or infection. It occurs when enough insulin is produced to prevent diabetic ketoacidosis but not to prevent severe hyperglycemia. Serum glucose levels may be 600 mg/dL or higher (Hudak & Gallo, 1994). Osmotic diuresis occurs as a result of the hyperglycemia, and extracellular fluid depletion follows. Fluids try to shift to the extracellular space, resulting in intracellular dehydration. Hypovolemia and shock may lead to seizures and coma.

HHNC, like diabetic ketoacidosis, is a medical emergency. Treatment requires greater fluid replacement than with diabetic ketoacidosis as the volume depletion is extreme. Intravenous fluids are initiated with 0.9% or 0.45% sodium chloride and infused at a rate of 6–20 L in the first 24 hours. The nurse must carefully monitor lung sounds, weight, vital signs, urine output and specific gravity, glucose level, and cardiac function. The volume of fluid replacement required places the client, especially the elderly client, at risk for cardiac complications and pulmonary edema. As with diabetic ketoacidosis, regular intravenous insulin infusion is given until the serum glucose level reaches 250 mg/dL, after which the sliding scale is used.

Hypoglycemia Hypoglycemia is defined by a fasting blood sugar of less than 50–60 mg/dL or when the client experiences hypoglycemic symptoms such as hunger, nausea, diaphoresis, and bradycardia. Symptoms occur when the glucose level falls below 60 mg/dL or when a high glucose level falls too rapidly (e.g. 300–180 mg/dL). Hypoglycemia can occur with too much insulin, too much exercise, or delayed eating. When in doubt, the client, family, or nurse should treat suspected hypoglycemia by giving the client sugar. Treatment of hypoglycemia has already been discussed.

Chronic Complications

Clients with either of type I or II DM are at risk for serious chronic complications of DM that occur as the disease progresses, especially when a normal blood sugar level is not consistently maintained. The following information details common chronic complications affecting the heart and vascular system, eyes, kidneys, and nervous system.

Angiopathy Angiopathy is a complication that occurs when blood vessels become damaged. Peripheral vascular disease with clotting abnormalities is a frequent cause of skin ulcerations, infection, gangrene, and amputation. Signs and symptoms of intermittent claudication include leg pain at rest, cold feet, loss of hair on the extremities, delayed capillary refill, and diminished pulses. The diagnosis is established by Doppler and angiographic studies to confirm the extent of vascular and microvascular damage. Treatment includes a comprehensive program to control cholesterol and triglycerides, treat hypertension, avoid smoking, and improve the management of DM. Antibiotics are given when an infection is present. Only some of these clients are candidates for vascular surgical repairs.

Diabetic Retinopathy Diabetic retinopathy occurs because of microaneurysms in the retinal vessels followed by hemorrhage and exudate formation. Retinopathy is a leading cause of visual loss and blindness in the United States and the leading cause of blindness in diabetics. Currently, 80% of clients who have been diabetic for at least 15 years suffer from retinopathy to some degree. Treatment consists of laser photocoagulation to stop the hemorrhage or vitrectomy to aspirate blood, membranes, and fibers from the inside of the eye. The ADA recommends that all diabetics have a yearly examination by a board-certified ophthalmologist. In addition, improved management of blood sugars using home monitoring and HbA_{1c} levels as parameters may decrease the incidence of blindness in diabetics. The diabetic is also at higher risk for cataracts and glaucoma.

Nephropathy Nephropathy is a kidney disease characterized by the development of degenerative lesions in the nephrons and may result in renal failure. The treatment for end-stage renal disease is dialysis. A kidney transplant may be performed if the client is a suitable candidate.

Neuropathy Neuropathy, the most common chronic complication of DM, is defined as any disease of the nerves. Clients frequently complain about pain and paresthesias (tingling, burning, itching) in their legs. The neuropathy is often worse at night. Clients frequently complain of lack of feeling in their extremities. For example, a blister may form and become infected, but the client will not feel any pain. A podiatrist is recommended for care of the foot and toenails. Nerve damage may occur in all tissues and organs. Therefore, complications may include abnormal gastric motility, erectile function, bladder function, and vascular tone. Impotence occurs in 30–60% of diabetic men as a result of nerve damage. A neurogenic bladder causes urine retention, difficulty in voiding, and a weak stream. These clients are at high risk for urinary tract infection. Additional chronic complications that may occur are ulcers and necrosis, in which the lesions are slow to heal. Clients with DM are prone to infections of many types, which are difficult to treat because of neuropathies and vascular insufficiency. Common infections include *Candida albicans*, boils, and furuncles.

$\mathcal{S}$UMMARY

An estimated 12% of Latinos over the age of 21 years have DM (American Diabetes Association, 1992).

Screening programs for DM will aid in the early diagnosis and improve the treatment of diabetics of all ages and cultures. Clients with DM must have good self-care skills to be able to adjust their diet, exercise, life style, and medications. The prevention and early treatment of complications require the comprehensive efforts of clients, families, and the DM health care team. Diabetic clients should be taught to monitor their glucose level, administer insulin or OHAs, and adjust their diet. They should know when to call the physician (e.g. glucose > 300 mg/dL). The nurse should teach clients what to do when fever, ketonuria, nausea, or vomiting occur. Treatment plans should be individualized with the goal of maintaining euglycemia to decrease the likelihood of complications. For example, because of stress, infection, or imminent surgery, the type II DM client may need to discontinue OHAs and administer insulin on a sliding scale for approximately 48 hours. Diabetic complications are classified into the two major categories of acute and chronic. Acute complications require emergency medical treatment. Support for the diabetic from the community, family, or significant other increases the likelihood of successful management and avoidance of chronic complications. The ADA provides excellent resources such as pamphlets, books, and the bimonthly magazine *Diabetes Forecast*. Monthly diabetic support groups facilitated by diabetic nurse educators are offered in most cities.

KEY WORDS

Counterregulatory hormones
Dawn phenomena
Diabetes mellitus
Diabetic ketoacidosis
Diabetic retinopathy
Glycosylated hemoglobin
Honeymoon phase
Hyperglycemia
Hyperglycemic hyperosmolar
  nonketotic syndrome
Hypoglycemia
Insulin
Ketonuria

Kussmaul's respirations
Lipodystrophy
Nephropathy
Neuropathy
Oral hypoglycemic agents
Peripheral vascular disease
Polydipsia
Polyphagia
Polyuria
Somogyi effect
Type I DM
Type II DM

QUESTIONS

Questions 1 and 2

Mrs. K. has type I diabetes mellitus and has been diagnosed with hyperglycemia and diabetic ketoacidosis.

1. Which of the following findings best describe the clinical manifestations of diabetic ketoacidosis?

    A. Polydipsia, malaise, and dry mucous membranes
    B. Anxiety, polyuria, and fatigue
    C. Lethargy, nausea, vomiting, and ketone or fruity-like breath
    D. Increased heart rate, hypotension, and malaise

2. Mrs. K. is admitted to the hospital, and the nurse notes that she is experiencing Kussmaul's respirations. These may be described as

    A. deep respirations with long expirations.
    B. shallow respirations alternating with long expirations.
    C. regular depth of respirations with frequent pauses.
    D. short expirations and inspirations.

3. In the client experiencing hypoglycemia, there is usually a sudden onset of symptoms. Most often the nurse or client would find a blood glucose level of

   A. < 5 mg/dL.
   B. < 50 mg/dL.
   C. < 75 mg/dL.
   D. < 100 mg/dL.

ANSWERS

1. *The answer is C.* Hyperglycemia is present; therefore the body uses fat and protein stores for energy. Fatty acids are transported to the liver, where the production of ketone bodies is accelerated. Ketone bodies accumulate in the blood (ketonemia) and spill into the urine (ketonuria). Ketones are an acid source, and metabolic acidosis occurs. The fruity odor to the breath results from the respiratory excretion of the acetone. Lethargy and coma result from the effects of acidosis and dehydration.

2. *The answer is A.* During ketosis, the respirations increase in rate and depth, and the breath has a "fruity" or acetone-like odor. This breathing pattern is the body's attempt to blow off carbon dioxide and acetone, thus compensating for the acidosis.

3. *The answer is B.* Clinical manifestations of hypoglycemia usually occur when the blood glucose level is around 50 mg/dL.

ANNOTATED REFERENCES

American Diabetes Association (ADA). (1997). Report of the expert committee on the diagnosis and classification of diabetes mellitus. *Diabetes Care 20*(7), 1183–1197.

This report highlights the changes in the diagnosis and classification of DM. In order to improve the quality of care of clients affected by DM, there have been initiatives to establish standards and consistency in the diagnosis and management of DM worldwide.

Hudak, C. M., & Gallo, B. M. (1994). *Handbook of critical care nursing.* Philadelphia: J. B. Lippincott.

A quick reference on assessment, diagnosis, and care of clients with acute illness. Extensive care plan for clients with diabetic ketoacidosis is included.

Karch, A. M. (1996). *Lippincott's nursing drug guide.* Philadephia: J. B. Lippincott.

Drug monograph, listed alphabetically give the nurse important clinical information. The guide includes drug-specific teaching points.

Lubkin, I. L. (1995). *Chronic illness impact and interventions*. Boston: Jones and Bartlett.

This text focuses on the many factors and issues that impact clients and families dealing with chronic conditions, including DM. It is intended for upper-level students and gives important information on how nurses can assist in developing self-management skills in the chronically ill client.

Lutz, C. A., & Przytulski, K. R. (1997). *Nutrition and diet therapy*. Philadelphia: F. A. Davis.

This is a comprehensive text on nutrition that covers a carbohydrate educational approach developed by the American Dietetic and Diabetic Associations.

Pagana, K., & Pagana, T. (1995). *Diagnostic and laboratory test reference*. St. Louis: C. V. Mosby.

This reference text presents tests alphabetically for quick reference. It includes normal and abnormal findings. There is patient education information for each test.

Phipps W., Cassmeyer, V., Sands, J., & Lehman, M. K. (1995). *Medical-surgical nursing concepts and clinical practice*. St. Louis: C. V. Mosby.

This text is an extensive treatment of the alterations in the body systems and nursing care for common problems in ill adults. The text gives a detailed review.

Zinman, B. (1997). Guidelines for the management of type II diabetes. In J. Olefsky (Ed.), *Current approaches to the management of type II diabetes: A practical monograph* (pp. 19–22). National Diabetes Education Initiative: Professional Postgraduate Services.

The National Diabetes Education Initiative reports on the clinical practice recommendations and position statements of the ADA in this publication for healthcare professionals.

INTERNET SITES FOR ADDITIONAL INFORMATION

Academy for the Advancement of Diabetic Research and Treatment:
  http://drinet.med.miami.edu

American Association of Diabetic Educators:
  http://aadenet.org

American Diabetes Association:
  http://diabetes.org

Children with Diabetes:
  http://castleweb.com/diabetes/index.html

1996 Diabetes Clinical Practice Recommendations of the ADA:
http://www.ada.judds.com/magazine/diabetescare/Supplement/SUP1/htm

Diabetes News:
http://www.diabetesnews.com

National Institute of Diabetes and Digestive and Kidney Diseases (NIDDK):
http://www.niddk.nih.gov/

THE ENDOCRINE SYSTEM

INTRODUCTION

The endocrine system facilitates functions of the body by synthesizing and releasing **hormones**. For a hormone to act, the tissue or cell must have a receptor that is susceptible to the hormone. Endocrine system disorders are either primary or secondary. In primary disorders, the defect is in the gland producing the hormones, as in glandular tumors, autoimmune disease antibodies attacking the gland, or inborn errors of metabolism. Secondary disorders are directly related to increased or decreased stimulation of the **endocrine gland** by the specific stimulating hormone, as in hypothyroidism caused by a lack of thyroid-stimulating hormone (TSH) secretion (Fig. 12-1).

The endocrine system is complex. Nurses must gain experience in assessing clients and using laboratory test data and pharmacological resources to improve their practice skills in endocrinology. Nurses must learn to care for clients in a variety of settings by developing history-taking and assessment skills to identify the objective and subjective data about the chief complaints and health status of clients regarding disorders of the endocrine system. The nurse should be alert for signs of common endocrine disorders, the appropriate diagnostic laboratory tests to perform, and the pharmacological agents prescribed in the treatment of these disorders. Since many endocrine disorders are monitored by serum or urinary hormone concentrations, it is helpful to have a laboratory resource available in the clinical setting. The nurse should also be able to identify the physiological changes that occur in the endocrine system as a result of the aging

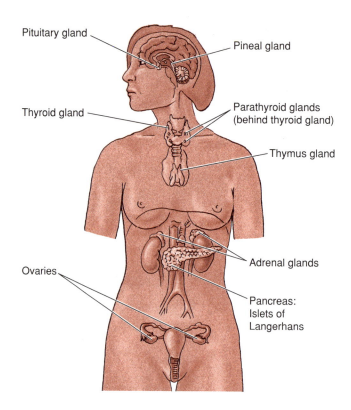

FIGURE 12-1

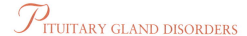

The location of the endocrine glands of the body.

process as well as the relationship between the endocrine system and other systems of the body.

*P*ITUITARY GLAND DISORDERS

Anterior Pituitary Gland Hyperfunction

The anterior pituitary gland secretes several hormones, one of which is growth hormone (Table 12-1). A benign pituitary adenoma can secrete excessive amounts of growth hormone. A growth-hormone secreting pituitary adenoma causes two major disorders: gigantism and acromegaly.

Gigantism Gigantism occurs in early childhood or puberty. When hypersecretion of growth hormone occurs in the pituitary, the client may grow to be 8 ft tall and may weigh over 300 lb. Many of these clients die in early adulthood.

Acromegaly Acromegaly occurs at 30–40 years of age. Hypersecretion of growth hormone results in enlargement of the hands, feet, nose, jaw, and forehead. The soft tissues also may be enlarged. The client complains of headaches and changes in vision. Hyperlipidemia, diabetes mellitus,

Hormone. A hormone is a chemical substance secreted by one cell or a group of cells. Hormones physiologically control other cells and organs of the body.

Endocrine Glands. The principal endocrine glands are the pituitary, pineal gland, thyroid, parathyroid, thymus, adrenal glands, pancreas, ovaries, and testes.

TABLE 12-1

ANTERIOR PITUITARY GLAND

Hormones	Functions
Growth hormone	Tissue growth and organic metabolism
Thyroid-stimulating hormone (TSH)	Synthesis and release of thyroid hormone from the thyroid gland
Adrenocorticotropic hormone (ACTH)	Secretion of corticosteroids from adrenal cortex
Gonadotropic hormones: follicle-stimulating hormone (FSH) and luteinizing hormone (LH)	Sex cell and hormone secretion
Prolactin or lactogen	Stimulation of milk production

increased excretion of urinary calcium, and an elevated blood phosphate concentration also may occur with acromegaly.

Diagnostic Studies The following actions should be taken to diagnose the endocrine disorder and its severity. The nurse should take a thorough history and physical examination, including height, weight, and measurement of head circumference and extremities. A plasma growth hormone concentration should be taken. Magnetic resonance imaging (MRI) with contrast is used to identify the tumor location. Other laboratory tests include fasting blood sugar (FBS), serum phosphate, 24-hour urinary calcium level, and cholesterol and triglyceride levels to identify hyperlipidemia.

Treatment Treatment consists of irradiating the adenoma or surgical excision (transsphenoidal pituitary surgery). The surgical options include a *hypophysectomy*, which is the removal of the entire anterior pituitary gland tissue, or an *adenectomy*, the removal of the pituitary adenoma (if the tumor is small). If a hypophysectomy is performed, the following medications must be taken for the duration of the client's life: glucocorticoid, thyroid hormone, and certain sex hormones. Pharmacological agents that may be used to return growth hormone levels to normal include a long-acting somatostatin analogue to suppress growth hormone secretion and bromocriptine (Parlodel), a dopamine agonist. Somatostatin and bromocriptine are used mainly when surgery and radiation are not successful.

Complications Complications of pituitary tumors include increased intracranial pressure (ICP) and compression of the optic chiasma or other brain tissues with resultant loss of vision. Postoperative **nursing care** includes monitoring for neurological complications every two hours or as ordered by the surgeon. Surgery may cause a disruption in the normal circulation of cerebrospinal fluid (CSF). Any signs of CSF leakage (glucose in nasal secretion), increasing temperature, or an increased white blood cell count may indicate meningitis and should be reported immediately. Sensory changes or other signs of increased ICP or neurological deficit also must be reported to the physician immediately. These clients often require an annual MRI to monitor the adenoma growth, and any deterioration in visual acuity should be reported to the physician for follow-up.

CASE STUDY: CLIENT WITH HYPERSECRETION OF THE ANTERIOR PITUITARY GLAND

Mr. S., 38 years of age, presents to an ambulatory clinic with the following symptoms: recurrent headaches unrelieved by over-the-counter (OTC) analgesics, diaphoresis, oily skin, peripheral neuropathy, and proximal muscle weakness. Upon examination, the physician notes enlargement of the feet, hands, and tongue. Laboratory test results are shown below. The normal parameters for adults are provided by Pagana & Pagana (1995).

Test	Client	Normal Laboratory Parameters: Adult
FBS	142 mg/dL	70–105 mg/dL
Insulin-like growth factor 1 (IGF-1)	186 mg/mL	42–110 mg/mL
Serum calcium	12 mg/dL	9.0–10.5 mg/dL
Serum phosphate	6 mg/dL	3.0–4.5 mg/dL

The client's vital signs are blood pressure, 158/98 mm Hg; temperature, 98.6°F; pulse, 82 beats/min; and 16 respirations/min. X-rays reveal that the sella turcica, mandible, and frontal sinuses are enlarged. MRI confirms the presence of a pituitary tumor, and a diagnosis of acromegaly is then made. To treat Mr. S.'s acromegaly, the physician performs a hypophysectomy.

Immediate postoperative **nursing care** involves monitoring the client's neurological status. The nurse must monitor the client's neurological signs every two hours or as ordered by the surgeon and report any changes in sensory or neurological condition. The client should be checked often for nasal drainage. If present, the drainage should be checked for the presence of glucose with glucose oxidase reagent strips. The presence of glucose may indicate a CSF leak, which must be reported immediately to the surgeon. A nasal sling is applied. A halo ring of drainage on the sling may also indicate a CSF leak. The sling should be changed as needed. If a CSF leak is present, report this to the surgeon, elevate the head of the bed, and keep the client on bedrest for 72 hours or until the leak ceases. The client must be instructed not to bend or lift heavy objects or strain during a bowel movement, as these activities can increase ICP. A stool softener should be given daily. The nurse also must administer intravenous antibiotics prophylactically to prevent infection and meningitis when a CSF leak is present or suspected. Other pharmacological agents including vasopressin (antidiuretic hormone [ADH], Pitressin) are given intramuscularly based on a urinary output of more than 900 mL/2 hr or of more than 200 mL/hr during the first 24 hours. The client must take hydrocortisone (Cortisol) for life (Lewis & Collier, 1996).

Antidiuretic Hormone (ADH). This is one of the major hormones secreted by the posterior pituitary, along with oxytocin, secreted during childbirth. ADH, also termed vasopressin, causes the kidneys to retain water. In high concentrations it causes vasoconstriction of blood vessels and elevates the blood pressure.

Anterior Pituitary Gland Hypofunction

Hypopituitarism is caused by a growth hormone or gonadotropin deficiency. Underlying causes include an autoimmune disorder, pituitary tumor, infection, hypothalamic dysfunction, viral hepatitis, and trauma. Dwarfism occurs as a result of the growth hormone or gonadotropin deficiency.

Pituitary Dwarfism This condition occurs in children. It is diagnosed by observing stunted growth below the third percentile, normal body proportions, and delayed puberty (due to decreased growth hormone levels). Adults with pituitary dwarfism exhibit short stature with decreased muscle mass, most likely because growth hormone basal levels have decreased.

Diagnostic Studies Diagnostic studies usually include measuring the serum hormone levels of the pituitary and target gland. Dwarfism results most commonly from a failure to secrete growth hormone. Therefore, gonadotropin, TSH, corticotropin, and prolactin also may be deficient. Decreased levels of serum cortisol, growth hormone, and target gland hormones occur. Levels of urinary cortisol are also decreased. To diagnose hypopituitarism, these laboratory results are combined with findings from the client's history and physical examination.

Treatment Treatment involves replacing growth hormone in prepubescent children. Surgical removal or irradiation of the pituitary tumor is performed if this is the cause of the anterior pituitary gland hypofunction. A well-balanced diet should accompany treatment, as nutrition is important along with growth hormone replacement for stimulating growth. Permanent hormone replacement with thyroid hormone, sex hormones, and corticosteroids is usually needed.

Posterior Pituitary Gland Hyperfunction

Malfunction in the posterior pituitary gland causes an excess of ADH to be produced. This may result in the syndrome of inappropriate anti-diuretic hormone (SIADH). SIADH can be caused by aberrant ADH production resulting from the following conditions: a tumor (e.g., oat cell lung cancer), head trauma, pulmonary disorder, Addison's disease, or subarachnoid hemorrhage.

SIADH   Clients with this disorder retain fluid in their cells and develop a serum (extracellular) sodium deficiency. Diagnostic studies include a serum sodium concentration of 100 mEq/L or less and a urinary sodium concentration above 20 mEq/L. Plasma osmolality is decreased, urine osmolality is increased, and urinary output is decreased. The client exhibits increased body weight, an absence of peripheral edema, and a urine specific gravity greater than 1.012 (1.005–1.020, adult normal laboratory parameters).

Treatment   The nurse should restrict the client's fluid intake to 800–1000 mL/day to facilitate the retention of sodium levels in the body. Furosemide (Lasix) is administered to increase diuresis. If a tumor is causing the SIADH, then radiation or surgery may be indicated. The nurse may administer a potassium supplement if it is ordered by the physician. Sodium chloride (NaCl) intravenous fluid (4.5%) may be required to increase the serum sodium concentration (Black & Matassarin-Jacobs, 1997).

CASE STUDY: HYPERSECRETION OF THE POSTERIOR PITUITARY GLAND

Mr. J., 55 years of age, presents to an emergency room with the symptoms of an 8-lb weight gain during the past week, headache, and fatigue. The significant medical history includes a hospitalization two weeks previously when the client was diagnosed with pneumonia. Diagnostic findings are as follows.

Test	Client	Normal Laboratory Parameters: Adult
Urine specific gravity	1.020	1.005–1.020
Urinary sodium	26 mEq/L	40–220 mEq/L
Serum sodium	115 mEq/L	135–145 mEq/L
Serum osmolality	280 mOsm/kg H_2O	285–295 mOsm/kg H_2O
Decreased urinary output	<1–2 mL/kg/hr	1–2 mL/kg/hr

Based on these laboratory values, a diagnosis of SIADH is made.

According to the plan of care, a nurse is assigned to Mr. J. upon his admission to the medical floor. The nurse notes the physician's order for fluid restriction to 900 mL/day and takes the following nursing actions: The nurse removes the water pitcher from the bedside and explains the rationale for doing this to Mr. J. The dietary department is also notified of the fluid restriction. The nurse instructs them to allow only 300 mL/day with meals, and the nursing staff to allow only 200 mL of extra fluid between meals per eight-hour shift. A sign is placed over the client's bed to warn staff and family that Mr. J. is on fluid restriction. Strict intake and output measurements are taken and documented during each eight-hour shift. The 24-hour totals are tabulated, documented, and reported to the physician. The nurse also discusses these instructions in detail with Mr. J.'s wife and family, as their support and cooperation in this plan of care are needed. The nurse discusses the physician's new orders with Mr. J. and instructs Mr. J. that he must eat nothing after midnight in preparation for laboratory work that will be performed early in the morning. The nurse explains to Mr. J. and his family that this type of endocrine condition occasionally worsens following an episode of pneumonia and that nothing he did caused this to happen. The nurse also reassures the client and family that the condition resolves by monitoring laboratory results and medically managing the illness.

Posterior Pituitary Gland Hypofunction

Diabetes Insipidus (DI) DI is caused by an ADH deficiency. This disorder is characterized by polydipsia (increased thirst) and polyuria (increased urination). The kidneys are prevented from reabsorbing water. Causes of DI include head trauma, central nervous system (CNS) infection, a vascular disorder, granulomatous disease, pituitary surgery, and any neurosurgery.

Diagnostic Studies The water deprivation test is used to diagnose DI. The client is given nothing by mouth for 8–16 hours, and two units of ADH diluted in saline solution are then given during a two-hour period. Plasma and urinary osmolality are then tested, and the disorder is determined to be nephrogenic, psychogenic, or pituitary in origin. Urinary osmolality is decreased in DI.

Clinical Manifestations The manifestations of DI include a urinary output of up to 20 L/day, with a decrease in the urine specific gravity, weight loss, hypotension, constipation, poor skin turgor, hypernatremia, and, eventually, shock.

Treatment The following plan of care is used to treat posterior pituitary gland hypofunction. Vasopressin (ADH, Pitressin) is administered to replace the deficiency and correct fluid and electrolyte imbalances. The hospitalized client's serum electrolyte levels should be measured daily. For chronic DI, desmopressin (dDAVP), a synthetic ADH, is given for its antidiuretic effect. The nurse must also institute dietary changes, such as lowering the amount of sodium and protein in the diet. The administration of thiazide diuretics increases chloride levels, allowing sodium and water to be reabsorbed in the proximal tubule of the kidney.

CASE STUDY: ADH DEFICIENCY

Mr. B., 42 years of age, presents to the emergency room with head trauma resulting from a motor vehicle accident (MVA). An MRI of the head is negative. He is admitted to the progressive care unit for 24-hour observation since he is alert and oriented. The nurses document an usually high amount of urinary output, 5000 mL, during the shift. The nurse notifies the physician, who examines the client and orders plasma and urinary osmolality and serum electrolytes. These studies are ordered to evaluate for DI.

Nursing care includes measuring and documenting fluid intake and output every two hours with notation of the urine specific gravity. Vital signs are assessed every four hours. The client should be instructed concerning the laboratory tests ordered by the physician, including daily electrolytes. Skin turgor, the condition of mucous membranes, and blood pressure are monitored for signs of dehydration. These include tenting of the skin, dry membranes, and lowered blood pressure. The client is weighed daily to monitor for weight loss. A dietitian should be consulted because the client is placed on a low-sodium and low-protein diet.

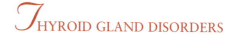

THYROID GLAND DISORDERS

T_3 and T_4. The thyroid gland secretes two major hormones, triiodothyronine and thyroxine, commonly termed T_3 and T_4, respectively. These hormones affect the body by increasing its metabolism.

The two primary hormones secreted by the thyroid gland are triiodothyronine (T_3) and thyroxine (T_4). The thyroid is a key organ controlling metabolism; thyroid disorders can result in disruption of normal body function (Fig. 12-2).

Hyperthyroidism

Hyperthyroidism is caused by the hypersecretion of thyroid hormones. The most common form of hyperthyroidism is Graves' disease.

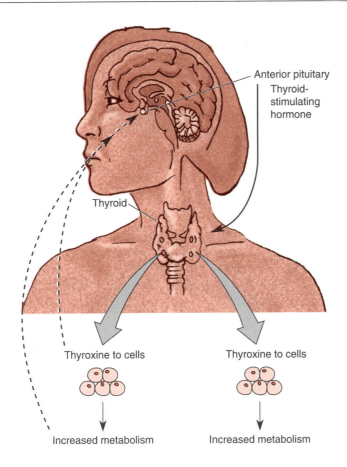

Thyroid-stimulating hormone

Anterior pituitary

Thyroid

Thyroxine to cells

Thyroxine to cells

Increased metabolism

Increased metabolism

FIGURE 12-2

Feedback regulation of thyroid hormone secretion.

Graves' Disease This is seen more often in women younger than 40 years of age. In this disorder, T_3 is elevated, T_4 is elevated, and TSH is decreased. TSH levels are decreased as a result of suppression by elevated thyroid hormone levels. A typical characteristic of Graves' disease is exophthalmos, the protrusion of the eyes as a result of fat and fluid behind the orbits. Graves' disease is thought to be an autoimmune disorder.

Goiter A goiter is an enlargement of the thyroid gland. Goiter formation is due to a hypertrophy of the thyroid gland that occurs when the pituitary gland secretes too much TSH in response to the decreased thyroid hormone in the blood (as in hypothyroidism). All physical examinations should include palpation of the thyroid gland to detect goiters or nodules. There are different types of thyroid goiters and nodules. Multinodular goiters are benign and usually are seen in women between 60 and 70 years of age. Thyroid nodules can be benign or malignant. The nodules form from an overgrowth of tissue caused by increased TSH stimulation and decreased T_3 and T_4 levels. Nuclear medicine thyroid scans and ultrasound are useful for the detection of goiters or nodules in the thyroid. When thyroid nodules are diagnosed, a surgeon is consulted. Treatment options include surgical removal of the goiter, and thyroid hormones are given to decrease TSH stimulation.

Thyroid-Stimulating Hormone (TSH). This hormone is secreted by the anterior pituitary gland. It stimulates the thyroid gland to secrete T_3 and T_4. Increased thyroid hormone levels in the fluids of the body decrease the secretion of TSH by the anterior pituitary. This is the feedback regulation of thyroid hormones.

Thyroid enlargement or nodules can be palpated on examination, and clients occasionally report difficulty swallowing or the sensation of a lump in the throat. Hard, painless nodules can be palpated in an enlarged thyroid. The nodules themselves are a sign of a thyroid disorder. The nodules need to be followed to exclude any disease requiring treatment. Radioactive iodine (RAI) uptake tests identify which nodules are benign or "hot" because they take up radioactive iodine. "Cold," or cancerous, nodules do not take up radioactive iodine, and serum calcitonin levels are elevated.

Clinical Manifestations Clinical manifestations of hyperthyroidism include fever, tachycardia, dysrhythmias, tremors, restlessness, loss of mental acuity, increased blood pressure, and increased respirations. Hyperthyroidism is potentially fatal if left untreated.

Diagnostic Studies There are several tests to determine the presence of hyperthyroidism. An elevated T_4, an elevated T_3, a low TSH, and a high free tyrosine index (FTI or T_7) indicate hyperthyroidism. Another measure is the thyroid-releasing hormone (TRH) stimulation test. In this test, pituitary TSH secretion is stimulated by hypothalamic TRH (Pagana & Pagana, 1995). This test would indicate the site of the defect (i.e., pituitary or thyroid gland). An electrocardiogram (ECG) may show tachycardia, atrial fibrillation, and altered P and T waves. In addition, MRI and ultrasound are used to detect thyroid tumors.

Treatment A regimen of drug therapy helps to stabilize the client. Even when surgical correction with thyroidectomy is indicated, the client must be stabilized initially. Antithyroid drugs, such as propylthiouracil (PTU) and methimazole (Tapazole), which block thyroid hormone synthesis, are therefore given. It takes 1–2 weeks to see results, and the medications peak in 4–8 weeks. The therapy is administered for six months to two years. Iodine blocks the release of T_3 and T_4. It is given prior to surgery and can only be given for ten days. Beta-adrenergic blocking agents (beta blockers) are the third category of drugs that are used to treat hyperthyroidism. Propranolol (Inderal) is frequently given to relieve the symptoms of hyperthyroidism. RAI is given orally to destroy thyroid tissue. The maximum effects occur in two to three months (Lewis, Collier, & Heitkemper, 1996).

Hyperthyroid Crisis When the client is experiencing a hyperthyroid crisis, thyroid storm, or thyrotoxicosis, emergency treatment is required. Interventions include intravenous fluids, oral PTU, intravenous iodine, intravenous dexamethasone (Decadron), a quiet and cool environment, and intravenous propranolol (Inderal) to stabilize the heart rate and blood pressure. A cooling blanket is used to combat hyperthermia.

Treatment Thyroidectomy, either a partial or a total removal of the thyroid, is occasionally performed for hyperthyroidism. A subtotal thyroidectomy involves the removal of 75–80% of the gland. In a total removal, 90–100% of the thyroid is excised. The resultant hypothyroidism requires that clients take thyroid medication daily for the rest of their lives.

Nursing Care Postoperative nursing care includes the following points. The nurse should check the neck for bleeding. The client should be kept in semi-Fowler's position, and a tracheotomy tray should be kept by the bedside for the first 48 hours after surgery, as bleeding or swelling may necessitate maintaining the airway via a tracheostomy tube.

Oxygen and suction should also be kept at the bedside; these may be required if the airway becomes obstructed from edema. The nurse must also be alert for laryngeal stridor, a harsh vibrating sound heard on expiration, which is a medical emergency. If the parathyroid glands are removed or damaged during surgery, tetany can result. Stridor may occur with respirations as a result of tetany, which causes laryngospasms. To treat tetany, calcium gluconate and calcium chloride should be kept available for intravenous administration. The nurse must also support the head and neck while turning the client to prevent tension along the suture line. Additionally, a high-calorie diet may be ordered. The nurse may need to consult with a dietitian.

Thyroiditis This is an inflammation of the thyroid gland. There are various etiologies and diagnostic types of thyroiditis. One type, de Quervain's thyroiditis, is caused by a viral infection. Hashimoto's thyroiditis, the most common type, occurs more often in women. It is thought to be a chronic autoimmune disorder that leads to hypothyroidism. Laboratory results reveal elevated levels of T_3 and T_4 in the acute stage of Hashimoto's thyroiditis. Recovery may occur spontaneously without treatment, weeks or months after the disorder is first seen. Clients may be treated symptomatically. For example, propranolol (Inderal) treats tachycardia and palpitations. Corticosteroids occasionally are used for Hashimoto's thyroiditis to decrease the inflammatory autoimmune response.

Hypothyroidism

Cretinism This congenital hypothyroidism occurs during the fetal or neonatal stage as a result of maternal iodine deprivation or congenital thyroid abnormalities. It can be treated at birth with thyroid medication. If not treated, cretinism can lead to irreversible mental retardation and defective physical development (dwarfism). Some characteristics of cretinism include a hoarse cry, squinting, respiratory problems, thick skin and lips, excessive sleeping, an umbilical hernia, and periorbital edema. Currently, the thyroid hormone levels of all newborns are screened automatically. This test helps to detect cretinism before permanent brain damage occurs.

Childhood Hypothyroidism This condition is caused by autoimmune thyroiditis. The child with hypothyroidism has normal intellectual development, but physical and sexual development are altered. The child should be referred to an endocrinologist and should undergo thyroid hormone replacement therapy.

Adult Hypothyroidism Also termed myxedema, this disorder slows the processes of the body. Clinical manifestations include personality changes, fatigue, and generalized interstitial, nonpitting edema. Myxedema refers to the puffy, mask-like face with swollen lips and thickened nose and periorbital edema that occurs with adult hypothyroidism. Other symptoms include impaired memory; slow speech; decreased initiative; cold intolerance; dry, coarse skin; muscle weakness; constipation; hair loss; weight gain; and brittle nails. Forgetfulness is an early sign of thyroid deficiency. Clients sleep long hours, and exhibit inattentiveness, lethargy, and mental sluggishness. Hypothyroidism occurs slowly, taking months to years to develop. If left untreated, hypothyroidism can affect multiple systems, including the cardiovascular, gastrointestinal, reproductive, and hematopoietic systems.

If myxedema is not controlled with synthetic thyroid hormone replacement, progressive deterioration can result. Marked impairment of consciousness or psychosis may occur. Treatment involves administering thyroid hormone replacement intravenously. Thyroid hormone replacement assists in normalizing the processes of the body and regulates the subnormal temperature, hypotension, and hypoventilation caused by myxedema.

Low levels of T_3 and T_4 indicate adult hypothyroidism. When the level of TSH is high, the defect is in the thyroid. When the level of TSH is low, the defect is found in the pituitary gland or hypothalamus. This condition is treated with thyroid hormone replacement for the remainder of the client's life. Levothyroxine (Synthroid) and norfloxacin (Noroxin) are the drugs of choice. These are initiated slowly and increased for 3–4 weeks. These medications potentiate the effects of anticoagulants, digoxin, and antidepressants. The nurse must therefore caution clients who are taking thyroid hormone replacement to notify the practitioner of this when he or she orders other medications; this prevents potential adverse drug interactions.

CASE STUDY: HYPOTHYROIDISM

Mrs. T., 50 years of age, has been complaining of forgetting appointments. She is very fatigued and sleeps 10–12 hours per night. She complains to her physician that this is very unusual for her, and she is worried. Her physician orders a thyroid panel to determine the levels of T_3, T_4, FTI, and TSH. Based on the resulting laboratory values, Mrs. T. is diagnosed with hypothyroidism.

The nurse should expect the following to occur: A low dose (25 μg) of levothyroxine (Synthroid) should be ordered and gradually increased after 3–4 weeks by 50 μg. Clients who receive thyroid hormone replacement must learn to take the medication each morning at approximately the same time before breakfast. Clients should be able to assess themselves to determine the effectiveness of therapy. Effective therapy increases energy, improves well-being, decreases puffiness, normalizes pulse rate, and improves temperature tolerance. The nurse should emphasize that thyroid hormone replacement is a life-long therapy. The client should be instructed to report if his or her pulse increases above 100 beats/min or if chest pain, palpitations, or anxiety occurs, as these symptoms may indicate that the dosage needs to be lowered. The client also should undergo periodic testing of T_3, T_4, FTI, and TSH levels (Wilson, Shannon, & Stang, 1998).

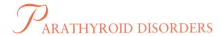

PARATHYROID DISORDERS

Hyperparathyroidism

Hyperparathyroidism, or increased parathyroid hormone (PTH), occurs when serum calcium levels are greater than 10 mg/dL and serum phosphorus levels are less than 3 mg/dL. PTH helps regulate calcium and phosphate levels by stimulating bone resorption and renal tubular reabsorption of calcium and activation of vitamin D. Primary hyperparathyroidism is caused by an adenoma. Secondary hyperparathyroidism is caused by a vitamin D deficiency or chronic renal failure. Tertiary hyperparathyroidism results from a complication of either a kidney transplant or chronic dialysis.

An imbalance of calcium and phosphate can lead to clinical sequelae. Increased calcium and phosphate levels in the urine may result in the development of calculi. Increased calcium levels may also cause increased production of gastrin and pepsin, resulting in peptic ulcer disease and a greater risk of pancreatitis.

Symptoms of hyperparathyroidism include anorexia, weakness, constipation, increased sleepiness, peptic ulcers, kidney stones (nephrolithiasis), and broken bones (from osteoporosis).

Parathormone (or Parathyroid Hormone). This major hormone, secreted by the parathyroid glands, is responsible for controlling the calcium concentration in the extracellular fluid. The parathormone targets three organs in controlling calcium: the absorption of calcium in the intestines, the excretion of calcium by the kidneys, and the release of calcium from the bone.

Treatment Treatment includes greatly increasing fluid intake, increasing ambulation, and limiting calcium intake. Plicamycin (Mithracin) is administered intravenously to treat hospitalized clients with hypercalcemia or hypercalciuria associated with advanced neoplasms. Plicamycin (Mithracin) lowers serum calcium levels in 48 hours, but toxic side effects such as bleeding and coagulation disorders may occur. Because these side effects are serious, plicamycin (Mithracin) is only given to clients with metastatic cancer of the parathyroid.

The client with hyperparathyroidism should be kept hydrated, and electrolyte balance should be maintained. Normal saline should be administered intravenously to correct fluid volume deficit. Furosemide (Lasix) is administered to decrease renal reabsorption of calcium, and propranolol (Inderal) is given to inhibit the action of catecholamines, which stimulate the release of PTH.

CASE STUDY: HYPERPARATHYROIDISM

Mr. W. has just returned to his hospital room after a subtotal thyroidectomy. The nurse notices that the muscles of his hand and feet are very tense and stiff. He exhibits positive Chvostek's and Trousseau's signs. The nurse notifies the physician.

After receiving orders from the physician, the nurse connects a rebreathing mask to the client. Hyperventilation and anxiety worsen hypocalcemia by inducing respiratory alkalosis that further lowers calcium levels. Intravenous calcium gluconate is administered slowly into a large vein. The intravenous injection solution can be given directly undiluted at a rate of 0.5 mL/min (Wilson, Shannon, & Stang, 1998). During the calcium administration, continuous cardiac monitoring is performed to assess for inverted T waves, a sign of hypercalcemia. Since other ions are also frequently depleted, magnesium and phosphorous levels should be determined. Vitamin D is administered. The client should be in a warm environment and be visible to the nurse at all times. A tracheostomy tray and intravenous calcium gluconate should be readily available. The nurse must stress the importance of following a low-phosphate diet. Follow-up therapy needs to be given if the tetany recurs.

Hypoparathyroidism

A decreased level of PTH is caused by hypomagnesemia (seen in alcoholism), malabsorption syndrome, or accidental removal of or damage to the parathyroid glands. Clinical manifestations include hypocalcemia, decreased PTH levels, and increased serum phosphate levels. Tetany is a complication of the hypocalcemia that accompanies hypoparathyroidism. It manifests in tingling lips, hands, or feet; progressive muscle tension; paresthesia; and stiffness. In severe cases of tetany, life-threatening dysphagia and laryngospasms can occur.

There are two assessment parameters the nurse must recognize, Chvostek's and Trousseau's signs, which are signs of tetany. *Chvostek's sign* is a facial muscle spasm elicited by tapping the facial nerves located below the temple in the region of the parotid glands. *Trousseau's sign* is a carpopedal spasm of the hand elicited by compressing the upper arm with a blood pressure cuff for 3 minutes. The disruption of arterial flow makes the distal nerves ischemic, eliciting the spasm (Fig. 12-3). Tetany is treated by the slow administration of intravenous calcium gluconate. Vitamin D must be replaced as well. A rebreathing mask prevents the hyperventilation and anxiety that further decrease serum calcium as a result of respiratory alkalosis (CO_2 loss from hyperventilation).

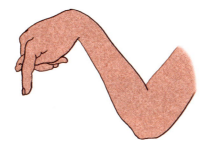

FIGURE 12-3

Trousseau's sign seen in tetany.

ADRENAL GLAND DISORDERS

Hypersecretion of the Adrenal Cortex

Hypersecretion of the adrenal cortex, or Cushing's disease, is caused by increased levels of glucocorticoids (Fig. 12-4). Cortisol is the primary glucocorticoid. High glucocorticoid levels can be caused by corticotropin-secreting tumors, adrenal cortex tumors, oat cell lung cancer, or the prolonged use of high doses of corticosteroids (iatrogenic Cushing's syndrome).

Clinical Manifestations The cortisol-secreting tumor causes hyperglycemia, protein wasting, and susceptibility to infection. Obesity in the trunk and abdomen, slender extremities, thin skin, moon face, and body image problems are common symptoms, and purple-red striae occur on the abdomen or buttocks. Premenopausal osteoporosis can also occur. In addition, the client may exhibit unexplained hypokalemia. Emotional changes range from depression to psychosis.

Diagnosis Diagnostic studies demonstrate an increased plasma cortisol level, decreased potassium, and increased FBS with glycosuria. Radiographs show osteoporosis, evidenced by porous bones and compression fractures of the vertebrae that cause a loss of height between vertebrae. A 24-hour urine test for free cortisol and a low-dose dexamethasone suppression test are performed to confirm the diagnosis.

Treatment Treatment for Cushing's disease includes surgical removal of the pituitary adenoma. For adrenal tumors or hyperplasia, an adrenalectomy is performed. In severe cases of Cushing's disease, total adrenalectomy (both adrenal glands) is performed. Administration of mitotane (Lysodren), a drug that suppresses cortisol production and kills adrenocortical cells, may be ordered. This is considered a medical adrenalectomy. The adrenal gland is irradiated in children.

It is worth noting that ketoconazole (Nizoral), an antifungal agent used to treat severe systemic infections, inhibits adrenal steroid secretion. However, acute hypoadrenalism is an adverse effect of this medication.

Adrenal Glands. These glands lie at the superior poles of both kidneys. Each gland is composed of two parts, the adrenal medulla and the adrenal cortex. The adrenal glands secrete the corticosteroids.

Cortisol. Cortisol is a hormone secreted by the adrenal cortex. It controls the metabolism of proteins, carbohydrates, and fats. Cortisol is the principal glucocorticoid.

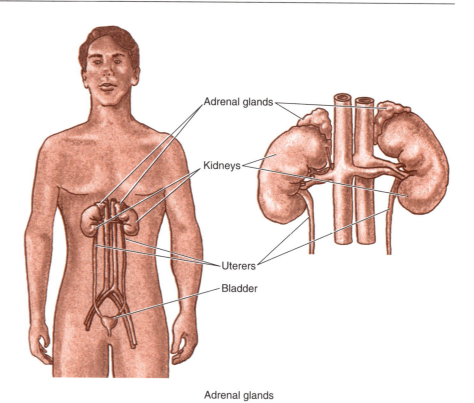

Adrenal glands

FIGURE 12-4

⬡

The adrenal glands.

Nursing Care Before the adrenalectomy, existing hypertension should be treated, and hyperglycemia and hypokalemia must be corrected. Electrolytes should be monitored closely, and abnormalities reported. The client should be given a high-protein diet.

Postoperative management for the first 24–48 hours consists of closely monitoring the client. High doses of cortisone are given intravenously during surgery and for two days thereafter to decrease blood pressure and maintain fluid and electrolyte balances. A nasogastric (NG) tube may be inserted. Vital signs are monitored for increased heart rate and blood pressure, dressings are examined for signs of hemorrhage, and the client is kept on bed rest until the blood pressure is stable. The nurse should provide a calm, stress-free environment for the client. Since the client will require lifelong corticosteroid replacement therapy, close follow-up and instruction concerning medication administration are essential.

Hyposecretion of the Adrenal Cortex

Addison's Disease. Medical treatment for Addison's disease focuses on replacing the deficient hormones; therefore, glucocorticoids and mineralocorticoids are replaced exogenously.

Adrenal cortex hyposecretion, or Addison's disease, causes decreased glucocorticoid, mineralocorticoid, and androgen levels. It is most likely an autoimmune disease in which adrenal tissue is destroyed. Many disorders cause this chronic adrenocortical insufficiency, including tuberculosis (TB), hemorrhage, fungal infections (coccidiomycosis), acquired immune deficiency syndrome (AIDS), and metastatic cancer. Other causes include the adverse effects of anticoagulant therapy and chemotherapy. Clinical manifestations include postural hypotension, progressive weakness, weight loss, and anorexia. Hyperpigmentation occurs in areas of the skin that are exposed to the sun and in palmar creases. Electrolyte imbalances also occur, including decreased sodium and increased potassium levels. Nausea, vomiting, and diarrhea are other symptoms of hyposecretion. Treatment for Addison's disease includes the administration of glucocorticoids to stabilize the blood pressure.

Corticosteroids. The corticosteroids are the mineralocorticoids, the glucocorticoids, and the androgen hormones.

Addisonian Crisis Also known as acute adrenal insufficiency, this life-threatening situation occurs when the decrease of adrenocortical hormones causes severe hypotension and mental confusion. An addisonian crisis can result from stresses such as trauma, surgery, infection, hemorrhage, and psychological trauma. Another cause of addisonian crisis is the sudden withdrawal of adrenal hormone therapy. This is why it is imperative to wean clients slowly from steroids rather than stopping their administration abruptly. Adrenal surgery and sudden pituitary destruction are also possible causes of addisonian crisis. Clinical manifestations include hypotension, confusion, hypovolemic shock, nausea, and vomiting. The three main goals in the treatment of clients with adrenal crisis are replacing fluid volume and correcting electrolyte imbalances, administering adrenal steroids to reestablish blood levels, and identifying and correcting the underlying illness that led to the crisis (Dennher, 1996).

Addisonian Crisis. When the client is in addisonian crisis, he or she may be given 10 or more times the normal quantity of glucocorticoids to prevent death.

Diagnosis The adrenocorticotropic hormone (ACTH) stimulation test is used to diagnose Addison's disease. A decreased ACTH level indicates Addison's disease. Other electrolyte changes that occur include a decreased chloride level, an increased potassium level, a decreased sodium level, decreased FBS, and increased blood urea nitrogen (BUN). A TB skin test is also performed for exclusion. A computed tomography (CT) scan of the adrenal gland may also be performed.

Treatment Treatment of Addison's disease includes the administration of hydrocortisone intravenously and the replacement of dextrose and sodium via intravenous fluids to restore electrolyte balance. The client should be monitored daily for weight loss and anorexia. The environment should be kept quiet, and the client should be informed of the treatment plan. If the TB test is positive, isoniazid (INH) is administered. These clients require steroid replacement therapy, and adjustments are required if the client also has influenza, undergoes tooth extraction, or has an infection. The practitioner should overcompensate when replacing steroids; insufficient steroid replacement can be life-threatening. Glucocorticoids are replaced by administering two thirds of the dose in the morning and one third in the evening. Mineralocorticoids are administered once a day in the evening to match circadian rhythms. The client needs to learn about addisonian crisis, and should have an emergency kit with 100 mg of intramuscular hydrocortisone and syringes available at all times (Kee & Hayes, 1997).

CASE STUDY: ADDISON'S DISEASE

Mr. H. has been complaining of progressive weakness, weight loss, and no appetite for the past four weeks. The nurse notes that the client is hypotensive and has hyperpigmentation on the palmar creases of his hands. The physician orders a serum cortisol test; the level is abnormally low. Based on this and the clinical findings, the physician diagnoses Mr. H. with Addison's disease.

The nurse should emphasize the following points to the client: Cortisol is administered to stabilize the blood pressure. The client must be cautioned that he or she can no longer tolerate any physical or emotional stress. The client should carry the emergency kit containing a hydrocortisone injection at all times. The nurse should emphasize that a person with Addison's disease can lead a fairly normal life with exogenous hormone therapy. Clients are taught to avoid stressful situations whenever possible and to follow a regimen of diet and rest to avoid hypoglycemia. The client should wear an identification tag that states that he or she has the disease and is on steroid therapy.

Disorders of Aldosterone Secretion

Primary hyperaldosteronism results from increased levels of aldosterone. This disorder is caused by an adrenal adenoma or bilateral adrenal hyperplasia. The clinical manifestations include the hallmark of hypertension with hypokalemia caused by the retention of sodium and the excretion of potassium. Symptoms include hypertension, headache, muscle weakness, fatigue, and cardiac dysrhythmia. If left untreated, the metabolic alkalosis that occurs can lead to tetany.

The diagnostic tests that are performed demonstrate increased levels of aldosterone. A 24-hour urine test for urinary sodium and potassium and CT scan of the adrenal glands are performed. Treatment consists of a unilateral adrenalectomy. Bilateral hyperplasia is treated by administering spironolactone (Aldactone) or amiloride (Midamor).

Disorders of the Adrenal Medulla

Disorders of the adrenal medulla are rare; the most common of these is pheochromocytoma.

Pheochromocytoma This benign neoplasm is usually located in the adrenal medulla. It is relatively rare and tends to occur in families.

Although the condition is potentially fatal, it can be managed well if detected at an early stage. The tumor causes increased catecholamine levels, which can result in extensive damage to the cardiovascular system. Clinical manifestations include episodic hypertension, increased FBS, hypermetabolism, throbbing headaches, facial flushing, sweating, blurry vision, and pallor. Diagnostic tests for pheochromocytoma demonstrate an increase in urinary metanephrines such as vanillylmandelic acid (VMA), and a CT or MRI localizes the tumor. Visualizing the tumor by CT or MRI differentiates the diagnosis from essential hypertension. Finally, surgical removal of the tumor by adrenalectomy is necessary for complete remission of pheochromocytoma.

CASE STUDY: PHEOCHROMOCYTOMA

Mr. J. arrives at the emergency room with a blood pressure of 300/175 mm Hg, pulse of 128 beats/min, and respiration of 24 breaths/min. The physician orders blood catecholamine levels and notes that they are markedly elevated. The x-ray studies that are ordered show a possible tumor of the adrenal gland. The preliminary diagnosis of pheochromocytoma is made. The nurse realizes that her role is to identify what precipitated the attack by questioning the client as to what he or she was doing prior to it. The nurse must also support the family and client. The nurse should realize that this is a life-threatening condition.

Summary

All bodily functions are regulated primarily by the nervous and endocrine systems. The endocrine system controls many of the different metabolic functions of the body. Some hormonal effects take place in seconds, while others last weeks or months. A few of the general hormones, such as growth hormone and thyroid hormone, initiate reactions in almost all of the body's cells. Other hormones affect only specific target tissues. For example, ACTH from the anterior pituitary specifically stimulates the adrenal cortex.

It is essential for the nurse to develop skills in the assessment, diagnosis, and treatment of clients with endocrine disorders. These disorders typically involve the hypo- or hypersecretion of a hormone. The delicate balance of hormones must be maintained for the client's continued health and well-being.

KEY WORDS

Acromegaly

Addison's disease

Addisonian crisis

Chvostek's sign

Cretinism

Cushing's disease

De Quervain's thyroiditis

Diabetes insipidus

Gigantism

Goiter

Graves' disease

Hashimoto's thyroiditis

Hyperparathyroidism

Hypophysectomy

Myxedema

Pheochromocytoma

Pituitary dwarfism

Primary hyperaldosteronism

Syndrome of inappropriate
   antidiuretic hormone (SIADH)

Tetany

Thyroid crisis

Thyroiditis

Trousseau's sign

QUESTIONS

1. A carpopedal spasm that occurs when arterial flow is interrupted by a blood pressure cuff for 3 minutes is

   A. Chvostek's sign.
   B. Murphy's sign.
   C. Trousseau's sign.
   D. Trollop's sign.

2. All of the following treatments should be ordered for a client with hyperparathyroidism except

   A. restriction of fluids.
   B. 80 mg of furosemide (Lasix) intravenously.
   C. limit calcium intake.
   D. normal saline intravenously.

3. Clinical manifestations of thyroid crisis include

   A. fever, tachycardia, hypertension, and restlessness.
   B. decreased respirations, subnormal temperature, and bradycardia.
   C. lethargy and decreased visual acuity.
   D. fatigue and sleeping more than ten hours per night.

4. Mrs. S. has just returned to her room after undergoing a subtotal thyroidectomy. Immediately following surgery, the nurse's first action is to

   A. check the incision site for infection.
   B. check for urinary output.
   C. monitor respiratory status for signs of obstruction (laryngeal stridor).
   D. check the neck for full range-of-motion status.

5. Mr. W. was diagnosed two years previously with Addison's disease that has been well managed. He suddenly presents to the emergency room with symptoms that the nurse correctly interprets as a possible addisonian crisis. The signs and symptoms that signal this crisis are

   A. hypertension, lethargy, and headache.
   B. hypotension, confusion, nausea, and vomiting.
   C. fatigue, dehydration, and fever.
   D. subnormal temperature, periorbital edema, and pedal edema.

6. Mr. B. is being treated for diabetes insipidus (DI). Which of the following orders from the physician should the nurse expect?

   A. Measure intake and output every 12 hours with routine vital signs.
   B. Measure intake and output every two hours, daily weight, and vital signs every four hours with daily electrolytes.
   C. Perform the urine specific gravity test every day.
   D. Perform the water deprivation test every day and measure intake and output every 12 hours.

ANSWERS

1. *The answer is C.* Trousseau's sign is a sign for tetany in which a carpal spasm of the hand can be elicited by compressing the upper arm with a blood pressure cuff, causing ischemia to the nerves distally.

2. *The answer is A.* Fluid intake should be encouraged (not restricted) to correct the fluid volume deficit. The other options are important for the treatment of hyperparathyroidism. Furosemide (Lasix) decreases the renal resorption of calcium, and normal saline intravenously corrects the fluid volume deficit.

3. *The answer is A.* The three other options describe the effects of hypothyroidism on the body's functions.

4. *The answer is C.* Tetany can occur as a complication of subtotal thyroidectomy if the parathyroid glands are damaged or removed. This causes laryngeal spasm and respiratory distress. Stridor may be the first sign exhibited by the client that warns of this postoperative complication.

5. *The answer is B.* Severe hypotension and vascular collapse are the hallmarks of addisonian crisis. In addition, gastrointestinal symptoms such as nausea, vomiting, cramping, and diarrhea are often present.

6. *The answer is B.* As a result of the extraordinary amount of fluids and electrolytes lost from DI, nursing care must include these measures.

ANNOTATED REFERENCES

Black, J. M. & Matassarin-Jacobs, E. (1997). *Medical-surgical nursing: Clinical management for continuity of care,* 5th ed. Philadelphia: W. B. Saunders.

This text is a comprehensive review of nursing care to provide continuity of care across various settings and situations.

Dennher, A. (1996). *Review of critical care nursing.* Philadelphia: W. B. Saunders.

This book of critical care nursing case studies is an important teaching tool for students and nurses. The book presents case studies with questions and answers that emphasize problem-solving and clinical decision-making.

Kee, J. & Hayes, E. R. (1997). *Pharmacology: A nursing approach,* 2nd ed. Philadelphia: W. B. Saunders.

This text provides nursing guidelines and instructions for clients for certain medications.

Lewis, S. M., Collier, I., & Heitkemper, M. M. (1996). *Medical-surgical nursing: Assessment and management of clinical problems,* 4th ed. St. Louis: C. V. Mosby.

This text provides extensive coverage of the nurse's role in the assessment and management of common medical-surgical health problems.

Pagana, K. & Pagana, T. (1995). *Diagnostic and laboratory test reference.* St. Louis: C. V. Mosby.

This clinical handbook lists laboratory tests alphabetically and provides the normal ranges for adults and children.

Wilson, B. A., Shannon, M., & Stang, C. (1998). *Nurses' drug guide.* Stamford, CT: Appleton & Lange.

This detailed drug guide provides important nursing information.

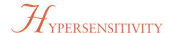

CARE OF THE CLIENT WITH AN IMMUNE DISORDER

HYPERSENSITIVITY

Immune disorders are classified into three types: hypersensitivities, auto-immune disorders, and immunodeficiency disorders. Hypersensitivities are further classified into four types. This classification primarily assists the nurse in examining the responses of the body to each of the initiating mechanisms of the immune system. Most often the immune system initiates a combination of these reactions. A **hypersensitivity** disorder is an overreaction of the immune system. The immune system initiates mechanisms that produce inflammation and tissue destruction. These mechanisms can be immunoglobulin E (IgE)–mediated, tissue specific, immune complex–mediated, or cell-mediated (Rote, 1994).

Type I Hypersensitivity Reactions

A type I hypersensitivity reaction is termed **anaphylaxis** (Lewis, 1996). It is the inappropriate release of histamine by mast cells in response to exposure to a substance. This type of immune disorder is generally referred to as an allergic reaction. A client experiencing hypersensitivity must have had previous exposure to the substance causing the reaction (Lewis, 1996). The presenting clinical manifestations may be localized or systemic. Local manifestations include hives, itchiness, flushing, nasal congestion, watery eyes, rhinorrhea, and tingling of the extremities. The manifestations of a

Hypersensitivity is an over-reaction of the immune system in which tissues become inflamed and eventually are destroyed.

Anaphylaxis is an immediate hypersensitivity response to an exogenous antigen.

systemic reaction include angioedema, a feeling of impending doom, bronchospasm, laryngeal edema, abdominal cramping, and diarrhea. The progression of this reaction from a local to a systemic response with resulting deterioration of the client's condition is termed *anaphylactic shock*. Anaphylactic shock is a life-threatening reaction with a very rapid onset. It is manifested by cardiovascular changes including lightheadedness, weakness, tachycardia, and hypotension. The fluid leakage from the capillaries and the resultant decrease in vascular resistance lead to circulatory shutdown. In addition to circulatory problems, the client also experiences increasing laryngeal edema that leads to laryngeal stridor and possible airway obstruction (Fig. 13-1).

FIGURE 13-1

▣

Anaphylactic reactions leading to anaphylactic shock.

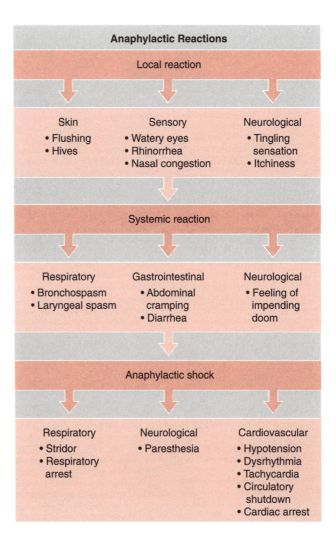

Care of the Client with an Anaphylactic Hypersensitivity Reaction The severity of the hypersensitivity reaction determines how the client should be treated. Consider the following scenario.

CASE STUDY: TYPE I HYPERSENSITIVITY REACTION

A 34-year-old man receives an intermittent infusion of ceftriaxone (third-generation cephalosporin) prior to undergoing surgery to repair a hernia. Within 5 minutes of the start of the medication, the client complains of itchiness and slight difficulty breathing. He also exhibits signs of mild anxiety. His chart lists an allergy to penicillin.

Assessment This man exhibits the clinical manifestations of an anaphylactic reaction. The ceftriaxone is the likely triggering substance. Penicillin and the cephalosporin agents are common triggers, but any substance can trigger a hypersensitivity reaction. Foods such as peanuts, strawberries, shellfish, and eggs are among the other common causes. Common substances such as dust, pollens, latex, and insect stings can also be triggering agents. It is important to take a thorough client history of any previous hypersensitivity reactions and the substances that triggered them.

In the case study, the client had an allergy to penicillin, which increased his risk of a reaction to the cephalosporin. After taking a thorough history, the nurse can take measures to reduce the risk of a reaction by preventing client contact with triggering substances, teaching the client what these substances are and how to avoid them, or proceeding with caution in exposing the client to possible triggering substances. Since the client in the case study is allergic to penicillin, it is the nurse's responsibility to administer a cephalosporin with caution. The order for the cephalosporin should be checked with the physician to verify that he or she is aware of the client's allergy to penicillin. Since some clients may be allergic to penicillin but not to cephalosporins, the physician may confirm his/her original order for the drug. Good planning prior to administering the cephalosporin should consist of having resuscitation medications and emergency equipment on hand. Most reactions leading to anaphylactic shock occur within the first hour of exposure; therefore, the client should be monitored closely during this time.

Allergic reactions to **latex** are becoming more common as a result of an increased exposure to products containing latex. Latex is found in many everyday products such as rubber bands, infant feeding nipples, dishwashing gloves, balloons, condoms, and telephone cords (Gold, 1994). Many medical products, including adhesive bandages, blood pressure cuffs, urinary catheters, intravenous catheters, injection ports on intravenous equipment, gloves, tourniquets, and rubber vial stoppers also contain latex (Gold, 1994). Therefore, it is important to determine if the client has an allergy to latex. Many of these products come in a nonlatex form, and

*Many everyday and medical products contain **latex**. Almost anything with a rubber-like texture contains latex. For persons with latex allergies, products made of vinyl or polyurethane can be substituted.*

most hospitals stock nonlatex products to use with clients with latex sensitivities. Other precautions can be taken to prevent the client's exposure to latex. Two methods of reducing the risk of client contact with latex include taping the latex ports on intravenous tubing and removing the rubber stoppers from vials before withdrawing medications. Silastic Foley catheters are an alternative to latex Foley catheters. Stopcocks offer an alternative to latex injection sites. Clients should wear a nonlatex band indicating their latex allergy while in the hospital and medical alert bracelets outside of the hospital to alert medical personnel to their latex allergy.

Nurses often develop sensitivities to latex as a result of overexposure to latex products. Therefore, it is important to recognize this risk and take precautions to prevent an allergic reaction. Generally nurses who become latex sensitive initially show a reaction to the gloves worn while caring for clients. A skin reaction on parts of the hand and arm covered by the glove is usually the first indication that the nurse is sensitive to latex. Latex reactions can be localized or systemic. Like any systemic allergic reaction, systemic latex reactions are potentially life-threatening. Vinyl gloves are available for nurses who are sensitive to latex. Although research suggests that latex gloves maintain their integrity better, vinyl gloves do provide good barrier protection and may reduce the risk of latex sensitivity (Korniewicz, Laughon, Butz, & Larson, 1989). Some glove manufacturers now make latex gloves that contain fewer latex proteins. This may help to lower the incidence of nurses experiencing latex sensitivity (Table 13-1).

Intervention Regardless of the triggering substance, clients who experience an anaphylactic reaction are treated primarily with epinephrine and antihistamines. Mild reactions such as a rash or itchiness that involve only a local response are usually treated with the antihistamine diphenhydramine (Benadryl). Systemic reactions are treated with 0.3–0.5 mL of **epinephrine** (1:1000 concentration) subcutaneously. Antihistamines may be administered intramuscularly or intravenously as well and, if the reaction progresses to anaphylactic shock, volume expanders, vasopressors, and bronchodilators may be required. Clients often receive a corticosteroid as well. The corticosteroid reduces the risk of a recurrence of the acute reaction, which can happen after the other agents are metabolized.

The client in the case study should receive a subcutaneous injection of epinephrine and either an intramuscular or intravenous injection of diphenhydramine (Benadryl). If the bronchospasm continues after the administration of these agents, the client should receive a second injection of epinephrine and an injection of hydrocortisone, a corticosteroid. If the client does not improve or goes into anaphylactic shock, an intravenous line should be started, and saline or a volume expander such as plasma or dextran should be administered. Aminophylline may be administered intravenously to decrease bronchospasm. The goals of therapy are to prevent vascular collapse resulting from blood vessels leaking fluid into the tissues and to prevent airway obstruction. Bronchospasm may progress to the extent that airway management is required. The insertion of an endotracheal tube may be necessary to establish and maintain an airway.

Epinephrine is the primary drug of choice for treating systemic anaphylactic reactions.

Common agents used in the treatment of an anaphylactic reaction include epinephrine, antihistamines, corticosteroids, bronchodilators, and vasopressors.

🞧

TABLE 13-1
SUBSTANCES THAT COMMONLY TRIGGER ANAPHYLACTIC REACTIONS

Drugs

Penicillins	Sulfonamides
Insulins	Aspirin
Tetracycline	Local anesthetics
Chemotherapeutic agents	Cephalosporins
Nonsteroidal anti-inflammatory agents	

Insect venoms

Hymenoptera[a]

Foods

Eggs	Milk
Nuts	Peanuts
Shellfish	Fish
Chocolate	Strawberries

Antitoxins

Tetanus antitoxin	Rabies antitoxin
Diphtheria antitoxin	Snake venom antitoxin

Treatment measures

Blood products (whole blood and components	Iodine-contrast media dye for IVP or angiogram test
Allergenic extracts in hyposensitization therapy	Latex

NOTE: From *Medical Surgical Nursing*, 4th ed. (p. 217), by Lewis, S. L., Collier, I. C., Heitkemper, M. M., 1996, St. Louis: C. V. Mosby. Reprinted with permission.
IVP = intravenous pyelography.
[a]Wasps, hornets, yellow jackets, bumblebees, and ants.

It is the nurse's responsibility to maintain airway clearance. Once an endotracheal tube is placed, the nurse should assess breath sounds in both lungs frequently. The client's level of oxygen saturation must be monitored by pulse oximetry; it should be in the range of 92–100%. The nurse should position the client with the head of the bed elevated 30 degrees. The nurse must also take steps to reduce the client's anxiety. An endotracheal tube prevents the client from speaking. This inability to communicate as well as the likely sensation of impending doom requires the nurse to soothe the fears of the client and make him/her comfortable.

In the case study, the client received 0.5 mL of epinephrine subcutaneously and 50 mg of diphenhydramine (Benadryl) intramuscularly. The client improved, and no wheezing was evident. The client was given an intramuscular injection of 100 mg of cortisol sodium succinate (Solu-Cortef), and a prednisone dose pack was initiated. The dose pack is an oral corticosteroid in which the dose is gradually decreased before therapy is completed.

It is important for people who are highly allergic to common substances to carry epinephrine injections with them at all times. The nurse should teach clients the proper use of these injections.

Each allergic reaction produced by an agent is generally more intense than the previous reaction; therefore, the client should avoid further exposure to the triggering substance. In the case study, the cephalosporin was discontinued. The client was informed of his allergy and instructed to carry a reminder that he is allergic to cephalosporins as well as penicillin.

Occasionally the triggering substance is so common that it is difficult to avoid. Bee stings are a good example. The nurse should teach clients who are allergic to common substances in their environment to minimize their risk of exposure. For example, persons who are allergic to bee stings should avoid wearing cologne and brightly colored clothing while outdoors, especially in the spring and summer months when bees are plentiful. If they must spend time outdoors, white or dark colors are more appropriate because these shades do not attract bees. Persons allergic to bee stings are likely to be allergic to bee pollen and honey as well. Clients should be aware of the risks involved if they are exposed to any substance containing bee pollen. Clients who are allergic to bee stings must be taught in advance how to self-inject epinephrine subcutaneously should they get stung. Epinephrine comes packaged as a kit with a prefilled syringe. To inject it, clients simply take the syringe out of the kit, remove the cap, and inject themselves in the arm or thigh (Table 13-2).

◈

TABLE 13-2

NURSING CARE RESPONSIBILITIES FOR
TYPE I HYPERSENSITIVITY REACTIONS

Assessment

Subjective:
   Known allergies
   Exposure to allergens
   Previous reactions
   Clinical manifestations
      Feeling of impending doom
      Itchiness
      Shortness of breath
      Numbness and tingling
        in the extremities
      Abdominal cramping

Objective:
   Clinical manifestations
      Skin reactions
      Respiratory distress
      Diarrhea
      Hypotension
      Tachycardia

Intervention

Airway management
   Head of bed elevated
   Oxygen
   Antihistamines
   Bronchodilators
   Corticosteroids

IV fluids
   Normal saline
   Volume expanders
   Blood products
   Vasoconstrictors

TABLE 13-2 *(continued)*

Prevention
Allergy testing
Avoidance of allergens
Antihistamines
Corticosteroids
Desensitization

Client Instruction
Avoidance measures
Importance of medical regimen
Wearing proper identification
Injection technique (subcutaneous epinephrine)

Some clients can become desensitized to allergens. The process of desensitization involves injecting minute amounts of the allergens into the client and then gradually increasing the doses for a prolonged period (Rote, 1994). **Nursing interventions** include assisting the physician in injecting the allergens and monitoring the client for anaphylactic reactions. The nurse must ensure that the client understands the risk involved and the signs and symptoms of an allergic reaction. Clients also should be told that desensitization is a lengthy process and that it is important to keep all of their scheduled appointments. The effectiveness of the series of injections planned by the physician is significantly decreased if the client does not receive all of the injections.

Type II Hypersensitivity Reactions

Type II reactions occur when an antigen on a cell's plasma membrane produces an antibody response within the body (Rote, 1994). Antigens are substances that induce antibody formation. The interaction between antigen and antibody forms the basis for an immune response. A type II reaction can occur in response to self–antigens as well as to environmental or other human antigens (Rote, 1994). As a result of these reactions, target cells are lysed, or cellular function is altered because antibodies (immunoglobulins) have bound to the cells. A hemolytic blood transfusion reaction is an example of a type II reaction.

Care of the Client with a Type II Hypersensitivity Reaction
Assessment In a hemolytic transfusion reaction, the antibodies in a client's body react to foreign antigens on the plasma membranes of transfused blood cells. This occurs when the transfused blood is not histocompatible with the client's blood. The clinical manifestations of this

reaction include urticaria, chills, fever, headache, low back pain, and wheezing. Hemoglobin is released into the plasma and urine as a result of the cytolysis that occurs during the reaction. The following case study illustrates this progression.

CASE STUDY: TYPE II HYPERSENSITIVITY REACTION

A 68-year-old woman is diagnosed with anemia secondary to gastro-intestinal (GI) bleeding. She is admitted to the intensive care unit (ICU) to receive a transfusion of packed red blood cells (RBCs). Blood is drawn for type and crossmatch. (Type and crossmatch refer to the laboratory determination of the donor's and recipient's ABO blood types and matching of some HLA indicators). The laboratory determines that her blood type is AB+. The nurse administers the first unit of packed RBCs. During the first 15 minutes of the infusion, the client complains of severe chills and dull pain in the lower lumbar region.

Hemolytic blood transfusion reactions generally occur as a result of ABO incompatibility between the client's blood and the donor's blood.

Nursing responsibilities for a client experiencing a hemolytic blood transfusion reaction are to:

- Stop the blood transfusion.
- Administer normal saline intravenously.
- Notify the physician.
- Notify the blood bank.
- Return the blood unit.
- Send two blood samples and a urine sample to the laboratory.
- Initiate supportive therapy for the client.

Intervention The nurse should deduce that the client in this case study is experiencing a cell-mediated reaction to the blood transfusion. Low back pain and severe chills are the typical signs of these reactions. This is a medical emergency caused by mismatching the client's and donor's ABO blood type. This client's AB+ blood type is uncommon, and thus it is likely that her blood is not ABO compatible with the donor's blood. The nurse's first action is to stop the transfusion. Normal saline should be infused in place of the donor blood, and fresh tubing should be used. Although packed RBCs are transfused with normal saline by Y-tubing, it is inadvisable to use the old tubing, since any remaining donor blood cells in it will be infused. The severity of the reaction is directly related to the amount of infused blood received.

The client should receive an infusion of normal saline and an antihistamine such as diphenhydramine (Benadryl). The nurse should be prepared to treat the impending shock that accompanies this type of reaction. Epinephrine may be required. The remaining blood and Y-tubing should be sent to the pharmacy for analysis to confirm that the reaction is related to the blood transfusion.

The nurse also should draw two vials of blood from a vein distant from the infusion site. The blood is then analyzed by the laboratory and blood bank. A urinalysis helps to determine if the reaction was hemolytic. Hemolysis of the RBCs releases hemoglobin into the plasma, which can lead to renal failure as a result of blood filtration in the kidneys and renal spasms. The hemoglobin will be found in the urine. The nurse should monitor the client for signs of hemoglobinuria. The client's intake and output, fluid status, blood urea nitrogen (BUN), creatinine, hemoglobin, hematocrit, and the presence of edema also should be monitored. An osmotic diuretic such as mannitol may be administered to prevent renal failure. A severe hemolytic reaction indicates a poor prognosis.

The best way to prevent a reaction is to ensure that the ABO blood types are compatible. This involves carefully identifying the ABO type of both the client and the blood product. The nurse should double-check all blood product transfusions with another licensed nurse and prepare only one transfusion at a time. In addition, the nurse must compare the client's name, medical record number, blood type, and donor blood expiration date with the client's arm band, blood unit identification tag, and label on the blood unit.

The blood should be infused slowly during the first 15 minutes. The nurse should take vital signs prior to the administration of the unit to serve as a baseline. Vital signs also should be checked 15 minutes after beginning the transfusion and should be monitored occasionally throughout the transfusion and from 30 minutes to 1 hour after the unit has been transfused. Throughout the transfusion, the nurse should frequently assess the client's comfort level.

Hemolytic reactions are not the only types of blood reactions. Febrile reactions are common reactions caused by leukocyte or thrombocyte incompatibilities between donor and client blood. The clinical manifestations of a febrile reaction include chills and fever that occur approximately 1 hour after the start of the transfusion, headache, flushing, and generalized weakness and discomfort. Persons with a history of multiple transfusions are susceptible to febrile reactions. This reaction is generally treated with an antipyretic medication such as acetaminophen (Tylenol). The physician's decision to continue or stop the transfusion depends on the severity of the reaction. Administering leukocyte-poor packed RBCs reduces the occurrence of febrile reactions. Leukocyte-poor cells are created either by a procedure termed "washing the cells" or by transfusing the donor blood through a filter that removes leukocytes.

Allergic reactions also can occur during a blood transfusion. Therefore, it is important to take a thorough history to determine whether the client has ever experienced an allergic reaction to any blood product. If the client is potentially allergic to blood products, the physician may decide to administer an antihistamine and a corticosteroid prior to the transfusion. Allergic reactions to blood products are treated in the same manner as allergic reactions to any other substance.

Type III Hypersensitivity Reactions

Type III reactions are immune complex–mediated. They are caused by antigen–antibody complexes that combine with immunoglobulins, making the complexes too small to be effectively removed by phagocytosis (Lewis, 1996). The complexes deposit in blood vessels of tissues, leading to tissue damage through inflammation and phagocytosis. Many autoimmune disorders are associated with this type of hypersensitivity. Unlike persons experiencing type I reactions, those experiencing type III reactions need not have been previously exposed to the antigen causing the reaction. Serum sickness is an example of this type of reaction. Horse antitoxin serum is a common triggering agent as well as penicillin and some other

Hemolytic blood transfusion reactions can be prevented by careful typing and crossmatching. Nurses should double-check all blood unit identification tags with the client's name, blood type, and medical record number.

In a **hemolytic reaction** blood cells are lysed while in a **nonhemolytic reaction** they are not. Hemolytic reactions occur as a result of ABO incompatibilities. Nonhemolytic reactions are a result of antibody–antigen reactions.

medications. Thus, some clients experience an allergic reaction to penicillin even without prior exposure.

Care of the Client Experiencing a Type III Hypersensitivity Reaction

Assessment and Intervention   The clinical manifestations of a type III reaction are similar to those of type I. A type III reaction also may manifest with lymphadenopathy, malaise, and joint pain. Nursing responsibilities for a client with a type III reaction are similar to those for type I.

Type IV Hypersensitivity Reactions

Type IV reactions are delayed reactions because they are cell–mediated. Cell-mediated reactions occur when sensitized T lymphocytes initiate a direct or indirect attack on antigens (Lewis, 1996). Macrophages and enzymes are released, causing tissue destruction. Some blood transfusion reactions also are delayed reactions. This is evident when the hemoglobin of the client decreases after a transfusion. The wheal and flare reaction that occurs in a positive tuberculosis test is an example of a cell–mediated reaction. Atopic dermatitis, another cell–mediated reaction, is a skin condition in which the client comes into direct contact with an allergen, resulting in skin lesions and redness. Other type IV reactions include reactions to poison ivy and transplant graft rejections.

Care of the Client with a Type IV Reaction Presenting as Graft Rejection

Clients who have undergone an organ transplant must constantly assess themselves for the signs and symptoms of **graft rejection**. Fatigue and tenderness over the graft site are the earliest signs of impending graft rejection.

Assessment and Intervention   The clinical manifestations of **graft rejection** include fever, malaise, fatigue, tenderness over the graft site, hypertension, an increased erythrocyte sedimentation rate (ESR), and increased enzyme concentrations. Graft rejections are treated with immunosuppressant medications. The presence of the Epstein-Barr virus (EBV) can complicate the treatment of graft rejection. Immunosuppressant medications promote the proliferation of EBV, which in turn leads to the development of cancer, in particular Burkitt's lymphoma. If drug therapy fails, insufficient vascularization of the tissues results in tissue necrosis, and the graft must then be removed. The client may or may not be eligible for another transplant.

$\mathcal{A}$UTOIMMUNITY

Autoimmunity is an abnormal condition in which the body initiates an immune response against its own tissues.

Tolerance to self-antigens sometimes breaks down, causing lymphocytes to react against their own tissue antigens. For unknown reasons, the body initiates an immune response against itself, an **autoimmune response**. One theory holds that bacterial or viral damage changes the shape of self-antigens, resulting in the initiation of an immune response (Lewis, 1996).

An autoimmune disorder may also develop when cells that have had no contact with circulatory and lymph system fluids, such as lens proteins or sperm, are released into these immune fluids during injury or surgery (Lewis, 1996). It has been documented that after 50 years of age the level of circulating autoantibodies increases (Lewis, 1996).

Autoimmune disorders are generally believed to be either organ specific or systemic (Lewis, 1996). Myasthenia gravis, type I DM, and pernicious anemia are examples of organ-specific autoimmune disorders. Some examples of systemic autoimmune disorders include rheumatoid arthritis, systemic lupus erythematosus (SLE), and scleroderma. Each disorder has different clinical manifestations and requires different therapeutic interventions. These disorders and the specific system involved in each are discussed in other chapters.

IMMUNODEFICIENCY

An immunodeficiency is an impairment of the immune system in which an invading organism produces an insufficient immune response. Immunodeficiencies result from genetic disorders such as severe combined immunodeficiency disease (SCID), chronic diseases, infections, nutritional deficiencies, or treatments such as chemotherapy. Immunodeficiencies are classified as primary or secondary. Primary disorders such as SCID arise from improperly developed immune cells (a defect in the immune mechanism itself). Secondary disorders such as acquired immunodeficiency syndrome (AIDS) arise from another disease process.

Infection

Infection is the invasion of the body by pathogens and the reaction of the body's cells to those pathogens. Infections are either acute or chronic, and acute infections may become chronic. A prolonged infection with methicillin-resistant *Staphylococcus aureus* (MRSA) is an example of an acute infection that becomes chronic. A person with a chronic infection such as herpes simplex can have episodes of acute exacerbation; that is, the condition periodically flares and then subsides.

Pathogens are transmitted either directly, through body-to-body contact, or indirectly, through contaminated food, water, air, soil, or vectors. Tuberculosis (TB) is an example of respiratory spread. The host must have a portal of entry such as the nose, mouth, urogenital tract, or a skin wound. For the pathogen to multiply, the host must be susceptible.

Immunity is a resistance that results from previous exposure to pathogens. It may be active, from a naturally acquired infection or from a vaccination that produces antibodies, or it may be passive, resulting from the transfer of antibodies from another person or animal. Natural **active immunity** forms during the disease process. In some instances, such as

Active immunity occurs when antibodies are formed within the person's body. Artificial active immunity occurs when an altered microbe, injected into the body, initiates antibody production.

chickenpox, the antibodies formed during the disease offer lifelong immunity. Artificial active immunity is acquired through intentional vaccination that stimulates antibody production. Persons inoculated with these vaccines occasionally require a revaccination or "booster shot" to sustain their antibody titer. Vaccines are prepared either as killed vaccines, live vaccines, or toxoids. Killed vaccines are developed from microbes and killed using heat or radiation prior to injection. When injected, they stimulate antibody production. The pertussis vaccine is a killed vaccine. Live vaccines are prepared from living, attenuated (weakened) microbes. They generally provide more protection than killed vaccines. The measles vaccine is a live vaccine. Toxoids are composed of inactivated bacterial toxins. The tetanus toxoid is an example of this type of vaccine.

Passive immunity is acquired when antibodies are transferred from an outside source. Natural passive immunity is acquired when antibodies are passed from the mother to the fetus. The mother's active immunity lends the infant immunity to certain diseases for the first few months of life. Artificial passive immunity is the injection of antiserum from an immunized source that produces immediate immunity. Two examples are diphtheria antitoxin and tetanus antitoxin. These are administered immediately after the client has been exposed to the pathogen. Many people are allergic to antiserums, especially horse antiserum.

Nursing Care of Clients with Infections For clients with infection, the goal is to resolve the infection and restore immune competence. Protecting against infection is the best way to meet these goals. Aseptic techniques for preventing transmission, increasing the host's ability to fight infections, and eliminating harmful pathogens are all necessary in caring for a client with an infection. The nurse must be familiar with these practices when caring for any client, because everyone is susceptible to infection.

Assessment It is imperative that the nurse take a thorough history and perform a thorough physical examination of any client with an infection. The nurse should attempt to identify any possible exposure to infectious pathogens. Possible sources of exposure include contact with others who have illnesses, travel in endemic areas, and contact with environments that likely contain harmful pathogens. Exposure to persons who have illnesses is a likely source of pathogen transmission if the illnesses are communicable. Chickenpox is an example of an illness that can be passed from one person to another. People tend to develop antibodies to the pathogens with which they commonly come in contact in their environment. When people travel outside of their usual environment, they may come in contact with pathogens they have not encountered previously and against which they have no antibodies. Even in their normal environment clients can still come in contact with harmful pathogens, such as those found during an influenza epidemic.

Persons exposed to harmful pathogens should be assessed for susceptibility to infections and for portals of entry. Protein deficiency and calorie malnutrition are common causes of immunodeficiency in geriatric clients

Passive immunity occurs when the body acquires antibodies from an outside source. Artificial passive immunity is acquired when the person receives antibodies from antiserum developed from an immunized source.

Factors that contribute to a person's susceptibility to infection include protein and calorie malnutrition, fatigue, aging, and stress.

(Joffrion & Leuszler, 1995). Elderly clients on a limited budget often consider payments for rent, utilities, and medications more of a priority than food and nutrition. The resulting malnutrition makes the elderly more susceptible to infections and anemia. Infections in such clients are also more difficult to treat, since protein and carbohydrates are necessary for more rapid healing. Stress and fatigue also can increase susceptibility to infections. Many changes occur as clients age that increases their susceptibility to infections. Skin becomes less elastic, the respiratory tract has fewer cilia, and urinary retention is more likely from a loss of bladder muscle tone as a result of neurological changes. Breaks in the integrity of the skin allow pathogens to enter the body. For this reason, it is important to assess the client's skin for open sores and cuts.

Checking baseline vital signs and white blood cell (WBC) counts and performing a culture and sensitivity analysis aid in diagnosing infections. The clinical manifestations of infection include fever, increased drainage, pus, and inflammation. Generally a person with an infection will have generalized body aches or tissue-specific pain. WBC counts rise during infections, but as the infection progresses in severity the counts may lower or "shift to the left." The nurse should examine the WBC count differential as this indicates the severity of the infection. During serious infections, as the body martials mature leukocytes in the immune response, the number of available leukocytes decreases. The body attempts to replace these cells with new ones, but the new leukocytes are immature. The WBC differential shows fewer mature leukocytes (neutrophils) and more immature leukocytes (bands). This is what is meant by a "shift to the left." Sepsis, a condition in which a client has an overwhelming systemic infection, often produces an abnormally low WBC count due to the body's inability to produce sufficient WBCs in response to the infection. The septic patient also may have an abnormally low body temperature. Sepsis can progress to shock.

Immunocompromised clients may not exhibit the expected signs of infection because they may not have enough immunocompetence to exhibit the signs of inflammation such as a fever. Protein malnutrition, certain medications such as steroids and chemotherapy, and disease states such as AIDS are causes of severe immunodeficiency. It is important to assess the immunocompromised client carefully for the signs of infection, as the symptoms may be subtle. Slight temperature elevations can signal severe infections. Pus formation is always a sign of an infection.

Intervention Nurses must be aware of the transmission routes of infectious pathogens. The **Centers for Disease Control (CDC)** list guidelines that health care providers should follow to ensure that proper precautions are taken when treating persons with infectious diseases. Hygiene and disinfection measures decrease the risk of pathogen spread. Proper hand washing is the single most important measure a nurse should practice to prevent the spread of infection. Disposing of infectious materials in biohazardous waste containers also is important to prevent the spread of pathogens.

In addition to the standard transmission routes of infection, it is necessary to understand the infectious pathogen itself and the body's response to

The predominance of immature lymphocytes in a WBC count differential indicates that an overwhelming infection is present.

The nurse must be astute to be able to discern an infection in clients who are immunocompromised. Signs of inflammation generally do not occur. Slight temperature elevations may be the only indication of a serious infection.

The **Centers for Disease Control** have published guidelines that show health care providers how to take proper precautions to prevent the spread of disease. Diseases are listed in alphabetical order and suggestions for reducing transmission are provided.

Currently, the presence of **multiple-drug resistant bacteria** in health care facilities is a primary concern. Thorough hand washing is the best way to prevent the spread of infection.

Nursing care for clients with fever includes antipyretic medications and tepid baths. If the fever is resistant to treatment, hypothermia blankets also are used. There is controversy over how high a temperature needs to be before treatment is initiated. Most sources recommend treating elevated temperatures after they reach 100.5°F–101.5°F.

it. Treatments are based on the type of pathogen that causes the infection. Bacterial infections are generally treated with antibiotics. However, more **antibiotic-resistant strains of bacteria** are emerging. Since these strains of bacteria are resistant to most antibiotics, it is imperative that the nurse avoid spreading bacteria from client to client. Thorough hand washing and contact isolation procedures help prevent this.

Nurses should frequently assess the vital signs of clients with infections. If they are experiencing temperature elevations of 101.5°F or greater, antipyretics such as acetaminophen (Tylenol) and tepid baths can help lower their body temperature. Temperatures greater than 102°–103°F may require a hypothermia blanket to lower the body temperature. Hypothermia blankets are fluid-filled mattresses that are placed under the client and connected to a unit that cools the fluid within the blanket. There should be no padding between the client's skin and the blanket, just a sheet or light bath blanket. Light covers should be placed over the client. The nurse must constantly monitor the client's body temperature while he or she is lying on the blanket. Most units are supplied with a rectal temperature probe that constantly measures the client's body temperature. Vital signs must be assessed frequently while the client is lying on the blanket. The fluid temperature should be set at or just below normal body temperature. The nurse should visually assess the client's skin frequently, as skin integrity may be lost as a result of the cooling action of the blanket (Fig. 13-2).

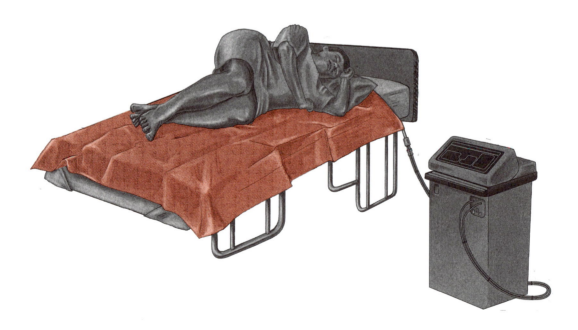

FIGURE 13-2 Hypothermia/hyperthermia mattress. (NOTE: From Phipps, Cassmeyer, Sands, & Lehman, (1995). *Medical-surgical nursing* (5th ed.). St. Louis: C. V. Mosby, p. 126.)

Fever and other components of the immune response deplete body fluids. Therefore, it is important to ensure that clients with infections maintain adequate fluid balance. Nutrition that is high in protein and carbohydrates also assists the client in fighting infections. Since these clients usually do not feel like eating, what they do eat must be nutritious. A number of medications can help stimulate a client's appetite if malnutrition becomes a problem while fighting an infectious disorder. Dronabinol is an example of one such agent. Rest also is helpful to bolster the immune system.

The nurse must teach the client self-care measures. Teaching the client to comply with therapy is an invaluable tool in fighting infections. Many people think that once they start to feel better it is safe to stop treatment. As a result, often the client experiences a resurgence of the infection. Clients also need to be taught that each infection is different and that a medication that is effective for one type of infection may not be effective for another, even if the symptoms are similar. Avoiding exposure to infections also is important. Once an infection has been resolved, it is important for clients to sustain their good health with proper nutrition and sufficient rest.

Client compliance with antibiotic therapy regimens concerns health care providers. Noncompliance leads to bacterial resistance to treatment and the growth of bacterial infections.

Human Immunodeficiency Virus (HIV) and AIDS

The invasion of HIV, a retrovirus, into the cells of the body results in HIV infection. The infection progresses from an asymptomatic stage to AIDS, in which a variety of life-threatening conditions such as cancers, opportunistic infections, and severe immunodeficiency occur. The infection progressively destroys the immune system, which results in decreased T4/CD4 cell counts. T cells are lymphocytes that have a major role in the body's defense against foreign substances. T4 cells are the T cells generally called T-helper cells. T4 cells induce the immune response. CD4 is an antigen of the cell membrane of the T4 cells. HIV invades the T4 cells by binding with the CD4 antigen (Lewis, 1996). The retrovirus responsible for this infection is transmitted through the exchange of body fluids that occurs during sexual activity, parenteral sharing of blood, and from mother to fetus or child (through the placenta or breast milk). The people most susceptible are those who are sexually active with multiple partners, intravenous drug users, and infants of HIV-positive mothers. The risk of transmission through sexual activity is increased even if only one partner has been sexually active with multiple partners. Consequently, sexual intercourse can no longer be considered as just between two people; it is between those two people and everyone else with whom they have been sexually intimate. The same principle applies to intravenous drug use. HIV is transmitted primarily by blood, semen, or vaginal fluid; these fluids are transmitted from an infected person to the bloodstream of an uninfected person (Flaskerud, 1995). Other types of body fluid are much less likely to transmit the retrovirus (Table 13-3).

✾

TABLE 13-3
RISK OF EXPOSURE TO HIV RELATED TO BEHAVIORS AND PRACTICES

Risk/Levels of Safety	Sexual Contact	Injection Drug Use	Perinatal Exposure
Absolutely safe	Abstinence Mutually monogamous with noninfected persons	Not using injection drugs	Abstinence Sterilization Non-infected mother
Very safe	Noninsertive sexual practices	Using sterilized injection paraphernalia	Birth control and abortion
Probably safe	Insertive sexual practices with use of condom	Cleaning injection paraphernalia with full-strength bleach	Use of condoms
Risky	Everything else	All other activities	Pregnancy if mother is HIV+ Breast-feeding

NOTE: From *HIV/AIDS: A Guide to Nursing Care,* 3rd ed., (p. 39), by Flaskerud, J. H., & Ungvarski, P. J., 1995. Philadelphia: W. B. Saunders. Reprinted with permission.

Care of the Client with HIV or AIDS Infection

Assessment HIV infection progresses from asymptomatic to life-threatening conditions in four distinct stages. Stage one occurs from 1 week to 6 months after exposure. The client may present with flu-like symptoms or no symptoms at all. The body is developing antibodies at this stage. From 2–18 weeks the HIV antibody test becomes positive; this is often referred to as the seropositivity stage. If symptoms are present, they include malaise, slight fever, swollen lymph glands, and body aches.

The client enters the second stage when the T4/CD4 counts fall below 500 cells per microliter. The constitutional symptoms of fever, night sweats, weight loss, diarrhea, swollen lymph glands, and recurrent candidiasis are common during this phase. These symptoms occur 6 weeks to 9 months after exposure if treatment has not been initiated.

Stage three occurs when the T4/CD4 cell counts fall below 200 cells per microliter. The client is now considered to have AIDS. Opportunistic infections and malignancies occur; common ones include *Pneumocystis carinii* pneumonia (PCP), cytomegalovirus, toxoplasmosis, Kaposi's sarcoma, recurrent TB, and candidiasis. At this stage, invasive cervical cancer is frequently present in women. Clients in the third phase may experience weight loss and severe diarrhea, commonly termed "wasting syndrome." HIV-related encephalopathy also occurs.

Stage four occurs when T4/CD4 counts fall below 50 cells per microliter. In stage four the immune system is so depleted that opportunistic infections and malignancies become life-threatening. This is the end-stage

Clients who are HIV positive must have their T4/CD4 counts monitored frequently. A count of less than 200 cells/μL indicates that the client has AIDS.

of AIDS. T-cell counts are so low that treatment options are less effective. Death occurs soon after the client progresses to this stage.

Clients with HIV infection can experience remissions. Current medications and better supportive therapy have made it possible for clients to regain high concentrations of T4/CD4. Thus, the T-cell levels of clients with AIDS may return to levels greater than 500 cells/μL. The occurrence of opportunistic diseases is directly related to the client's concentrations of T4/CD4 cells (Table 13-4; Fig. 13-3).

The nurse should take a complete history and perform a thorough physical examination of clients at risk for HIV infection. Information concerning possible risk factors should be obtained during the client history. Nurses commonly make assumptions about which clients are the "type" to be infected with HIV. This is not wise, considering how many people are infected and the fact that this disease crosses all barriers of gender, sexual preference, age, race, and geographical location. Any client with a history of frequent infections should be assessed for possible past exposure to the HIV retrovirus. Indeed, clients are often first diagnosed with HIV while being seen for an opportunistic infection. This is unfortunate because the earlier the client is diagnosed the easier it is to slow the progress of the disease.

A number of tests are used to detect the presence of HIV. The **enzyme-linked immunosorbent assay (ELISA)** and **Western blot** are the most common tests. Both of these assays test for the presence of antibodies to the HIV retrovirus. The ELISA is generally performed first. If it detects antibodies, a Western blot test is then performed to confirm the results. False-positive and false-negative results are possible. One problem with both of these tests is that antibodies must be present for the test to be sensitive to, and thus detect, the infection. There is a "window period" between the

The **ELISA** and **Western blot assays** detect antibodies to HIV. Antibodies must develop before these tests are positive for infection. There is a period of time after infection but before antibody development when the test will be negative.

TABLE 13-4
STAGES OF HIV/AIDS

Stage	Symptoms
Asymptomatic	Body begins to develop antibodies. HIV test is positive when the body seroconverts. May experience no symptoms. Some people experience malaise, slight fever, swollen lymph glands, and body aches. People may remain in this stage without the appearance of symptoms for 9–10 years.
Early symptomatic	T4/CD4 cell counts drop below 500 cells per microliter. Constitutional symptoms of fever, night sweats, weight loss, diarrhea, swollen lymph glands, and recurrent candidiasis occur.
Late symptomatic (AIDS)	T4/CD4 cell counts drop below 200 cells per microliter. Life-threatening opportunistic infections and malignancies occur. Wasting syndrome occurs.
Advanced disease	T4/CD4 cell counts drop below 50 cells per microliter. Opportunistic infections and malignancies frequently occur. Severe wasting syndrome occurs. This marks end-stage disease.

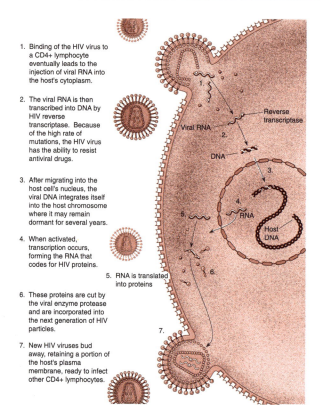

1. Binding of the HIV virus to a CD4+ lymphocyte eventually leads to the injection of viral RNA into the host's cytoplasm.

2. The viral RNA is then transcribed into DNA by HIV reverse transcriptase. Because of the high rate of mutations, the HIV virus has the ability to resist antiviral drugs.

3. After migrating into the host cell's nucleus, the viral DNA integrates itself into the host chromosome where it may remain dormant for several years.

4. When activated, transcription occurs, forming the RNA that codes for HIV proteins.

5. RNA is translated into proteins

6. These proteins are cut by the viral enzyme protease and are incorporated into the next generation of HIV particles.

7. New HIV viruses bud away, retaining a portion of the host's plasma membrane, ready to infect other CD4+ lymphocytes.

FIGURE 13-3

◙

Destruction of the body's defenses by human immunodeficiency virus (HIV). (NOTE: From Kenny, P. (1996). Managing HIV infection: How to bolster your patient's fragile health. *Nursing '95* (August), p. 31.)

The **wasting syndrome** associated with AIDS is defined as the loss of 10% or more of body weight with any of the following constitutional symptoms: fatigue, malaise, diarrhea, anorexia, and weakness.

time when the virus infects the client's T cells and when the body develops antibodies to the virus during which antibody-testing assays give a false-negative result. Several examinations test for the retrovirus itself; however, these tests are performed infrequently because they are expensive and not readily available.

During the client's physical examination the nurse should assess for signs of HIV infection including swollen lymph glands, malaise, body aches, and other generalized flu-like symptoms. The presence of recurrent infections such as yeast or thrush also needs to be assessed. These symptoms, in addition to a positive history of potential exposure to HIV, suggest that the client may be HIV positive. In certain stages of the disease, the client may develop leukoplakia (small, white patches) in the oral cavity. These patches are similar to thrush but do not flake off with a tongue blade. The condition is usually painless. The presence of these patches suggests HIV infection.

Kaposi's sarcoma is a common opportunistic malignancy in HIV-positive clients. This malignancy presents as a skin disorder. The lesions that appear on the skin look like bruises. They are irregularly shaped and usually have a bluish-red color. They can appear anywhere on the body, disappear over time, but reappear later in random locations.

Vomiting and diarrhea are common in the later stages of this disorder. Most clients become anorectic and weak as well. When patients start to lose weight and muscle mass as a result of the symptoms of diarrhea and anorexia, they are experiencing a **wasting syndrome**, as described previously. Therefore, it is important for the nurse to take a complete history of the client's diet, exercise habits, sleep, and any weight loss. Since the client may be losing a large amount of fluids from vomiting and diarrhea, it is important to assess for the clinical manifestations of dehydration, including poor skin turgor, dry mucous membranes, thirst, and warm, dry skin. In addition, the client should be assessed for the signs of malnutrition such as weight loss, poor muscle tone, poor wound healing, and fatigue.

HIV-induced encephalopathy is common. Therefore, it is important for the nurse to question the client concerning memory loss or confusion. Family members may be of assistance in ascertaining if the client is experiencing memory loss or seems disoriented at times. The nurse can perform simple neurological examinations to test for cognitive ability. One elementary test involves having clients recall verifiable incidents of their life such as the year they were born. This tests long-term memory. A good test of short-term memory is to have clients state a short list of common items such as a pencil, book, clock, and coin, and then ask them to recall the items 10 or 15 minutes later. Cognitive ability also can be tested by examining their ability to perform analytical and mathematical analyses. Two examples of a test of cognitive ability include asking the client to explain the adage "birds of a feather flock together" or having them count to 70 by increments of seven. The nurse can determine disorientation by assessing if the client is oriented to person, place, and time.

It is important to assess the HIV-positive client for any signs of infection or immune compromise. The nurse also should check if there have been opportunities for infections to occur, such as exposure to illnesses, skin breakdown, mucosal lesions, or client susceptibility. Measuring the WBC and T4/CD4 counts is important as these laboratory tests are the best indications of the severity of the disease.

Intervention Consider the following case study.

CASE STUDY: HIV INFECTION

A 44-year-old man presents to an ambulatory care center with flu-like symptoms. He is sexually active with two women. He states that he uses recreational drugs on occasion. Because of his positive history of risk factors, an HIV screening is done. Both the ELISA and Western blot tests are positive for the HIV virus.

Nursing care goals for a client who has AIDS or is HIV positive include the maintenance or restoration of normal body temperature, fluid balance, normal bowel function, skin integrity, neurological function, and adequate caloric intake, as well as protection from infection. It is important to assist the client in coping with the disease. Maintaining hope is a high priority. Another important nursing responsibility is to teach clients how to function optimally in their environment. Clients also must learn how to avoid transmitting the disease to others.

The goals of nursing care for HIV-positive clients include the maintenance or restoration of normal body temperature, fluid balance, bowel function, skin integrity, neurological functioning, and adequate protein and calorie intake, as well as protection from infection.

Pre-and post-test counseling are important for clients who suspect they may have HIV or who test positive for the HIV virus.

The nurse needs to instruct the client concerning the test procedures. When a client is tested, counseling should be included. Even if the test is negative, the client needs counseling for the behaviors that brought him or her in to be tested. It is also advisable that the client be retested in 3 months if he or she engages in high-risk behavior (Flaskerud, 1995). Any client who tests seropositive for HIV must undergo post-test counseling, which includes referral to an early intervention program and, if needed, to a partner notification program (Flaskerud, 1995). The client in the case study should be referred to both programs. Client referrals to a support group and other community agencies that offer assistance also are appropriate. Above all, the nurse must be an advocate for the client.

HIV-positive clients need information to protect themselves from infection. It is important for these clients to get adequate nutrition and rest. Teaching clients fatigue-relieving measures such as time management, stress reduction strategies, and how to balance rest and activity assists in preventing the onset of new infections. Clients with AIDS may need assistance with activities of daily living (ADL). Providing support during periods of severe exacerbations of their illness helps these clients to manage their overall illness.

The client in the case study is experiencing mild symptoms of HIV infection. He is most likely in the first stage of the disease. Assisting him in developing and maintaining good health habits may slow the progression of the disease. The client requires counseling for his recreational drug use, as this habit greatly weakens the ability of his immune system to fight the disease. The nurse also should instruct the client that a good balance between rest and activity as well as optimal nutrition serve to postpone the development of AIDS.

It is difficult for clients with AIDS to get adequate nutrition. Consuming foods that are high in protein and calories helps clients to maintain or restore immune competence. Clients should make every calorie count; in other words, they should be able to take in adequate nutrients without having to increase greatly the amount of food eaten.

Clients with AIDS-related diarrhea should be taught to follow a diet high in protein and calories and low in residue. A low-residue diet has decreased fiber and no products that contain lactose.

For clients experiencing wasting syndrome, getting adequate nutrition is even more of a challenge. The nurse should suggest drinking fluids between instead of during meals to prevent satiety as a result of fluid intake. Since diarrhea is a common problem for clients with wasting syndrome, reducing odors in the environment is a necessity. Clients should be able to eat in a pleasant environment without noxious odors. If they are experiencing diarrhea, it is better for them to consume foods that are low in bulk. Generally these patients should be on a diet that is high in protein and calories and low in residue. Low residue refers not only to the bulk in food but also to the residue that food leaves in the digestive system. Milk and milk products such as cheese are not allowed on a low-residue diet. If the client is experiencing stomatitis, cold food may be better tolerated. Medications can help stimulate a client's appetite. Dronabinol (Marinol) and megestrol are two examples of appetite stimulants. Occasionally it is necessary to include enteral or parenteral nutritional support (Table 13-5).

Maintaining a proper fluid balance can be difficult for clients suffering from wasting syndrome. Clients need to be counseled concerning the need

TABLE 13-5
NUTRITIONAL MANAGEMENT

Dietary Recommendation	Intervention

Diarrhea
  Lactose-free,
   low-fat, low-fiber,
   and high-potassium
   foods
	Avoid dairy products, red meat, margarine, butter, eggs, dried beans, peas, raw fruits and vegetables. Cooked or canned vegetables will provide needed vitamins. Encourage potassium-rich foods such as bananas and apricot nectar. Discontinue foods, nutritional supplements, and medications that may make diarrhea worse (e.g., Ensure, antacids, stool softeners). Avoid gas-producing foods. Serve warm, not hot, foods. Plan small, frequent meals. Drink plenty of fluids between meals.

Constipation High-fiber foods	Eat fruits and vegetables (e.g., beans, peas) and cereal and whole wheat breads. Gradually increase fiber. Drink plenty of fluids. Exercise.
Nausea and vomiting Low-fat foods	Avoid dairy products and red meat. Plan small, frequent meals. Prepare non-odorous foods. Eat dry, salty foods, serve food cold or at room temperature. Drink liquids between meals. Avoid gas-producing, greasy, and/or spicy foods. Eat slowly in a relaxed atmosphere. Rest after meals with head elevated. Antiemetics may be taken 30 min before meals.
Candidiasis Soft or pureed foods	Serve moist foods. Drink plenty of fluids. Avoid acidic and spicy foods. Use straw and tilt head back and forth when drinking. To decrease discomfort, eat a soft diet, such as puddings and yogurt.

Fever
  High-calorie,
   high-protein foods
	Use nutritional supplements. Increase fluid intake.

Altered taste Diet as tolerated	Try herbs and spices. Marinate meat, poultry, and fish. Serve food cold or at room temperature. Drink plenty of fluids. Add salt or sugar. Introduce alternative protein sources.
Anemia High-iron foods	Eat red meat, organ meats, and raisins. Drink orange juice when taking iron supplements to facilitate absorption.
Fatigue High-calorie foods	Cook in large quantities and freeze in meal-size packets. Use microwave and convenience foods. Use easy-to-fix snack foods. Encourage social support system to assist with meal planning and preparation. Provide in-home homemaker services. Access community Meals-on-Wheels programs.

NOTE: From *Medical-Surgical Nursing*, 4th ed., (p. 247), by Lewis, S. L., Collier, I. C., Heitkemper, M. M., 1996, St. Louis: C. V. Mosby. Reprinted with permission.

to increase their fluid intake. Fluid intake and output must be strictly measured. Observing for clinical manifestations of dehydration is also important. If dehydration occurs, intravenous fluid replacement may become necessary. The nurse should monitor the client's electrolytes, because potassium losses are common as a result of diarrhea from the wasting syndrome.

Special care must be taken of the client's skin during wasting syndrome. Decubiti form easily on clients who do not get the proper nutrition and have skin irritants such as constant diarrhea. Friction and pressure from spending too much time in bed also can contribute to the development of decubiti. Keeping the skin clean and dry is a priority. Superfatted soaps, which will not strip the skin of natural moisture, are recommended to clean the skin (Ungvarski & Schmidt, 1995). Skin protectants such as emollients and lubricants also help protect against skin breakdown. Padding bony prominences and frequently repositioning the client are good skin protective measures. If the skin does develop sores or ulcers, occlusive dressings such as Op-Site and Duoderm are contraindicated for immunocompromised clients (Ungvarski & Schmidt, 1995). Nonocclusive dressings such as saline-soaked gauze are recommended.

The client in the case study is angry because he feels that contracting HIV was very unlikely. He does not think he has been promiscuous nor does he feel that he has a "hard core" drug habit. He claims that life is so unfair and asks why he is being punished. It is the nurse's role to help the client examine his feelings. He may require further counseling. Anger is an appropriate coping mechanism at this stage of his acceptance of the disease.

Alterations in **self-concept** are likely with this disorder. Clients need to be allowed to verbalize their feelings without fear of judgment. They need to explore ways to keep hope alive. Complementary therapies may provide the client with a renewed sense of control over the disease. Many HIV-positive clients claim that nontraditional therapies that include herbs and special diets, biofeedback, acupuncture, and shark cartilage are very helpful. The nurse should encourage the client to discuss the use of complementary therapies. In this way the client's primary provider can evaluate the interactive effects of complementary and traditional therapies.

HIV-related encephalopathy is a neurological disorder caused by HIV infection. The nurse should be aware of any incidences of increasing confusion and disorientation and report any neurological abnormalities to the primary provider. A client who has encephalopathy needs to be periodically reoriented to time, place, and person, and requires additional protection from injury. The nurse also must assist the client's family and caregivers in understanding the disease and teach them how to protect the client.

Disease transmission is a primary concern. Clients should be taught about how to prevent disease transmission. Clients who are sexually active must be taught safe-sex practices. The best way to prevent transmission is to use a condom with spermicidal gel each time the client has sexual intercourse. A surprisingly large number of people do not know how to use a condom correctly. Spermicidal gel, which may have some viricidal function, should be applied to the inside tip of the condom prior to placing it on the head of the penis. Leave room at the tip of the condom, then gently roll it down the shaft of the penis. Once the man has ejaculated, the condom should be grasped at the base of the penis (to keep ejaculate within the condom) before withdrawal. The condom should then be removed and discarded (Fig. 13-4).

Once clients learn to live with HIV, they need to be taught how to prevent disease transmission. It is inappropriate to instruct a client to forego intimacy. The nurse should recommend being honest with partners and taking precautions to prevent viral transmission. Clients also require assistance in learning about the progression of the disease and what can be done to lessen its effects.

Prior to using occlusive dressings such as Op-Site or Duoderm, the nurse must determine if the client is immunocompetent.

Self-concept issues are a constant concern for clients with HIV or AIDS, especially in light of the public response to the disease. Additionally, several opportunistic diseases and malignancies are disfiguring or debilitating.

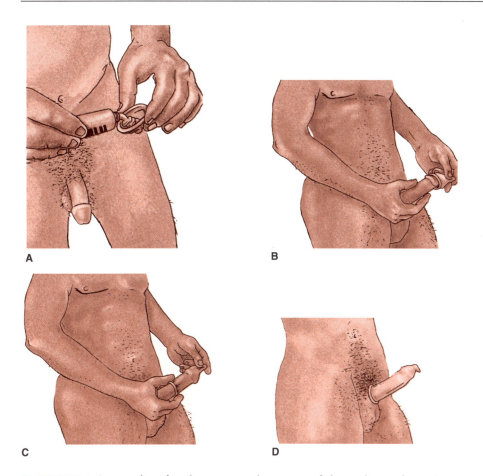

FIGURE 13-4 Steps taken for the correct placement of the male condom. *A* Spermicidal gel is placed in the tip of the condom. *B* Air is removed from the reservoir, and the condom is placed over the erect penis. *C* and *D* The condom is rolled over the shaft of the penis to the hairline. (NOTE: From Lewis, C. L., Collier, I. C., & Heitkemper, M. M. (1996). *Medical-surgical nursing* (4th ed.). St. Louis: C. V. Mosby, p. 248.)

The primary goal of **nursing care** for clients with HIV is protection from infection. New drug therapy combinations show great promise in protecting the client from progression of the disease and reducing the virus to almost undetectable levels in the body. Reverse transcriptase and protease inhibitor agents help clients to regain high T4/CD4 cell counts. The reverse transcriptase agents also assist in preventing the spread of the retrovirus to new cells. However, they do not interfere with viral replication within the infected cells. The most commonly used agents of this category are zidovudine (AZT, Retrovir), didanosine (Videx), zalcitabine (Hivid), and lamivudine (Epivir). The protease inhibitors reduce the viral load within cells. Currently the protease inhibitors are still in the experimental stages but are being prescribed more often in combination with the

Antiretroviral drug agents cause severe depression of bone marrow cell production. For this reason clients should have their blood counts monitored frequently. The agents also are difficult to tolerate. As a result medication dosages are changed and different combinations of therapies are administered to make clients more comfortable.

reverse transcriptase agents to help increase T-cell counts. The FDA-approved protease inhibitors include saquinavir (Invirase), indinavir (Crixivan), and ritonavir (Norvir). The antiretroviral agents have a number of adverse effects including severe bone marrow depression, nausea, fatigue, headache, insomnia, and pancreatitis.

Clients always should be aware of their T4/CD4 counts. The client in the case study had a count of 385 cells per microliter upon his first visit. He later became proficient at monitoring the adverse effects of lowered counts. The client kept a log of his cell counts and planned his activities based on these levels. This provided him a greater amount of control over his disease.

During times when the T4/CD4 counts are low, clients should take precautions to avoid exposure to infectious pathogens. Avoiding people who are ill and refraining from travel may be necessary. However, most of the infections that HIV-infected people contract are opportunistic and thus unavoidable. The best preventive measures include meeting nutritional needs and getting adequate rest.

A number of medications are used to treat opportunistic infections. Viral infections are treated with acyclovir (Zovirax), foscarnet, or ganciclovir. Acyclovir (Zovirax) treats the herpes simplex virus. Foscarnet and ganciclovir are used to treat cytomegalovirus. These medications must be infused for 1 hour, and the client should be well hydrated prior to receiving them. As the drugs are nephrotoxic, the nurse must monitor the client's BUN and creatinine concentrations.

For the treatment of fungal infections, nystatin, clotrimazole, fluconazole, and amphotericin B are used. Nystatin and clotrimazole are used to treat oral candidiasis. Nystatin can be frozen for better oral retention, and clotrimazole is available as a lozenge. Client compliance is difficult to obtain with clotrimazole as it must be taken five times a day for 14 days and causes oral irritation. Fluconazole is used for cryptococcal meningitis. It is nephrotoxic and causes gastrointestinal distress. **Amphotericin B** is a powerful agent used to treat cryptococcal meningitis and histoplasmosis. It must be infused over a period of 6 hours. To prevent precipitation, amphotericin B must be diluted in 5% dextrose in water (D5W), never in normal saline. As it is light sensitive as well, the bottle should be covered to protect the infusion from light. There is a high risk that clients may develop hypersensitivity or phlebitis. The nurse must monitor the client for severe hypokalemia as well.

PCP is a type of pneumonia that commonly affects clients with AIDS. It is treated with **sulfamethoxazole-trimethoprim (Bactrim)** or pentamidine. Clients who take sulfamethoxazole-trimethoprim (Bactrim) must be well hydrated, and those clients taking it orally should drink a full glass of water beforehand. The client must be made aware that the drug causes photosensitivity. If clients who take this medication do not protect themselves from sunlight, they can develop serious rashes over their entire body. The client's fluid intake and output should be monitored. Blood dyscrasias are a common adverse effect of this medication. **Pentamidine 300** is administered in aerosol form. It alters the deoxyribonucleic acid (DNA) of the body; therefore, it should be administered in an environment where only the patient can inhale the aerosol spray. Pentamidine 300 can-

Because antiviral agents are nephrotoxic, it is necessary to monitor BUN and creatinine levels of clients receiving these agents. The client should be well hydrated prior to receiving these medications.

Clients often do not comply with the antifungal therapies because of the necessity of a lengthy treatment and the irritation that the medications cause.

Amphotericin B is a powerful antifungal agent that is very difficult for clients to tolerate. It must be diluted in D5W and infused over 6 hours. Clients on amphotericin B are at high risk for developing hypersensitivity and phlebitis (see Fig. 13-2). It causes the client to become very weak and hypokalemic.

Sulfamethoxazole-trimethoprim (Bactrim) causes a generalized, serious rash on skin that has been exposed to the sun. The client needs to be well hydrated before taking this medication.

not be mixed with normal saline because precipitates will form. It should be mixed in sterile water using a protective ventilation hood to prevent accidental inhalation. The adverse effects of pentamidine 300 include severe hypotension, hypoglycemia, bone marrow depression, and kidney and liver damage.

Clients with PCP are at risk for contracting TB infections. TB is treated with isoniazid, amikacin sulfate, and rifampin. TB requires a long treatment phase, often 9 months to 2 years. As TB is highly contagious, respiratory isolation is necessary if the client is hospitalized. Otherwise, the client needs to be taught to cover nose and mouth when coughing or sneezing. AIDS clients especially are at risk because drug-resistant TB is prevalent. The adverse effects of TB treatment include hepatotoxicity, peripheral neuropathy, and GI upset. **Rifampin** discolors all body fluids to a reddish-orange color that stains clothes and contact lenses. Since alcohol decreases the effectiveness of these medications, clients must abstain from drinking. It is likely that clients will not comply with therapy. Some public health departments have resorted to direct therapy in which a health department official actually witnesses the client taking his or her medication once per day. Accordingly, the dosages of the medications are adjusted so that they only need to be taken once per day in an attempt to improve compliance and help stop the spread of TB (Table 13-6).

The client in the case study has had two episodes of PCP. Both times the client was treated and responded well to sulfamethoxazole-trimethoprim (Bactrim) administered intravenously. The client currently is taking sulfamethoxazole-trimethoprim (Bactrim) as well as zidovudine and didanosine.

Pentamidine 300 is an aerosol form of medication that alters DNA. Therefore, the nurse should be sure that only the client inhales the agent during treatment.

Client compliance with TB treatment is a concern because of frequent episodes of GI distress and the lengthy treatment required. The drugs also are expensive, but many communities have resources to help pay for this treatment.

Rifampin discolors all body fluids a reddish-orange hue. This discoloration stains contact lenses and clothing.

TABLE 13-6
DRUG THERAPY FOR HIV/AIDS AND OPPORTUNISTIC DISEASES

Classification	Disease(s)	Drug Agents
Reverse agents	HIV/AIDS	Zidovidine (AZT, Retrovir), didanosine (ddl, Videx), stavudine (Zerit), lamivudine (Epivir), and zalcitabine (ddC, Hivid)
Protease inhibitor agents	HIV/AIDS	Saquinavir (Invirase), indinavir (Crixivan), and ritonavir (Norvir)
Antiviral agents	Herpes simplex, varicella zoster, and cytomegalovirus	Acyclovir (Zovirax), ganciclovir (Cytovene), and foscarnet (Foscavir)
Antifungal agents	Candidiasis and histoplasmosis	Nystatin (Mycostatin), clotrimazole (Mycelex), fluconazole (Diflucan), and amphotericin B
Antiprotozoan agents	*Pneumocystis carinii*, toxoplasmosis	Sulfamethoxazole-trimethoprim (Bactrim), and pentamidine (Pentam 300)
Antimycobacterial agents	Tuberculosis	Isoniazid (INH), rifampin, and amikacin sulfate (Amikin)

He states that he constantly battles oral thrush. The client boasts of being relatively healthy and continues to be able to work and enjoy a full life.

Clients experiencing opportunistic diseases are generally very sick. They need support and intervention to fight the disease as well as to rebuild their immune system. Confidentiality is an important issue, as many people have experienced prejudice as a result of their HIV-positive state. Fear of losing family, friends, jobs, and health insurance are real concerns for clients with HIV infection. All 50 states have mandated that AIDS must be reported to the CDC. It varies by state whether HIV-positive clients who do not have AIDS need to be reported. Most states have ruled that only those people who have a need to know should be informed of a person's HIV-positive state.

Summary

Disorders of the immune system include hypersensitivities, autoimmunities, and immunodeficiencies. Hypersensitivities are disorders in which the person's immune system has overreacted. Autoimmunities occur when the body fails to recognize self-antigens and therefore releases an immune response against itself. Immunodeficiencies are disorders in which the immune system cannot initiate an effective response to invading pathogens.

The **nursing care** of clients with an immune disorder depends on the type of disorder. Hypersensitivities generally are treated immediately. Care must be taken to prevent the client from going into shock. Maintaining the airway and adequate circulation are the primary goals for treating clients who are experiencing a hypersensitivity reaction. Autoimmune disorders are treated primarily with corticosteroids to decrease the immune response. It is also important to provide supportive therapy. There are two goals for treating patients with an immunodeficiency: to bolster the immune system to fight invading pathogens, and to give supportive therapy to decrease the effects of invading pathogens.

KEY WORDS

ABO incompatibility
Active immunity
Anaphylaxis
Autoimmunity
Enzyme-linked immunosorbent assay
Hemolytic blood transfusion reactions
Hypersensitivity
Immune competence

Immune deficiency
Nonhemolytic blood transfusion reactions
Passive immunity
Retrovirus
T4/CD4 cells
Wasting syndrome
Western blot

QUESTIONS

1. A 24-year-old male client presents to the emergency room complaining of shortness of breath, itchiness, and anxiety. He states that he was just stung by a bee and that he has had a previous allergic reaction to a bee sting. Which of the following medications should the nurse administer to the client first?

   A. Atropine sulfate (Atropine)
   B. Ipratropium (Atrovent)
   C. Epinephrine
   D. Alprazolam (Xanax)

2. Which of the following procedures is most effective for preventing hemolytic blood transfusion reactions?

   A. Administering the blood through 5% dextrose in water (D5W)
   B. Administration of a steroid prior to the transfusion
   C. Careful identification of the client and the blood product
   D. Using a leukocyte-poor filter during the transfusion

3. An early sign that a client with a kidney transplant is beginning to reject the organ is:
   A. abdominal distention
   B. flank tenderness
   C. hypotension
   D. shortness of breath

4. A client with AIDS is experiencing diarrhea related to the wasting syndrome. Which of the following nutritional changes should the nurse suggest to the client to ease the diarrhea?
   A. Avoid potassium-rich foods
   B. Eliminate lactose from the diet
   C. Increase fiber in the diet
   D. Restrict fluids

5. A 45-year-old male client who is HIV positive states that he no longer sees his friends. He is afraid they will not accept him now that he is HIV positive. He has not informed any of his friends or his employer of his HIV-positive status. His T4/CD4 counts are 765 cells per microliter. Which of the following nursing diagnoses is most appropriate for this patient?
   A. Anxiety related to fear of death
   B. Denial related to an asymptomatic stage of HIV infection
   C. High risk for opportunistic infections related to a low T-cell count
   D. Social isolation related to fear of rejection

6. Patient teaching for a client who is taking zidovidine (AZT) should include which of the following instructions?

A. Complete blood counts need to be monitored.
B. The drug is to be taken for 10–14 days.
C. The drug should be taken with milk.
D. Tolerance to the drug increases over time.

ANSWERS

1. *The answer is C.* Epinephrine at a concentration of 1:1000 is the first medication administered for the systemic symptoms of anaphylaxis. It acts as a vasoconstrictor and bronchodilator, reducing the effects of bronchospasm and circulatory shutdown associated with anaphylaxis. Atropine sulfate (Atropine) reverses bradycardia. Patients experiencing anaphylaxis do not experience bradycardia. Ipratropium (Atrovent) is a bronchodilator but does nothing to reverse the symptoms of shock associated with anaphylactic reactions. Alprazolam (Xanax) relieves anxiety, but this client's anxiety is a result of the neurological reaction that is part of anaphylaxis. Treating the anaphylaxis is the first priority.

2. *The answer is C.* Hemolytic transfusion reactions result from ABO incompatibility between the client's and donor's blood. Careful determination that the client is receiving the right unit of blood is vital to prevent these reactions. Blood should be administered through normal saline, not D5W. However, fluid choices are not related to hemolytic reactions. Administering a steroid and transfusing through a leukocyte-poor filter helps prevent nonhemolytic reactions, not hemolytic reactions.

3. *The answer is B.* Tenderness over the site of the transplanted organ is one of the earliest symptoms of graft rejection. Kidney transplant rejections do not manifest as abdominal distention or hypotension. The client may become hypertensive. Shortness of breath is a late sign of graft rejection as a result of developing congestive heart failure from kidney failure.

4. *The answer is B.* Clients with AIDS who are experiencing diarrhea should avoid milk and milk products because of the irritating effect these foods have on their digestive systems. The client will need potassium-rich foods as a result of potassium losses from diarrhea. Increasing fiber will further irritate the gastrointestinal tract of AIDS clients. Restricting fluids will only serve to dehydrate the client further.

5. *The answer is D.* This client is experiencing social isolation from his fear of rejection by his friends. The client is not exhibiting the symptoms of anxiety and is not denying his condition. The client is not at risk for opportunistic diseases at this time because his T-cell counts are close to normal.

6. *The answer is A.* AZT causes severe depression of bone marrow cell production; therefore, complete blood counts need to be monitored. The drug must be taken for much longer than 14 days. The drug does not need to be taken with milk. It does not cause gastrointestinal irritation, but the milk may irritate the gastrointestinal tract if the client is experiencing diarrhea related to AIDS. Tolerance, a problem with this agent, will not decrease over time. The drug is discontinued if the client is not able to tolerate it.

ANNOTATED REFERENCES

Flaskerud, J. H. (1995). Health promotion and disease prevention. In J. H. Flaskerud & P. J. Ungvarski (Eds.), *HIV/AIDS: A guide to nursing care* (3rd ed., pp. 30–63). Philadelphia: W. B. Saunders.

Flaskerud and Ungvarski are recognized experts on the issues of caring for HIV-infected persons. This chapter in their book gives a summary of the risk factors and available testing procedures for HIV/AIDS. It discusses the need for counseling for clients who are HIV positive.

Gold, J. (1994). Ask about latex. *RN*, 32–34.

This article discusses the new issues involving the common use of latex. It explores caring for clients and health care providers who are allergic to latex and suggests ways to avoid coming into contact with latex.

Joffrion, L. P. & Leuszler, L. B. (1995). The gastrointestinal system and its problems in the elderly, with nutritional considerations. In J. Stanley & B. G. Beare (Eds.), *Gerontological nursing* (pp. 241–254). Philadelphia: F. A. Davis.

This is a good resource for information on caring for the elderly. This chapter describes the effects of protein and caloric malnutrition, a common cause of immune deficiency.

Korniewicz, D. M., Laughon, B. E., Butz, A., & Larsen, E. (1989). Integrity of vinyl and latex procedure gloves. *Nursing Research, 38 (3)*, 144–146.

This research article examines the differences in integrity between vinyl and latex gloves. Both offer barrier protection.

Lewis, S. L. (1996). Nursing role in management of altered immune responses. In S. L. Lewis, I. C. Collier, & M. M. Heitkemper (Eds.), *Medical-surgical nursing: Assessment & management of clinical problems* (4th ed., pp. 207–234). St. Louis: C. V. Mosby.

This chapter covers nursing care for persons with immune disorders. Lewis, Collier, and Heitkemper are recognized leaders in medical-surgical textbooks. Dr. Lewis is an expert on the effects of immune disorders.

Rote, N. S. (1994). Alterations in immunity and inflammation. In K. L. McCance & S. E. Huether (Eds.), *Pathophysiology: The biological basis for disease in adults and children* (2nd ed., pp. 268–298). St. Louis: C. V. Mosby.

This chapter provides an overview of the pathophysiology involved in immune disorders. It discusses and classifies the different types of hypersensitivity disorders.

Ungvarski, P. J. & Schmidt, J. (1995). Nursing management of the adult client. In J. H. Flaskerud & P. J. Ungvarski (Eds.), *HIV/AIDS: A guide to nursing care* (3rd ed., pp. 134–184). Philadelphia: W. B. Saunders.

This text covers the health instructions that clients with HIV/AIDS should receive. It also gives a brief description of the current research involving HIV/AIDS.

INTERNET SITES FOR ADDITIONAL INFORMATION

AIDS Resources:
http://www.zumacafe.com/pocaf/aids.html

CDC Wonder:
http://wwwonder.cdc.gov/

Delaware Valley Latex Allergy Support Network, Inc.:
http://www.latex.org/

National Institute of Allergy and Infectious Diseases
http://www.niaid.nih.gov/

𝒩EOPLASTIC DISORDERS

𝒟EVELOPMENT OF NEOPLASTIC DISORDERS

Neoplastic disorders are conditions of uncontrolled and progressive cellular proliferation. Neoplasms are either benign or malignant and develop as a result of two cellular dysfunctions. The first is a dysfunction in **cellular differentiation**. Normal stem cells of a particular tissue differentiate into mature functioning cells of that tissue (Bender, Yasko, & Strohl, 1996). The cells differentiate in an orderly process from an immature to a mature state. Differentiation is controlled by proto-oncogenes that dictate the mature functioning state of cells. In the development of neoplasms, the normal function of cellular differentiation is lost. Haphazard differentiation occurs in which some cells of a tissue or organ dedifferentiate into less mature cells. In malignant tumors, cellular dedifferentiation occurs as a result of exposure to carcinogens, oncogenic viruses, genetic alterations, or genetic mutations (Fig. 14-1).

Abnormal cellular proliferation is the second cellular malfunction that leads to neoplastic development. Cells are normally controlled by an intracellular mechanism that determines when cellular proliferation is necessary (Bender, Yasko, & Strohl, 1996). Dynamic equilibrium is achieved when cellular proliferation equals cellular degeneration (Bender, Yasko, & Strohl, 1996). New cell growth occurs in response to a physiologic need for more cells. Cell growth stops in response to **contact inhibition**. This is an internal mechanism within tissues that triggers cells to stop proliferating because there is no room to expand. The rate of cellular proliferation differs for each tissue. Bone marrow cells proliferate frequently and rapidly

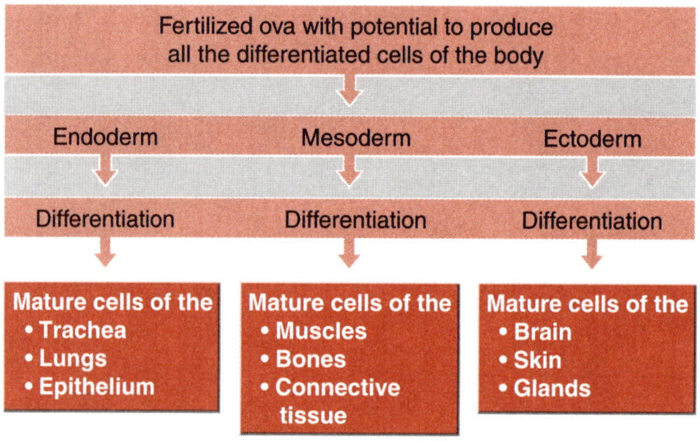

FIGURE 14-1

Normal cellular differentiaton.

Cellular differentiation is the normal process in which the body's cells progress from an immature embryonic state to a differentiated, specialized state. Microscopically, fully differentiated cells resemble the mature cells of the specific tissue or organ.

Contact inhibition is a normal process within tissues that triggers cells to stop reproducing because there is no space left to expand.

A **benign tumor** does not have infiltrative or metastasizing properties, but a **malignant neoplasm** does.

because blood cells have a short life cycle. Conversely, liver cells proliferate infrequently and slowly. Cell death within the liver seldom occurs, and the body cannot regenerate liver cells as fully as tissues with rapid regeneration such as bone marrow. Neoplastic cells may proliferate at the same rate and manner as the normal cells of the tissue from which they arise (Bender, Yasko, & Strohl, 1996). However, these cells divide indiscriminately and haphazardly, and the tissues lose contact inhibition. The neoplastic tissue becomes expansive and, in the case of malignant tissues, infiltrative as well.

Benign tumors neither infiltrate the tissue of origin nor spread to other tissues. **Malignant tumors** expand and infiltrate the tissues of origin and can spread or metastasize to other areas of the body. Cancerous tumors are malignant (Table 14-1).

Theory of Cancer Development

Several theories exist concerning the development of cancer. The theory of initiation and promotion has gained the most acceptance. This theory

⌖

TABLE 14-1
COMPARISON OF BENIGN AND MALIGNANT TUMORS

Characteristic	Malignant Tumor	Benign Tumor
Encapsulated	Rarely	Usually
Differentiated	Poorly	Partially
Metastasis	Frequently present	Absent
Recurrence	Frequent	Rare
Vascularity	Moderate to marked	Slight
Mode of growth	Infiltrative and expansive	Expansive
Cell characteristics	Abnormal, less like parent cells	Fairly normal cells, similar to parent cells

NOTE: From "Nursing Role in Management," by C. M. Bender, J. M. Yasko, and R. A. Strohl, 1996, in *Medical-surgical nursing: Assessment and management of clinical problems* (4th ed., p. 264), edited by C. L. Lewis, I. C. Collier, and M. M. Heitkemper, St. Louis: C. V. Mosby. Reprinted with permission.

states that cancer develops progressively. The first stage of cancer development is *initiation*, an irreversible alteration in the cell's genetic structure resulting from the actions of a chemical, physical, or biological agent (Helman & Thiele, 1991). The second stage of cancer development is termed *promotion*. **Initiators** may only cause single-strand breaks in the host's deoxyribonucleic acid (DNA). These single-strand breaks do not cause enough mutations to result in cancer. At least one more mutation must occur in the cells in which a mutation has already occurred. **Promoters** cause reversible proliferation of the altered, initiated cell. As the initiated cell population grows, the likelihood of a second cellular mutation occurring also increases (Helman & Thiele, 1991). Promoters that increase this likelihood are reversible life-style habits such as cigarette smoking, a high-fat diet, and alcohol consumption.

Progression is the next stage of cancer development. At this phase the growth rate of the tumor increases, and invasion and metastasis are likely to occur (Helman & Thiele, 1991). The tumor cells may begin to produce their own growth factor as a result of genetic changes (Helman & Thiele, 1991). The tumor grows and expands at this stage. Symptoms begin to appear during progression.

The last stage of cancer development is **metastasis**. Malignant cells spread to regions surrounding the tumor or to other tissues of the body. There are three generally accepted theories of metastatic spread. One route is through the vascular system; malignant cells pass from the lymph nodes into the venous system. The malignant cells are released into the bloodstream, and the cell aggregates are trapped in the capillaries of tissues and organs (Bender, Yasko, & Strohl, 1996).

A second route may be through the lymphatic system. Lymphatic vessels drain all of the body's intracellular fluid spaces. Cancer cells that break free from the initial tumor mass almost always become trapped in the lymph nodes (Bender, Yasko, & Strohl, 1996). Therefore, it is likely that the lymphatic system carries cancer cell aggregates to other areas of the body from the intracellular spaces within tissues drained by the lymphatic vessels.

The third route of metastasis is implantation. Implantation occurs through serosal or surgical seeding. Malignant cells may cause the DNA of normal cells to break down through the use of enzymes and migration. The malignant cells attach to and enter the normal cell through the cell membrane (Bender, Yasko, & Strohl, 1996). This occurs in three stages. The first stage is the attachment of malignant cells to the extracellular matrix (Helman & Thiele, 1991). These cells initiate a local degradation of the extracellular matrix (Helman & Thiele, 1991). Finally, the malignant cells invade normal cells through the degraded matrix (Helman & Thiele, 1991). This is the attach, degrade, and conquer theory of metastatic progression. Most cancer deaths result from metastatic disease (Figs. 14-2 and 14-3).

The immune system is intricately involved in cancer development. When malignant cells invade the body, an immune response is initiated. However, some tumor cells have the ability to change their cell surface antigens, making them more effective in avoiding an immune response. This may occur through a number of mechanisms. Malignant cells may slip through as a result of weakened cell antigens that are incapable of initiating an immune response (Bender, Yasko, & Strohl, 1996). The tumor may have the ability

Initiators, generally known as carcinogens, are irreversible factors that damage DNA. Examples include radiation, drugs, pesticides, and certain foods. **Promoters** are reversible factors that accelerate DNA damage within the body. Examples include the life-style factors such as smoking, excess dietary fat, and alcohol consumption.

Metastasis is the spread of malignant cells to regions surrounding the tumor or other tissues of the body. Once cancer has metastasized, it is at an advanced stage and is difficult to treat.

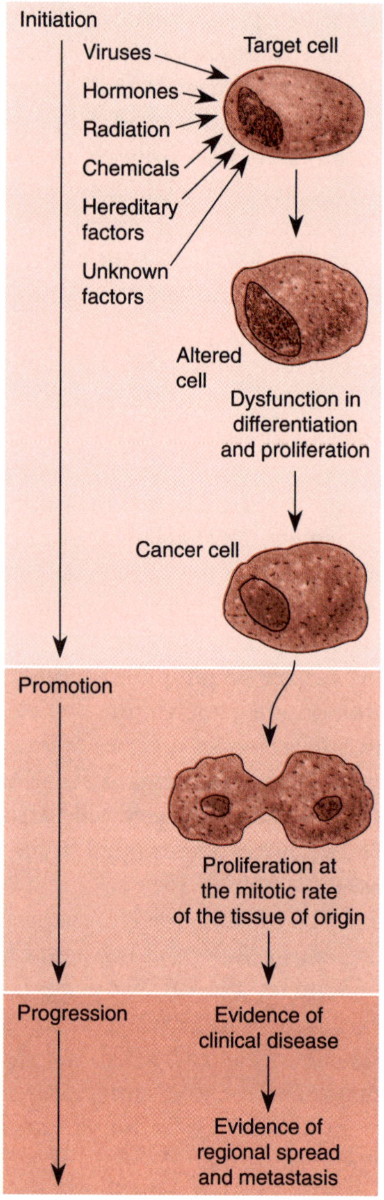

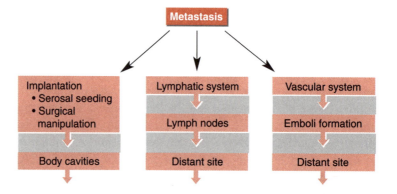

Initiation

Viruses
Hormones
Radiation
Chemicals
Hereditary factors
Unknown factors

Target cell

Altered cell

Dysfunction in differentiation and proliferation

Cancer cell

Promotion

Proliferation at the mitotic rate of the tissue of origin

Progression

Evidence of clinical disease

Evidence of regional spread and metastasis

FIGURE 14-2

Process of cancer development.

FIGURE 14-3

Routes of metastases.

Metastasis

Implantation
• Serosal seeding
• Surgical manipulation

Body cavities

Lymphatic system

Lymph nodes

Distant site

Vascular system

Emboli formation

Distant site

to change or lose antigenic determinants, thereby rendering the immune response ineffective (Bender, Yasko, & Strohl, 1996). Alternatively, the body may be flooded with tumor cell antigens that bind to antibodies or receptors on the lymphocytes, preventing them from recognizing cancer cells (Bender, Yasko, & Strohl, 1996). The tumor-associated antigens can then bind with T-cells, preventing immune system recognition of the antigen (Bender, Yasko, & Strohl, 1996). In cellular **dedifferentiation,** the cells return to an embryonic or fetal state; therefore, the body does not recognize the cells as foreign (Bender, Yasko, & Strohl, 1996).

In **dedifferentiation,** tumor cells return to an embryonic state. It is difficult to determine the tissue of origin of these cells from a biopsy specimen. Dedifferentiation is a defense mechanism of malignant cells.

Classification of Cancer

Cancer can be classified according to anatomical site, histological analysis, and extent of the disease. Classification according to anatomical site involves a description of the tissue of origin. Cancers that arise from embryonic tissue are classified as embryonal tumors. A blastoma is an example of this type of cancer. A neuroblastoma is a malignant cancer of the embryonic tissues of the nervous system. Tumors that arise from the lymphatic tissues are termed lymphomas. Tumors that arise from the white blood cell–forming organs are termed leukemias. Cancers that arise from connective or supportive tissues such as bone, cartilage, fat, and nerves are termed sarcomas. Carcinomas include any cancer that derives from epithelial tissue such as the skin or lining of body cavities. Carcinoma of glandular tissue such as the breast or prostate is termed adenocarcinoma. Using this classification, colon cancer is classified as colon carcinoma.

Cancers also can be classified by histological analysis. This type of classification is known as **grading**. The process of grading involves examining the tissue of origin microscopically. This determines whether tumor cells are malignant. A biopsy specimen with histological analysis is the only definitive method of diagnosing cancer. The examiner must determine the amount of differentiation in the tumor tissue. A client with cancer has a better prognosis if the tumor tissue closely resembles the tissue of origin. In other words, the prognosis is better for the client if the tumor cells are well differentiated. The levels of grading are I–IV. Grade I tumor cells differ slightly from normal cells. Grade II tumor cells are more abnormal. Grade III tumor cells are very abnormal. Grade IV tumor cells are immature and primitive, and it is difficult to determine their tissue of origin (Table 14-2).

Grading determines whether tumor cells are present. Microscopic analysis determines the primary site of the tumor.

Cancer also is classified according to the extent of the disease. This classification is known as **staging**. There are several types of staging criteria. In one type, the extent of the disease is classified by a numerical system of stages 0–4. Stage 0 is cancer in situ, meaning that the cancer is almost invisible. The Pap smear often aids in diagnosing cervical cancer in situ. Stage 1 means that the extent of the tumor is limited to the tissue of origin. Stage 2 indicates that the tumor has limited local spread. In stage 3, the tumor has extensive local and regional spread. Tumors in stage 4 have metastasized. Many physicians use this staging procedure for lymphomas, but in addition, they denote whether the patient has experienced unexplained weight loss and fever or night sweats within 6 months preceding the diagnosis.

Staging classifies the extent of the disease.

◙

TABLE 14-2
HISTOLOGICAL ANALYSIS CLASSIFICATION

Grade I: Cells differ slightly from normal cells (mild dysplasia) and are well differentiated.

Grade II: Cells are more abnormal (moderate dysplasia) and are moderately differentiated.

Grade III: Cells are very abnormal (severe dysplasia) and are poorly differentiated.

Grade IV: Cells are immature and primitive (anaplasia) and are undifferentiated; the cell of origin is difficult to determine.

The **TNM staging criteria** are (T) tumor size, (N) nodal involvement, and (M) the presence of metastasis.

This is denoted with an A if these constitutional symptoms are absent or a B if these symptoms are present. For stage 4 lymphomas, most physicians denote biopsy-documented involvement of tissue and organs with letters. For example, an M denotes marrow involvement, an H denotes liver (hepatic) involvement, and an L denotes lung involvement (Table 14-3). The **tumor node metastases (TNM)** method is used to stage some cancers. This method classifies by tumor size, degree of regional spread, and the absence or presence of metastasis. T, tumor size, refers to the size of the primary tumor at the time of diagnosis. The classification ranges from Tis (for carcinoma in situ) to T4 (for the largest tumors). The N (N0–N4) denotes evidence of tumor cells in the regional lymph nodes. The client may have a tumor without lymph node involvement (N0) or extensive lymph node involvement (N4). M denotes the presence or absence of metastasis. The classification M0 means there is no evidence of metastasis. M1–M4 denote ascending degrees of metastatic involvement (Table 14-4). The following case study illustrates tumor staging.

◙

TABLE 14-3
STAGING CLASSIFICATION

Stage 0: The cancer is in situ.

Stage I: The tumor is limited to the tissue of origin, and there is tumor growth.

Stage II: There is limited local spread.

Stage III: There is extensive local and regional spread.

Stage IV: Metastasis occurs.

NOTE: From "Nursing Role in Management," by C. M. Bender, J. M. Yasko, and R. A. Strohl, 1996, in *Medical-surgical nursing: Assessment and management of clinical problems* (4th ed., p. 270), edited by C. L. Lewis, I. C. Collier, and M. M. Heitkemper, St. Louis: C. V. Mosby. Reprinted with permission.

⊠

TABLE 14-4
TNM CLASSIFICATION SYSTEM

Primary Tumor (T)
T0   No evidence of primary tumor
Tis   Carcinoma in situ
T1–4 Ascending degrees of increasing tumor size and involvement

Regional Lymph Nodes (N)
N0   No evidence of disease in the lymph nodes
N1–4 Ascending degrees of nodal involvement
Nx   Regional lymph nodes cannot be assessed clinically

Distant Metastases (M)
M0   No evidence of distant metastases
M1–4 Ascending degrees of metastatic involvement of the host, including distant nodes

NOTE: From "Nursing Role in Management," by C. M. Bender, J. M. Yasko, and R. A. Strohl, 1996, in *Medical-surgical nursing: Assessment and management of clinical problems* (4th ed., p. 271), edited by C. L. Lewis, I. C. Collier, and M. M. Heitkemper, St. Louis: C. V. Mosby. Reprinted with permission.

CASE STUDY: TUMOR STAGING

A 58-year-old woman undergoes a breast biopsy. Histological examination of the biopsy specimen reveals a nonencapsulated, malignant carcinoma of the breast, a grade II, T2N1M0 tumor.

Based on the TNM classification, the client has a malignant breast cancer with moderately differentiated cells. The tumor is not encapsulated but has only moderate local spread (as denoted by the T2 classification). Some regional lymph nodes are involved (denoted by the N1 classification). The M0 classification denotes that the tumor has not metastasized. In light of this analysis, the client has a moderately good prognosis. The prognosis would be better if the tumor were encapsulated, smaller, or without nodal involvement. It would be worse if the tumor were larger, had more extensive lymph node involvement, or had metastasized. The client's physician will most likely recommend that she undergo a modified radical mastectomy of the affected breast, including removal of the lymph nodes in the ipsilateral axilla. The client will also most likely undergo radiation or chemotherapy to prevent a recurrence of the carcinoma.

Prevention and Detection

Cancer development can be prevented to some extent by reducing or avoiding exposure to known or suspected carcinogens and cancer-producing agents. Eating a well-balanced diet of vegetables, fresh fruits, whole grains, and fiber and avoiding fats and preservatives help to reduce the

A healthy diet, weight control, avoiding exposure to known carcinogens, and reducing stress may help to prevent cancer.

risk of developing cancer (Fig. 14-4). Adequate rest and exercise also are recommended. Clients must learn to reduce the stress in their lives and to cope with unavoidable life-style stressors.

Regular health examinations and screenings also are recommended to reduce the risk of developing cancer. The American Cancer Society has created the CAUTION acronym to help people recognize the seven warning signs of cancer (Bender, Yasko, & Strohl, 1996) (Table 14-5). Clients need to learn and practice self-examination techniques. The early detection of cancer is a positive factor in a client's prognosis. Clients who practice good self-examination techniques and seek immediate medical care if cancer is suspected are more likely to have a good prognosis.

There are specific **screening procedures** to detect different kinds of cancer, such as mammography and digital prostate examinations. The diagnosis is made based on the client's health history and identified risk factors, a physical examination, and specific diagnostic tests. Risk factors for cancer include a family history of the disease, exposure to known carcinogens, prolonged irritation of tissues, poor dietary habits, and a stressful life style.

The physical examination should include the musculoskeletal system, neurological system, and respiratory system. The skin and rectum should be examined for changes; spleen, liver, and lymph nodes should be palpated. Cancer commonly occurs in the reproductive system, in the testes and prostate of men and in the breasts, cervix, and uterus of women. Hemoccult tests assess abnormal colon bleeding, which is an indicator of a possible cancer. The nurse should ask if clients have any pain, abnormal swelling, unusual discharge, or have noticed any significant change in their body.

A number of diagnostic tests assist the practitioner in determining the presence of cancer. Specific cancers are diagnosed with blood tests such as a complete blood count (CBC) or carcinoembryonic antigen (CEA). CBC detects leukemia. CEA detects embryonic tumors, especially colon cancer.

Several **screening procedures**, including examinations, mammograms, Pap smears, hemoccult analysis, and skin assessments, detect cancer.

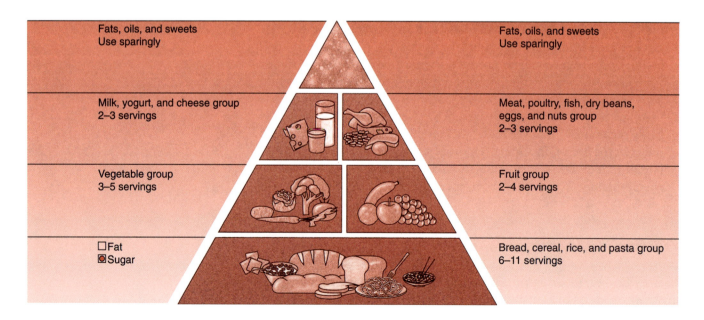

FIGURE 14-4 The food pyramid guide.

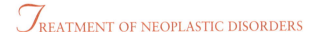

TABLE 14-5
SEVEN WARNING SIGNS OF CANCER

Change in bowel or bladder habits

A sore throat that does not heal

Unusual bleeding or discharge from any body orifice

Thickening or a lump in the breast or elsewhere

Indigestion or difficulty in swallowing

Obvious change in a wart or mole

Nagging cough or hoarseness

NOTE: From "Nursing Role in Management," by C. M. Bender, J. M. Yasko, and R. A. Strohl, 1996, in *Medical-surgical nursing: Assessment and management of clinical problems* (4th ed., p. 274), edited by C. L. Lewis, I. C. Collier, and M. M. Heitkemper, St. Louis: C. V. Mosby. Reprinted with permission.

The Pap smear, a cytology examination, helps to determine the presence of cervical cancer. Proctoscopic examinations assist in the diagnosis of prostate and colon cancer. The prostate can be palpated for enlargement and abnormal firmness. Radiologic examinations such as mammography, magnetic resonance imaging (MRI), and computed tomography (CT) scans also help to determine the presence of cancer. A nuclear medicine bone scan is very useful in detecting bone metastases. The definitive test for cancer remains a **biopsy** with histological analysis.

> A biopsy of a tumor with histologic analysis of the biopsy specimen is the definitive test for cancer.

TREATMENT OF NEOPLASTIC DISORDERS

Cancer is generally treated with surgery, chemotherapy, radiation therapy, or a combination of these three techniques. When treating cancer, the goal is either **cure**, **control**, or **palliation**. Factors that determine the treatment modality include the histologic type of the cancer, the location and size of the tumor, and the extent of disease. The client's physiological and psychological status and expressed desires also are important in determining the treatment plan.

> The treatment goals for cancer are **cure**, **control**, or **palliation**.

As a result of new developments, cancer is now treated as a chronic rather than a terminal disorder. Currently a number of cancers are curable. Some leukemias and lymphomas have excellent cure rates. The goals for clients who are in remission are rehabilitation and prevention of further cancer development. Some cancers cannot be cured, but it is possible to control the disease. The client initially undergoes treatment and is then treated with maintenance therapy to control cancer proliferation. For these clients, the goal is to improve their quality of life. Some types of cancer require palliative therapy. **Nursing goals** for these clients include relieving their discomfort and allowing them to die with dignity.

Surgery

Most clients with cancer are surgical candidates; however, some tumors are deemed inoperable. Inoperable tumors cannot be removed from the body. These tumors are either too large, too infiltrated into the tissue to remove effectively without extensive damage, or too inaccessible. **Surgery** can effectively cure and control some cancers and can also be used for palliative care. Cure and control are affected by tumor size, rate of growth, and infiltration. Tumors that are encapsulated without spread into surrounding tissues are the easiest to remove. Tumors with slow rates of growth have a better cure rate because it is easier to ensure that all cells have been removed. To cure or control tumor growth, a margin of surrounding normal tissue must be resected at the time of surgery (Pfeifer, 1997). This prevents any tumor cells from being left in the remaining tissue. These measures reduce the risk of seeding tumor cells into healthy tissues.

Some examples of surgical procedures include colostomies to relieve tumor obstruction of the bowel and the insertion of feeding tubes for clients with cancer of the neck. Surgery is used for rehabilitative purposes as well. For example a breast reconstruction after a mastectomy lessens the effects of an altered body image.

Radiation Therapy

Radiation therapy can shrink and control the spread of malignant tumors. Treatment can be accomplished by either an external or an internal source of radiation. Clients treated externally are placed within a machine that emits radiation at the tumor. Internal radiation therapy involves implanting radioactive seeds within the tumor. Radiation primarily works by the interaction of free radicals with the DNA, ribonucleic acid (RNA), and enzymes of cells. Radiation often produces a double-strand break in the chromosome, which is lethal to both normal and malignant cells.

The radiation treatment plan is based on an estimate of the radiosensitivity of the tumor cells. The goal is to kill the tumor cells with minimal damage to normal cells. Cells that regenerate rapidly are more radiosensitive than those with slower regeneration times. Therefore, cells within the bone marrow, ovaries, testes, and lymphatic tissue are more sensitive to radiation therapy than cells in the muscle, tendons, and nerves. Knowing this information makes it easy to predict that cancer within the bone marrow would be easier to treat with radiation than cancer within muscle.

The radiation oncology specialist attempts to determine the therapeutic ratio to predict the success of radiation therapy. The **therapeutic ratio** is the relationship between the radiation dose that normal tissues can tolerate and the radiation dose necessary to destroy tumor cells (Bender, Yasko,

---

Surgery is used to cure, control, or palliate cancer symptoms.

To cure or control tumor growth, a margin of surrounding normal tissue must be resected at the time of surgery.

*The **therapeutic ratio** refers to the relationship between the radiation dose tolerated by normal tissues and the dose necessary to destroy tumor cells.*

& Strohl, 1996). A therapeutic ratio of greater than one is more indicative of success than a ratio of less than one.

Care of the Client Receiving Radiation
The client in the case study underwent a modified radical mastectomy to remove the cancerous breast and regional lymph nodes. Her oncologist has recommended radiation therapy to treat any tumor cells in the remaining lymph nodes. Lymphocytes are generally radiosensitive. The muscle, tendons, and nerves in the area are usually less radiosensitive. Since the therapeutic ratio is in the client's favor, radiation therapy is used to treat her cancer. The physician believes this client can be cured.

Radiation can cure, control, or palliate. It can be used alone or, as in the case study above, in combination with other therapies. It is often used to reduce the size of a tumor prior to resection. For inoperable tumors, radiation reduces tumor size to control growth, to relieve pain from pressure caused by the tumor, or to relieve obstruction. Cancer-related conditions that are relieved by radiation include pain from bone and brain metastases, neurological symptoms from brain metastases, spinal cord compression, intestinal obstruction, superior vena cava obstruction, bronchial or tracheal obstruction, and bleeding. For the client in the case study, it is used postoperatively to control regrowth.

Radiation therapy has a number of adverse effects. One of these, the sloughing (shedding) of cells, results in thin, denuded, or ulcerative tissues. As a result mucositis, nausea, vomiting, diarrhea, and cystitis commonly occur. The adverse effects are related to the area receiving radiation. For example, radiation of the head and neck results in mucositis of the mouth and throat. The client with breast cancer in the case study mentioned previously is likely to experience lung fibrosis as a result of receiving radiation to the chest wall. When normal cells begin to repair cellular damage, additional adverse effects occur. These include alopecia, leukopenia, thrombocytopenia, and sterility. These effects, again, are directly related to the area that has received radiation. Less radiosensitive tissues in the path of the radiation undergo capillary damage that results in edema, inflammation, atrophy, fibrosis, and necrosis. Skin reactions commonly occur from external radiation. The skin in the irradiated area becomes dark and may blister and crack. It usually becomes very dry and irritated.

Skin reactions occur more commonly from **external radiation therapy**. Linear accelerators emit x-rays that penetrate the skin; however, some of the x-rays are scattered by the skin, causing a skin reaction. The skin, once irradiated, permanently darkens. The client may have an altered body image. This should be of concern, especially if the area is clearly visible (such as the face or neck). Clients should be taught to treat skin reactions by keeping the skin clean and dry, reducing friction, and avoiding irritation from factors such as chemicals or the sun. During external radiation therapy, the skin must be free of lotions, creams, ointments, and powders because a number of these skin protectants contain metallic particles that can scatter the x-rays.

The client in the case study receives external radiation. Her skin is marked with an indelible dye that indicates the area to be irradiated. These markings

---

Radiation can cure, control, or palliate.

The adverse effects of external radiation therapy are typically related to the area receiving radiation. Fatigue, however, is a generalized adverse effect of radiation therapy.

External radiation therapy often causes skin reactions. The irradiated areas of skin should be kept clean and dry, and creams, lotions, and ointments should not be applied as they may contain metallic particles that may scatter the x-rays.

are carefully placed and must not be removed. Marking the area may be uncomfortable for clients because of the awkward positions in which they may be placed and the hard surface of the radiation device (Fig. 14-5).

The client should be aware that radiation is silent, invisible, and painless. The client's awkward position and the hard, flat treatment table are generally the only discomforts of radiation therapy. The client also needs to know that once the machine is turned off, radiation is no longer emitted. The client commonly believes (wrongly) that he or she is now **radioactive**. Additionally, the number of radiation treatments given does not reflect the severity of the disease or the likelihood of cure.

Internal radiation is used to treat some cancers. There are two types of internal radiation, mechanically placed sealed therapy and unsealed therapy. Sealed therapy involves placing a radiation source in an external mold. The mold is then placed over the skin or inserted into a body cavity. These molds can be applicators, seeds, wires, or tubes. Some are implanted permanently, such as the gold grains (radioactive seeds) that are inserted into the abdomen during a radical prostatectomy. Other molds are temporary, such as the radioactive wires that are inserted into the cervix to treat cervical cancer. All radioactive materials have a half-life, during which their radioactivity decreases to half of its original value. Thus, even permanently placed materials eventually lose their radioactivity (Fig. 14-6).

In unsealed radiation therapy, the client consumes radioactive material. The material is administered either orally or intravenously, or it can be instilled into a specific body cavity. For example, oral radioactive iodine is given to clients with thyroid goiters. The iodine comes in the form of a pill that the client can easily swallow.

Safety Precautions Several safety precautions should be followed with clients who are receiving internal radiation. A radiation safety officer (RSO) must be available to help monitor the levels of radiation that are emitted. The RSO informs the staff of the safety interventions that are required. A private, preferably lead-lined, room is necessary. The client should be placed on radiation precaution isolation, and a sign must be posted that informs everyone in contact with the client of his or her radioactivity. A written list of instructions and precautions should be placed on the client's chart. Additionally, with internal sealed radiation, a

---

Clients who receive external radiation therapy are not **radioactive** afterward. It is necessary to take radiation precautions with these clients only when they are actively receiving treatment.

Clients who receive internal radiation therapy **are** radioactive. Radiation precautions should be taken with these clients.

Radioactive particles that become dislodged from the client should not be handled. The RSO should be notified, and the materials should be removed with forceps and placed in a lead-lined container.

FIGURE 14-5

◙

The linear accelerator delivers supervoltage treatment.

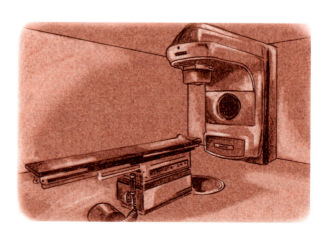

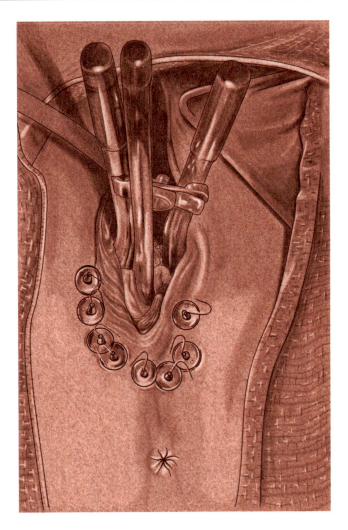

FIGURE 14-6

Internal sealed radiation. Wires and applicator implanted into the perineum and vagina are used to treat cervical cancer after a hysterectomy.

lead-lined container and long forceps should be kept in the room to replace the radiation source should it become dislodged. Persons less than 18 years of age and anyone who is pregnant should be restricted from the client's room. Caregivers should wear radiation monitors or film badges to measure their cumulative absorption of radiation. The amount of radiation emitted daily should be measured with a Geiger-Müeller detection device.

The principles of **time, distance,** and **shielding** aid in protecting others from radiation. Time is the period that a person can safely spend in the same room with the radioactive client. Time is dependent on distance and shielding, but usually it is recommended that no more than 15 minutes be spent in the presence of a radioactive person. Caregivers should attempt to spend as little time as possible in the client's room. This protective measure also unfortunately serves to isolate the client. Therefore, it becomes necessary to assist the client in finding diversionary activities.

Distance is the amount of space between the client and the other person. Radiation loses its intensity according to the inverse square law. For example, a person who is two times farther from the source will receive one-fourth the amount of radiation that is emitted. Visitors should remain at least 6 feet away from the source of radiation. Direct-care providers should remain at a distance of 3 feet or more from the client (Fig. 14-7).

The principles of **time, distance,** and **shielding** should be used when caring for clients who are radioactive.

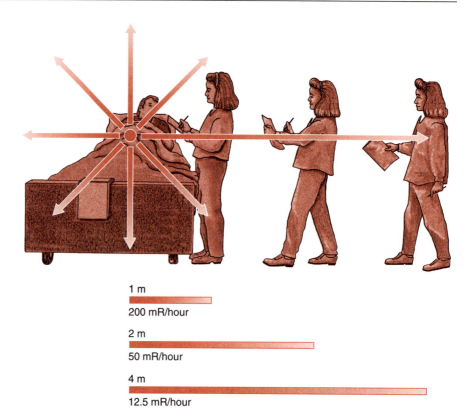

1 m
200 mR/hour

2 m
50 mR/hour

4 m
12.5 mR/hour

FIGURE 14-7

◙

The principle of distance. The nurse nearest the source of radioactivity (patient) is exposed to more radioactivity.

Shielding involves the use of a lead shield. The shield is placed between the client and the visitor. This practice is controversial because it is believed that the amount of time the caregiver spends in the room may be increased as a result of awkward maneuvering around the shield. It is somewhat effective in reducing the risk of exposure to family and friends. However, the visitor must not be tempted to prolong his or her stay in the room because of the presence of the shield. Visitors must be informed that lead shields cannot totally protect them.

Internal unsealed therapy is cause for another concern not shared by any other therapy: body fluids may be contaminated by the radioactive source. In unsealed therapy, the client's saliva, perspiration, blood, vomitus, and urine are radioactive. Precautions are taken for 24–96 hours after therapy to prevent others from exposure to the radioactive material. Food trays are made of paper, and all serving materials are disposable. Linens are generally stored until the Geiger-Müller counter shows that radiation is within safe limits. Urine may be disposed of in the toilet, but the toilet should be flushed several times following urination.

Chemotherapy

Chemotherapy cures, controls, and palliates.

Chemotherapy treats cancer systemically. Chemical agents are specially developed for their cell-killing properties. Chemotherapy treats many types of solid tumors and is the primary therapy for leukemia and lymphoma. There are two categories of chemotherapeutic agents, cell-cycle specific and cell-cycle nonspecific. Cell-cycle–specific agents affect cells during the process of replication and proliferation. Some of these agents are even more specific in that they only affect cells in certain phases of the cell cycle. Plant alkaloid agents, for example, are only effective on cells during the metaphase stage of mitosis. Cell-cycle–nonspecific agents affect cells in all phases of the cell cycle (Fig. 14-8).

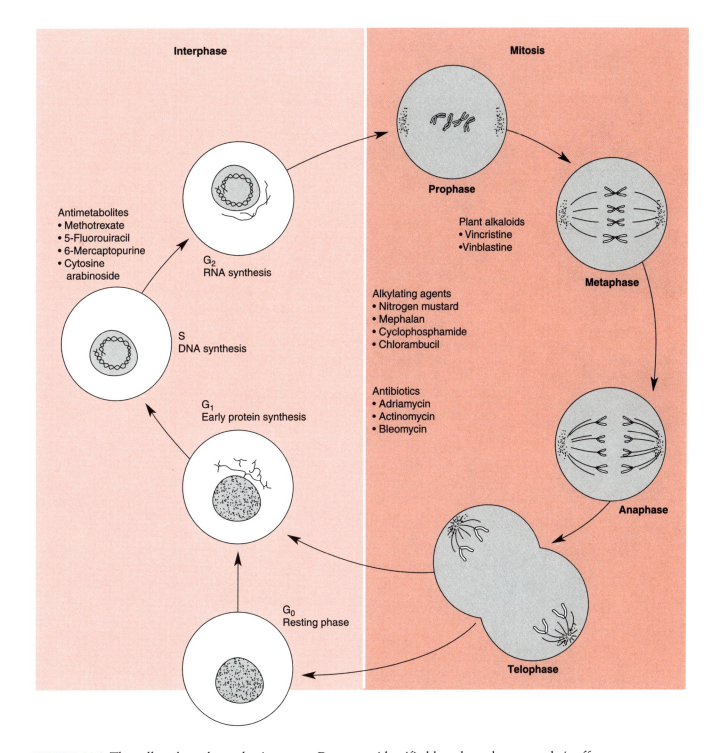

FIGURE 14-8 The cell cycle and neoplastic agents. Drugs are identified by where they exert their effect.

Patients are usually treated with a combination of chemotherapeutic agents. This kills more cells because the therapy is effective during different stages of the cell cycle. In addition, a combination of agents causes more cell death with lower doses of individual agents. Chemotherapeutic agents often have dose-related adverse effects. Adjuvant therapy should be part of the chemotherapy protocol, as some of these agents potentiate the effect of the chemotherapeutic agent. For example, steroids may alter the cell membrane so that chemotherapeutic agents penetrate the tumor cell more effectively. Therefore, dexamethasone is given intravenously prior to some chemotherapy treatments. Some adjuvant agents are administered to prevent toxic effects of a chemotherapeutic agent. For example, the uroprotectant mesna (Mesnex) is given prior to the administration of cyclophosphamide to prevent hemorrhagic cystitis (Table 14-6).

> The **cellular response to chemotherapy** is affected by the cellular mitotic rate, the age of the tumor, the location of the tumor, the presence of resistant tumor cells, and the physiological and psychological status of the client.

Factors that affect the **cellular response to chemotherapy** include the cellular mitotic rate, the age of the tumor, the location of the tumor, the presence of resistant tumor cells, and the physiological and psychological status of the client. Rapidly growing tumors respond better to chemotherapy because the most effective agents work during cellular proliferation and replication. Younger tumors have a better cell response to chemotherapeutic agents because they contain more proliferating cells. As tumors age, their growth rate generally slows. In addition, they build vascular networks that protect them from chemotherapeutic agents. The anatomical location of some tumors protects them from chemotherapeutic agents. Very few agents are able to cross the blood–brain barrier; thus brain tumors are difficult to reach. In addition, malignancies can mutate, resulting in a biochemical response that renders the cells incapable of converting the chemotherapeutic agent to an active form. Another factor that affects the response to chemotherapy is the health and well-being of the client. Weakened clients have difficulty tolerating the adverse effects of chemotherapeutic agents. Clients who are not committed to therapy may have trouble complying with the treatment regimen because of these adverse effects. Even when chemotherapy is successful, the problem of drug-resistant resting cells and nonproliferating cells remains.

Administration of Chemotherapeutic Agents   Chemotherapeutic agents are administered by the oral, subcutaneous, intramuscular, topical, intra-arterial, intracavitary, intraperitoneal, intrathecal, and intravenous routes (Langhorne, 1997). The nurse most commonly administers chemotherapeutic agents intravenously. Therefore, the nurse must be thoroughly versed in how to administer chemotherapy safely. The nurse usually undergoes a chemotherapy inservice and competency assessment before being allowed to administer chemotherapy independently. A consent form needs to be signed by the client before chemotherapy can be administered.

> For peripheral infusion of chemotherapeutic agents, a vein large enough to accommodate the infusion without irritating the intima should be selected. The catheter should be as small as possible to promote venous blood flow around the angiocatheter.

Several safety precautions must be taken before administering chemotherapy intravenously. The nurse should begin the intravenous infusion with normal saline or 5% dextrose in water (D5W) through a small lumen catheter. The nurse should avoid using an extremity with venipuncture sites proximal to the intravenous site or with poor lymphatic drainage. The vein that is selected should be large enough to accommodate

TABLE 14-6

CHEMOTHERAPY PHARMACOLOGY

Classification	Action	Cell Cycle	Examples	Adverse Effects
Antimetabolites	Inhibit DNA synthesis by substituting erroneous metabolites in DNA metabolism	S phase cell-cycle specific	Cytosine arabinoside (Ara-C), 5-fluorouracil (5-FU), methotrexate	Occur in the hematopoietic and gastrointestinal (GI) systems
Antitumor antibiotics	Inhibit RNA and DNA synthesis by altering nucleic acid synthesis and functioning	Cell-cycle nonspecific	Doxorubicin, bleomycin, mitomycin	Occur in the hematopoietic, GI, reproductive, and cardiac systems. Doxorubicin is extremely vesicant, has a lifetime dose limitation from cardiac toxicity, and is termed the "red devil." Bleomycin causes pulmonary fibrosis and is highly likely to cause anaphylaxis.
Alkylating agents	Cause single- and double-strand breaks in DNA; inhibit RNA, protein, and DNA synthesis	Cell-cycle nonspecific	Cyclophosphamide, cisplatin, busulfan, nitrogen mustard, ifosfamide	Occur in the hematopoietic, GI, and reproductive systems. Cyclophosphamide and ifosfamide are highly likely to cause hemorrhagic cystitis. Cisplatin is a nephrotoxic and ototoxic heavy metal.
Vinca alkaloids	Destroy the mitotic spindle, resulting in metaphase arrest that inhibits RNA and protein synthesis	M phase cell-cycle specific	Etoposide, vinblastine, vincristine, teniposide	Occur in the hematopoietic, integumentary, neurological, and reproductive systems. Etoposide causes severe hypotension if rapidly infused.
Nitrosureas	Interfere with DNA replication and repair; can cross the blood–brain barrier	Cell-cycle nonspecific	Carmustine, lomustine, chlorozotocin, dicarbazine	Occur in the hematopoietic and GI systems. Delayed myelosuppression occurs.
Hormones	Either have a direct effect on the tumor or suppress the body's hormones that feed the tumor	Cell-cycle nonspecific	Androgens, estrogens, corticosteroids, progestins, estrogen antagonists	Occur in the reproductive system. Some hormones affect the hematopoietic and GI systems.

509

the infusion without irritating the intima. The client should be instructed to report any changes in sensation, especially burning or stinging. A blood return confirms that the catheter is still in the vein; this is checked before infusing the chemotherapeutic agent. If there is no blood return, a new catheter should be placed in a different vessel.

Some chemotherapeutic agents are classified as irritants. These irritate the vessel but do not lead to tissue necrosis if they infiltrate surrounding tissues. If the client complains of burning and stinging but a good blood return is evident, it is safe to continue administering an irritant. If the agent being infused is classified as a **vesicant**, meaning that tissue necrosis will occur if the agent infiltrates surrounding tissues, the infusion must be discontinued if the client experiences burning or stinging (Table 14-7).

If a vesicant does infiltrate the surrounding tissues, the condition is termed an extravasation and is treated as follows: The intravenous line must be stopped immediately, and the physician should be notified. The physician may order an antidote for the chemotherapeutic agent. The intravenous tubing should be removed from the catheter hub, and the catheter should be left in place. If an antidote is ordered, it should be injected into the angiocatheter and injected a number of times subcutaneously into the skin surrounding the catheter site. The catheter can then be removed. A topical corticosteroid cream may be applied as well, and the site should be

> If a client complains of burning or stinging during the infusion of a vesicant chemotherapeutic agent, the infusion should be stopped immediately.

◙

TABLE 14-7
IRRITANT AND VESICANT CHEMOTHERAPY AGENTS

Agents with Irritant Potential	Agents with Vesicant Potential
Carmustine	Amasacrine
Etoposide	Bisantrene
Mitoguazone	Dacarbazine
Plicamycin	Dactinomycin
Streptozocin	Daunorubicin
Teniposide	Doxorubicin
Vindesine	Epirubicin
	Esorubicin
	Idarubicin
	Mechlorethamine
	Menogaril
	Mitomycin
	Mitoxantrone
	Piroxantrone
	Vinblastine
	Vincristine
	Vinorelbine

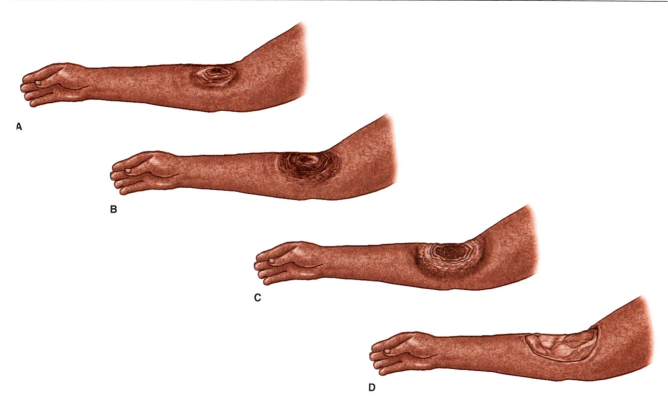

FIGURE 14-9 *A* Cutaneous effects of vesicant extravasation; note central necrosis and surrounding erythema and induration. *B* Lateral progression of initial cutaneous effects, which occurs over a period of weeks. *C* Eschar requiring surgical debridement eventually develops. *D* Wide surgical excision of involved area on forearm.

elevated. In addition, a cold compress should be applied for 24–48 hours unless a vinca alkaloid agent has extravasated; if it has, heat should be applied to the site. The extravasation should be documented and the site monitored closely for several days. Any sign of worsening skin integrity needs to be reported to the physician. An extravasation report should be filed according to agency policy (Fig. 14-9).

Vesicant agents should be administered through central venous catheters (CVCs) after verifying placement and good blood return. Central venous access devices are now widely used. CVCs are inserted into the subclavian vein, and the distal tip rests at the opening of the right atrium (Fig. 14-10). They promote the rapid dilution of the chemotherapeutic agent and decrease the incidence of extravasation. They also reduce the need for multiple venipuncture sites. The CVCs used most often are tunneled long-term silastic catheters, right atrial catheters, peripherally inserted central catheters (PICCs), and implanted infusion ports. Right atrial catheters are inserted into the chest wall and tunneled into the subclavian vein. Short-term CVCs, usually made of polyurethane, are inserted at the bedside. These catheters have a single, double, or triple lumen and are made to stay in place for a few weeks. Long-term right atrial catheters such as the Groshung, Hickman, and Broviac catheters are made of

If a vinca alkaloid chemotherapeutic agent has extravasated, warm compresses should be used instead of the cool compresses used with other chemotherapy extravasations.

The central venous access devices that are used most often include tunneled long-term silastic catheters, peripherally inserted central catheters (PICCs), implanted infusion ports, and right atrial catheters.

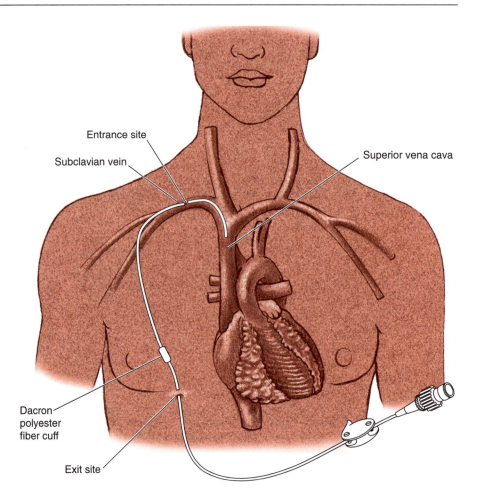

Entrance site

Subclavian vein

Superior vena cava

Dacron polyester fiber cuff

Exit site

FIGURE 14-10

◙

Tunneled long-term silastic catheter placement.

silicone rubber, can be used for months, and have a single or double lumen (Fig. 14-11). They are surgically placed.

PICC lines are inserted into one of the large, superficial veins in the antecubital space, through the subclavian vein, and into the superior vena cava with the tip at the right atrium. Their flexibility allows the client to maintain the use of his or her arm. These devices usually are inserted by specially trained registered nurses at the bedside. They are widely used in home health care.

Implanted infusion ports are accessed with a beveled-tip needle that prevents coring of the diaphragm.

Implanted infusion ports are central catheters attached to a reservoir. The reservoir is implanted under the skin to prevent the catheter from exiting through the skin. The tip is located at the opening of the right atrium like the PICC. These are placed surgically and remain patent for a long time. They are cosmetically more appealing as the catheter is hidden under the skin. These catheters are accessed through the skin with a special needle called a Huber needle, whose beveled tip prevents it from coring the diaphragm of the reservoir. Huber needles are either straight or bent at a 90° angle to provide better access to the device (Fig. 14-12).

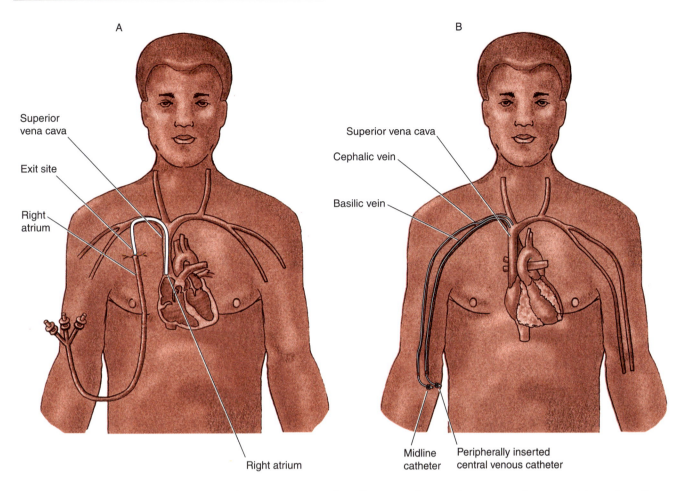

A
Superior vena cava
Exit site
Right atrium
Right atrium

B
Superior vena cava
Cephalic vein
Basilic vein
Midline catheter
Peripherally inserted central venous catheter

FIGURE 14-11 *A* Right atrial catheter placement. *B* Peripherally inserted central venous catheter (PICC) and midline catheter (MLC).

Central catheters can cause the following **complications**: clotting, sepsis, bleeding, thrombosis, technical problems, catheter migration, air emboli, and local infections (Viall, 1990). **Nursing care** for these catheters includes a periodic aseptic cleansing of the site. The site is dressed with a gauze or occlusive dressing such as Tegaderm. Implanted infusion devices must have a dressing over the site only when the device is being utilized. Agency policy determines how often the site should be cleansed. For long-term catheters without an implanted infusion port, the endcaps must be changed every 72 hours to decrease the risk of infection (Viall, 1990).

Each lumen of the catheter must be flushed with heparinized saline when not receiving an infusion. Generally 1–3 mL of fluid are enough to clear the catheter. The implanted infusion device is an exception, as the reservoir and catheter usually hold approximately 3–5 mL of fluid. The type of device dictates how often the catheter must be flushed. Each lumen of the short-term CVCs should be flushed every 8–12 hours (Viall, 1990). The long-term tunneled catheters and PICC lines generally are flushed once per week, and implanted infusion ports are flushed once per month

The **complications** associated with central catheters include clotting, local infections, bleeding, thrombi, air emboli, catheter migration, technical problems, and sepsis.

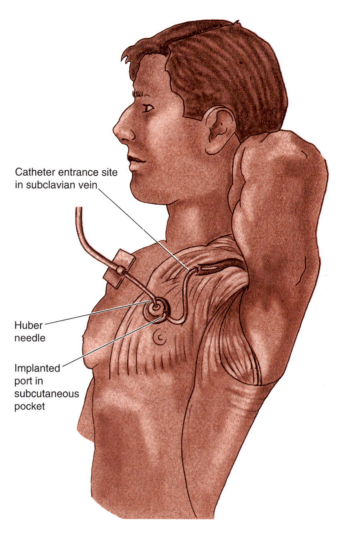

Catheter entrance site
in subclavian vein

Huber
needle

Implanted
port in
subcutaneous
pocket

FIGURE 14-12

Implanted infusion reservoir and
noncoring needle.

Groshung catheters should be
flushed with normal saline
instead of heparinized saline.

(Viall, 1990). The exception to this recommendation is the **Groshung
catheter**, which has a special design and should be flushed with normal
saline (5 mL) instead of heparin (Viall, 1990). All of the devices should be
flushed after an infusion has been completed.

Safety Precautions Chemotherapy adversely affects normal tissues. The
chemotherapeutic agents have a cytotoxic effect on normal cells just as
they have on cancer cells. As a result, it is important for the nurse to handle these agents safely. Protective garments should be worn to prevent the
agent from spilling on the nurse or his or her clothing. **Latex gloves** always
should be worn when handling these agents. If splashing or inhalation of
the agents is likely to occur, the nurse should wear a moisture-protective
gown and mask. Most importantly, splashing and inhaling the agents
should be avoided. Only a licensed pharmacist using a protective laminar
air hood should mix these agents.

Latex gloves always should
be worn when handling
chemotherapeutic agents.

A spill kit always should be within reach in case a chemical spill
occurs. The spill kit contains the spill until personnel trained in the
proper cleanup of a spill can be notified. The spill kit includes latex

gloves, a moisture-protective gown with elastic cuffs, a mask, absorbent materials to contain the spill, signs to warn others of the spill, and tools to safely remove the spill. Any item contaminated with chemotherapeutic agents during a spill must be washed thoroughly in hot water. If the item is not washable, it must be destroyed. Clients receiving chemotherapy like to have personal objects with them while they receive infusions for reasons of comfort. If these items are not washable, the nurse should take steps to protect them from possible spills. All disposable items used in administering the chemotherapeutic agents need to be discarded in an Occupational Safety and Health Administration (OSHA)–approved, leak-proof container. The waste container must then be discarded in an approved incinerator.

The only nurses who should administer chemotherapy are those who have been trained in how to handle these agents. It is essential that the "five rights" of medication administration—right patient, right drug, right dosage, right route, and right time—be implemented. The agents must be administered exactly as ordered. This includes the order of adjuvant agents as well as the chemotherapeutic agents. Pregnant or lactating women should not administer these agents. The workload of the unit should be distributed to minimize employee contact with the agents. Personnel who routinely infuse chemotherapeutic agents should undergo periodic health screenings to detect possible complications of exposure. Any known exposure should be documented.

Management of the Adverse Effects of Chemotherapy One must be able to differentiate between the toxic effects of the chemotherapeutic medications and the progression of the malignancy. It is also important to differentiate between the tolerable side effects of the medications and the acute toxic effects. To address these concerns, the nurse must know the typical effects of the specific cancer undergoing treatment and the agents being used to cure or control the cancer.

Chemotherapeutic agents commonly cause leukopenia and anemia. All chemotherapy medications have a time period, termed the **nadir**, when they have the most destructive effect on the blood cells. Since leukopenia results in a high risk of infection, the nurse should monitor for the nadir effect. During recent years, medications have been developed to decrease the effect that chemotherapy has on blood cells. These agents, termed **colony-stimulating factors** (CSFs), stimulate the production of new blood cells. Three common agents of this type are epoetin alfa (Epogen, Procrit), which stimulates red blood cell production; filgrastim (Neupogen), which stimulates neutrophil production; and sargramostim (Leukine), which stimulates bone marrow production.

The adverse effects of CSFs include hypersensitivity reactions, fever with possible chills and rigors, fatigue, flu-like symptoms, gastrointestinal (GI) distress, chest pain, and renal toxicity. The fatigue and diarrhea associated with these agents may limit the dose that can safely be used. It is important to monitor the electrocardiogram (ECG) and oxygen saturation of clients who experience chest pain. The client's blood urea nitrogen (BUN) and

The client's personal mementos that cannot be washed in hot, soapy water should be protected from chemotherapy spills.

Disposable equipment used to infuse chemotherapeutic agents should be discarded in a leak-proof container and burned in an approved incinerator.

Chemotherapy protocols should be followed exactly as ordered by the physician. The order of the agents can be changed only with the physician's consent.

The **nadir** refers to the time period when the chemotherapeutic agent will have the most destructive effect on the body's blood cells.

Colony-stimulating factors stimulate the production of new blood cells. Since they elicit an immune response, hypersensitivity is a common adverse reaction.

creatinine levels should be monitored as well. If the client is experiencing fever or muscle or joint pain, a mild antipyretic such as acetaminophen (Tylenol) may be administered. Chills associated with rigors are treated with intravenous meperidine (Demerol). The nurse must frequently monitor the client's vital signs as well as intake and output. Steroids should not be given because they interfere with the CSF response of these agents.

Some chemotherapeutic agents frequently cause nausea, vomiting, and anorexia. In anticipation of this, antiemetics should be administered on a scheduled basis rather than as needed. Excellent antiemetic results have been seen with serotonin blockers such as granisetron (Kytril) and ondansetron (Zofran). After chemotherapy, these medications should be continued orally; the duration of therapy depends on the chemotherapeutic agent that was administered. Meals should consist of foods that are least irritating to the GI system. Most clients prefer light meals that are low in protein during this time. They should be served in a pleasant environment free of noxious odors. One simple way to decrease a client's nausea is to remove the lid of the food tray before taking the food to the client. This allows food odors to dispel somewhat before the client receives the meal. Favorite foods should not be given if the client is nauseous and vomiting; this only encourages aversions to foods that later may help the client gain weight.

Chemotherapy causes ulcerations of the mucosal lining of the GI tract. Clients with ulcerations are best able to tolerate a bland, moist, and soft diet. Local anesthetics that have no sugar, alcohol, or dyes, such as Ulcerase, are used to relieve the pain caused by oral ulcerations. A goal of **nursing care** is to prevent candidiasis from developing. To prevent this infection, clients must rinse their mouth and brush their teeth immediately after eating foods with a high sugar content. Frequent saline mouthwashes and soft, sponge-like toothbrushes will help to prevent infection. Mycostatin (Nystatin) is the preferred drug for the treatment of candidiasis.

Neurological problems commonly occur after the administration of chemotherapeutic agents. The most frequently reported complications are constipation, foot drop, and jaw pain. For constipation, the nurse should instruct the client to keep an accurate record of bowel movements. Stool softeners help to lessen constipation. Foot drop is a neurological condition in which the foot remains in extension instead of in a normal flexed position. Foot drop usually is a transient effect that resolves after the treatment is discontinued. The client requires assistance from the nurse in positioning the extremity to facilitate recovery. The foot should be supported in the flexed position, and passive range-of-motion exercises should be performed frequently. Jaw pain is temporary and can be relieved by chewing. The client must be told that chewing will lessen the pain, not increase it.

Some chemotherapeutic agents, such as cyclophosphamide (Cytoxan) and ifosfamide (Ifex), cause hemorrhagic cystitis. In this emergency condition, the bladder hemorrhages as a result of irritation caused by the chemotherapeutic agent. The medication must be stopped immediately. Hemorrhagic cystitis can be prevented by increasing the client's recommended daily fluid intake by 1–1.5 times. Intake and output should be carefully monitored, and the client should be instructed to urinate often to

Clients who are receiving chemotherapy generally prefer light meals that are low in protein. Cooled fruit is generally tolerated well by clients.

Local anesthetics used to ease stomatitis pain should be free of sugar, dyes, and alcohol. The client risks aspirating food if the oral cavity is anesthetized during meals. Encourage the client to rinse his or her mouth with saline before meals to alleviate the pain of eating.

decrease the time that the medication remains in the bladder. These agents ideally should be administered during the day. The uroprotectant mesna (Mesnix) often is administered to prevent hemorrhagic cystitis.

Alopecia is another common adverse effect of chemotherapy. The client should be warned **before** the medication is administered that the agent may cause loss of hair. This allows the client time to have a wig made that matches his or her hair color. The amount of hair lost depends on the chemotherapy dose, the duration of treatment, and the physiological status of the client. Nothing can prevent hair loss. The nurse needs to be aware of the severe effect that alopecia has on the client's self-image. The client must be told that hair loss is temporary, and when the treatments are completed, hair will regrow. Post-treatment hair, however, may have a different texture and possibly a different color. Many clients after chemotherapy have hair that is coarse, abundant, and curlier than before.

Chemotherapy also alters the client's sexual and reproductive functions. Sterility may be temporary or permanent depending on the medication and the client's physiological status. Women may require vaginal lubricating agents after chemotherapy. A water-based lubricant such as Astroglide that contains no dyes, perfumes, or alcohol should be used. The client often may not feel energetic enough to be sexually intimate. The nurse should encourage other forms of physical contact to maintain a sense of intimacy in the client's relationships. Men and women should use birth control for up to 2 years after treatment. Genetic counseling also is recommended.

There are other common side effects of chemotherapy. One of the most common is the sensation of feeling cold all of the time. Clients currently receiving chemotherapy tend to be sensitive to slight temperature changes and require extra warmth in their environment. Another common side effect is insomnia or nightmares. Reassure the client that these are expected side effects and that they should resolve after treatment. It is important for the nurse to teach clients to manage the adverse effects of chemotherapy (Table 14-8).

> Common side effects of chemotherapy are feeling cold all the time and experiencing insomnia and nightmares.

Bone Marrow Transplantation

Bone marrow transplants are performed to cure cancer or to boost the client's immune system after he or she has undergone a course of cell-destroying therapy. The transplant procedure involves identifying a compatible donor by human leukocyte antigen (HLA) histocompatibility matching. There are three types of bone marrow matches. With an **allogenic match**, the client's bone marrow is matched with another person's bone marrow. The other person usually is a sibling, because the client's brothers and sisters are most likely to have a compatible match. With **autologous matches**, a portion of the client's own bone marrow is removed, chemotherapy or radiation is then performed, and the bone marrow is implanted back into the client. The third type of bone marrow match, a **syngeneic match**, involves the donattion of bone marrow from an identical twin.

> There are three types of bone marrow matches. An **allogenic match** is a histocompatible match between two people. In an **autologous match** the client's own marrow is implanted. A **syngeneic match** is the match between identical twins.

(text continues on 522)

TABLE 14-8

Teaching the Client to Manage Side Effects of Chemotherapeutic Drugs

Side Effects	Points to Cover
Aches and Pains **Nursing action:** assess location, quality, and duration of pain.	Pain medication should be taken regularly. Side effects are constipation, dry mouth, and drowsiness. Strategies for rest and relaxation include music, progressive relaxation exercise, distraction, and positive imaging.
Alopecia • Hair loss: adriamycin, cyclophosphamide, daunorubicin, dacarbazine, vinblastine, mitoxantrone, taxol. • Hair thinning: 5-fluorouracil, methotrexate, bleomycin, vincristine, etoposide, edatrexate. **Nursing action:** discourage scalp tourniquets for clients with diseases that originate with or metastasize to the scalp.	Hair loss occurs 10–21 days after drug treatment. Hair loss is temporary; it grows back when the drug is stopped. Hair loss may be sudden and in large amounts. Select wig, cap, scarf, or turban before hair loss occurs. Avoid hair dryers, curling irons, and harsh or frequent shampoos. Keep head covered in summer to prevent sunburn and in winter to prevent heat loss.
Anorexia **Nursing action:** assess dietary history and monitor serum albumin and transferrin levels.	The client should eat with others in an attractive, pleasant area with soft music. Freshen up before meals. Practice good oral hygiene and exercise regularly. Eat small, frequent meals (5–6 meals daily). Avoid drinking fluids with meals; this prevents feeling full. Concentrate on eating high-protein foods such as eggs, milk products, peanut butter, tuna, beans, and peas. Breakfast may be the least difficult to consume; try to consume one-third of daily calories with this meal. Monitor and record weight weekly and report weight loss.
Constipation • Vincristine, vinblastine, narcotics. **Nursing action:** determine normal bowel habits; advise the client not to strain with bowel evacuation and to respond immediately to the urge to defecate.	Increase the intake of high-fiber foods such as whole grain products, bran, fresh fruit, raw vegetables, and popcorn. Increase fluid intake to 2–8 quarts of liquids daily; drink fresh fruit juices, prunes, or hot liquids on waking. Follow prescribed use of stool softener. Follow prescribed medications if no bowel movement occurs for 3 days or more.
Cystitis • Cyclophosphamide, ifosfamide. **Nursing action:** observe the color and amount of urine and assess frequency of voiding; advise the client to take oral cyclophosphamide early in the day.	Increase fluid intake to 3 quarts daily. Empty bladder at least once every 4 hours, especially at bedtime and at least once during the night. Report increasing symptoms of painful, frequent, or bloody urination, pain, fever, and chills promptly to the physician.

TABLE 14-8 *(continued)*

TEACHING THE CLIENT TO MANAGE SIDE EFFECTS OF CHEMOTHERAPEUTIC DRUGS

Side Effects	Points to Cover
DIARRHEA **Nursing action:** monitor serum fluid and electrolytes and the number, frequency, and consistency of diarrhea stools.	Avoid consuming high-roughage, greasy, and spicy foods, alcoholic beverages, tobacco, and caffeine products; avoid using milk products (can use boiled skim milk). Eat a bland diet. Increase fluid intake to 3 quarts of liquid daily (weak, tepid tea, bouillon, grape juice). Record the number and consistency of daily bowel movements and report information to the physician. Follow prescribed medication schedule if the problem persists for more than 1 day. Cleanse the rectal area after each bowel movement.
DEPRESSION **Nursing action:** assess for change in mood and affect.	Set small goals that can be achieved daily. Participate in enjoyable and diversionary activities such as music, reading, and outings. Express feelings and concerns to others.
FATIGUE **Nursing action:** assess for possible causes (anemia, chronic pain, stress, depression, and insufficient rest or nutritional intake).	Conserve energy and rest when tired: plan rest periods. Plan for gradual accommodation of activities into life style. Monitor dietary and fluid intake daily.

HEMATOPOIETIC CHANGES

Side Effects	Points to Cover
• Leukopenia: most myelosuppressive agents produce a nadir in the white blood cell count 7–14 days after drug administration. Myelosuppression is severe and prolonged with increased dosage of: Busulfan 2–6 g Carboplatin 2–4 g Cyclophosphamide 5–10 g Cytarabine 3–6 g Etoposide 2–4 g Methotrexate 2–6 g **Nursing action:** monitor the white blood cell count and differential; change equipment as indicated such as the oxygen delivery system and intravenous lines; teach sexual hygiene. • Thrombocytopenia: drugs associated with a delayed cumulative effect: mitomycin, nitrosureas	Avoid sources of infection [people with bacterial infections, colds, sore throats, flu, chicken pox, measles, and cold sores, people recently vaccinated with live attenuated viruses (Measles/Mumps/Rubella, Diphtheria/Pertussis/Tetanus)]. Avoid having fresh fruit, plants, and flowers near the bedside. Avoid cleaning animal litter boxes. Maintain good personal hygiene: bathe daily, wash hands before eating and preparing food, cleanse thoroughly after bowel movements, keep nails clean and clipped short and straight across. Maintain adequate fluid intake. Conserve energy; get adequate rest and exercise. Prevent trauma to skin and mucous membranes. Avoid elective dental work or surgery. Avoid enemas, rectal suppositories and thermometers, and rectal catheters. Use toothettes or nonabrasive dental cleaning devices.

TABLE 14-8 *(continued)*

TEACHING THE CLIENT TO MANAGE SIDE EFFECTS OF CHEMOTHERAPEUTIC DRUGS

Side Effects	Points to Cover
Nursing action: monitor platelet counts; observe bleeding precautions; apply firm pressure to venipuncture site for 3–5 minutes; monitor the number of pads used by menstruating women; make sure there are no sharp objects near the client.	Report the following signs and symptoms of infection immediately to the physician: fever of 38°C or greater, cough, sore throat, a shaking chill, painful or frequent urination, and vaginal discharge.
	Avoid using a straight-edge razor or power tools, and avoid any physical activity that may cause injury.
	Avoid drugs containing aspirin.
• Anemia	Humidify the air; use lotion and lubricants on the skin and lips.
	Avoid invasive procedures; no intramuscular injections.
Nursing action: monitor hematocrit and hemoglobin levels, especially during the drug nadir.	Discourage bare feet when ambulatory.
	Use sanitary pads, not tampons.
	Report the following signs and symptoms immediately to the physician: bleeding gums, increasing bruising; petechiae, purpura, hypermenorrhea, tarry stools, blood in the urine, or coffee-ground emesis.
	Plan periods of rest.
	Report the following promptly to the physician: fatigue, dizziness, shortness of breath, and palpitations.
NAUSEA AND VOMITING	
Nursing action: premedicate with an antiemetic before nausea begins, usually 30 minutes before meals; patient may require routine antiemetics for 3–5 days following some chemotherapy protocols; monitor fluid and electrolyte levels.	Eat frequent, small meals. Avoid greasy and fatty foods and very sweet foods and candy.
	Avoid unpleasant sights, odors, and tastes.
	Cold foods, salty foods, dry crackers, and dry toast may be more tolerable.
	If vomiting is severe, restrict the diet to clear liquids and notify the physician.
	Consider diversionary activities such as music therapy and relaxation techniques. Use strategies that were successful during times of stress.
	Report weight loss to the physician.
MUCOSITIS, RECTAL	
Nursing action: monitor for electrolyte imbalance and granulocyte count; monitor the number, consistency, and amount of bowel movements and urinary output; assess for rectal bleeding.	Eat low-residue and easily digestible foods.
	Increase liquid intake.
	Follow the prescribed medication schedule of anti-diarrheal and pain-control drugs.
	Wash the rectal area with soap and water following each bowel movement; pat or air-dry skin.
MUCOSITIS, VAGINAL	
• Symptoms occur 3–5 days after chemotherapy and subside 7–10 days after treatment.	Report pain, ulceration, or bleeding of the mucous membranes lining the perineum and vagina to the physician.
	Sitz bath with warm salt water may relieve vaginal itching and odor.

TABLE 14-8 *(continued)*

TEACHING THE CLIENT TO MANAGE SIDE EFFECTS OF CHEMOTHERAPEUTIC DRUGS

Side Effects	Points to Cover
	Use hydrogen peroxide (one-quarter strength) with warm water after voiding to rinse perineal area. Avoid commercial douches, tampons, and scented pads or liners.
PHARYNGITIS AND ESOPHAGITIS • The first symptom is often difficulty or pain on swallowing, which may progress to ulceration and infection. **Nursing action:** monitor for inability to swallow.	Eat a soft puréed or liquid diet. Follow the prescribed medication schedule to relieve discomfort. Report to the physician any symptoms that persist for more than 3 days.
SKIN CHANGES **Nursing action:** perform ongoing skin assessments.	Maintain good personal hygiene: wash underclothes and clothing in contact with skin with mild detergent. Topical preparations to minimize itching. Avoid perfume and perfumed lotion. Avoid scratching to prevent infection. Avoid wearing rough fabrics and tight-fitting clothes (panty hose and jeans).
STOMATITIS (ORAL) • Symptoms occur 5–7 days after chemotherapy and persist for up to 10 days post-treatment.	Continue brushing regularly; use a soft toothbrush. Use a nonirritating mouthwash such as a salt, soda, and water solution at least four times daily (¼ tsp salt, 8 oz H_2O, pinch of soda). Avoid irritants to the mouth such as tobacco, alcoholic beverages, spices, and commercial mouthwashes. Avoid wearing dentures until mouth soreness heals. Maintain good nutritional intake; eat soft or liquid foods high in protein; add sauces or gravies to make food easier to ingest. Follow prescribed medication schedule to eradicate infections like oral candidiasis. Report persistent symptoms and any white patches that occur on the tongue, back of throat, or gums to the physician promptly.
TASTE ALTERATIONS • Many chemotherapeutic agents affect the client's sensation of taste. Cisplatin, a heavy metal, commonly causes a metallic taste in the mouth. **Nursing action:** assess for the presence of taste alterations.	Experiment with a variety of foods to determine the most palatable. Occasionally food that the client has not liked in the past may now be the most palatable. Eating with plastic utensils and drinking fluids from nonmetallic containers may decrease the metallic taste in the mouth.

NOTE: From "Chemotherapy Administration," by S. E. Otto, 1993, in *Pocket guide to intravenous therapy* (2nd ed., pp. 499–501), edited by J. C. LaRocca and S. E. Otto, St. Louis: C. V. Mosby. Reprinted with permission.

Prior to bone marrow transplant, cytoreduction using high-dose chemotherapy and radiation produces a totally immunosuppressed state. Once the body is free of cancer cells, the donated or autologous bone marrow is transplanted into the client. The goal is to prevent complications while the transplanted bone marrow begins to rebuild the body's immune system and replace its cells.

A serious complication from bone marrow transplantation is **graft-versus-host disease**. In this physiological process, donated bone marrow mounts an immune response to the client's cells. This occurs because the donor's antigens do not match the client's antigens. Graft-versus-host disease is treated with steroids and immunosuppressant agents. If this complication is not successfully stopped, the transplantation fails.

Infection is another common complication from bone marrow transplants. The client is at high risk for developing an infection because of the immunocompromised state that is required before the transplant. Interstitial or nonbacterial pneumonias are common and pose a risk for clients until their bodies can begin to replace granulocytes. These clients must be kept in a protective environment until they have mounted a sufficient immune response to either prevent an infection or fight one that may develop.

Nursing care for clients who have had a bone marrow transplant includes assisting the client to practice meticulous personal hygiene to prevent infection and skin breakdown. The nurse must prevent anorexia and malnutrition. In addition, a strict protective environment must be maintained using laminar flow to sterilize the air surrounding the client. Since clients who undergo bone marrow transplants have lengthy hospitalizations, it is important to find diversionary activities for them and to help them not feel too isolated.

*In **graft-versus-host disease** the donor's marrow mounts an immune response to the client's antigens.*

COMPLICATIONS OF CANCER

CASE STUDY: COLON CANCER

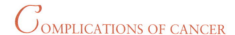

A 62-year-old man has been diagnosed with colon cancer. He undergoes a partial bowel resection, and the surgeon reports that only a portion of the tumor was removed because of infiltration into the intestine. The client must undergo palliative chemotherapy. The physician orders the chemotherapy agent 5-fluorouracil (5-FU) with leucovorin (Wellcovorin). There is no evidence that the tumor has metastasized.

It is the nurse's responsibility to monitor the client for the most common side effects of the 5-FU infusion, including fatigue, anorexia, nausea, vomiting, leukopenia, thrombocytopenia, photosensitivity, stomatitis, and alopecia. The nurse also must monitor for complications from the client's colon carcinoma. Infection is a common complication as a result of the client's immunocompromised state and the accompanying anorexia. Common sites of infection include the lungs, mouth, GI system, rectum, and peritoneal cavity. Sepsis is another possible complication. The nurse should explain to the client in the case study that there is a risk of infection caused by the cancer and ensuing treatment. The client must be taught to monitor for early signs of infection such as a generalized achy feeling and slight fever. The client must be encouraged to fight the anorexia also caused by the disease and its treatment. Appetite stimulants may be indicated.

Oncological Emergencies

Paraneoplastic syndromes, another frequent complication of cancer, cause physiological effects that result from the release of certain hormones. These syndromes are usually seen in clients who are in an advanced stage of disease. Some examples include Cushing's syndrome, which is related to the secretion of adrenocorticotropic hormone (ACTH); hyponatremia, which is related to the syndrome of inappropriate antidiuretic hormone (SIADH); hypoglycemia, which is related to the secretion of insulin; and hypercalcemia, which may be related to a parathyroid hormone–like substance. Venous thrombosis also occurs, possibly related to hypercoagulability. The client in the case study does not have as high a risk for developing a paraneoplastic syndrome as clients with other types of cancers. However, it is important for the nurse to monitor for signs of the venous thrombosis that may occur with colon carcinoma.

Some cancers may eventually cause infarction or organ failure. Infarctions result from the formation of thrombi composed of tumor cells. Necrosis occurs as these thrombi occlude the vessels of major organs, typically the lung, heart, and brain. Organ failure may occur as a result of tumor invasion of the organ. Bowel obstructions are common complications of colon cancer. Radiation often can relieve these obstructions by shrinking the tumor over time. Occasionally adjuvant therapies are initiated to combat the tumor's effects on the organ. If bowel obstruction becomes a problem, a colostomy may be performed to bypass the obstruction.

Spinal cord compression is another common complication of certain cancers. The tumor compresses nerves of the spinal cord, causing severe pain, parasthesia, and other neurological dysfunctions such as paralysis. Radiation often is used to reduce the tumor to relieve the compression. This is a frequent complication of breast cancer metastases. To manage this complication successfully, the nurse must be alert for early changes in the client's neurological status and must notify the physician immediately of even slight changes, as compression is a medical emergency.

Cardiac tamponade, or pericardial effusion, is another medical emergency associated with cancer. This complication occurs most commonly with lung and breast tumors but can occur with certain lymphomas, GI carcinomas, sarcomas, and melanomas (Schweid, Etheredge, & Weiner-McCullough, 1994). Clients experiencing cardiac tamponade often complain of chest pain and shortness of breath. A paradoxical pulse (pulsus

Malignant neoplasms cause several **medical emergencies,** including paraneoplastic syndromes, infarction, organ failure, cardiac tamponade, superior vena cava syndrome, and spinal cord compression. The nurse must carefully assess for the presence of early symptoms of these emergencies.

paradoxus) and jugular venous distention are signs of this disorder. Pulsus paradoxus is the fading of a pulse sensation during inspiration. Muffled heart sounds may be heard during auscultation. Pericardial friction rubs are frequently heard. Cardiac tamponade is treated with pericardio-centesis, the removal of accumulated fluid in the pericardium, either by a pericardial tap or by pericardial fenestration. The client should be made aware of the signs of impending pericardial effusion.

Superior vena cava syndrome is a third medical emergency associated most commonly with clients with lung cancer. This syndrome results from superior vena cava obstruction. Dyspnea, facial edema, and edema of the hands are the most common manifestations. Edema in the upper extremities but not in the dependent areas of the body is another indication of this condition. The blood pressure in these clients is higher in the arms than in the legs. Headache and a decreased level of consciousness also can occur. Superior vena cava syndrome is treated with radiation. **Nursing care** goals during treatment should consist of maintaining the client's oxygenation and preventing thrombi from forming.

Pain as a Complication of Cancer

Fatigue and **pain** are the most debilitating effects of cancer.

Pain and **overwhelming fatigue** are the most debilitating complications of cancer. Unfortunately pain from cancer often is not alleviated because of health providers' ignorance of pain-management methods. The Agency for Health Care Policy and Research (AHCPR) has published guidelines for the treatment of cancer pain (McCaffery & Ferrell, 1994). These guidelines describe the consequences of inadequate pain control, including suffering, anxiety, fear, depression, isolation, anger, and immobility (McCaffery & Ferrell, 1994). The agency recommends that pain medications should be used on a scheduled basis rather than as needed to control pain. The World Health Organization (WHO, 1990) recommends a three-step analgesic ladder of nonopioid analgesics, opioid analgesics, adjuvant agents, and combinations of these three treatment options (Table 14-9). The three-step ladder represents increased levels of medication for pain management based on the intensity of the client's pain. Inadequate pain control presents more of a problem for these clients than overdoses of pain medications.

Pain is subjective. To manage pain adequately the nurse should listen to and trust the client. If the client states that the pain is not being adequately controlled, measures must be taken to reduce the pain to manageable levels. Health care workers often inadequately manage the pain of clients who are being treated for cancer.

The non-narcotic agents that are preferred for managing cancer pain include salicylates, acetaminophen, and nonsteroidal anti-inflammatory drugs (NSAIDs). The opiates of choice are codeine, hydromorphone (Dilaudid), and morphine. Adjuvant agents—antidepressants, antiemetics, and stimulants—are given to enhance the analgesic effects of the other agents.

Opiates are recommended to successfully manage cancer pain.

Several routes are available to administer pain medication to cancer patients, but the oral route is preferred (as long as it is effective), because it is cost-effective and noninvasive, and compliance is simple. The disadvantages of the oral route include a slow onset and incomplete absorption. The rectal and transdermal routes often are good choices if the client cannot tolerate oral medications as a result of vomiting or not being given

TABLE 14-9
WHO Three-Step Analgesic Ladder

Third step:

opioid analgesics for moderate
to severe pain ± nonopioid
analgesics and ± adjuvant
agents

Second step:

opioid analgesics for mild to
moderate pain; nonopioid
analgesics ± adjuvant
agents

First step:

nonopioid analgesic
± adjuvant agents

anything by mouth. The intramuscular route is not used because of the muscle deterioration from cancer-induced malnutrition. For pain that is resistant to treatment through other routes, the subcutaneous and/or intravenous routes are used. Although invasive, it is an easy route for administration and provides good blood levels of the drugs. Narcotic infusions can be administered by subcutaneous pump, intravenous patient-controlled analgesia (PCA), intravenous drip, or the epidural or intrathecal route. These infusions offer the best control for severe, intractable pain but are expensive and require training to perform them properly.

Nonpharmacological therapies also exist for pain management, including attention diversion, relaxation or meditation techniques, guided imagery, hypnosis, biofeedback, and cutaneous stimulation (massage). Heat or cold therapy also can be effective. In contralateral cold stimulation, ice is applied to the unaffected side of the body. This has been very effective in relieving the pain caused by bone marrow aspirations. Transcutaneous electrical nerve stimulation (TENS) uses the gate theory of pain control and has effectively relieved pain. All of these therapies are accepted pain-control treatments. They should, however, be used in conjunction with pharmacological measures if they do not provide sufficient pain control.

The client with colon cancer in the previously mentioned case study should be treated like someone with a chronic disorder. A cure is not likely, but with careful supportive therapy the client may be able to experience quality, pain-free time despite the cancer. Pain management is a significant factor in the client's treatment. Currently he is experiencing more postoperative pain than cancer pain. As a result of his recent bowel resection, he can take nothing by mouth until peristalsis returns. He uses a PCA pump that infuses 1 mg of meperidine (Demerol) on demand every 10 minutes. He also is receiving a basal dose of 1.5 mg/hr. He reports level 2 pain on the visual analog scale (VAS) of pain. The client may begin to experience pain associated with the cancer as the disease progresses. The WHO recommendations help customize the pain management program for his individual needs.

The complications from the analgesics can be managed effectively. Narcotics cause constipation, nausea, vomiting, drowsiness, sedation, and respiratory depression. Constipation is treated with laxatives and controlled with stool softeners. The nurse should assist the client in recognizing the signs of approaching constipation. Increasing fluid and fiber intake helps to prevent constipation.

Nausea and **vomiting** are controlled with antiemetics. Morphine and hydromorphone (Dilaudid) do not cause these symptoms as often as codeine and meperidine (Demerol). Administering antiemetics on a set schedule can eliminate the nausea and vomiting associated with cancer and chemotherapy. It may be necessary to try a number of different agents to find the one best tolerated by the client.

The sedation and respiratory depression associated with narcotics are more pronounced at the beginning of therapy and usually resolve in 2–5 days after a stable therapeutic dose is reached. Drinking beverages with caffeine during the day can help relieve these side effect until they resolve. The narcotic-induced respiratory depression usually is not serious enough to limit the dose until the respiratory rate is less than 10 breaths/min. Narcotics can be reversed with naloxone (Narcan) if the client is over-medicated. However, nurses must use caution with naloxone (Narcan) as clients revive rapidly and with pain. Since naloxone (Narcan) does not last as long as most narcotics, it is necessary to monitor the client until the effects of the pain medication have worn off. The nurse must monitor the client for signs of a narcotic overdose. Nurses cannot let their fear of causing an overdose prevent them from treating a client's pain effectively. As addictions to the medications used for managing cancer pain are almost nonexistent, clients should not be concerned about developing one.

Administering antiemetics on a set schedule can eliminate the nausea and vomiting associated with cancer and chemotherapy.

SUMMARY

Clients with cancer may fear pain, disfigurement, emaciation, financial drain on resources, loss of independence, abandonment, and death. Their family members also may fear what they do not know. The nurse can promote a more positive outlook for the client no matter what the stage of the cancer. Understanding how cancer develops and affects the body allows the nurse to assist the client in exploring and choosing treatment. The nurse also monitors the client for the adverse effects from both the cancer and the treatment. The goals of treatment are cure, control, or palliation. Surgery, radiation, and chemotherapy in combination with supportive therapy are used to treat cancer.

Health care providers must be taught ways to manage cancer pain. Cancer treatment is now based on rehabilitation and support. The client must be made comfortable by minimizing pain. It is imperative that the nurse work with the client, the family, and health care providers to manage the disease successfully.

There are multiple adverse effects both of cancer itself and the therapies used to treat it. Malignant tumors invade tissues and develop a vascular system to protect them from the treatments used to kill the tumor cells. Thus, obstruction and bleeding are common effects of cancer. Organ failure occurs as the tumors mature. The treatments contribute to the deterioration of the client's overall condition. Normal body cells are damaged by the treatments used in the care of clients with cancer. Maintaining body functions is a major treatment goal for patients with malignant tumors.

Maintaining a hopeful attitude may be the client's greatest challenge. The nurse, being available for the client and having a caring attitude, can positively influence the client's outlook. The nurse should listen attentively to the client's fears and concerns. Client education is of utmost importance in managing cancer. The nurse must assist the client in setting and meeting realistic goals. Caring for clients with cancer can be heartbreaking, but the rewards of the emotional and cognitive investments made are well worthwhile.

KEY WORDS

Benign
Biopsy
Bone marrow transplantation
Chemotherapy
Colony-stimulating factor
Differentiation
Grading
Histocompatibility

Irritant
Malignant
Metastasis
Neoplasm
Radiation
Staging
Vesicant

QUESTIONS

1. A 78-year-old man with lung cancer is treated with platinol (Cisplatin). The client complains of a metallic taste in his mouth. This alteration in taste is an adverse effect of platinol (Cisplatin) because the medication is a heavy metal. He asks the nurse to give him something to reduce the taste. Which of the following is correct?

A. He may find it more palatable to eat with plastic utensils and avoid drinking fluids from metal containers.

B. He will not be able to avoid this taste; thus he should learn to accept it and force himself to eat.

C. Medications can be administered prior to a meal to anesthetize the oral cavity. These decrease the taste and should be administered.

D. Since this taste alteration is a sign of platinol (Cisplatin) toxicity, the medication should be stoppped immediately.

2. A 42-year-old woman receives external radiation to treat her ovarian cancer. The client is at risk of developing which of the following adverse effects from the direct effect of her radiation treatments?

A. Alopecia

B. Chest pain

C. Diarrhea

D. Dyspnea

3. A 64-year-old woman with breast cancer is treated with cyclophosphamide (Cytoxan). The client is at risk for developing hemorrhagic cystitis as a result of bladder irritation. Which of the following adjuvant agents helps prevent this adverse effect?

A. Furosemide (Lasix)

B. Leucovorin (Wellcovorin)

C. Mesna (Mesnex)

D. Phenazopyridine (Pyridium)

4. An 82-year-old man complains of level 8 pain on the visual analog scale (VAS). His respiratory rate is 24 breaths/min. The client's pain is associated with the progression of liver carcinoma. The client has a patient-controlled analgesic (PCA) pump that infuses 1 mg morphine sulfate every 10 minutes on demand. He has been using the PCA appropriately. What should the nurse do first to alleviate the client's pain?

A. Administer lorazapam (Ativan) to relieve the anxiety associated with his pain.

B. Discontinue the PCA and administer morphine intramuscularly.

C. Instruct the client to perform guided imagery to reduce the focus on his pain.

D. Ask the physician to add a bolus dose and a basal dose to the PCA infusion.

5. A client with oral carcinoma is treated with external radiation. He fears that his family is being exposed to radiation while caring for him at home. What should the nurse tell this client about his therapy?

A. The client can reduce the risk to his family by sleeping in a separate room.

B. A home health care agency should care for him instead of his family.

C. If the client's linens are washed separately and the toilet is flushed each time he urinates, exposure to others will be minimal.

D. Clients receiving external radiation pose no radiation risk to others.

6. A 76-year-old woman with multiple myeloma complains of shortness of breath and chest pain. The nurse believes that the client is developing cardiac tamponade. Which of the following manifestations is a classic sign of this disorder?

   A. Bounding pulse
   B. Cyanosis
   C. Pulsus paradoxus
   D. S3 heart murmur

ANSWERS

1. *The answer is A.* Platinol (Cisplatin) is a heavy metal and leaves a metallic taste in the mouth. Nothing will eliminate it, but it can be reduced by using nonmetallic utensils and drinkware. The oral cavity should not be anesthetized (even locally) before eating as it may increase the risk of aspiration. A metallic taste is an adverse effect but not an indicator of toxicity.

2. *The answer is C.* The direct effects of external radiation depend on the site being irradiated. Because the client is radiated in the lower pelvic area, diarrhea is common from radiation damage to the mucosal lining of the intestine. Alopecia is likely to occur only if the head has been treated. Dyspnea and chest pain are likely only if the upper thorax, breast, or chest area has been treated.

3. *The answer is C.* Mesna is a uroprotectant that decreases the irritating effects of cyclophosphamide (Cytoxan). Leucovorin (Wellcovorin) is a folic acid that protects against methotrexate (Mexate) toxicity and potentiates the effect of 5-fluorouracil (5-FU; Adracil). Furosemide (Lasix) is a diuretic that depletes the client's hydration status, perhaps worsening the condition. Phenazopyridine (Pyridium) is a topical agent that exerts an analgesic effect on the urinary tract. It does not protect against the irritating effects of cyclophosphamide (Cytoxan) that cause the bladder to hemorrhage.

4. *The answer is D.* A pain level of 8 cannot be managed effectively with tranquilizers and nonpharmacological measures. Morphine administered intramuscularly may be more effective to prolong pain relief, but it is more irritating to the tissues. Additionally, this client would require frequent injections to sustain pain relief. Clients with PCA infusions often complain of a cycle that consists of pain, injection, sleep, and pain. Clients in this state feel that they are not receiving relief because their alert moments are filled with pain. This client has a high level of pain and requires an immediate dose (bolus). Adding a basal rate sustains the client's relief, except during exertion when he can use the intermittent dose.

5. *The answer is D.* The client is never radioactive during external radiation therapy. Answers A, B, and C falsely assume the client is radioactive.

6. *The answer is C.* Pulsus paradoxus occurs when the intensity of the pulse decreases on inspiration. It is a classic sign of cardiac tamponade resulting from the compression of the great vessels when the inflamed tissues are stretched during inspiration. The pulse may be less pronounced, but it is

not bounding. Since this condition does not affect the valves of the heart, murmurs are not heard. Cyanosis only occurs in pulmonary involvement. Cardiac tamponade affects the pericardium and cardiac muscle; any pulmonary involvement would be a secondary condition.

ANNOTATED REFERENCES

Bender, C. M., Yasko, J., M., & Strohl, R. A. (1996). Nursing role in management: Cancer. In Lewis, S. L., Colier, I. C., & Heitkemper, M. M. (Eds.), *Medical-surgical nursing: Assessment and management of clinical problems* (4th ed., pp. 261–315). St. Louis: C. V. Mosby.

Lewis, Collier, and Heitkemper are recognized experts in medical-surgical nursing. This chapter provides an excellent overview of the pathophysiology and etiology of cancer.

Helman, L. J., & Thiele, C. J. (1991). New insights into the causes of cancer. *Pediatric Clinics of North America, 38* (2), 201–217.

This article presents clearly the current theories of cancer development and the stages of metastasis.

Langhorne, M. (1997). Chemotheraphy. In Otto, S. E. (Ed.), *Oncological nursing* (3rd ed., pp. 530–572). St. Louis: C. V. Mosby.

This chapter explains how chemotherapy acts on cells. It also gives practical information for administering chemotherapeutic agents. It lists safety precautions and includes important points for client instruction.

McCaffery, M., & Ferrel, B. R. (1994). How to use the new AHCPR cancer pain guidelines. *American Journal of Nursing* (July), 42–46.

These authors have written extensively on how to manage cancer pain. In this article they discuss some common myths concerning pain medications. A case study and question-and-answer format are used to discuss the AHCPR cancer pain guidelines.

Pfeifer, K. A. (1997). Surgery. In Otto, S. E. (Ed.), *Oncological nursing* (3rd ed., pp. 471–502). St. Louis: C. V. Mosby.

This chapter discusses the issues involved in the surgical treatment of cancer. The entire textbook is an excellent source for the practicing oncology nurse.

Schweid, L., Etheredge, C., & Weiner-McCullough, M. (1994). Will you recognize these oncological crises? *RN* (September), 23–28.

This article utilizes case studies to describe how to recognize oncological emergencies and treat clients who are experiencing them. The guidelines discussed in this article are obtained by dialing 1-800-4-CANCER.

Viall, C. D. (1990). Your complete guide to central venous catheters. *Nursing 90* (February), 34–41.

This article discusses the different types of central venous catheters and provides a good description of how to use and care for them.

World Health Organization (1990). *Cancer pain relief and palliative care.* Geneva, Switzerland.

This organization has defined a protocol for managing cancer pain. The three-step approach is the worldwide standard for clients with cancer pain.

INTERNET SITES FOR ADDITIONAL INFORMATION

CancerNet
  http://icicsun.nei.nih.gov

Cancer Pain Page
  http://www.mdacc.tmc.edu/~acc

National Cancer Institute
  http://rex.nci.nih.gov/

Oncolink
  http://www.oncolink.upenn.edu/

❧ Clients with Burns

*I*ntroduction

The burn client represents a trauma model with a myriad of medical, nursing, and psychosocial needs and challenges. The purpose of this chapter is to provide a basic understanding of the methods required to care for these complex cases. The *burn care team* of health care professionals is composed of the physician, psychiatrist, nurse, physical therapist, social worker, occupational therapist, recreational therapist, dietitian, psychologist, and family and spiritual support staff. Care of the client with a burn injury focuses on a holistic and comprehensive approach to medical and nursing management and involves multisystem treatment. Many programs and organizations are dedicated to education of the public to prevent burn injury, yet two million Americans each year require medical care for burn injuries (Thelan, Davie, Urden, & Lough, 1994).

The outermost layer of skin, the epidermis, is thickest on the soles of the feet and palms of the hand and functions as a protective layer. The second layer, the dermis, is really composed of two layers, which contain the blood vessels, sweat glands, and sebaceous glands, hair follicles, nerves, and sensory fibers for pain, touch, and temperature. The third layer, the hypodermis, contains fat and smooth muscle and acts as a heat shield, shock absorber, and storage for nutritional agents (Fig. 15-1). When a person is burned, loss of the normal function of the skin results in a constellation of physiologic changes. These include loss of the protective barrier, loss of body fluids, alteration in temperature control, and destroyed sensory receptors, sweat glands, and sebaceous glands.

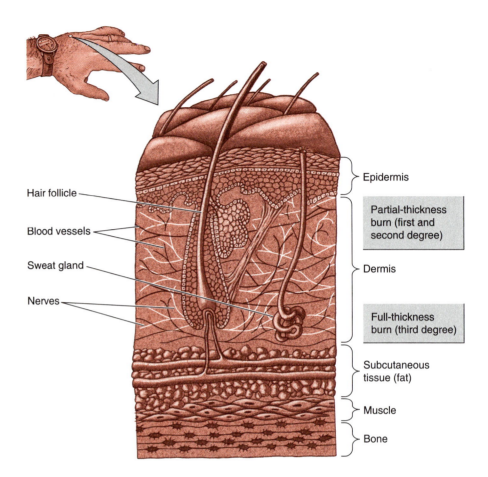

FIGURE 15-1

▨

Anatomical diagram of layers and structures of the human skin that are affected by burn injuries.

Hypovolemia. Hypovolemia is a loss of circulatory fluid volume resulting from loss of blood cells. Loss of fluid in the blood cells themselves (intracellular) and loss of fluid in the surrounding tissues (extracellular) occur in conditions such as burns.

Hypovolemic Shock. This type of shock occurs with inadequate perfusion/oxygenation of tissues and cells from massive or sudden loss of circulatory fluid volume. Signs and symptoms include weak and rapid pulse; hypotension; change in sensorium; restlessness; pale, clammy skin; rapid, shallow breathing; and decreased urinary output.

Etiology of Burns

The degree of the burn depends on the causative agent and the duration of exposure to the agent. Once the protective barrier of the skin is damaged, the capillaries dilate, and plasma escapes into the surrounding tissues. This rapid loss of fluid produces an intravascular fluid volume deficit and causes the first of the two stages that occur with burns, the **hypovolemic stage**. The hypovolemia, in addition to other physiologic changes, causes a decrease in cardiac output, and the major organs and tissues do not receive the fluid and oxygen they normally require. This rapid loss and shift of fluid can lead to **hypovolemic shock**.

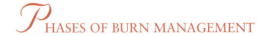
HASES OF BURN MANAGEMENT

Emergency or Shock Period of Burn Management

The hypovolemic stage that occurs in the first 24–48 hours requires immediate intervention. In a severe burn, most of the fluid loss may not be visible, but fluid seeps deep into the wounds and adjacent tissues. The fluid that seeps into the deeper tissues may constitute over half of the extracellular fluid. **This emergency period** of shock and hypovolemia after the injury lasts until capillary integrity and fluid and electrolyte balance are restored. Replacing fluid and electrolytes (i.e., fluid resuscitation) is initiated as soon as the severity of the burn is assessed and the airway is secure. Immediate care must include frequent assessment of lung sounds for evidence of increased fluid in the lungs, a complication called *pulmonary edema.*

Acute Period of Burn Management

The acute period begins after the first 24–72 hours at the end of the emergency period once the fluid and electrolyte balance is restored and diuresis of interstitial space fluid begins. This marks the second stage of burns, the *diuresis stage*. The diuresis stage requires continued acute management. It ends with the closure of the wound, but the length of time before the burn wound is healed varies according to the thickness and extent of the burn. In a severe full-thickness burn, the acute period may last for months.

Rehabilitative Period of Burn Management

Rehabilitation starts with the client's admission and continues throughout the course of treatment until functional and psychosocial deficits are restored and scars are managed. This period may last for weeks, months, or even the rest of the client's life.

CLASSIFICATION OF BURNS AND OTHER ASSESSMENTS OF CLIENTS WITH BURNS

In addition to the other routine assessments, the burn client requires immediate assessment of the depth and severity of the burn injury. Historically, first-, second- or third-degree burns were the terms used to classify burns, but these terms were not descriptive of the actual injury. A more accurate description of the damage to the tissue is used today, in the classification into partial-thickness and full-thickness burns. Initial assessment of the burn client requires classification according to the size and depth of the burn as given below.

Size of Burns

For adults, the size of the burn is determined with the "rule of nines" body chart. In adults, the body parts are divided into surface areas of multiples of 9% (Fig. 15-2). At initial assessment, the burned area of the body is shaded into the drawing, and the amount of body surface damaged by

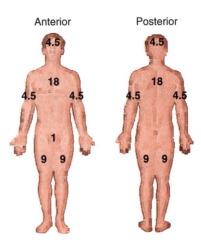

FIGURE 15-2

The "rule of nines" body chart is used for adults to determine the size of the burn. Body parts are divided into surface areas of multiples of 9%.

the burn is calculated. For infants and children, a separate chart is used because of the relatively larger head and smaller body parts of children as compared to adults. The calculations for adults are as follows:

Anterior head	=	4½%	Posterior arm	=	4½%
Posterior head	=	4½%	Perineum	=	1%
Anterior trunk	=	18%	Anterior leg	=	9%
Posterior trunk	=	18%	Posterior leg	=	9%
Anterior arm	=	4½%			

Depth of Burns

The depth of the burn is assessed according to the varying depths of skin and tissue destruction (Fig. 15-3). *Partial-thickness* (includes first- and second-degree) *burns* are characterized by damage to part of the epidermal and dermal layers of the skin. A *full-thickness* (third-degree) *burn* is defined as injury to the epidermis, dermis, and other tissue layers, which include subcutaneous, muscle, and nerve tissue. The depth of tissue injury is further classified as *superficial*, involving only the epidermis, and *deep*, involving the dermis as well.

Superficial Partial-Thickness, or First-Degree Burns These burns are characterized by erythema and mild discomfort. A common example is sunburn. These burns usually heal within a week, and treatment consists of increasing fluids and pain relief with mild analgesics.

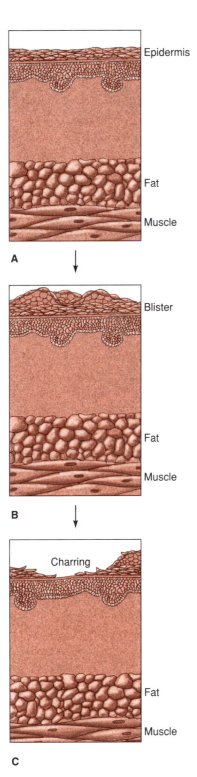

FIGURE 15-3 *A.* Superficial partial-thickness burns. The skin is reddened. A common example is sunburn. *B.* Deep partial-thickness burns. The skin surface is red with white areas and blisters. *C.* Full-thickness burns with eschar. The burn appears brown and leather-like. The burn extends through all layers of the skin, including the subcutaneous layers.

Mr. Johnson, age 24 years, was burned on the posterior right arm and part of the back of his torso by hot water. His weight is 80 kg. His health history is negative for any preexisting illness, and he describes his general health as good. After examination, the nurse determines that the burn should be described as a superficial partial-thickness burn, which involves 15% of the body surface area (BSA).

This client would probably be treated on an outpatient basis since superficial partial-thickness burns up to 15% BSA in an otherwise healthy young adult can be managed in that setting. The burn would appear red, as if sunburned. The immediate health needs would be to relieve discomfort and replace fluids that shifted into the burn area in the first 24–30 hours. Wound healing is completed in 1 week.

Moderate Partial-Thickness, or Second-Degree Burns These burns are characterized by bright-red or mottled skin. They may be weeping fluid and are very sensitive to touch or to air currents. Blisters may form. These burns usually heal within 1–6 weeks, depending on the depth of injury.

Deep Partial-Thickness, or Second-Degree Burns These burns are characterized by a red skin surface with white areas in deeper parts that may change to yellow with healing. They usually require surgical intervention and skin grafting and take up to six weeks to heal. These burns may progress to full-thickness burns when infection occurs.

Full-Thickness, or Third-Degree Burns These burns extend through all layers of skin including the subcutaneous tissue layer. They appear white, red, or brown and leather-like. Because of the damage to the nerve endings, they do not cause pain and are not sensitive to touch or air currents. They usually require skin grafting and are susceptible to infection. The client is at risk for electrolyte and metabolic imbalances.

CASE STUDY: FULL-THICKNESS BURN

Mrs. Hernandez, age 69 years, presented to the emergency room with a hot water, full-thickness burn, which involved her entire face and anterior right arm (9% BSA).

This type of client usually requires hospitalization in a burn unit with comprehensive care delivered by a burn team. The age of the client and body area involved (face) require emergency care in which airway management is a priority. The burn will appear white, red, or brown with leather-like texture. The initial complaint would not be of pain.

Age of the Client

Age is an important part of the clinical assessment because it reflects on the severity of a burn; the size of the burn in relation to the BSA; the developmental and psychological adjustments; and management considerations with preexisting health problems. Infants under two years of age and adults over 60 years of age have a higher mortality rate than clients in other age groups (Phipps, Cassmeyer, Sands, & Lehmar, 1995).

Area of Burn Injury

It is important to note which body part has been damaged when assessing the severity of a burn and the potential needs for recovery and rehabilitation. Burns of functional areas such as the hands or cosmetic areas such as the face require a longer recovery than other burn areas for both physical and emotional reasons. Burns of the head, neck, or chest may compromise respiratory function and require emergency attention for maintenance of the airway. Burns of the perineum are at greater risk for infection due to contamination. Encircling burns of an extremity, chest, or trunk may cause a constricting contraction, producing a tourniquet effect that may compromise circulation or respiration.

Burn Agent or Mechanism

The nature of the causative agent has a direct impact on the prognosis and treatment of the client. Thermal burns are the most common burns, frequently the result of household accidents with hot water, steam, or direct contact with fire.

Radiation burns are uncommon. These are usually localized. Although they may appear to be of the thermal type, they are actually due to exposure to high doses of radiation and do not appear for days to weeks after exposure. Radiation burns may occur as a complication of radiation therapy or as a wound from an explosion (e.g., bombs in war).

Electrical burns are seen mostly in men after exposure to a low- or high-voltage current. Included in this category are lightning strikes (mortality is 25%) and occupational accidents (Phipps, et al., 1995).

Chemical burns resulting from contact with strong acids or alkalis are commonly seen in industry. Examples of chemical burns also include accidents with household substances such as drain cleaner, paint remover, or disinfectant. Chemical splashes to the eyes and face occur in both domestic and industrial accidents. Tar and asphalt burns are chemical burns, with injury to the hands accounting for 70% of this type of burn. Alkali burns usually are the most serious (Phipps, et al., 1995).

Inhalation burns signal a high risk for airway obstruction and may be life-threatening. Obstruction is usually caused by airway edema, resulting in occlusion.

Medical History of the Client

The medical history of the burn client can be overlooked in the immediate rush of emergency care, with tragic results. Obtaining a complete medical history is vital when caring for a burn client. Co-morbid, or preexisting, conditions such as diabetes mellitus, heart disease, renal disease, or central nervous system (CNS) disorders may further complicate an already complex injury.

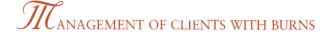

$\mathcal{M}$ANAGEMENT OF CLIENTS WITH BURNS

Triage

Triage criteria for burn clients are essential to access the appropriate level of health care. Minor burn injuries can be treated on an outpatient basis. These include partial-thickness (second-degree) burns affecting less than 15% BSA in an adult or full-thickness (third-degree) burns affecting less than 2% BSA. Hospitalization is necessary for partial-thickness (second-degree) burns affecting 15–20% BSA or full-thickness (third-degree) burns affecting 2–10% BSA in an adult.

Major burn injuries require hospitalization in a burn unit. These comprise partial-thickness (second-degree) burns affecting more than 25% BSA or full-thickness (third-degree) burns of more than 10% BSA in an adult. Smaller burns with complicating features (co-morbid conditions) or burns at the extremes of age, such as in infants and geriatric clients, likewise require hospitalization in a burn unit (Phipps, et al., 1995).

Airway Management

Airway management is essential, especially in cases of burns on the face and neck or smoke inhalation. Clients should be observed for signs of respiratory distress such as tachypnea, anxiety, agitation, hoarseness, stridor, or wheezing. If the burn client displays any signs of respiratory distress or has suspected smoke inhalation, endotracheal intubation may be necessary to maintain respiratory function and oxygenation. Even when intubation is not required, the burn victim who has any inhalation injury should be given oxygen by mask. Respiratory management of the burn client should include monitoring arterial blood-gas levels of pH, oxygen, and carbon dioxide.

Fluid Resuscitation

Once a patent airway and oxygenation have been assured, circulation management is the next critical intervention. All jewelry should be removed to prevent the tourniquet effect that can severely restrict circulation. Ideally, rapid fluid replacement should commence within an hour of the burn injury to deter hypovolemic shock. The Parkland formula is the most widely used fluid replacement formula: 4 mL Ringer's lactate (RL) solution × body weight in kilograms (kg) × percentage of BSA of the burn = the 24-hour fluid requirements (Thelan, et al., 1994). For example, the fluid replacement calculation for a woman of 60 kg with a 25% BSA burn is as follows:

$$4 \text{ mL} \times 60 \text{ kg} \times 25\% \text{ (BSA)} = 6000 \text{ mL in 24 hours}$$

Fluid replacement should be administered via two large-caliber peripheral angiocaths or a central venous catheter. Blood volume falls most rapidly, and edema increases rapidly within the first eight hours. Thus, one-half of the replacement of fluids and electrolytes must be given within the first eight hours. During the second eight-hour period, one-fourth of the total amount is given, and during the third eight-hour period the remaining one-fourth is administered (Phipps, et al., 1995). For example, in the calculation above, for a requirement of 6000 mL in 24 hours, the client would be given 3000 mL in the first eight hours, and 1500 mL during the second and third eight-hour periods. RL solution, usually the fluid of choice, is administered rapidly to help restore normal cardiac output and maintain oxygenation. Hypokalemia and hyponatremia also may occur, and the rapid replacement of fluids with RL helps to prevent electrolyte imbalances. Colloids such as albumin or fresh frozen plasma may also be given.

Renal Management

Acute renal failure may occur if fluid replacement is not adequate. A Foley, or indwelling, catheter is inserted to monitor hourly urinary outputs. Urinary output should be 30–50 mL/hr (Thelan, et al., 1994). *Hyperkalemia* can occur when cells excrete potassium due to cell damage (hemolysis), metabolic acidosis, or renal failure. *Hypokalemia* can occur due to massive loss of fluids and electrolytes. Urinalysis is followed closely to detect myoglobinuria (dark, port-wine urine color) due to passage of the end products of the hemolyzed cells through the glomeruli. As muscle cells die, potassium myoglobin (muscle pigment) is given off within six hours of injury. These end products passing through the glomeruli can cause massive tubular destruction. Treatment includes the administration of mannitol, an osmotic diuretic, to force diuresis. Other diuretics are avoided to preserve intravascular volume. Urine specific gravity, which measures the concentration of the urine, is checked frequently for indications of hypovolemia.

Gastrointestinal Management

Clients with burns over more than 20% BSA are prone to developing paralytic ileus and ulcers. Nasogastric (NG) tubes are often placed for gastric decompression for 24–48 hours (Thelan, et al., 1994). Curling's ulcers, or stress ulcers, may occur as a result of decreased perfusion to the gastrointestinal (GI) tract. Bowel movements must be documented and tested for occult blood. In recent years, the incidence of ulcers in burn clients has decreased with the prophylactic use of histamine (H_2)-receptor antagonists such as cimetidine (Tagamet), ranitidine (Zantac), famotidine (Pepcid), or nizatidine (Axid), which decrease stomach acid.

Pain. Pain is a subjective experience and should be defined by the client's individual experience. Pain is caused by stimulation of sensory nerve endings. Therefore, clients with full thickness burns with destruction of nerve endings may not experience pain sensations. Since pain includes both physical and emotional responses of the body, the burn victim may exhibit or verbalize pain in a variety of ways.

Pain Management

Small doses of intravenous morphine sulfate or a continuous morphine drip are usually given. If the client is intubated, other sedative medications may be given in conjunction with morphine. Total full-thickness burns are rare; a mixture of partial-thickness and full-thickness burns are more common. A client with this type of burn experiences severe **pain** and anxiety. Drug regimens that combine morphine with diazepam (Valium) or other antianxiety agents are often effective. The nurse must monitor any client receiving morphine for signs of respiratory depression. If the client is on a ventilator, use of the paralyzing agent pancuronium (Pavulon) with morphine is often necessary. As the client improves, alternative comfort methods such as guided imagery, biofeedback, and **hydrotherapy** may provide relief (Fig. 15-4).

Hydrotherapy. Because of the properties of water related to buoyancy and cleansing action, water is an ideal agent for burn wound care. The burn is cleaned and debrided while the client soaks in the hydrotherapy tub (Hubbard tank). Gentle massage by the warm water is also therapeutic. Programs of exercise are often implemented in the hydrotherapy tub.

Tissue Oxygenation

Frequent assessment of peripheral pulses (extremity pulse assessment) is important to evaluate arterial blood flow and edema under the **eschar** since edema may obstruct venous return (Fig. 15-5). Ischemia, necrosis, and gangrene are complications that may develop. The nurse should assess for diminished capillary refill, diminished peripheral pulses, paleness, cyanosis, pain, and paresthesia as warning signals of ischemia. If the eschar and swelling compromise arterial blood flow, an escharotomy, an incision made through the eschar to release fluid and allow for swelling without constricting tissue oxygenation, may be necessary.

Eschar. This is slough or nonviable tissue produced by a burn. Eschar needs to be removed because it is a medium that can foster infections, and it also can cause constriction of the circulation. Eschar is typically thick and leather-like.

FIGURE 15-4

⌧

A hydrotherapy unit is used to provide relief for a burn patient and to clean and debride burn wounds.

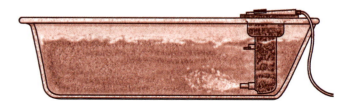

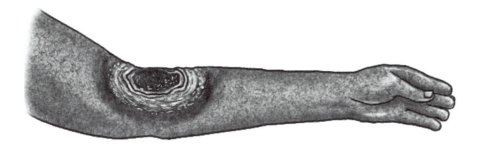

FIGURE 15-5

Eschar, the nonviable tissue produced by a burn, is shown.

Skin Integrity

The integrity of the skin is restored by the following physiologic changes that occur in a three-stage process of healing. The first phase, the *inflammatory phase,* occurs from the time of the burn injury to day 3–4. This phase includes vascular and cellular changes as the body responds to isolate the wound. The wound is isolated from the external environment by the following changes: platelets aggregate, blood coagulates, smooth muscle contracts, and the lumens of vessels narrow, preventing blood loss and entry of bacteria. Vasodilation occurs during day 2–4, increasing the blood flow to the wound, which, in turn, causes erythema, edema, and tenderness. The immune system responds by increasing phagocytes to clean the wound.

The second phase, the *proliferative phase,* occurs from day 4 postburn to day 20. Fibroblasts synthesize collagen and provide strength to the wound. Epithelial cells form over the wound and pull the wound edges toward the center. This phase is known as *wound contraction.*

The third phase of wound healing, the *maturation phase*, occurs 20 days postburn to scar tissue formation. Collagen deposits form scar tissue, but the resultant scar is never as strong as regular tissue.

Wound Management

There are three methods of wound care:

1. **Open method.** A wound is left open to air with the application of a topical agent.
2. **Semi-open method.** A topical agent is applied to the wound, using gauze to keep the topical agent in place.
3. **Closed method.** A topical agent is used on the wound with adaptic or xeroform and covered with kerlix.

General principles of infection control require that the nurse adhere to scrupulous sterile technique in the care of the burn client. Reverse isolation is recommended in the general hospital setting without a special burn unit to decrease the likelihood of infection. Aseptic technique is used during all dressing changes. Eschar, when present, should be removed as it acts as a media for bacterial growth. Hydrotherapy, in conjunction with the physical therapy department, is often used. Daily cleansing of the burn and debridement assist in wound healing and removal of eschar. Hydrotherapy facilitates the removal of medications before the next application; it is also the most comfortable method of removing dressings. The hydrotherapy solution may be plain water, normal saline, or an electrolyte solution (Phipps, et al., 1995). Hydrotherapy is usually done once or twice daily, and the nurse must ensure that the client does not get chilled. Hydrotherapy is contraindicated during the acute phase if the client is unstable or has sudden changes in temperature, pulse, or respirations. Hypothermia may occur, and fluid warmers or hypothermia blankets may be used.

Drugs Used for Wound Care

Topical agents applied to the burn wound decrease infection and promote healing. An outline of the commonly used drugs is included here. In clinical practice, the various drugs and their side effects, the client's wound condition, and any cultures must be reviewed daily.

Mafenide acetate (Sulfamylon) is a topical, white cream that penetrates the eschar and is bacteriostatic. It is applied with sterile gloves on the surface of the wound, and gauze may be placed over the area. The wound is cleansed prior to the next application once or twice daily. The drug is discontinued once healing is noted.

Silver sulfadiazine (Silvadene) is a white cream with bactericidal action. It is applied to the wound once or twice daily on a saturated gauze or with a sterile gloved hand. It is not used in clients with a history of renal disease. This drug may cause depression in white blood cell (WBC) formation, with a decrease from the normal of 5000 mm^3 to as low as 1500 mm^3. If the number of WBCs stays low for more than 12 hours, the physician should be notified, and a different topical agent prescribed.

Povidone-iodine (Betadine) is a red-brown ointment with broad antimicrobial action. It is applied to the wound three times a day with a sterile gloved hand or on gauze.

Silver nitrate in a 0.5% solution is saturated on sterile gauze sponges, applied to the wound, and kept continually moist. It has a bacteriostatic action. Dressings are removed every 12–24 hours by soaking the client in a tepid saline solution in a hydrotherapy tub or by soaking the dressed area, depending on the extent of the burn.

Skin Grafting

Skin grafts are applied to cover the wound, promote healing, and prevent infection and contractures. The burn team, consisting of health professionals in nursing, surgery, plastic surgery, physical therapy, nutrition, and psychology, contributes to the care of the burn client who requires skin grafting. A brief definition of the various types of grafts is given below. In clinical practice, specific needs of the client with various types of grafts are managed by the burn team. Definitions of the various grafts are as follows:

Autograft. A skin graft made from the client's own body.

Homograft. A skin graft harvested from cadaver skin generally acquired 6–24 hours after death. However, best results are obtained if homografts are acquired within four hours of death. Homografts are temporary grafts that are rejected after two weeks. They are usually dressed with a nonadherent agent; the dressing should not be changed for 24–48 hours. Grafts are usually taken from the abdomen, thigh, or back. It is a partial-thickness graft, and it has the appearance of sunburn.

Heterograft (xenograft). A skin graft harvested from skin from another species, such as a pig. Heterografts last for 3–4 days.

Synthetic skin. A man-made synthetic substitute for skin.

Homografts, heterografts, and synthetic skin provide temporary coverage as the burn heals. These temporary coverings are gradually rejected and are easily removed from the newly healed skin (Phipps, et al., 1995).

CASE STUDY: FULL-THICKNESS BURN

Mr. H. is a 28-year-old man who has sustained a 40% BSA full-thickness burn as a result of an explosion in the paint factory where he is employed. The paramedics in the ambulance and the emergency room staff have stabilized Mr. H. by intubating him, starting intravenous therapy with Ringer's lactate, placing an indwelling catheter in his bladder, inserting a NG tube, and offering simple explanations to Mr. H. regarding his treatment. The burn injury is observed to be a 40% BSA full-thickness burn on his face, both arms, and the posterior portion of both thighs.

Mr. H. is transported by helicopter to the regional burn center approximately three hours after the explosion. At time of admission to the burn unit, he has received 5000 mL of Ringer's lactate. His urine output is stable at about 40 mL/hr since catheterization. Further nursing assessment reveals Mr. H. to be alert and oriented; his lungs are clear to auscultation; respirations are 20 via the ventilator; and the cardiac monitor demonstrates normal sinus rhythm at 84 beats/min. Bowel sounds are hypoactive with the NG tube on low, intermittent suction draining a small amount of greenish-brown gastric liquid. There is marked swelling and tightness of the skin around the eyes, arms, and hands. Mr. H.'s ring and watch have been removed in the emergency room.

Fluid resuscitation is achieved in the first 24 hours after the burn injury by using the Parkland fluid formula. By the third day, Mr. H. is demonstrating stable blood gases and laboratory values, and he is weaned from the ventilator and extubated. The burn treatment consists of cleansing the area twice a day in the hydrotherapy tub in the physical therapy department. Analgesia is given 30 minutes before each burn cleansing treatment. The cleansing and debridement are followed by application of the antibiotic cream sulfadiazine (Silvadene) to his arms, hands, and thighs. The burn is treated by an open method.

Mr. H.'s bowel sounds return to normal, and he begins eating on the fourth day. He is evaluated by a dietitian for his caloric needs, and he receives three meals and two snacks daily consisting of high-protein, high-calorie food sources. His nutritional intake is supplemented with vitamins and Ensure. Mr. H. is weighed daily.

Grafting procedures on his arms are begun on postburn day 10. A series of grafting procedures are performed over the next two weeks, with excision and grafting to the face and thighs. Mr. H. has adherence and viability of all his grafts, with no infection.

Physical therapy begins on the day of admission. Passive exercises are performed for the first few days, and activity advanced to ambulation of short distances by postburn day 8. Mr. H. is expected to perform his activities of daily living (ADL) at this stage of his rehabilitation. With the nurses and physical therapists, he performs active range of motion exercises.

Mr. H. is seen weekly by the burn unit psychologist to assist in the development of coping skills. He becomes more open in the expression of his fears, and he is especially worried about his future job opportunities. Vocational counseling and retraining are available during the rehabilitation period.

Laboratory Assessment

Blood and urine chemistry give critical information concerning the impact of the burn on the client's organs and cell function. Electrolytes, blood chemistry, and hematocrit should be monitored carefully. The complete blood count (CBC) is checked for signs of sepsis (WBC count elevated above 10,000 mm^3) or depression of WBC formation (WBC count decreased below 5000 mm^3). Urinalyis, blood urea nitrogen (BUN), and serum creatinine should be followed to monitor renal function.

Total Parenteral Nutrition (TPN). Parenteral nutrition is administration of nutrition into the vascular system as opposed to through the digestive system. "Total" refers to the need to provide all of the total daily nutritive needs for the client, which include caloric requirements, carbohydrate, protein, fat, vitamins, and trace elements needed every 24 hours.

Nutritional Management

Nutritional demands are increased to maintain a state of hypermetabolism until wounds are 90% healed. Depending on the BSA involved, the client's metabolic rate may be elevated 40–100%. The daily protein requirement is also greater than normal due to the negative nitrogen balance. A dietary consult is always obtained to calculate the protein and caloric requirements for the client. Initial nutrition needs are supplied by **total parenteral nutrition** (TPN) with lipids until GI motility is restored. Once enteral feeding is started, the nurse should establish some of the client's food preferences that will meet his or her protein and caloric requirements. Daily caloric intake should be maintained at 3500–5000 calories. Vitamins, dietary supplements, and zinc should be given daily to meet the client's nutritional demands and promote wound healing. The client's weight should be measured daily. Initially, weight gain occurs due to fluid retention, but weight decreases following the diuresis phase.

Promoting Mobility and Prevention of Contractures

A comprehensive program of splinting, positioning, exercise, ambulation, and regaining ADL should begin immediately. Contractures are common complications of burn injuries. Occupational and physical therapists are involved in the client's care from the time of admission. Keeping the client flat assists in preventing contractures.

Patient Education Management

Nurses should teach **coping mechanisms** to both client and family. The nurse must encourage the client to develop a realistic self-image. Techniques to prevent skin breakdown in which the client can be involved must be identified, as a loss of control is frequently experienced. Exercise programs to prevent and control contractures and to maintain current functional ability provide some sense of control.

$\mathcal{S}$UMMARY

In conclusion, the nursing assessment and management of the burn client require a comprehensive and multidisciplinary approach. Once the client's burn area is assessed, the surface area and depth of the wound are determined. It is essential to maintain an airway and adequate oxygenation, especially for the client with a facial burn or smoke inhalation. The oxygen saturation should be monitored closely by pulse oximeter or blood gases. Because of the large fluid losses and fluid shifting in a burned area, nursing care to prevent and treat hypovolemia and shock is initiated immediately. Intravenous fluids are replaced according to the Parkland formula. The nurse must accurately monitor intake and output hourly. Assessment for signs and symptoms of hypovolemia includes observing for decreased sensorium, tachycardia, hypotension, decreased urine output, and pale, clammy skin. The nurse administers analgesics to provide comfort, especially 30 minutes before dressing changes. Because of the extensive emotional demands on a burn client, the client and family must be kept well informed of the progress and plan of care. Mutual goal setting with the burn team, client, and family is needed. Initially, the nurse

Coping Mechanisms. This is a term used to describe the efforts or strategies by which an individual adjusts to the environment and life's demands. Coping mechanisms are especially needed after a serious burn. Examples of coping strategies needed during the recovery phase of burns include identifying client and family strengths, developing a realistic body image, reintegrating the client into previous roles as much as possible, and demonstrating self-care in exercise and skin care programs.

should document the appearance, extent, and cause of the burn wound. The wound should be assessed on each shift for signs of infection and the stage of healing. The nurse should offer reassurance and support to the client and family and encourage positive coping skills.

KEY WORDS

Autograft

Burn care team

Coping mechanisms

Diuresis of interstitial space fluid

Eschar

Fluid resuscitation

Full-thickness burns

Heterograft

Homograft

Hydrotherapy

Hypovolemia

Inhalation burns

Partial-thickness burns

Respiratory distress

Total parenteral nutrition

QUESTIONS

1. The setting that is most suitable for the treatment of the client with a superficial partial-thickness burn is
   A. admission to a burn unit.
   B. admission to a medical unit.
   C. treatment in an emergency room or ambulatory care setting.
   D. home health care.

2. A superficial partial-thickness burn wound would appear
   A. red, as if the client were sunburned.
   B. bright red and weeping fluid.
   C. mottled without weeping fluid.
   D. brown and leather-like.

3. The *immediate* health needs that the nurse must address in a client with superficial partial-thickness burns are
   A. airway management and hypovolemic shock.
   B. moderate discomfort and minor fluid loss.
   C. pain management with intravenous morphine.
   D. renal management with insertion of a Foley, or indwelling, catheter.

4. A superficial partial-thickness burn should heal in
   A. one week.
   B. three weeks.
   C. six weeks.
   D. two months.

5. The setting that is most suitable for the treatment of a client with a full-thickness burn is

   A. admission to a burn unit.
   B. admission to a medical unit.
   C. treatment in an emergency room or ambulatory care setting.
   D. home health care.

6. A full-thickness burn wound would appear

   A. red, as if the client were sunburned.
   B. bright red and weeping fluid.
   C. mottled and not weeping fluid.
   D. brown and leather-like.

7. In a patient with a full-thickness burn of the face, the nurse must immediately address

   A. airway management and hypovolemic shock.
   B. moderate discomfort and minor fluid loss.
   C. pain management with intravenous morphine.
   D. wound care.

8. A full-thickness burn of the face should heal in

   A. one week.
   B. three weeks.
   C. six weeks.
   D. months.

ANSWERS

1. *The answer is C.* Superficial partial-thickness burns of up to 15% of the body surface area (BSA) in an otherwise healthy young adult can be treated on an outpatient basis.

2. *The answer is A.* Superficial partial-thickness burns appear red, as if the client were sunburned. Bright red or mottled wounds describe moderate partial-thickness burns, and brown or leather-like wounds describe full-thickness burns.

3. *The answer is B.* Moderate discomfort and minor fluid loss into the burn area that occurs within 24–32 hours are the two major health needs that the nurse should address with a superficial partial-thickness burn. Treatment usually consists of increasing oral fluids and pain relief with mild oral analgesics. The position of most comfort for the client while horizontal is prone.

4. *The answer is A.* Healing of a superficial partial-thickness burn usually occurs within a week.

5. *The answer is A.* Full-thickness burns usually require hospitalization in a burn unit with comprehensive care by a burn team. The age of the client and the body area involved determine the need for emergency attention.

6. *The answer is D.* A full-thickness burn appears white or brown and leather-like.

7. *The answer is A.* Airway maintenance is a priority in a full-thickness burn of the face, as swelling may cause airway obstruction. The nurse must observe the client for tachypnea, anxiety, agitation, hoarseness, stridor, or wheezing as signs of respiratory distress. Fluid resuscitation requires intravenous lactated Ringer's solution to be started in the ambulance or the emergency room. These burns usually require skin grafting, but this is not a priority in the emergency management period.

8. *The answer is D.* A long period of recovery would be expected with a full-thickness burn. These burns usually require skin grafting and are susceptible to infection. Plastic surgery may be needed during the rehabilitation phase.

ANNOTATED REFERENCES

Phipps, W., Cassmeyer, V., Sands, J., & Lehman, M. K. (1995). *Medical-surgical nursing concepts and clinical practice.* St. Louis: C. V. Mosby.

This text gives extensive information on alterations in the body systems and nursing care for common problems in ill adults. It is useful for a more detailed review.

Thelan, L. A., Davie, J. K., Urden, L. D., & Lough, M. E. (1994). *Critical care nursing: Diagnosis and management.* St. Louis: C. V. Mosby.

This is a specialty nursing text that contains information on the emergency and acute periods of care for clients with burns as well as nursing care of adults with other conditions requiring critical care.

INTERNET SITES FOR ADDITIONAL INFORMATION

National Rehabilitation Information Center (NARIC).
NARIC has information on all aspects of disability rehabilitation:
gopher://www.cais.net:80/hGET%20/naric/home.html

Emergency Nurses Association
http://www.ena.org

First Aid Online
http://www2.vivid.net/~cicely/safety

𝒯HE INTEGUMENTARY SYSTEM

𝒥NTRODUCTION

The skin is the largest organ of the body and is the first line of defense against infectious agents. The skin protects the body from pathogens and prevents the penetration of microorganisms. It also contains secretions that have antibacterial properties. The normal flora of the skin provides additional protection by producing antibacterial substances and competing for essential nutrients. Periodically, the skin also sheds the top layer of dead cells that contain bacteria (Schaffer, Garzon, Heroux, & Korniewicz, 1996). Intravenous catheters or other devices, burns, and breaks in the skin from a surgical incision or wound disrupt the integrity of the skin which renders the client susceptible to infection.

𝒲OUND HEALING

A wound is a bodily injury that disrupts the normal continuity of structures and tissue. A wound usually involves a break in the integrity of the skin. A contused wound, such as a bump on the head, is a wound in which the skin remains unbroken. The restoration of integrity to the skin or tissues starts immediately after the injury. Factors affecting wound healing are age, nutritional status, general state of health, obesity, smoking, diabetes mellitus (DM), steroid therapy, severity of the wound, location,

Body Defense Mechanisms. The body has three major types of defense mechanisms against organisms: mechanical, biological, and chemical.
The skin is the first line of mechanical defense. It protects the body from the constant bombardment of organisms (Schaffer, Garzon, Heroux, & Korniewicz, 1996).

extent of injury to the tissues, and available body reserves for the regeneration of tissue.

Nursing care of a client with a wound always begins with frequent assessment of the progress of wound healing. Inspection of the wound includes assessment for signs of bleeding in or around the wound. Discoloration or swelling of the skin adjacent to a surgical or traumatic wound may indicate a pooling of blood as in a hematoma and should be reported. Bleeding in and around a wound and clot formation can delay healing. Accumulation of serosanguineous fluid or purulent drainage also must be assessed and reported to the physician. If a drain has been placed in a wound to remove excess fluid, the color, amount, odor, and consistency of the drainage must be recorded. Dressings covering a wound must also be inspected frequently.

General parameters to monitor in a client with a wound include temperature, pain, white blood cell (WBC) count, and electrolyte levels. An elevated temperature and WBC count can signal local or systemic infection. The presence of purulent drainage should be reported immediately, as infection is likely. In a surgical wound, a discharge of serosanguineous drainage on the fourth or fifth day postoperatively must always be investigated as a possible sign of failure of wound healing.

Nursing care of a client with a wound also includes monitoring nutritional status. Virtually every nutrient plays some role in the healing process. Supplemental vitamins, dietary supplements, or total parenteral nutrition may be needed. Early ambulation and exercise assist in providing adequate circulation of blood to the wound. Depending on the location of the wound, positioning may also be very important to avoid prolonged pressure to the wound area. Adequate rest is also needed to facilitate healing.

When the integrity of a client's skin is impaired, for whatever reason, the wounds heal by primary, secondary, or tertiary intention. For any type of wound, nursing care involves documenting the size, location, depth, and shape of the wound, as well as the presence of exudate or odor and granulation tissue.

Primary Intention

In this process, the edges of the wound are brought together surgically and approximated to allow healing to take place. An example of this is a laceration that has been sutured. Most surgical wounds heal by primary intention, especially when the surgical incision is a clean, straight line in which the layers of muscle, tissue, and skin are well approximated by suturing. The first four days after suturing, the wound is erythematous, warm to the touch, painful, and indurated (swollen). From the seventh to ninth day, a healing ridge of collagen forms along the wound edges. If a wound is not healing properly according to the above-mentioned steps, infection may be present, characterized by wound drainage, increased temperature, increased WBC count, odor, and increased redness at the site of the wound. Sterile dressings must always be used for wounds healing by primary intention.

Secondary Intention

Secondary intention is the process of granulation in which the tissue color changes from pink to red as the wound heals from the inside out. A wound that heals by secondary intention should not have exudate or odor. Wounds such as ulcers, where it is difficult to approximate the defined edges, heal by secondary intention. These types of wounds are more susceptible to infection. A wound that is healing abnormally by secondary intention appears excessively dry or contains moist granulation tissue with exudate or odor. Sterile, wet-to-dry, coarse mesh dressings moistened with sterile saline are typically used. Occasionally transparent dressings such as Op-Site or Duoderm are used. When a transparent dressing is used, it is usually maintained until pink tissue forms underneath.

When drainage or any other sign of infection is evident, a wound culture and sensitivity should be performed. If the culture is positive for gram-negative organisms, the dressing should be changed frequently. Exudate that accumulates under the occlusive dressing should be evacuated with a sterile needle, and a patch of occlusive dressing should then be applied to the wound.

Tertiary Intention

Wounds heal by tertiary intention when a delay occurs between injury and treatment. The wound may eventually heal by secondary intention when it is left open or by primary intention when it is approximated. These wounds are highly susceptible to infection, since more microorganisms than usual have penetrated the wound before it is treated.

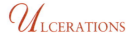

ULCERATIONS

These are wounds without clearly defined edges that are difficult to approximate surgically. Pressure sores and venous stasis ulcers are common types of ulcerations. Pressure sores can occur on any area of the body, but they are most common over the coccyx, heels, and elbows. This is because pressure on the soft tissue covering these bony prominences results in injury and skin breakdown. Venous stasis ulcers are usually located in the lower legs. Malnutrition, immobility, anemia, and moisture are risk factors for pressure sores. Smoking, chronic venous insufficiency, severe varicose veins, and DM are risk factors for venous stasis ulcers. Ulcerations are classified into stage I through stage IV as described below.

Nurses have a major responsibility in the prevention and treatment of ulcerations. While other health team members such as physical therapists, dietitians, and physicians contribute to the client's care, nurses are primarily responsible for preventing pressure sores and managing skin breakdown. Nurses must begin any prevention program by first identifying

Braden Scale. The prevention of pressure sores is a critical index of quality nursing care. Dr. Barbara Braden has developed a valid assessment tool named the Braden Scale that is used widely to predict the risk of pressure sores. The client is scored in areas of activity, mobility, nutrition, and friction, and shear. In addition, Dr. Braden taught Dr. Roux more than 25 years ago. Dr. Braden is regarded as an excellent nurse role model and researcher by Dr. Roux.

high-risk clients when they are admitted to a facility or during the intake interview for home care. The **Braden Scale** is an example of a pressure sore risk assessment tool (Bergstrom, Braden, & Smith, 1988; Armstrong, Bergstrom, Braden, Norrell, & Waltman, 1991; Bergstrom, Boynton, Braden, & Bruch, 1995; Bergstrom, Braden, Champagne, Kemp, & Ruby, 1996). Currently, many institutions have developed skin care protocols for nurses based on research and national standards. An example of a wound or skin care protocol that any facility can use is given in Appendix 1 (Reeves & Blair, 1995). This example emphasizes early and continual daily wound assessment, consistent intervention by caregivers, and the use of a variety of different products for wound management. More research and information sharing concerning client outcomes based on these practice guidelines will improve the care of clients with impaired skin integrity.

Stage I

These sores occur underneath an intact epidermis. Pressure ulcers, minor skin tears, or abrasions are all examples of stage I ulcerations. These sores usually occur over bony prominences. They appear as reddened areas and do not blanch. **Nursing treatment** should focus on protecting the sore and preventing it from progressing to the next stage. The nurse should turn the client on a regular schedule, improve the client's hydration and nutrition, increase mobility if possible, and have the physical therapist provide exercise if needed.

Stage II

Stage II sores are a partial-thickness skin loss involving the epidermis or dermis. The sores appear as blisters, abrasions or shallow breaks in the skin, and exudate may be evident. **Nursing treatment** involves protecting the skin, preventing the sore from worsening, and maintaining a moist wound bed to promote granulation tissue. The nurse should treat all stage II ulcerations the same as those in stage I and refer to the wound care protocol for treatment guidelines (Appendix 1).

Stage III

Stage III sores are a full-thickness skin loss involving subcutaneous tissue that may extend to or involve the fascia. These sores form deep craters that may or may not undermine adjacent tissue. There is moderate to heavy exudate. **Nursing care** focuses on preventing the wound from progressing to stage IV. Treatment goals include maintaining a moist wound bed, absorbing excess exudate, and preventing infection.

Stage IV

In stage IV sores, there is full-thickness skin loss with extensive damage to the tissue that may involve muscle, bone, tendon, joint, or joint capsule. Tunneling may be evident. **Nursing care** goals include maintaining a moist wound bed, absorbing excess exudate, preventing infection, and eliminating tunneling and extension of the ulceration.

CASE STUDY: STAGE III ULCERATION

Mrs. W. was diagnosed and hospitalized with a stage III ulceration over her coccyx area. She has been confined to her bed, and her daughter has been caring for her at home. Her health history reveals that she has had type I DM the past ten years. Her last fasting blood sugar (FBS) was 78 mg/dL. Her ulceration measured 6 cm in diameter and was 3 mm deep. The copious serous exudate draining from the ulceration had an odor.

No tunneling is noted. The surrounding edges are composed of pink granulation tissue, and the bed of the wound is red. The nurse notes that the Op-Site occlusive dressing covering the wound is stretched by drainage that has accumulated underneath. According to the hospital's pressure ulcer protocol, the following actions should be performed:

1. Using a sterile technique, a needle (18 gauge or wider) and syringe are used to drain the excess exudate from the middle of the dressing. The entry puncture is then covered with a small piece of occlusive dressing. This maintains the sterility of the dressing and allows the wound bed to be viewed.
2. A turning schedule should be followed to take pressure off the ulcerated area. The client should be turned every two hours.
3. Fluid intake should be increased unless contraindicated. The nurse should auscultate the lungs frequently.
4. The nurse should encourage the client to increase his or her nutritional intake, and caloric intake should be coordinated with the physician and dietitian. The nurse should understand that healing demands more calories than normal, and there should be an increase in vitamin C and zinc. The client may need to be monitored on a daily calorie count. Nutritional supplementation may be needed.
5. The client's blood sugar level should be checked upon awakening and at bedtime, and insulin should be administered according to the established sliding scale. Regular insulin is given to lower any increased blood sugar levels as needed.
6. The ulceration should be assessed daily for size, exudate, odor, the presence of granulation tissue, the status of the wound bed and surrounding tissue, and the depth and presence of any

tunneling or undermining of skin edges to document healing. The physician should be notified if progress is not noted. The nurse must promptly treat any other pressure sores that are noted to prevent progression to a higher stage. Air mattresses (as well as other types of mattresses) are used to prevent the development of additional pressure areas.

7. Excellent personal hygiene should be provided to facilitate increased circulation to promote healing.

8. The client is encouraged to perform as many activities of daily living (ADL) as possible to maintain or raise his or her current level of functioning.

9. Emotional support helps the client and family to develop coping mechanisms. The nurse can inform the daughter of the support systems and other help that is available to assist her with turning and caring for Mrs. W. after her discharge.

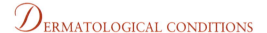

$\mathcal{D}$ERMATOLOGICAL CONDITIONS

Common skin problems result from a primary condition or from a response or reaction to infectious agents, medications, sun exposure, or environmental agents. The following section describes the skin lesions and the required nursing care for these common dermatological conditions. It is very helpful to have resources such as a dermatology color atlas readily available for reference in the clinical area. Even experienced physicians and nurses need to use these resources to diagnose and treat dermatological conditions.

Pruritus

Pruritus is defined as an itching of the skin that leads to the motor response of scratching. Pruritus is considered either a diagnosis or a symptom of an underlying condition such as poison ivy, poison oak, or poison sumac dermatitises, or chicken pox. **Nursing care** focuses on improving the client's level of comfort and preventing him or her from scratching, which can cause further skin excoriation and increase the risk of infection. Treatment consists of cold applications, tepid baths containing oatmeal, cornstarch, or baking soda; or the application of an emollient lotion. Pharmacological treatment includes applying a topical corticosteroid ointment and administering antihistamines or tranquilizers, especially at night.

Acne Vulgaris

This common skin condition is seen in adolescents and some adults. The various causes of acne include genetics, hormonal changes, nutritional status, and skin and hair hygiene. Comedomes, commonly referred to as blackheads, are often the first sign of acne. The skin becomes shiny and oily, and papules, pustules, nodules, and cysts can occur. The large lesions that occur can cause scarring. Medical management usually involves washing the face twice a day with benzoyl peroxide, applying vitamin A, and using antibiotic therapy. Common antibiotic regimens include erythromycine ethylsuccinate (EES) and minocycline hydrochloride (Minocin). These are used for long-term, low-dose antibiotic therapy. For adolescent girls 15 years of age or older, oral contraceptives (such as Ortho Tri-Cyclen) are now acceptable to use in the treatment of acne vulgaris. Nurses must teach clients to comply with treatment and practice good personal hygiene (especially with skin and hair) and general positive health behaviors. These adolescents must also be encouraged to maintain a positive self-image; this is an area of major concern.

Dermatitis

Dermatitis manifests on the skin as erythema, localized edema, and vesicle formation with exudate that crusts and scales. Contact dermatitis is frequently caused by environmental agents such as poison ivy and poison oak. Weeping uninfected lesions occur. Crusts and scales that form should be allowed to drop off. Systemic and topical corticosteroids and calamine lotion are used. Nurses must prevent any further contact with the causative environmental agent and teach the client about this disease. Clients should use a mild soap such as Ivory during the acute stage of dermatitis. Contact dermatitis is not communicable.

Eczema

Atopic dermatitis, or eczema, is linked to both a genetic predisposition and allergies. Many clients with eczema develop hay fever or asthma. The major symptom is pruritus, which causes the itching that leads to eczematous lesions. Scarring does not usually result. These clients usually have dry skin, and changes in temperature and humidity affect this disease. Lesions are noted on the neck, eyelids, behind the ears, on the wrists, and in the antecubital and popliteal areas. Erythema is also present. Eczema is treated by applying topical corticosteroids and cool compresses to the affected areas. Clients with recurrent dermatitis are frequently referred to an allergist. If allergy testing reveals that they are allergic, pharmacologic agents may help their condition. Antihistamines, antibiotics, and systemic corticosteroids may be necessary.

Psoriasis

This common, chronic skin condition is caused by an unusual mitotic rate (cell division) of the skin cells. While the usual turnover time for normal skin is 28 days, in psoriasis the formation and sloughing of cells is accelerated to 4–7 days. Psoriatic lesions (papules) are raised, erythematous, and scaling. They commonly occur on the elbows, scalp, legs, and trunk. Nails may also be pitted. Topical keratolytic agents or steroids with Op-Site or wet dressings may be used. The topical medication should be applied in a thin layer over the lesions and a thicker coat over any plaques. Ultraviolet light therapy is used in severe cases. Since this skin condition is chronic, nurses should focus on helping the client to develop strategies and coping mechanisms for living with the disease. Most clients with psoriasis are treated on an ambulatory basis, but the condition often fluctuates between periods of exacerbation and remission. Currently there is no cure for this genetically linked skin condition. Clients should be cautioned that they may have difficulty adapting to temperature extremes and should compensate by adding or removing layers of clothing. The client also should avoid sunbathing and washing the skin frequently, as these actions cause scaling and soreness.

$\mathcal{S}$KIN INFECTIONS

Invading organisms frequently cause infections in the skin. The major classes of skin infections—parasitic, fungal, viral, and bacterial—are discussed below.

Parasitic Infections

The major parasitic infections are pediculosis and scabies.

Pediculosis Pediculosis is an infestation of lice. Lice eggs are found on hair shafts and clothing and are gray, glistening, oval-shaped bodies. Pediculosis commonly infects children of all socioeconomic backgrounds. Parents should be taught to recognize lice eggs and other symptoms. The importance of detecting and treating pediculosis must be emphasized to all caregivers. To decrease embarrassment, they should also be reminded that this is a common infection among children. Pediculosis is diagnosed by observing the eggs, small raised macules, erythema, and pruritus. Lice infest humans in three areas of the body: the head, body, and pubic area. Head lice are most common among young schoolchildren. Pubic lice are transmitted by sexual contact, sheets, and towels. A lice infestation is treated with topical lindane (Kwell or Scabene), pyrethrin (RID), or another pediculocide. Instructions for application differ according to the product; therefore, the nurse must give clear instructions to the client and parents concerning the specific use of a specific pediculocide. The nurse also must teach the client how to prevent the infection from spreading. The entire family may need to be treated prophylactically as well, as lice are highly contagious and can transfer rapidly to members of the same household. Sheets and towels should be washed in hot water, and other precautions against contagion should be observed. For example, combs, brushes, towels, and hats should not be shared.

Scabies This parasitic infection is caused by the female itch mite. The scabies parasite penetrates and lays its eggs in the skin. The most common symptom is wave- or thread-like brown lines that appear on the wrists, hands, elbows, axilla, nipples, belt line, gluteal creases, and male genitalia. Treatment consists of lindane or another type of pediculocide. Nurses must include several major points when educating clients in the prevention and treatment of scabies. The client and all family members must be treated, even if some do not appear to be infected. The cream or lotion should be applied to the entire body from the neck down. The nurse must emphasize that clothes, towels, and sheets must be laundered in hot water. Precautions against contagion must be taken, and underclothing, sheets, and towels should be laundered the day of treatment. The specific instructions for each type of medication should be followed carefully, as many require a second application.

Fungal Infections

These infections include fungus, mold, and yeast.

Candida Albicans C. *albicans* is a yeast-like fungus that commonly presents in the vagina, mouth, GI tract, perineal area, or under the breasts. When the fungus grows in the mouth, the condition is known as thrush. Candidiasis results from an overgrowth of C. *albicans* on the skin or mucous membranes. This organism thrives in warm, moist areas. The infection is treated with nystatin (Mycostatin), which is available in the form of tablets, powder, or vaginal suppositories. Clotrimazole (Mycelex), ciclopirox (Loprox), and ketoconazole (Nizoral) also are effective. Fluconazole (Diflucan) is a fungistatic drug that treats oropharyngeal, systemic, and vaginal candidiasis. Candidiasis causes the skin to appear red, shiny, and edematous. The nurse should educate the client concerning candidiasis and assess him or her often to ensure early detection. Fungal infections in the webs between the fingers are caused by constant immersion of hands in water and insufficient drying. If a client has a fungal infection, the nurse and client must be alert for the presence of underlying conditions such as acquired immunodeficiency syndrome (AIDS) or diabetes that immunocompromise the client.

Tinea Tinea is a superficial fungal infection (dermatophytosis) of the skin. It occurs on various areas of the body. When the infection appears on the scalp, it is termed *tinea capitis*. If the body or pubic area is affected, a diagnosis of *tinea corporis* is made. Common sites of infection are the feet and the webs between the toes; this is diagnosed as *tinea pedis*. Most clients have infections that can be managed successfully with topical antifungal drugs such as miconazole (Monistat) and tolnaftate (Tinactin).

Ringworm, another tinea infection, occurs almost exclusively in school-children. The disease consists of round, erythematous lesions with scaling and pustules at the edges. This infection is treated with the antifungal drug griseofulvin (Grisactin). The infection resolves after several weeks. **Nursing care** should focus on medical management of the infection, encouraging personal hygiene, and wearing cotton clothing that will absorb moisture.

Bacterial Infections

Impetigo Impetigo is a bacterial infection of the skin caused by staphylo-cocci or β-hemolytic streptococci. This infection is seen most commonly in the summer or early fall. Lesions on the skin manifest as vesicles that weep and form a honey-colored crust. The lesions are treated applying warm saline compresses. Topical antibiotics are used three times per day, and systemic antibiotics may be required. Children are most susceptible to impetigo. **Nursing care** should focus on educating the family extensively concerning cleanliness and **hand washing**. Family members should wash their hands after any contact with the children, use separate towels, and wash linens frequently.

Hand Washing. Clients and nurses both risk infection from inadequately washing their hands or not washing their hands at all. Not practicing this aseptic technique results in the spread of microorganisms from nurses to clients and from one client to another.

Folliculitis This infection of the hair follicle is caused by staphylococci. Common sites of folliculitis include the eyelid and the face. Furuncles and carbuncles are folliculitis in deeper layers of the skin. Treatment involves practicing good personal hygiene using soapy water, applying warm compresses, and using topical antibiotics such as neomycin and polymyxin B (Neosporin) or bacitracin. In severe cases, such as a diabetic client with extensive folliculitis, systemic antibiotics are needed. **Nursing care** should focus on teaching the client about personal hygiene, complying with medical management, and preventing the spread of the disease to other persons.

Viral Infections

Warts Warts are viral infections on the skin. They are benign and painless and look like papules. Warts usually disappear over time without treatment, but the client may seek treatment for cosmetic reasons. Warts can be cauterized, cryosurgically excised, or removed by a topical application of acidic compounds. The nurse should focus on preparing clients for medical intervention if it is required.

Herpes Simplex Virus (HSV) HSV is a viral infection that is divided into two major categories, type 1 and type 2. Type 1 occurs on the face and mouth (cold sores or fever blisters), eyes (keratitis), and in the brain (encephalitis). HSV is frequently seen as recurrent lesions with burning and pruritus, erythema, and vesicles, especially on the face and mouth.

Lesions appear on the face and mouth more often after exposure to direct sunlight. HSV type 2 is a sexually transmitted virus that manifests as painful lesions in the genital area that crust over and heal in approximately ten days. The presence of the virus is diagnosed by a Tzanck smear. General health behaviors that prevent the recurrence of HSV include getting proper nutrition and adequate rest, and successfully managing stress. Pharmacological treatments include antivirals such as acyclovir (Zovirax) and famcyclovir (Famvir). Nurses should provide information concerning the sexual transmission of HSV type 2, emphasize the use of condoms during all sexual contact, and encourage the client to avoid sexual contact during periods when lesions are present.

Herpes Zoster Also known as shingles, this virus manifests as vesicle clusters that form in a line and are usually unilateral. The virus follows the dermatome pathways; thus the vesicles never cross the midline of the body. However, nerves on both sides of the midline may be involved. A rash develops first, followed by the vesicles. Fever, lethargy, itching, and pain may precede the vesicles. If vesicles develop within 1–2 days after the pain, then the course of the disease usually lasts 2–3 weeks, but if they develop over 7 days, the course may be prolonged. Pain may be intermittent or constant and may last for weeks or months. Pharmacological treatment includes antiviral medication, analgesics, and occasionally, steroids. Antiviral medications commonly used include famcyclovir (Famvir) and acyclovir (Zovirax). Analgesic treatment may be needed, as the level of pain varies widely from mild burning to a deep, visceral pain. Calamine lotion may relieve the occasional itching. The nurse should focus on teaching the client about the course of the disease and how to prevent the spread of chickenpox (caused by the varicella-zoster virus) to other clients. People who are exposed to herpes zoster and who have not previously had chickenpox can develop this disease. Only persons who have already had chickenpox should care for these clients. Extreme caution should be taken if a client has not yet had chickenpox and is immunocompromised with another condition such as cancer or AIDS.

Infection Control Precautions for Herpes Zoster. Herpes zoster, or shingles, is communicable only to people who have not previously had chickenpox. Infection control precautions should be maintained until all vesicles have crusted over.

TUMORS OF THE SKIN

Corns and calluses are thickened skin lesions on the feet that cause pain when the client walks. Clients with corns or calluses should seek podiatric care on a regular basis.

Keratoses

Seborrheic Keratoses These are large, dark lesions that resemble warts. Most of these lesions do not require treatment but are worth documenting to ensure that they do not undergo suspicious changes. **Nursing care**

should focus on thoroughly assessing the client's skin and teaching the client to report any change in the lesion.

Actinic Keratoses These lesions are brown, gray, or red in color, round or irregularly shaped, and dry or scaly. They should be removed by curettage and cautery, because one-fourth develop into squamous cell carcinoma. Nurses should focus on performing a thorough skin assessment and educating clients to assess and report any inflammation or growth of the lesion.

Leukoplakia Leukoplakia is a premalignant lesion that manifests as a thickened white patch on the mucous membranes. These cells may develop into squamous cell carcinoma. People who smoke or chew tobacco or who have poorly fitting dentures are at higher risk for developing oral cancer. An examination of the oral mucous membranes should be included in all physical and dental examinations. When any suspicious white or red patches are found, the client should be referred immediately for diagnosis and intervention.

Pigmented Nevi

Pigmented nevi are commonly referred to as moles. Many people have only one nevus; some may have multiple nevi. Moles are not a health problem unless they develop into malignant melanomas. Nurses should thoroughly assess the skin and teach the client the warning signs of precancerous moles. The Skin Cancer Foundation has created a mnemonic device to assist in the identification of changes in moles that require immediate attention. The following list details the "ABCD" of identification of possible malignant changes in moles: A = asymmetric; B = borders: uneven; C = color: multiple shades; D = diameter: > 6 mm. If A, B, C, and D are present, the client should be referred to a dermatologist. In general, the client and nurse need to report any changes in a mole to the physician immediately.

Squamous Cell Carcinoma

Squamous cell carcinoma is a malignant tumor of the epidermis usually resulting from exposure to sunlight. The American Cancer Society (ACS) has diligently held public health campaigns to encourage people to use sunscreen, educate parents to use sunscreen on their children, and to diminish the importance of a tan as an indicator of beauty. Chemosurgery is used to remove most of these tumors. **Nursing care** should focus on encouraging compliance with the ACS guidelines for sunscreen prevention, immediate assessment of lesions, medical management, and prevention of further lesions.

Basal Cell Carcinoma

This occurs on hairy areas of the body. The lesions are translucent, with pink or red telangiectatic vessels running across the surface. Basal cell carcinomas are treated by curettage, cautery, surgical excision, radiation, or chemosurgery. These lesions tend to grow slowly; however, clients should seek medical attention as soon as they are noticed.

Malignant Melanoma

This is one of the most serious and deadly malignant skin tumors. The lesions are seen most often on the head, neck, and lower extremities. They have an irregular border; are yellow, blue, or black in color; and have surrounding erythema. Metastasis occurs frequently. The seriousness of the metastasic spread depends on the depth of the lesion prior to diagnosis. Early diagnosis is the goal of treatment; therefore, nurses must focus on educating clients and the public to notify the nurse practitioner or physician of any changes in a mole or lesion. The nurse can help the client to develop coping mechanisms to prepare for surgical excision of the lesion. When metastasis occurs, the client is treated by an oncologist, and he or she undergoes chemotherapy.

Kaposi's Sarcoma

Once uncommon in the United States, Kaposi's sarcoma is now seen more commonly, as it is one of the manifestations of AIDS. The sarcoma manifests as red, purple, or dark plaques or nodules on the skin or mucous membranes. Kaposi's sarcoma spreads slowly. Radiation therapy, chemotherapy, and immunotherapy are used to treat this disease. The nurse must teach the client about the disease and help him or her to develop coping mechanisms. A detailed description of nursing care for a client with AIDS is given in Chapter 13.

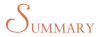

Summary

The skin is the largest organ of the body and is directly involved in the prevention of infection. The nurse should be aware of the normal healing patterns of skin. This will assist in the rapid assessment and intervention strategies required when a skin wound is present. Because the population is living longer and more emphasis is being placed on providing quality care at a lower cost, standardized pressure sore risk assessments and skin care protocols should be in place in every institution.

The nurse must be aware of various skin conditions such as infections, dermatitis, and tumors that require astute observation, documentation, and referral. Resources such as a color atlas of dermatology should be readily available so that nurses can easily cross-reference changes observed in the clients' skin. Any client with a mole that has changed in color, size, border, or symmetry should be referred to a dermatologist immediately. Prevention remains the primary defense against skin cancer and oral cancer. Nurses must continuously provide public health education precautions concerning these conditions.

KEY WORDS

Acne vulgaris	Primary intention
Actinic keratosis	Pruritus
Atopic dermatitis	Psoriasis
Basal cell carcinoma	Scabies
Candidiasis	Seborrheic keratosis
Contact dermatitis	Secondary intention
Folliculitis	Squamous cell carcinoma
Herpes simplex	Stages I, II, III, IV ulcerations
Herpes zoster	Stasis dermatitis
Impetigo	Tertiary intention
Kaposi's sarcoma	Tinea capitis
Leukoplakia	Tinea corporis
Malignant melanoma	Tinea pedis
Pediculosis	Warts
Pigmented nevi	

QUESTIONS

1. Herpes zoster, or shingles, manifests as a cluster of small vesicles usually occurring on the back, face, or scalp. One major problem with this condition is

    A. there is pain.
    B. there is no effective therapy.
    C. it is not contagious.
    D. reverse isolation is needed.

2. Mr. D. has been diagnosed with psoriasis. The nurse instructs the client to prevent scaling and soreness by doing all of the following *except*

    A. wearing warm clothing in cold temperatures.
    B. avoiding exposure to sunlight whenever possible.
    C. bathing frequently to prevent infection.
    D. adding clothing in the winter and removing clothing in the summer.

3. If the client with psoriasis complains about pruritus, the nurse should suggest using

   A. drying soaps or agents.
   B. hot water when bathing.
   C. emollient lubricants.
   D. a towel to provide vigorous drying after bathing.

ANSWERS

1. *The answer is A.* The herpes zoster virus follows nerve pathways. Discomfort and pain are the major problems. The pain may vary from burning and tingling to deep, visceral pain. The pain may be intermittent or constant and may last from weeks to months.

2. *The answer is C.* Hydration and softening of the skin are goals in the treatment of psoriasis. Frequent bathing and overuse of soap may dry the skin further.

3. *The answer is C.* Applying lotions with emollients in a thin layer over the skin and a thick layer over plaques usually is helpful with psoriasis. Psoriasis is not curable and fluctuates between periods of exacerbation and remission. Avoiding sunburn, infections, extremes of temperature, drying soaps, and stress are suggested ways to manage psoriasis.

ANNOTATED REFERENCES

Armstrong, N., Bergstrom, N., Braden, B., Norrell, K., & Waltman, N. (1991). Nutritional Status, pressure sores, and mortality in elderly patients with cancer. *Oncology Nursing Forum, 18*(5), 867–873.

This research study examines the relationship of nutritional status, the presence of pressure sores, and the incidence of mortality in elderly cancer clients. The Braden Scale is used as the risk assessment tool. The results demonstrate a significant relationship between nutritional status and the risk of pressure sores and support the validity of the use of the scale in clinical practice.

Bergstrom, N., Boynton, P., Braden, B., & Bruch, S., (1995). Using a research-based assessment scale in clinical practice. *Nursing Clinics of North America 30*(3), 539–551.

This research study uses the Braden Scale as a risk assessment tool to increase the clinical application of using a skin protocol for the prevention, early identification, and treatment of pressure sores.

Bergstrom, N., Braden, B., Champagne, M., Kemp, M., & Ruby E., (1996). Multi-site study of incidence of pressure ulcers and the relationship between risk level, demographic characteristics, diagnoses, and prescription of preventive interventions. *Journal of American Geriatrics Society, 44*, 22–30.

This is a research study that uses multiple sites to study pressure ulcers and effective interventions.

Bergstrom, N., Braden, B., & Smith, C. (1988). Paving the way to research in nursing homes. *Geriatric Nursing*, 38–41.

This research study uses a delphi survey among the nursing home staff to determine what the staff felt were their most important nursing care issues, and what could be done about them. From this survey, pressure sores, with their various assessment and treatment questions, are identified as the priority for nursing research. Based on this initial survey, the research team has continued the years of development, testing, and clinical utilization of the Braden Scale.

Reeves, C. & Blair, D. (1995). *Impaired skin or tissue integrity protocol and standards of practice.* Wichita Falls, TX: Bethania Regional Healthcare Center.

This skin risk assessment and treatment protocol was developed by two nurses from the Education department of the facility. All nursing and other multidisciplinary staff were educated concerning the protocol. All facilities are encouraged to use skin risk assessment and treatment protocols, either adopted from other authors or agencies or written specifically by their own agency.

Schaffer, S., Garzon, L., Heroux, D., Korniewicz, D. (1996). *Infection prevention and safe practice.* St. Louis: C. V. Mosby.

This pocket-sized book provides CDC guidelines and the latest recommendations for infection prevention.

INTERNET SITES FOR ADDITIONAL INFORMATION

Dermatology in the Cinema:
http://itsa.ucsf.edu/~vcr/Dermcin.html

Dermatology Online:
http://www.rrze.unierlangen.de/docs/FAV/fakultaet/med/
kli/derma/bilddb/db.htm

APPENDIX 1:
IMPAIRED SKIN OR TISSUE INTEGRITY PROTOCOL

Developed by Charlene Reeves, M.S.N., R.N., C.N.S., and Denise Blair, R.N., this is an example of a risk assessment tool and intervention guidelines for skin and wound care. All agencies must be accountable for the early identification and treatment of any impairment in the client's skin integrity.

INSTRUCTIONS FOR PRESSURE ULCER ASSESSMENT

1. Complete the client's admission record. If the existing pressure ulcer or skin breakdown score is more than 8, an *Initial Pressure Ulcer Assessment Sheet* (Fig. 16-1) **must** be completed by the admitting nurse.
2. An individualized treatment plan must be completed by the nurse and placed with the chart within 24 hours of admission, containing the physician's orders and nursing care per the skin protocol.
3. The daily reassessment of the pressure ulcer(s) must be performed by the client's primary care nurse (designate shift). The nurse's assessment must be documented on the *Pressure Ulcer Daily Flow Sheet* (Fig. 16-2).
4. A referral must be made to Education Services if a pressure ulcer is identified. An additional referral must be made to the Physical Medicine and Respiratory Therapy departments for stages III and IV pressure ulcers.
5. The physician must be notified when any break in skin integrity is identified or tissue integrity is compromised. The physician must give orders immediately concerning what treatment should be administered.

THE STANDARDS OF PROFESSIONAL PRACTICE: CARE OF THE CLIENT WITH IMPAIRED SKIN OR TISSUE INTEGRITY

Desired Client Outcome

Wound management services are designed to achieve the following outcomes with the client and family:

1. The client's skin or tissue integrity must be improved.
2. The client must demonstrate, if possible, a positive self-concept evidenced by active participation in the program.

3. The nurse must emphasize the importance of good nutrition, adequate hydration, compliance with treatment, the need for daily skin inspections, and increased mobility.

4. The nurse must initiate appropriate pressure-relieving measures to prevent shear and friction on the skin or tissue surfaces. These measures work to improve or maintain skin or tissue integrity.

5. With proper education, the client and significant other should be able to demonstrate an understanding of how to prevent skin breakdown.

6. The client's expected outcome at the time of discharge consists of the attainment of intact skin or tissue, no further breakdown, no pressure and risk factors to compromise wound healing further, and no signs or symptoms of local or systemic infection.

7. The client should have an enhanced quality of life through improvement or restoration of skin or tissue integrity.

8. The client should be discharged home with a home health care or social services consult if the client is unable to take care of him- or herself or if no support system is available.

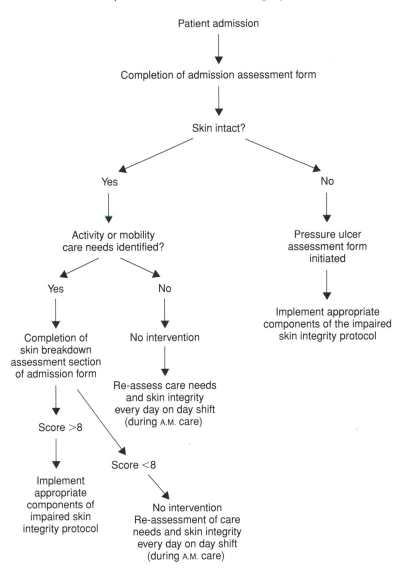

FIGURE 16-1

Components of Impaired Skin or Tissue Integrity Protocol
(Use with open wounds managed without surgery)

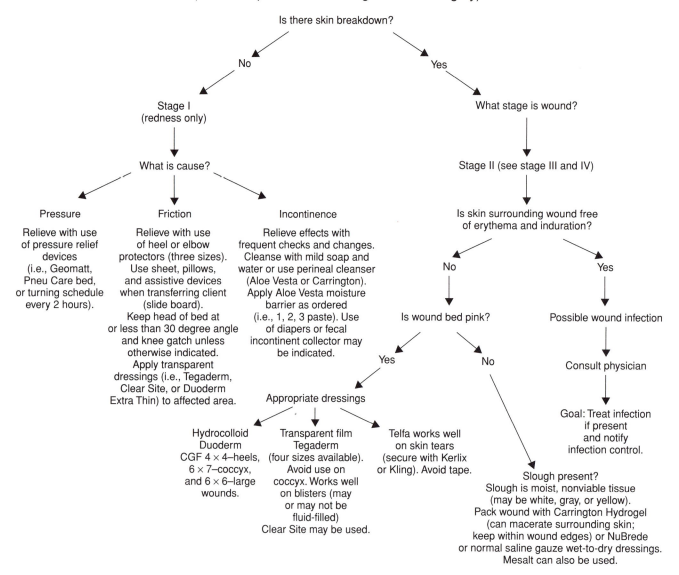

FIGURE 16-2

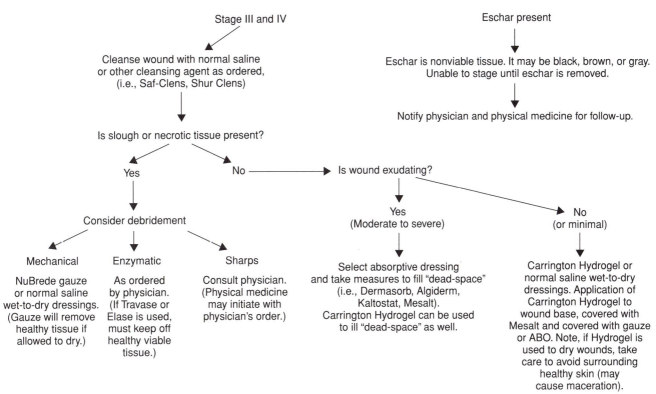

Stage III and IV

Cleanse wound with normal saline
or other cleansing agent as ordered,
(i.e., Saf-Clens, Shur Clens)

Is slough or necrotic tissue present?

Yes

No → Is wound exudating?

Consider debridement

Mechanical
NuBrede gauze
or normal saline
wet-to-dry dressings.
(Gauze will remove
healthy tissue if
allowed to dry.)

Enzymatic
As ordered
by physician.
(If Travase or
Elase is used,
must keep off
healthy viable
tissue.)

Sharps
Consult physician.
(Physical medicine
may initiate with
physician's order.)

Yes
(Moderate to severe)

Select absorptive dressing
and take measures to fill "dead-space"
(i.e., Dermasorb, Algiderm,
Kaltostat, Mesalt).
Carrington Hydrogel can be used
to ill "dead-space" as well.

No
(or minimal)

Carrington Hydrogel or
normal saline wet-to-dry
dressings. Application of
Carrington Hydrogel to
wound base, covered with
Mesalt and covered with gauze
or ABO. Note, if Hydrogel is
used to dry wounds, take
care to avoid surrounding
healthy skin (may
cause maceration).

Eschar present

Eschar is nonviable tissue. It may be black, brown, or gray.
Unable to stage until eschar is removed.

Notify physician and physical medicine for follow-up.

Product	Change
Duoderm	Q 3 days
Tegaderm	Q 3 days
Tella	Daily
Caarrington Hydrogel	Daily
NuBrede or normal saline wet-to-dry	Q shift
Mesalt	Daily
Enzymatic agents	As ordered
Dermasorb	Daily
Algiderm	Daily
Kaltostat	Daily

APPENDIX

LIST OF ABBREVIATIONS

α	Alpha
β	Beta
γ	Gamma
ABC	Airway, breathing, and circulation
ABG	Arterial blood gas
ACE	Angiotensin-converting enzyme
AChR	Acetylcholine receptors
ACOG	American College of Obstetrics and Gynecology
ACS	American Cancer Society
ACTH	Adrenocorticotropic hormone
ADA	American Diabetic Association
ADH	Antidiuretic hormone
ADL	Activities of daily living
AHA	American Heart Association
AHCPR	Agency for Health Care Policy and Research
AIDS	Acquired immunodeficiency syndrome
ALL	Acute lymphocytic leukemia
ALT	Alanine aminotransferase
AML	Acute myelogenous leukemia
APTT	Activated partial thromboplastin time
ARDS	Acute respiratory distress syndrome

ARF	Acute respiratory failure
ASA	Aspirin
AST	Aspartate aminotransferase
ATG	Antithymocyte globulin
ATP	Adenosine triphosphate
AVM	Arteriovenous malformation
AWHONN	Association of Women's Health, Obstetric, and Neonatal Nursing
BPH	Benign prostatic hypertrophy
BRP	Bathroom privileges
BSA	Body surface area
BSE	Breast self-examination
BUN	Blood urea nitrogen
CA^{2+}	Calcium
CABG	Coronary artery bypass graft
CAD	Coronary artery disease
CBC	Complete blood count
CBI	Continuous bladder irritation
CDC	Centers for Disease Control and Prevention
CEA	Carcinoembryonic antigen
CHF	Congestive heart failure
CIE	Counterimmunoelectrophoresis
CIN	Cervical intraepithelial neoplasia
Cl^-	Chloride
CML	Chronic myelogenous leukemia
CMTS	Color, movement, temperature, and sensation
CMV	Cytomegalovirus
CNS	Central nervous system
CO_2	Carbon dioxide
COPD	Chronic obstructive pulmonary disease
CPAP	Continuous positive airway pressure
CSF	Cerebrospinal fluid
CT	Computed tomography
CVA	Cerebrovascular accident
CVC	Central venous catheter
CVP	Central venous pressure
D5½ NS	5% dextrose in half normal saline
D5RL	5% dextrose in Ringer's lactate
D5W	5% dextrose in water
DES	Diethylstilbestrol
DIC	Disseminated intravascular coagulopathy
DKA	Diabetic ketoacidosis
DM	Diabetes mellitus
DNA	Deoxyribonucleic acid
DTR	Deep tendon reflexes
DTs	Delirium tremens
DVT	Deep vein thrombosis
EBL	Estimated blood loss
EBV	Epstein-Barr virus
ECF	Extracellular fluid

ECG	Electrocardiogram
EEG	Electroencephalograph
EES	Erythromycin ethylsuccinate
EGD	Esophagogastroduodenoscopy
ELISA	Enzyme-linked immunosorbent assay
EMG	Electromyography
ENT	Ear, nose, and throat
ER	Emergency room
ERCP	Endoscopic retrograde cholangiopancreatography
ESR	Erythrocyte sedimentation rate
ESRD	End-stage renal disease
FBS	Fasting blood sugar
FDA	Food and Drug Administration
FEV	Forced expiratory volume
GCS	Glasgow coma scale
GERD	Gastroesophageal reflux disease
GFR	Glomerular filtration rate
GI	Gastrointestinal
H_2 receptor	Histamine receptor
HAV	Hepatitis A virus
HbA_{1c}	Glycosylated hemoglobin
HBIG	Hepatitis B immunoglobulin
HbS	Sickled hemoglobin
HBsAg	Hepatitis B surface antigen
HBV	Hepatitis B virus
HCl	Hydrochloric acid
HCV	Hepatitis C virus
HDAg	Hepatitis D antigen
HDL	High-density lipoprotein
HDV	Hepatitis D virus
HEV	Hepatitis E virus
HHNC	Hyperglycemic hyperosmolar nonketotic coma
HIDA	Hepatobiliary iminodiacetic acid analogue scan
HIV	Human immunodeficiency virus
HLA	Human leukocyte antigen
HPV	Human papilloma virus
HRT	Hormone replacement therapy
HSV	Herpes simplex virus
HSV-2	Herpes simplex virus-2
IABP	Intra-aortic balloon pump
IBS	Irritable bowel syndrome
IBW	Ideal body weight
ICF	Intracellular fluid
ICH	Intracerebral hemorrhage
ICP	Intracranial pressure
ICU	Intensive care unit
IDDM	Insulin-dependent diabetes mellitus
IgE	Immunoglobulin E
IGF-1	Insulin-like growth factor-1
IgG	Immunoglobulin G

INH	Isoniazid
INR	International normalized ratio
IOP	Intraocular pressure
ITP	Idiopathic thrombocytopenia purpura
IUD	Intra-uterine device
IVP	Intravenous pyelogram
K^+	Potassium
KVO	Keep vein open
LDH	Lactate dehydrogenase
LDL	Low-density lipoprotein
LEEP	Loop electrodiathermy excision procedure
LES	Lower esophageal sphincter
LFT	Liver function tests
LGI	Lower gastrointestinal
LLQ	Left lower quadrant
LOC	Level of consciousness
LP	Lumbar puncture
LUQ	Left upper quadrant
MAOB	Monoamine oxidase B
MAOI	Monoamine oxidase inhibitors
MCH	Mean corpuscular hemoglobin
MCHC	Mean corpuscular hemoglobin concentration
MCT	Midchain triglyceride
MCV	Mean corpuscular volume
Mg^{2+}	Magnesium
MI	Myocardial infarction
mL	Milliliter
MRI	Magnetic resonance imaging
MRSA	Methicillin-resistant *Staphylococcus aureus*
MS	Multiple sclerosis
MUGA	Multi-gated acquisition scan
MVA	Motor vehicle accident
Na^+	Sodium
NaCl	Sodium chloride
NCI	National Cancer Institute
NG	Nasogastric
NGT	Nasogastric tube
NGU	Nongonococcal urethritis
NIDDM	Non–insulin-dependent diabetes mellitus
NIH	National Institutes of Health
NPH	Neutral Protamine Hagedorn
NS	Normal saline
NSAID	Nonsteroidal anti-inflammatory drug
O_2	Oxygen
OHA	Oral hypoglycemic agent
ORIF	Open reduction and internal fixation
OTC	Over-the-counter
PAC	Premature atrial contractions
Pa_{CO_2}	Arterial carbon dioxide partial pressure
PACU	Postanesthesia care unit

Pa$_{O_2}$	Arterial oxygen partial pressure
Pap	Papanicolaou
PAP	Pulmonary artery pressure
PAT	Paroxysmal atrial tachycardia
PCA	Patient-controlled analgesia
PEEP	Positive end-expiratory pressure
PET	Positron emission tomography
PICC	Peripherally inserted central catheters
PID	Pelvic inflammatory disease
PJC	Premature junctional contractions
PMS	Premenstrual syndrome
PNS	Parasympathetic nervous system
PRBC	Packed red blood cells
PSA	Prostate specific antigen
PT	Prothrombin time
PTCA	Percutaneous transluminal coronary angioplasty
PTH	Parathyroid hormone
PTT	Partial thromboplastin time
PTU	Propylthiouracil
PUD	Peptic ulcer disease
PVC	Premature ventricular contractions
PZI	Protamine zinc insulin
RAI	Radioactive iodine
RAS	Reticular activating system
RBC	Red blood cell
RDW	Red blood cell distribution width
REM	Rapid eye movement
RIND	Reversible ischemic neurological deficit
RL	Ringer's lactate
RLQ	Right lower quadrant
RNA	Ribonucleic acid
ROM	Range of motion
RPR	Rapid plasma reagin
RSO	Radiation safety officer
RUQ	Right upper quadrant
SA	Sinoatrial
SAH	Subarachnoid hemorrhage
SCA	Sickle cell anemia
SCID	Severe combined immunodeficiency disease
SDAT	Senile dementia of the Alzheimer's type
SIADH	Syndrome of inappropriate antidiuretic hormone
SLE	Systemic lupus erythematosus
SNS	Sympathetic nervous system
SSRI	Selective serotonin reuptake inhibitors
STD	Sexually transmitted diseases
SVT	Supraventricular tachycardia
TENS	Transcutaneous electrical nerve stimulation
TIA	Transient ischemic attack
TMJ	Temporomandibular joint

TNM	T = tumor size and extent; N = nodal size and location; and M − presence of distant metastasis
TPA	Tissue plasminogen activator
TPN	Total parenteral nutrition
TRAM	Transverse rectus abdominus myocutaneous flap reconstruction
TRH	Thyroid-releasing hormone
TSE	Testicular self-examination
TSH	Thyroid-stimulating hormone
TSS	Toxic shock syndrome
TUIP	Transurethral incision of the prostate
TURP	Transurethral resection of the prostate
UGI	Upper gastrointestinal
UTI	Urinary tract infection
V/Q	Ventilation–perfusion ratio
VAS	Visual analog scale
VDRL	Venereal Disease Research Laboratories
VMA	Vanillylmandelic acid
WBC	White blood cell
WHI	Women's Health Initiative
WHO	World Health Organization

INDEX

Page numbers followed by a t or an f indicate tables or figures, respectively.

ISBN 0-07-105480-4

90000

9 780071 054805

REEVES/MED-SURG
NURSING (U.S.)